You and Your Health
Volume 3
More Diseases
First Aid
Emergencies

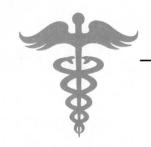

VOLUME 3
New Edition

You and Your Health

More Diseases
First Aid
Emergencies

In three volumes, illustrated

Harold Shryock, M.A., M.D., and
Mervyn G. Hardinge, M.D.,
Dr.P.H., Ph.D.

In Collaboration With 28 Leading Medical Specialists

Published jointly by

PACIFIC PRESS PUBLISHING ASSOCIATION
Boise, ID 83707
Oshawa, Ontario, Canada
Montemorelos, N. L., Mexico

REVIEW AND HERALD PUBLISHING ASSOCIATION
Washington, DC 20039-0555
Hagerstown, MD 21740

CONTENTS

Volume 1—More Abundant Living

Volume 2—The Human Body; Diseases; Symptoms

Volume 3—More Diseases; First Aid; Emergencies

INTRODUCTION

The descriptions of organ systems and their diseases are completed in volume 3 of *You and Your Health*. In section I the body's control systems (the glands and the nervous system) are considered. Section II pertains to the special sense organs and their diseases. Of particular interest here is chapter 7, devoted entirely to pain and the meanings of various kinds of pain.

The next three sections (III, IV, and V) are concerned with diseases that affect any part of the body or even the entire body—the systemic diseases. Here we find discussions of the characteristics and manifestations of cancer, the deficiency diseases, the disorders of regulation, and allergy. The six chapters devoted to systemic infections are arranged according to the various disease-producing organisms.

The final two sections of volume 3 consist of five chapters of "What to Do" instructions for handling accidents, poisonings, sudden illnesses, and care in the home for someone ill.

At the back of volume 3, as is true also of volumes 1 and 2, the reader will find a complete General Index for the entire three volumes of *You and Your Health*. It will direct the reader to items such as Obesity in volume 3, Peptic ulcer in volume 2, or Smoking as a cause of disease in volume 1. Also at the back of volume 3 a series of four-color anatomical illustrations has been included, several of them transparent plates, with organs numbered and labeled for easy identification.

SECTION I

The Glands and the Nervous System

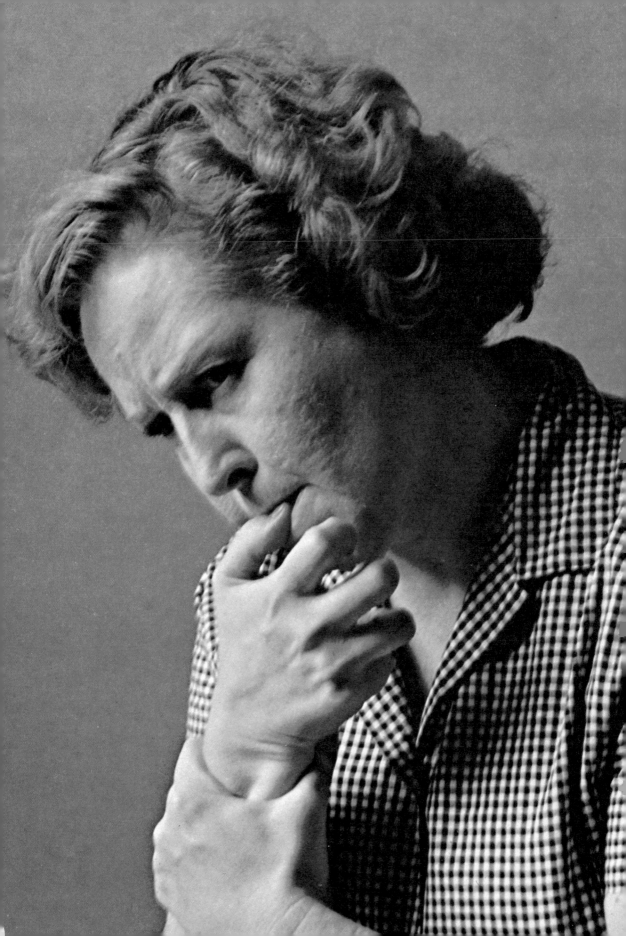

The Glands

The human body is a community of organs and tissues. Each vital part performs its specific task and thus contributes to the welfare of the whole.

The organs of the human body may be compared to various facilities found in a typical city. The brain, for instance, might be compared to the library and city hall. The skeleton is like the product of a construction company which builds the framework of buildings. The digestive organs are the city's food markets and eating places. The organs for eliminating the body's wastes may be compared to a disposal company. The lungs may be likened to air conditioning equipment. The nerves compare favorably to the communication system of a telephone company. The heart and blood vessels are like the utilities for gas, power, and water.

And now we come to the glands of the body, which may be compared to small manufacturing plants located here and there throughout a city.

The body has many glands with many different jobs to do. A gland is an organ containing highly specialized cells which produce a chemical substance materially important to some other part of the body.

Two Kinds of Glands

The body's glands may be divided into two general groups: exocrine and endocrine. The exocrine glands produce fluid secretions delivered by ducts (small tubes) either to the body's surface (as in the glands of the skin) or to an interior passageway of the body such as the esophagus, the trachea, the stomach, or the intestine. Endocrine glands produce chemical substances classed as hormones, which are delivered directly to the blood instead of through a duct. The transfer takes place as the blood passes through the gland.

The exocrine glands (those with ducts) are closely related to the organs and systems of which they form parts. These are therefore described in the chapters dealing with those respective systems. For example, the sweat glands and oil glands of the skin are described in chapter 24, volume 2, which pertains to the skin.

The breasts, largely glandular in nature, are described in chapter 28, volume 2, which deals with the reproductive organs. Incidentally, the breasts are composed of modifications of the structures belonging to the skin, adapted in this case to produce milk. It should be noted that the glands of the breasts are typically exocrine in that their secretion is a fluid delivered to the surface by small ducts which open at the nipple.

Exocrine glands of another group are found in the moist membranes of the

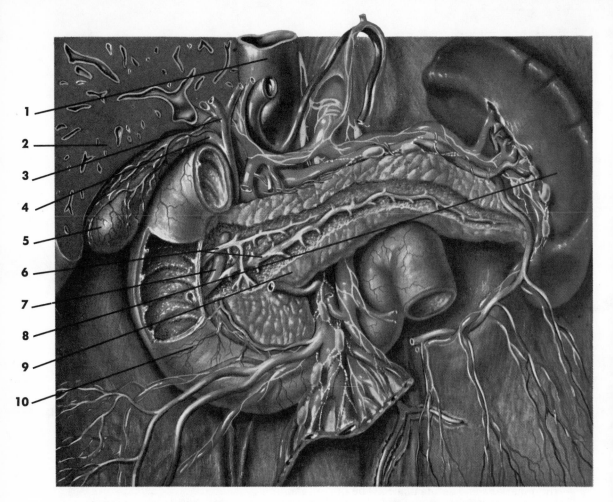

1 Inferior vena cava
2 Liver
3 Hepatic duct
4 Cystic duct
5 Gallbladder
6 Pancreatic ducts
7 Common bile duct
8 Spleen
9 Pancreas
10 Duodenum

Anatomical relationship of the duodenum, pancreas, and gallbladder. (For still greater detail see Trans-vision plates V and VI at the back of this volume.)

body. These secrete the fluids and mucus which keep the membranes in good condition. The large salivary glands in the walls of the mouth belong to this group. The saliva which they produce contains water and mucus and a digestive enzyme called ptyalin which aids in the digestion of starch.

Also belonging to the glands in the moist membranes are those in the esophagus, the stomach, and the intestines. These are discussed in chapter 16, volume 2, which deals with the digestive organs. Although the function of many of these glands is to keep the membranes moist and in good condition, some of them are adapted to produce digestive enzymes.

The glands located in the membranes that line the air passages also belong to the general exocrine group. They produce secretions with a high content of mucus, which serves not only to keep the membranes moist but also to trap the small particles of dust and foreign material inhaled along with the breath. These glands are discussed in chapter 12, volume 2, which deals with the organs of breathing and speaking.

Other glands of this general type are located in the membranes which line some of the organs of reproduction, discussed in chapter 28, volume 2.

Their secretions keep the membranes moist and well lubricated and also help to control the balance between acidity and alkalinity of the membranes.

The liver is often classed as one of the exocrine glands because, among its many functions, it produces bile, a fluid conveyed away from the liver through the hepatic duct and the common bile duct. Making connection with these ducts is the duct of the gallbladder, in which the bile is stored as necessary. As the bile leaves the common bile duct, it enters the duodenum, where it aids in the emulsification, and thus the digestion, of fats.

The pancreas is an interesting gland but difficult to classify because part of it functions as an exocrine gland and part as an endocrine gland. We will therefore include it in our description of the endocrine glands. One of the functions of the pancreas is to produce pancreatic juice, which is carried by a system of ducts to the interior of the duodenum where it assists in the digestion of food. This exocrine function of the pancreas is mentioned in chapter 18, volume 2.

The Endocrine Glands

The endocrine glands, which produce hormones and deliver them to the blood, constitute a system of their own. The endocrine organs individually perform separate and unique functions, but by interrelations they influence one another and thus cooperate in regulating the body's various physiological processes. The remainder of this chapter will deal with the various endocrine glands. These include the pituitary, the adrenals, the thyroid, the parathyroids, that part of the pancreas

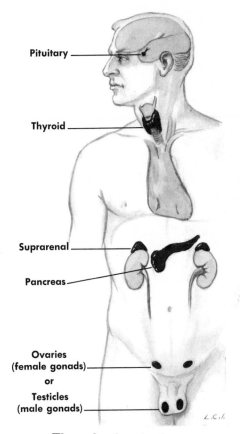

The endocrine glands.

which functions as an endocrine gland, and the sex glands of both male and female.

The Pituitary Gland (Hypophysis)

The functions of the endocrine glands are very much interrelated. Several of the hormones produced by them serve only to alter the functions of other endocrine glands. The more we learn about the endocrine glands, the better we understand the purpose for these interrelationships. They serve as double checks and automatic controls—a fortunate arrangement, because it makes unnecessary any conscious control of the functions of certain organs.

The pituitary gland occupies an important place in this relationship. In fact, it plays a dominant role. As can be

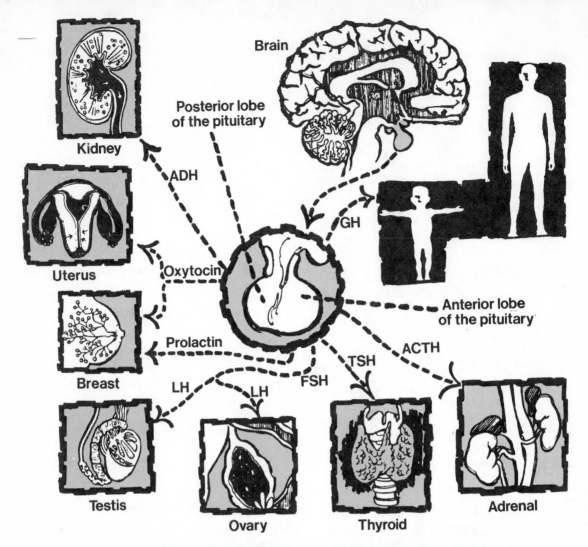

The Pituitary and Its Hormones. Reading clockwise: Somatotropin (GH) promotes the growth and development of the entire body; Corticotropin (ACTH) stimulates the cortex of the adrenal glands to produce certain steroid hormones; Thyrotropin (TSH) stimulates the thyroid to produce its hormones; Follicle-stimulating hormone (FSH) prepares the follicles of the ovaries to produce female sex cells and, in the male, stimulates the production of male sex cells by the testes; Luteinizing hormone (LH) collaborates with FSH and stimulates the ovaries to produce estrogen and the testes to produce testosterone; Prolactin stimulates the female breasts to produce milk; Oxytocin causes (a) contraction of the uterus (only during pregnancy) and (b) ejection of milk during suckling; and Vasopressin (ADH) conserves the body's water.

seen from the accompanying drawing, the pituitary's functions, for the most part, are to regulate the activity of other glands. One observer has said it this way: The pituitary gland is the conductor of the endocrine orchestra.

Even its location in the body suggests its importance. Placed at the center of the head, it is closely associated with the base of the brain. It is only a little larger than an ordinary garden pea, but it is protected by a bony capsule which surrounds more than half of its surface. The blood supply to this gland cares adequately for the needs of its cells and transports their hormones to all parts of the body. From the standpoint of both structure and of function, the pituitary is conveniently divided into two parts: an anterior lobe and a posterior lobe. We will now consider the hormones produced by each of these lobes:

The Hormones of the Anterior Lobe of the Pituitary Gland. One of the hormones produced by the anterior lobe of the pituitary is somatotropin, the growth hormone (GH). It influences those organs and tissues concerned with the process of growth. In promoting growth, this hormone works in collaboration with hormones produced by the thyroid gland, by the endocrine portion of the pancreas, and by the testes. For a discussion of the disorders of growth, see the sections on "Gigantism and Acromegaly," page 24, and on "Pituitary Dwarfism," page 25, in the following chapter.

A second hormone produced by the anterior lobe of the pituitary is corticotropin, also called the adrenocorticotropic hormone (ACTH). This hormone, although carried by the blood throughout the entire body, influences primarily the cells in the cortex portion of the adrenal glands, promoting their well-being and stimulating them to produce some of the steroid hormones, mentioned in this chapter under "The Adrenal Glands," pages 18 and 19.

A third hormone produced by the anterior lobe of the pituitary is thyrotropin, the thyroid-stimulating hormone (TSH), which influences the thyroid gland to produce the thyroid hormones.

The anterior lobe of the pituitary produces two hormones known as gonadotropic hormones because they influence the activities of the sex organs (gonads). These hormones occur in both males and females, but their effects in the bodies of women differ from those in the bodies of men. They are known as (1) the follicle-stimulating hormone (FSH) and (2) the luteinizing hormone (LH).

In women the follicle-stimulating hormone (FSH) encourages the development of structures within the ovaries which produce and liberate the female sex cells (ova). The same hormone, circulating in the blood of a man, stimulates his testes to produce male sex cells (spermatozoa).

In women, the luteinizing hormone (LH) collaborates with the FSH to complete the liberation of the female sex cells (ova). In addition, it encourages the development of a gland structure (the corpus luteum) that develops in the empty follicle of the ovary after the female sex cell has been liberated. It also stimulates the ovary to produce the estrogenic hormones which maintain the feminine characteristics. In a man, this same hormone stimulates the interstitial cells of the testes to produce testosterone—the hormone which maintains the masculine characteristics.

The anterior lobe of the pituitary also produces the hormone prolactin. The primary function of prolactin is to stimulate the female breasts to produce milk. Interestingly, small amounts of this hormone are produced continuously in both men and women. At the time of pregnancy the production of prolactin in a woman increases as much as twenty times. Production of milk is inhibited during pregnancy by the high concentration of estrogen at this time. Following delivery of the child, the estrogen level declines, allowing the breasts under the influence of prolactin to produce milk in abundance for several months. For a discussion of the disorders of prolactin secretion, see the item on "Galactorrhea" in the following chapter, pages 23 and 24.

Hormones Released by the Posterior Lobe of the Pituitary. The posterior lobe of the pituitary is responsible for the release of two hormones: (1) vasopressin, the antidiuretic hormone (ADH), and (2) oxytocin.

Vasopressin acts on the cells in the

17

tubules of the kidneys to decrease the amount of water allowed to pass into the urine. When the body fluids become too dilute, the production of vasopressin is decreased so that more water is allowed to escape from the body. Reciprocally, when the body fluids become too concentrated, production of vasopressin is increased to conserve the amount of water in the body.

Oxytocin has no demonstrable effect in a man's body, but in a woman it has two effects, both of which are related to childbearing. It causes a contraction of the muscle of the uterus, but this effect is limited to the time of childbirth. Second, it acts on the breasts during the time of lactation to aid in the release of milk.

The Adrenal Glands
(Suprarenal Glands)

There are two adrenal glands, a right and a left, each of which caps the corresponding kidney. The adrenal glands are sometimes called the suprarenal glands. Each gland consists of a central portion, the medulla, which is surrounded by the cortex. Inasmuch as the gland is somewhat flat as it caps the kidney, the medulla is placed like the filling of a sandwich between two layers of the cortex.

The two parts of the adrenal gland (medulla and cortex) function quite differently and independently. Thus we might say that each adrenal gland is two glands in one. The cortex is essential to life; and if, through disease or removal, a person is deprived of the hormones which the cortex normally produces, he will die unless he receives these hormones by artificial means. The adrenal medulla, by contrast, is not essential to life.

Many spectacular forms of illness occur when disease or malfunction involves the adrenal glands. These are discussed in the following chapter.

The Hormones Produced by the Adrenal Cortex. The hormones produced by the adrenal cortex are designated by

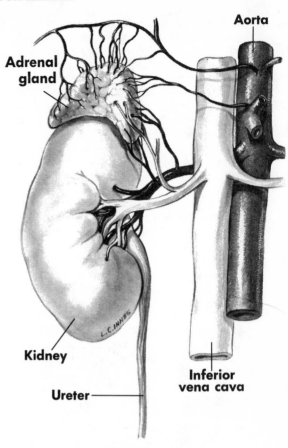

An adrenal gland, an odd-shaped organ with a rich blood supply, is capped over the upper part of each kidney.

the chemist as steroids, sometimes collectively called the "adrenal corticoids."

Cortisone and hydrocortisone affect many different cells throughout the body (particularly liver cells, muscle cells, and fat cells) to bring about the conversion of protein and fat to carbohydrate. These two corticoids are therefore called glucocorticoids.

Aldosterone, another one of the "adrenal corticoids," has the effect of changing the ability of various cells to absorb certain of the mineral ions which circulate in the body's fluids. It is therefore called a mineralocorticoid. Specifically, aldosterone acts on the kidneys to favor the elimination of po-

18

tassium and the retention of sodium.

A fourth steroid produced by the cortex of the adrenal gland is an adrenal androgen, which is a masculinizing hormone. When it is produced in excessive amounts in a woman, there develop certain physical characteristics normally typical of the male.

In the preceding section on the pituitary gland it was stated that corticotropin (ACTH), produced by the anterior lobe of the pituitary, stimulates the cortex of the adrenal gland to produce steroid hormones. This influence from the pituitary gland seems to be more effective in stimulating the production of glucocorticoids and sex hormones than of the mineralocorticoids. Many of the symptoms of masculinization in women are due to ACTH.

The Adrenal Medulla. This central portion of the adrenal gland is unique among the endocrine glands of the body in that it functions as an integral part of the sympathetic division of the autonomic nervous system. This means, first, that being under the control of the nervous system, it produces hormones in response to nervous impulses received from the brain. It means, in addition, that the hormones produced here have the same effect throughout the body as do the nerves of the sympathetic division of the autonomic nervous system. Thus the adrenal medulla is part of the body's alarm system and serves, along with parts of the nervous system, to prepare the body to meet an emergency. It does this very effectively because its hormones are circulated by the blood and therefore reach all tissues of the body.

The adrenal medulla produces two hormones: (1) epinephrine (commonly called adrenaline) and (2) norepinephrine. For our present purpose, we will consider that the effects on the body of these two hormones are so similar as to be identical. They have the effect of declaring a state of emergency throughout the body. They limit such activities as digestion that can be postponed for a little while until the emergency is over. They increase the amount of blood available to the body tissues by speeding up the heart rate and at the same time raising the blood pressure. They provide tissue fuel by influencing the liver and other tissues where carbohydrate is stored so that the amount of glucose in the circulating blood is increased to meet the possibility of sudden activity by the muscles. They increase the rate of metabolism so as to make energy available more quickly.

The Thyroid Gland

The thyroid gland, located in the neck, fits closely around the front and sides of the trachea (windpipe) just below the larynx (voice box). It is shaped something like a set of saddle bags, with a narrow portion connecting them in front of the trachea and a rather large lobe on each side. The thyroid gland receives an abundant supply of blood both to nourish its own cells and to carry away the hormones it produces.

The thyroid is composed of thousands of small "follicles," each consisting of a single layer of cells on the outside with a core of gelatinous substance on the inside. The core material serves as a storage reservoir for excess hormones. Surrounding each follicle are blood capillaries. The cells which form the shell of the follicle can direct the hormones which they produce into either the blood or the central storage reservoir, depending upon the body's needs at the moment.

The thyroid gland produces three hormones: thyroxine, triiodothyronine, and calcitonin. The first two affect the tissues of the body in about the same way, and so we will not need to give separate descriptions of what they do.

It will be recalled that the body's need for thyroid hormones is monitored by the anterior lobe of the pituitary gland, which produces thyrotropin (TSH) as needed to regulate the activity of the thyroid gland.

Several manifestations of poor health result when the thyroid gland does not function properly, some of them quite

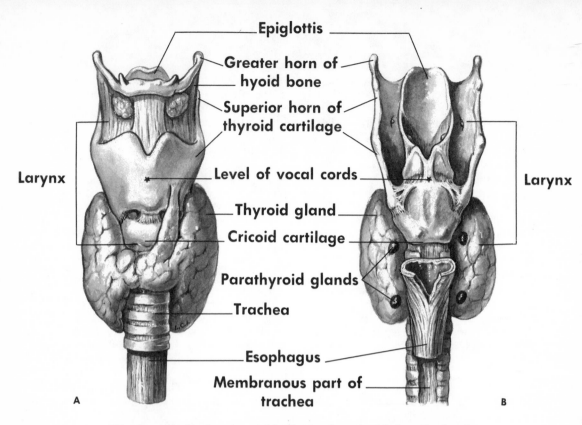

Epiglottis

Greater horn of hyoid bone

Superior horn of thyroid cartilage

Larynx

Level of vocal cords

Thyroid gland

Cricoid cartilage

Parathyroid glands

Trachea

Esophagus

Membranous part of trachea

Larynx

A

B

The thyroid gland rests astride the trachea, just below the larynx. A. Anterior view. B. Posterior view, showing the parathyroid glands located against the back surfaces of the lobes of the thyroid gland, usually two on each side.

spectacular. They are described in the following chapter.

The normal effects of thyroxine and triiodothyronine on the body may be summarized as follows: (1) They increase the consumption of oxygen by most of the body's tissues. This means that the rate of metabolism (the rate at which oxidation in the body's cells occurs) is under the control of the thyroid gland. (2) They improve a person's ability to think. When they are in short supply, thinking is retarded, sometimes extremely. An overproduction may make a person irritable and restless. (3) Adequate amounts of these thyroid hormones are also needed for normal growth and skeletal development in a child. In this latter function they operate in conjunction with the growth hormone (GH) produced by the anterior lobe of the pituitary gland.

Calcitonin, the other one of the three

hormones produced by the thyroid gland, is manufactured by cells lying between and among the follicles mentioned above. Calcitonin has an influence on the amount of calcium which circulates in the blood. It is antagonistic to the parathyroid hormone produced by the parathyroid glands and therefore helps in maintaining a precise balance between the amount of calcium in the blood and that which is stored in the body's bones.

The Parathyroid Glands

The parathyroid glands are very small organs, usually four in number, located on the back surfaces of the lateral lobes of the thyroid gland. They produce the parathyroid hormone, which controls the amounts of calcium and phosphate which circulate in the blood serum. This control is very important, so much so that a person cannot survive after the removal of his parathyroid glands unless he receives therapeutic doses of vitamin D. This vitamin maintains a proper level of calcium in the blood serum even though this calcium may have to be derived from the bones.

The Pancreas

As mentioned earlier, the pancreas contains two kinds of tissue, both of them glandular; but one kind functions as an exocrine organ and the other as an endocrine organ. Here we will discuss the pancreas as an endocrine organ.

The pancreas is located in the abdominal cavity, close to the stomach and duodenum. That part of its tissue which performs an endocrine function consists of many scattered islands of tissue (the islets of Langerhans). These contain different types of cells and have no connection with the system of ducts that carries the pancreatic juice to the duodenum.

One kind of cells within the islets of Langerhans produces insulin; another produces glucagon. These two hormones have an opposite effect in regulating the use of glucose (blood sugar) by the various tissues of the body. The two hormones, therefore, counterbalance each other.

When the amount of glucose in the blood plasma increases, the production of insulin is correspondingly increased, with the result that the entry of glucose

A microscopic view of an islet of Langerhans surrounded by the type of gland tissue within the pancreas which produces "pancreatic juice." Notice that there are many blood capillaries within the islet of Langerhans, but no provision for carrying the hormones away through a duct.

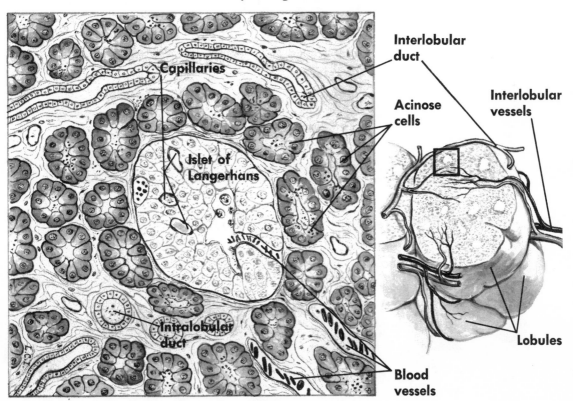

into muscle and other tissues is made easier, and the storage of glucose in the liver is facilitated.

In the absence of a sufficient amount of insulin, the level of glucose in the blood increases to such high levels that the excess is eliminated through the kidneys. Such a condition occurs in the disease diabetes mellitus. (See chapter 13, volume 3.) The condition may become so severe that, if untreated, the patient becomes unconscious and may die because of damage to his nervous system.

Too much insulin is detrimental in that it brings about such a lowering of the blood sugar that the body tissues are unable to receive their essential requirements. This, too, can lead to unconsciousness and death. Thus we see that insulin is a vital hormone and also that its quantity must be precisely controlled.

Glucagon, the other hormone produced by the islets of Langerhans, brings about in emergency situations a release of the stores of blood sugar throughout the body. This release enables the system to maintain as long as possible a proper level of glucose in the blood plasma.

The Ovaries as Endocrine Organs

The functions of the ovaries as well as those of the other female sex organs are under the control of the hormones produced by the anterior lobe of the pituitary gland. Under stimulation from the pituitary the ovaries produce important hormones of their own. Estradiol is the outstanding one of the several estrogens produced by the ovary. Progesterone, another, is produced by the cells which develop in an empty follicle after an ovum has been released.

Estradiol has two effects: (1) it regulates the functions of the reproductive organs and the desire for sexual activity; and (2) in the adolescent girl it stimulates the development of the feminine characteristics.

Progesterone is produced not only by the corpus luteum of the ovary but also, in smaller amounts by the cortex of the adrenal gland and by the placenta. Its function is to stimulate the lining of the uterus (except during pregnancy) so that it will be prepared to receive and nourish the cells which will develop into a child if pregnancy occurs. This preparation of the lining of the uterus takes place each month. Then, if no pregnancy occurs, most of this lining tissue is eliminated at the time of menstruation.

The Testes as Endocrine Organs

The testes have two functions: to produce male sex cells and to produce the male hormones called androgens. Androgens are produced mostly by the interstitial cells, which lie in clumps between the tubules which produce the male sex cells.

The principal androgen produced by the testes is testosterone, a steroid hormone. It has the effect, in an adolescent boy, of stimulating the development of the secondary male characteristics and, in a man, of maintaining these characteristics. It also stimulates desire for sexual activity and, other factors being favorable, promotes a feeling of well-being and aggressiveness.

Endocrine Gland Disorders

The endocrine glands belong to the body's control system. The hormones which they produce help to regulate the functions of cells and tissues throughout the body. It is reasonable to expect, then, that when the endocrine glands are affected by disease or when they do not function normally, there will be telltale symptoms even in remote parts of the body.

The present chapter is concerned with the various disturbances of the pituitary, the adrenals, the thyroid, the parathyroids, the islets of the pancreas, and the sex glands. It also deals with the systemic symptoms which such disturbances produce and with the available treatments for the ailments.

Pituitary Disorders

The location, structure, and normal functions of the pituitary gland are discussed in the preceding chapter.

DIABETES INSIPIDUS

In diabetes insipidus, a rare chronic disorder, large quantities (up to 20 quarts [20 liters] per day) of dilute urine are produced. It is accompanied, of course, by the symptom of severe thirst. The urine in this disorder does not contain glucose (sugar), as is the case in diabetes mellitus. The fundamental difficulty is a failure of the posterior lobe of the pituitary to release the normal amount of vasopressin (ADH), which acts on the cells of the kidney tubules in such a way as to favor the resorption of water from the kidney tubules.

Care and Treatment

A person with a mild case of diabetes insipidus may choose to tolerate the symptoms of excessive thirst and frequent urination rather than be bothered with the frequent administration of the vasopressin medication which serves as a replacement for the deficient antidiuretic hormone. Without therapy, however, the person with diabetes insipidus faces the ever-present danger of dehydration. The medication presently most successful is a synthetic product (desmopressin acetate), administered as a nasal spray one to three times a day.

GALACTORRHEA (ABNORMAL MILK PRODUCTION)

An overproduction of the hormone prolactin (produced in the anterior lobe of the pituitary) occurs sometimes in patients with pituitary tumors. The out-

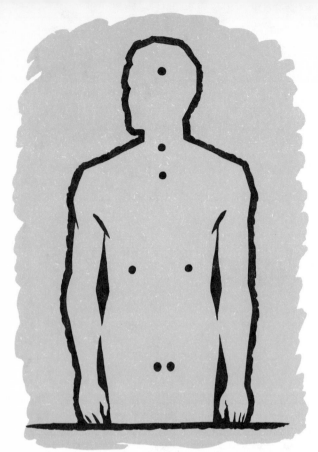

Location of main endocrine glands.

The vital pituitary gland is located at the base of the brain deep inside the head. The diagram shows its main parts.

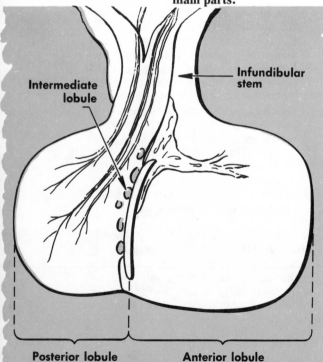

standing symptom is activation of the breast tissue to produce milk (galactorrhea). This may occur in men as well as in women (unrelated to a pregnancy). The amount of milk may be so small as to be observed only when the nipple is compressed. In a woman there may also be a cessation of menstruation; and in a man, impotence.

GIGANTISM AND ACROMEGALY

The disorders termed gigantism and acromegaly are characterized by an overproduction of somatotropin, the growth hormone (GH), produced by cells in the anterior lobe of the pituitary. The overproduction usually results from the development of a tumor in the pituitary gland, the cells of which manufacture an excess of this hormone. The tumor may be either slow growing or fast growing. If the overproduction occurs during childhood, gigantism results, with an adult height ranging from six and a half feet upward. If the overproduction of hormone begins after adult growth has been attained, acromegaly is the result. In acromegaly no apparent further increase takes place in height, but the hands and feet gradually enlarge. An exaggeration of facial features also occurs, with the jaw, lips, nose, and ridges above the eyes becoming prominent.

Care and Treatment

The treatment of gigantism or acromegaly requires the destruction of the overactive tumor. Such a case deserves the supervision of highly trained specialists who will decide on the treatment best suited for the individual. Radiation treatment or some form of surgery are the usual methods of therapy.

PANHYPOPITUITARISM (very rare)

Panhypopituitarism is a condition in which all the secreting cells of the anterior lobe of the pituitary fail to produce adequate quantities of their respective hormones. In view of the close

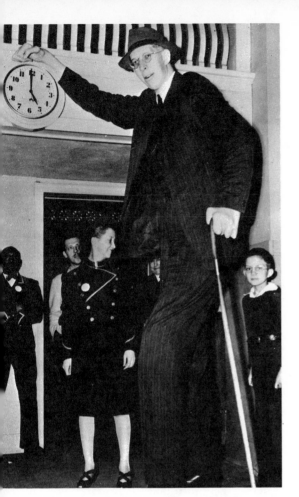

Gigantism stems from an excess of
the growth-promoting hormone.

relationship between the pituitary and
the other endocrine glands, these other
glands are affected also. In the mildest
form of the disease, there is atrophy of
the sex organs, with a reduction in axillary and pubic hair and a tendency to
premature aging. In more severe cases,
symptoms include also weakness, low
blood pressure, low blood sugar, low
body temperature, and loss of appetite.
One of the most common causes is
bleeding into the pituitary after delivery (Sheehan's syndrome).

Care and Treatment

**Treatment requires "replacement
therapy"—the administration of
many hormones to replace those
found deficient. Treatment should be
under the direction of a specialist in
endocrinology.**

PITUITARY DWARFISM

Hormones from several of the endocrine organs, including the pituitary,
the thyroid, the adrenals, and the sex
glands, influence the rate and the extent of growth. Deficiencies cause various kinds of dwarfism. But here we
speak of the kind of short stature
caused primarily by a decrease in production of somatotropin, the growth
hormone (GH) produced by the anterior lobe of the pituitary gland. The
body's proportions are relatively normal. Dwarfs of this type have become
famous circus performers, and some
have become wealthy. Sexual development is often deficient in this type of
dwarfism.

Care and Treatment

**To be effective, treatment of pitu-
itary dwarfism must be begun in
early childhood. It consists of administering somatotropin (growth hormone) of human origin. This medication is very expensive. Treatment
should be planned by specialists at a
medical center.**

Adrenal Disorders

ADDISON'S DISEASE

Addison's disease is the name given
to a serious condition caused by atrophy or destruction of the cortexes of
the adrenal glands. In the majority of
cases the atrophy of the functioning
cells is part of an autoimmune disorder
in which white blood cells invade the
functioning tissue of the adrenal cortex. The other cases are caused by a
progressive destruction of the functioning tissue by a disease such as tuberculosis or cancer, or by an inflammatory
process. Symptoms of Addison's disease usually do not develop until about
90 percent of the tissue of the adrenal
cortexes has been incapacitated.

The symptoms of Addison's disease
include chronic fatigue, exhaustion,
low blood pressure, and usually a loss
of sodium chloride and water from the
blood and tissues. The patient has poor

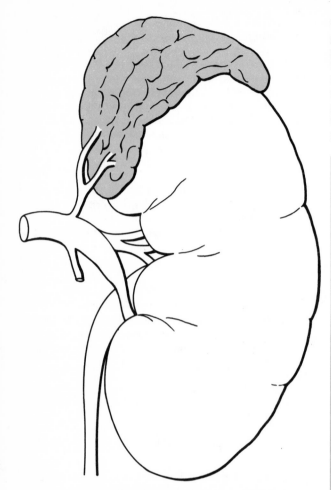

Adrenal gland rests on kidney.

tal condition, it is no longer so. Given good medical supervision and intelligent cooperation by the patient, an active and comparatively normal life is now possible for most persons with this affliction. However, a continuous program of daily hormone replacement therapy must be followed meticulously for the remainder of life.

Care and Treatment

The physician's task of evaluating a case of Addison's disease is made more difficult if it happens that the patient has received steroid medication within the year. If such should be the case, the patient should, by all means, mention it to his doctor.

The essence of treatment consists in supplementing the hormones and chemical substances now in short supply in the patient's body.

For the treatment of an "addisonian crisis" the patient must receive promptly, by intravenous injection, a large volume of physiologic sodium chloride solution together with hydrocortisone. For routine maintenance he must take daily doses of both hydrocortisone and fludrocortisone—the latter to replace the aldosterone hormone which he now lacks. He must have an abundance of water. His doctor must give prompt attention to any aggravating condition such as injury, surgery, or infection.

Patients with Addison's disease should wear an identifying bracelet, so that if they are injured or become unconscious, medical personnel could be alerted.

appetite and frequent attacks of nausea, vomiting, and diarrhea. In about half the cases there is an increase in the pigmentation of the skin in the body creases (especially those of the palms), over pressure areas, and around the areolae of the nipples. The person with Addison's disease is in continuous danger of "addisonian crisis," a life-threatening condition in which he goes into a form of shock in response to such stresses as vomiting, injury, or infection.

The disease may be accompanied by many and varied complications. It demands expert study and medical guidance. While the malady was once a fatal

ADRENAL VIRILISM

In this condition a tumor or an increase in the number of functioning cells in the adrenal cortex causes an overproduction of the masculinizing hormone androgen. When the condition develops in early childhood there is a hastening of the changes characteristic of adolescence—an early onset of sexual maturity. When the condition begins in adulthood, masculine characteristics become accentuated in both men and women.

Care and Treatment

The treatment for severe cases is the surgical removal of the adrenal glands if a tumor is present, or suppression of pituitary ACTH with cortisol or similar glucocorticoids if any enzyme defect in the adrenals has led to excessive ACTH from the pituitary. Following either treatment there must be precise follow-up care with replacement hormone therapy.

CUSHING'S SYNDROME

Cushing's syndrome, a rare ailment occurring more commonly in women than in men, is caused by an overabundance of glucocorticoids—hormones normally produced in the cortexes of the adrenal glands. Cushing's syndrome can result (1) from an overproduction of the pituitary hormone corticotropin (ACTH) which, in turn, stimulates the adrenals, even though normal, to excess activity; (2) from disease in an adrenal gland (usually a tumor) which causes an overproduction of the glucocorticoids; or (3) from the taking of excessive amounts of glucocorticoid hormone (such as cortisone) as a medication.

The usual symptoms are obesity (involving the face and trunk), muscular weakness, excessive growth of hair on the face and chest, atrophic changes in the skin, elevation of blood pressure, suppression of menstruation in women and decrease of sex desire in men, and a thinning of bone structure. Often there is an associated development of diabetes mellitus.

Care and Treatment

The plan of treatment must be based on a careful study of the cause of the ailment in the individual case—whether it be tumor of the pituitary gland, tumor of one adrenal gland, or excess medication with glucocorticoid hormone. In the first two instances, specialized surgical removal of the tumor or of the entire adrenal gland(s) or the pituitary tumor may be indicated. Surgical cases usually require precise follow-up care with replacement hormone therapy.

HYPERALDOSTERONISM (CONN'S SYNDROME)

In hyperaldosteronism there is an excess of aldosterone produced in the cortexes of the adrenal glands. The normal function of this hormone is to control the retention of sodium and the elimination of potassium as takes place in the kidneys and certain of the body's exocrine glands. The condition is typically caused by a tumor of one of the adrenal glands, but in some cases it is due to a mere increase in number of the cells which produce this hormone.

In mild cases the only symptom is a mild to moderate increase in blood pressure. In more severe cases occasions of weakness, abnormal skin sensations, and come-and-go weakness of muscles will also occur.

Care and Treatment

In the usual case the treatment requires the locating and surgical removal of the adrenal tumor.

PHEOCHROMOCYTOMA

The pheochromocytoma is a life-threatening tumor which develops in the medullary portion of an adrenal gland. It produces an excess of the same hormones as are normally produced in the adrenal medulla. The outstanding symptom is an excessively high blood pressure, with associated sweating, a rapid pulse, and other signs of excessive adrenalin production.

Care and Treatment

Early recognition and prompt removal of this tumor gives a good prospect of a favorable outcome.

Thyroid Disorders

The thyroid gland produces three hormones: thyroxine, triiodothyronine, and calcitonin. Thyroxine is the principal hormone and the one to which we

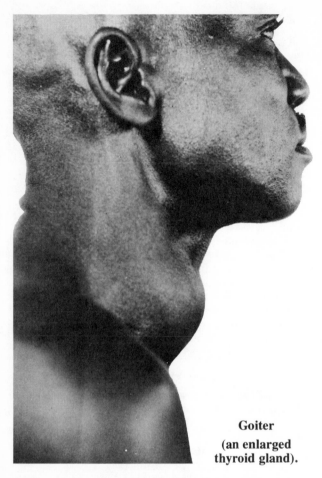

Goiter

(an enlarged thyroid gland).

give attention here. The effects of all three of the hormones are summarized in the preceding chapter.

GOITER

An enlarged thyroid gland is called a goiter, whatever the cause of enlargement. In some goiters an excess of thyroxine is produced, and in others a reduced amount. An overabundance of thyroxine causes a speeding up of many body activities. The relative activity of the thyroid gland can be determined by a laboratory procedure in which the thyroid hormones in the blood are measured.

GOITER, NONTOXIC

In this condition the thyroid gland enlarges, but it does not produce more than the normal amount of its hormones. In fact, in some cases of nontoxic goiter there may even be a deficit of hormone production.

The basic cause of the nontoxic goiter is some interference with the mechanism for producing thyroxine. Because thyroxine is now in short supply, the thyroid gland enlarges (under the overruling stimulation of the pituitary gland) in an effort to compensate for the deficiency. Factors which may provoke this condition are (1) a shortage of iodine, one of the constituents of thyroxine (now extremely rare in the U.S.A.); (2) the excessive use of the thyroid-depressing drugs; and (3) inherited defects of the body's enzyme system. One of the most common causes now is Hashimoto's disease in which autoantibodies (antibodies against one's own body) damage the thyroid.

In former decades nontoxic goiter was much more common than now because iodine was in short supply in the food and water of certain geographic areas. This deficiency has been corrected by the widespread use of iodized salt.

Care and Treatment

The essential treatment for nontoxic goiter is the administration of thyroxine as a medication. This compensates for the reduced amount of the hormone produced by the thyroid gland and thus removes the stimulus for the gland to function beyond its normal capacity.

HYPERTHYROIDISM

Hyperthyroidism, as the term implies, is a condition in which the thyroid gland is more active than normal. The condition is usually due to overproduction of both of the hormones thyroxine and triiodothyronine. There are several manifestations of hyperthyroidism. We will discuss the two most common: (1) thyrotoxicosis (Graves' disease) and (2) toxic nodular goiter.

A. *Thyrotoxicosis (Graves' disease,*

exophthalmic goiter). Thyrotoxicosis is more common in women than in men at the ratio of three to one. It may occur at any age but is most frequent between the ages of ten and fifty. The predisposition to the disease often runs in families. The basic cause is now assumed to be a disturbance in the body's immune system.

The symptoms of thyrotoxicosis may develop suddenly or gradually. Sudden onset often follows some injury, a severe infection, or some psychic upset. The usual symptoms are nervousness, intolerance for heat, rapid heartbeat, weight loss, tiredness, increased appetite, excessive thirst, difficult breathing, weakness of the muscles, fine tremor, frequent urination, and diarrhea. A goiter (enlargement of the thyroid gland) is usually obvious, although in a few cases the thyroid may remain normal in size. A prominent symptom in about 70 percent of the cases is a "staring expression" of the eyes so that the eyes may even appear to bulge. It is this appearance of the eyes that prompted the term exophthalmic goiter (goiter with protruding eyes).

Care and Treatment

Every person with thyrotoxicosis should be under the care of a physician. The excess production of thyroid hormones causes all tissues of the body to function beyond their normal rate, as though operating under a condition of perpetual emergency. The outlook for untreated cases is unfavorable, eventual death being caused by problems of nutrition or by heart failure.

Many cases respond favorably to the use of "antithyroid" drugs which have the effect of suppressing the excess activity of the thyroid gland. But these may produce unfavorable side effects and therefore must be used only under careful professional supervision.

The administration of radioactive iodine is being used successfully in many clinics. The thyroid gland absorbs and retains the iodine which,

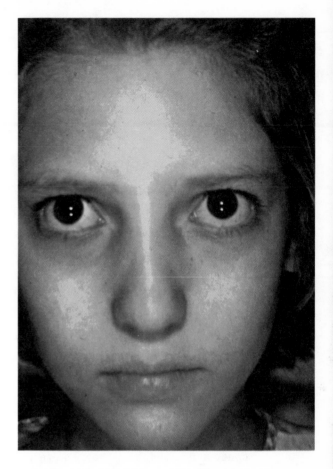

Abnormally prominent eyes, appearing to bulge, characterize thyrotoxicosis (Graves' disease).

because of its radioactivity (it emits beta rays), destroys many of the overactive cells in the gland. In about 40 percent of the cases thus treated the radioactive iodine destroys so many of the functioning cells that the remaining ones do not produce as much thyroxine as the person needs. Thus the patient must take supplementary thyroxine by mouth as a medication for the rest of his life.

Surgical removal of part of the hyperactive thyroid gland is still used occasionally for cases in which other methods of treatment are inadequate.

B. *Toxic Nodular Goiter.* Although

29

an excess of thyroid hormones is produced in this type of goiter, as in thyrotoxicosis, it has a different background of origin. Toxic nodular goiter usually occurs as a late complication of nontoxic goiter. In such a case isolated areas of tissue within the thyroid gland become unresponsive to the body's normal checks and balances and proceed to produce excesses of hormones.

Toxic nodular goiter usually develops later in life than thyrotoxicosis. The symptoms always come on more slowly and are not so extreme. Bulging of the eyes (exophthalmos) does not occur. In neglected cases damage to the heart may develop.

Care and Treatment

The treatment for toxic nodular goiter is either surgery or radioactive iodine. The response to the use of radioactive iodine is usually good.

HYPOTHYROIDISM

In hypothyroidism the thyroid gland secretes less than the normal amount of thyroxine; however, rather surprisingly, the gland may in some cases be considerably enlarged. The most extreme cases of hypothyroidism are the congenital or childhood type, known as cretinism, and the later-developing type, myxedema.

A. *Cretinism*. Children with this condition do not grow as rapidly or symmetrically as they should. Their minds develop slowly. No abnormality may be seen at birth, but within a few weeks the skin begins to thicken, and the cry becomes hoarse. The tongue becomes large, and the facial expression, piglike. The teeth are late in developing. If not treated, cretins become and remain deformed, feebleminded dwarfs, for whom little improvement is possible after the usual growing years are past.

Now that adequate treatment is available for cretinism, it is urgent that the condition be recognized in early infancy and treatment begun promptly.

There is the unhappy possibility that this condition may not be recognized in an infant until permanent damage has already been done. Best results are obtained when treatment is begun even before the classic symptoms develop. There is growing interest, therefore, in screening programs by which all newborn infants are tested (by chemical examination of small blood samples) so as to detect any deficiency of the thyroid hormone.

Care and Treatment

The remedy for congenital hypothyroidism, or for cretinism if it has already developed, consists of the administering of thyroxine to make up for the deficiency in what the child's own thyroid gland is producing.

B. *Myxedema*. In myxedema the production of thyroxine is below normal, oxidation in the body is decreased, and all the chemical activities of the body are slowed down. The heartbeat and breathing become slower, and the heart action becomes weaker. The heart may become dilated. Perspiration is scanty, and susceptibility to infection is increased. The temperature is below normal. The patient feels chilly and asks for more clothing, especially bedclothing. A peculiar type of tissue swelling follows, which may occur in any or all of the body tissues. It changes the skin, causing it to become puffy, rough, and thickened. The hair becomes dry and falls out easily. The nails are brittle and cracked. The body as a whole appears fat and soggy. The voice often sounds hoarse and harsh, hearing is impaired, and the victim appears mentally dull.

Myxedema is, typically, a disease of adults and occurs whenever the production of thyroid hormones is greatly reduced. Myxedema may occur in a case in which there has been intensive treatment for hyperthyroidism. In such an instance, the treatment has caused the production of thyroid hormones to be reduced below the normal level. This problem may be prevented if patients treated for hyperthyroidism have periodic blood tests and, as soon as they become hypothyroid, are treated with thyroxine. Development of this complication does not necessarily mean that the treatment of the hyperthyroidism was faulty. The treatment may have been the means of saving the patient's life. In such a case in which the thyroid gland is no longer producing as much hormone as it should, it is relatively easy for the physician to arrange to make up for the deficiency by prescribing thyroxine medication.

Care and Treatment

The treatment of myxedema consists of administering thyroxine.

THYROID MALIGNANCY (CANCER OF THE THYROID)

Although still a relatively rare disease, cancer of the thyroid has shown a marked increase in recent years. Some instances occur in persons who have had a goiter for many years. Others seem to occur independent of any previous thyroid disease. It is important, however, for a person with goiter to report promptly to his doctor should he notice a sudden enlargement or pain in an existing goiter or should he suddenly develop difficulty in breathing or notice a change in the quality of his voice.

The use of radioactive iodine in the treatment of goiters in adults does not predispose to cancer of the thyroid. However, cancer of the thyroid is more common in persons who, during childhood, received X-ray treatments to the tonsils or other tissues within the neck. A person with such a history should inform his physician.

Care and Treatment

The treatment of thyroid malignancy is surgical removal of part or all of the thyroid gland.

Following surgery, some clinics use radioactive iodine in the hope that this will seek out and destroy any remaining islands of malignant thyroid tissue or of malignant tissue that has migrated (metastasized) to some other part of the body.

After removal of part or all of the thyroid gland it is always advisable for the patient to take appropriate doses of thyroxine for the remainder of life in order to restore the amount of thyroid hormone which the body requires and to suppress TSH in an attempt to prevent growth of any remaining thyroid tissue.

THYROIDITIS

Thyroiditis is an unfortunate name for a small group of conditions which involve the thyroid gland; the members of the group seem not to be related to each other.

A. *Acute Thyroiditis*. This is a rare condition in which the thyroid gland becomes inflamed because of the invasion of bacteria. In this case the term *thyroiditis* is justified because of the presence of acute inflammation. The infection reaches the thyroid from surrounding tissues of the neck or because a cyst of the thyroid has become infected. The patient suffers from fever and pain in the neck and notices an enlargement in the area of the thyroid gland.

Care and Treatment

The treatment of acute thyroiditis consists of eradicating the infection by the use of antibiotic medications as prescribed by a physician.

B. *Subacute Thyroiditis*. In this inflammatory condition a painful enlargement of the thyroid gland occurs which persists over a period of weeks or months. It is caused, presumably, by a virus. In mild cases the illness subsides spontaneously after days or a few weeks. In the severe cases, if untreated, there may be remissions and relapses over a period of one or two years.

Care and Treatment

The severe cases respond favorably to the administration of a corticosteroid medication, which should be tapered off within a period of one

31

month. Such medication, of course, should be under the direct supervision of a physician.

C. *Chronic Thyroiditis.* This is really not an inflammatory condition at all, in spite of the implication of the term *thyroiditis. (Itis* usually means "inflammation.") The term embraces a small group of chronic diseases in which the thyroid becomes enlarged to various degrees and in which the functioning tissue of the thyroid is gradually replaced by connective tissues and, sometimes in part, by lymphocytes.

Hashimoto's thyroiditis is the outstanding member of the group. This disease is twenty times more frequent in women than in men. Its usual occurrence is between the ages of thirty and fifty. Typically it results in a reduction of the normal function of the thyroid gland. Patients complain of fatigue. The thyroid gland may be two or three times its normal size and is of firm consistency.

Care and Treatment

The treatment consists of administering thyroxine to make up for what the gland is no longer producing on its own.

Parathyroid Disorders

The parathyroid glands produce a hormone which controls the amounts of calcium and phosphorus which circulate in the blood. The principal disorders are (1) hypoparathyroidism (in which an insufficient amount of hormone is produced) and (2) hyperparathyroidism (in which an excess of the hormone is produced).

HYPERPARATHYROIDISM
Hyperparathyroidism occurs more commonly than hypoparathyroidism. It is characterized by a high level of calcium in the blood serum and in the urine. This may be responsible for the development of kidney stones (because of the large amount of calcium being eliminated through the kidneys) and for

fatal damage to the kidneys by deposits of calcium within their tissues. There also occurs a rarefaction of the bones, as observed by X-ray, on account of the withdrawal of calcium salts. The symptoms include excessive thirst, excessive urination, pains in the back and in various bones and joints, and loss of appetite sometimes accompanied with nausea and vomiting.

Usually, the cause of hyperparathyroidism is the development of a benign tumor within one or more of the parathyroid glands. Increased function of the parathyroid glands can also develop in association with chronic kidney disease and in rickets. Certain malignant tumors in other parts of the body apparently may produce a hormone with function similar to that of the parathyroid hormone, even to the extent of producing symptoms of hyperparathyroidism.

Care and Treatment

When hyperparathyroidism is caused by the development of a tumor within the parathyroid glands, surgical removal of the involved tissue is necessary.

HYPOPARATHYROIDISM
In this disorder the amount of calcium in the blood serum is low, the amount of phosphorus, high. When it begins in childhood, a stunting of growth takes place, with malformation of the teeth and a deficiency in mental development. In the acute phase of the disorder there are cramps of the muscles (especially the abdominal muscles), difficult breathing, sensitivity to light, and convulsions. When the condition becomes chronic, there is a tendency to the formation of cataracts of the eyes and permanent brain damage.

Cases of hypoparathyroidism that develop spontaneously are rare. The usual circumstance that causes hypoparathyroidism is the removal of the parathyroid glands when thyroid surgery is performed. Persons who have had this kind of thyroid surgery should therefore be alert to the possibility of the presence of hypoparathyroidism.

Care and Treatment

Cases of hypoparathyroidism respond favorably to a carefully regulated program of therapy. This requires the administration of salts of calcium (by vein in acute cases) and of a special type of vitamin D preparation. Dairy products should be avoided because of their high content of phosphorus. Frequent laboratory checkups must be made to keep track of the patient's response to the treatment and thus to avoid recurrence of the symptoms.

Pancreatic Islet Cell Disease

Scattered throughout the substance of the pancreas are "islets" of cells that function collectively as an endocrine organ and produce the hormone insulin. The notable example of a disorder in which these islets function abnormally is diabetes mellitus, which is considered in chapter 13, volume 3.

Male Sex Gland Endocrine Disorders

Testosterone is the masculinizing hormone. It is produced in the testes by cells that lie between the sex-cell-producing tubules. During fetal life testosterone is responsible for the development of the external male sex organs. At adolescence and thereafter it is testosterone that stimulates and maintains a man's secondary sex characteristics.

The production of testosterone by the testes is stimulated by luteinizing hormone (LH) of the anterior lobe of the pituitary. Insufficient production of testosterone accounts for absence, reduction, or loss of male characteristics—male hypogonadism. Excess production accounts for male sexual precocity.

HYPOGONADISM, MALE

In hypogonadism production of testosterone and/or male sex cells (sper-matozoa) is diminished or absent. We are concerned here with cases suffering from a deficiency in the production of testosterone. The condition may be caused by disease of the pituitary in which the luteinizing hormone (LH) is deficient or by disease within the testes.

When the condition develops before adolescence, the individual fails to experience the normal transition from boyhood to manhood. He continues to grow in height, but remains slender; his voice remains high-pitched; his arms and legs are relatively longer than normal for his height; he does not develop a beard; and his external sex organs remain infantile.

When hypogonadism develops during adulthood, the secondary masculine characteristics regress and sexual impotence develops.

Care and Treatment

Restoration of testosterone can be accomplished by (1) the administering of chorionic gonadotropin (to stimulate the testes to produce their own testosterone) or (2) by the direct administration of synthetic testosterone. For the adolescent patient, the dosage should be moderate at the beginning and then gradually increased.

MALE SEXUAL PRECOCITY

An excess of testosterone may be produced in three conditions: (1) premature activation of the testes by pituitary hormones so that a boy develops adult masculine characteristics at an earlier-than-normal age, (2) overproduction of male hormones, and (3) the development of a type of tumor within one testis which produces an excessive amount of testosterone.

Care and Treatment

Treatment requires attention to the underlying cause, whether it be premature activation of the testes or overproduction of male hormones (overactivity of the pituitary, the adrenals, or the testis). In cases where a tumor is affecting the hor-

33

CHAS. PFIZER & CO., INC.

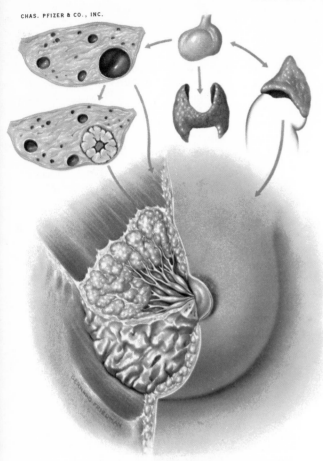

Interrelationship between the endocrine glands and the growth and development of the breast.

mone-producing cells within a testis, removal of the involved testis is indicated.

Female Sex Gland
Endocrine Disorders

The ovaries, the essential female sex glands, produce two hormones: estrogen and progesterone. Estrogen, which consists of a closely related group of hormones in which estradiol is outstanding, is the feminizing hormone and is responsible for the development and maintenance of the body features and functions characteristic of womanhood. Progesterone is concerned with pregnancy and serves to ready the uterus for the event of pregnancy and to prepare the breasts during pregnancy for their function of producing milk.

The production of estrogen by the ovaries is stimulated by the luteinizing hormone (LH) of the anterior lobe of the pituitary.

HYPOGONADISM, FEMALE

The condition in which the characteristics of womanhood do not develop at the time of adolescence or in which these characteristics wane after having once developed is called female hypogonadism. It can be caused (1) by insufficient stimulation of the ovaries by the pituitary hormone, (2) by poorly formed or poorly functioning ovaries, or (3) by the absence of ovaries, as when they have been removed by surgery.

When a teenage girl's ovaries fail to produce a sufficient quantity of estrogen, her sex organs, both internal and external, fail to develop beyond their childhood status; her breasts remain undeveloped; her figure conforms to the childhood pattern; and she does not menstruate.

When a woman's ovaries are removed during her prime of life after they have previously functioned normally, she experiences changes similar to what occurs in an older woman at the time of the menopause: her monthly menstruation ceases, she is no longer capable of pregnancy, her uterus and vagina become smaller, she experiences hot flashes, and her breasts tend to become pendulous.

Care and Treatment

Replacement therapy, using oral estrogen, to provide the lacking hormone, is the mainstay of treatment. Inasmuch as the functions of the endocrine glands are very much interrelated, it is advisable to consult a physician trained in the speciality of gynecology or endocrinology.

The Nervous System

The human body may be likened to a large industrial plant—not because it manufactures anything commercially, but because, as in a factory, each department works harmoniously with all the others. In order for an industrial plant to maintain such harmony it must be controlled by an adequate communication system and a central office. The superintendent in charge must receive reports from all departments and send back instructions on how operations are to proceed.

Elsewhere in these volumes we have noticed how hormones influence the functions of certain tissues and how the DNA molecules in each of the cells throughout the body have a controlling influence on events within the cells. In the present chapter we take up the nervous system, which exerts the highest order of control throughout the body and is able to modify this control in ways suitable to a person's chosen activities.

Just as in an industrial plant not all reports find their way to the superintendent in charge, so in the human body, not all activities are controlled directly by the brain. Various minor nerve centers exercise a degree of control over small parts of the body. But even these are subject to the overruling control of the brain, just as in an industrial plant the boss of a department has

to take orders from the superintendent in charge of the plant.

Nerve Cells and Nerves

Like other parts of the body, the nervous system is composed of cells, millions upon millions of them. These are of two kinds: nerve cells and supporting cells. The nerve cells are highly specialized for their own particular work.

As shown in the accompanying illustration (next page), a typical nerve cell has a cell body which contains its nucleus, several short branches called dendrites, and one long branch called an axon. Nerve impulses pass through a nerve cell in only one direction. Entering through one of the dendrites, an impulse passes through the cell body and then into the axon. At the end of the axon it is transferred either to another nerve cell or to some functioning tissue which this nerve cell influences. Some axons are short and simply carry nerve impulses to another nerve cell located close by. Others are many inches in length.

The point at which the axon of one nerve cell contacts a dendrite or the body of another nerve cell is called a synapse. A nerve impulse, in going from its starting point to its terminal point, may cross several synapses. A nerve "pathway" is composed of a se-

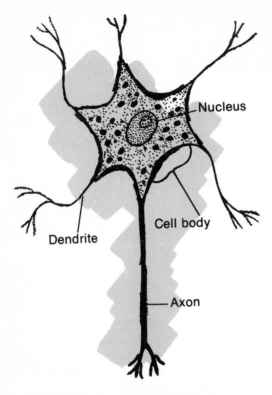

View of nerve cell and its parts.

ries of nerve cells which pass the nervous impulse from one to the next in sequence.

Some nerve cells have the job of carrying nerve impulses toward the spinal cord or the brain. These impulses may originate in the skin, in some internal structure of the body, or in one of the organs of special sense like the eyes or ears. Other nerve cells simply carry nervous impulses from one part of the spinal cord or the brain to some other part of the spinal cord or brain. Still others carry impulses from the brain or spinal cord to the muscles, to the internal organs, to the glands, or to the blood vessels. We see, then, that it is the nerve cells which form the body's communication system, keeping the brain informed of what is going on in various parts of the body and then carrying messages back from the brain to regulate the activity of the various tissues and organs.

The axons going to or from a certain

part of the body are bundled together to form a "nerve," just like the wires that carry telephone messages to the houses in a certain section of town are bundled together to form a telephone cable. Some of the axons in a nerve will be carrying nervous impulses toward the spinal cord or brain and others will be carrying impulses away from the spinal cord or brain.

A little earlier we mentioned that there are two kinds of cells in the nervous system: nerve cells and supporting cells. The supporting cells do not carry nervous impulses but, as their name implies, help to hold the nerve cells and their axons in place.

The Spinal Cord

The spinal cord is a long, slender cable of nerve tissue which extends lengthwise through the vertebrae of the spinal column. At the upper end it connects with the brain through an opening in the floor of the skull. It extends downward almost to the level of the hips. It is well protected by the vertebrae, whose bony processes join together to form a canal within which the spinal cord is located.

Attached to the spinal cord are thirty-one pairs of nerves in which are axons that carry nerve impulses to and from the spinal cord. These spinal nerves reach out to all parts of the body except the head. Some of them go down the arms and legs as far as the fingers and toes. Others supply the tissues of the chest wall and of the abdominal wall.

Inside the spinal cord are many nerve cells as well as bundles of axons. Some of the nerve cells specialize in receiving the nerve impulses from the various parts of the body. Others carry some of these impulses up to the brain. Still other nerve cells in the spinal cord have axons which extend out through the spinal nerves to the muscles and blood vessels and glands.

Spinal Reflexes

Many of the nerve cells in the spinal cord are organized to provide a simple

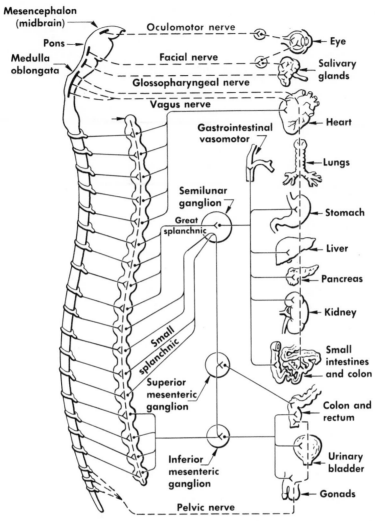

Autonomic nervous system, showing the different organs whose functions are regulated by the nerves of the sympathetic (solid lines) and parasympathetic (broken lines) divisions.

type of control for a certain part of the body to which they are linked. For example, when one's finger touches something hot, a nervous impulse is carried from the finger to the spinal cord. Connections made there transfer the impulse to the nerve cells that control certain muscles in the arm and forearm which jerk the hand away from the hot object.

At the same time connections are also made with nerve cells carrying impulses up to the brain. These register a sensation of heat from the finger and indicate that the hand has been pulled away from the hot object. The action of pulling the hand away took place before the brain became aware of it.

A nervous pathway which operates automatically without having to wait for directions from the brain is called a reflex. Many such reflex circuits operate throughout the body, and because they can operate automatically, they increase the efficiency of the nervous system.

Let us take another example. When a person has stood in the same spot for a while, particularly when his feet are close together, he may tend to lean either to the right or to the left. As he does this, the muscles on the opposite side of his legs are stretched a bit. The stretching sends off nervous impulses to the spinal cord. There they make reflex connections with nerve cells which cause the muscles being stretched to contract enough to bring the person back into an erect position.

It is this kind of reflex which the doctor tests, during a physical examination, when he checks the patient's "knee jerk." By tapping on the tendon just below the kneecap, he sets off a reflex mechanism which, if the nerves and spinal cord at this level are working normally, causes the muscles in the patient's thigh to produce a quick kick. If the patient does not respond this way or if the knee jerk on the left is different from that on the right, the doctor knows that something is wrong with the nerve connections.

Many of the things you do "because I cannot help it" are caused by the reflex connections built into your nervous system. When you stumble over the edge of the rug, you automatically extend your arms in the direction of your fall. You do not have time to think about it, but you are automatically stimulated to act by complicated reflex circuits.

The Brain

We recognize the brain as the headquarters of the entire nervous system. The physiologist sometimes speaks of it as a complicated "monitoring apparatus," but it is more than this.

The brain receives nerve impulses from all parts of the body, including the sense organs. Thus it is kept constantly informed of conditions within and without the body. On the strength of this information it controls the body's activities.

We mentioned earlier that the spinal cord is in communication with the outlying parts of the body through thirty-one pairs of spinal nerves. The brain, in turn, is in communication with the spinal cord and thus with the areas served by the thirty-one pairs of spinal nerves. In addition, the brain is served by twelve pairs of so-called cranial nerves which connect with it through openings in the skull. These serve the region of the head, and some of them even pass deeply into the chest and the abdominal cavity, where they make contact with the organs located there.

The brain has four principal parts: the brainstem, the cerebellum, the interbrain, and the cerebrum.

The Brainstem contains many axons passing between the spinal cord and the parts of the brain. Like the spinal cord, it also has many nerve cells of its own. These are concerned with some of the body's more complex reflex mechanisms. Here we have the control areas for breathing, for influencing the rate of the heartbeat, for the regulation of blood pressure, for swallowing, for coughing, for sneezing, and for vomiting. Also within the brainstem we have the nerve-cell connections that take care of the automatic and voluntary components of eye movements and of the movements of the body as these enable a person to keep his balance.

Even though we speak of certain of the functions just listed as being controlled in the brainstem, we must recognize that the cerebrum, operating at a higher level of control, can, within certain limits, overrule the brainstem. That is, when a person so desires, he can take control of such activities as breathing, swallowing, and moving the eyes. For example, a person can hold his breath if he chooses until he becomes unconscious. Then, with the cerebrum being no longer able to function, the brainstem takes over again and breathing resumes so that the person soon regains consciousness. The same with moving the eyes. A person can deliberately move his eyes to the right or to the left by overruling the automatic controls contained in the brainstem.

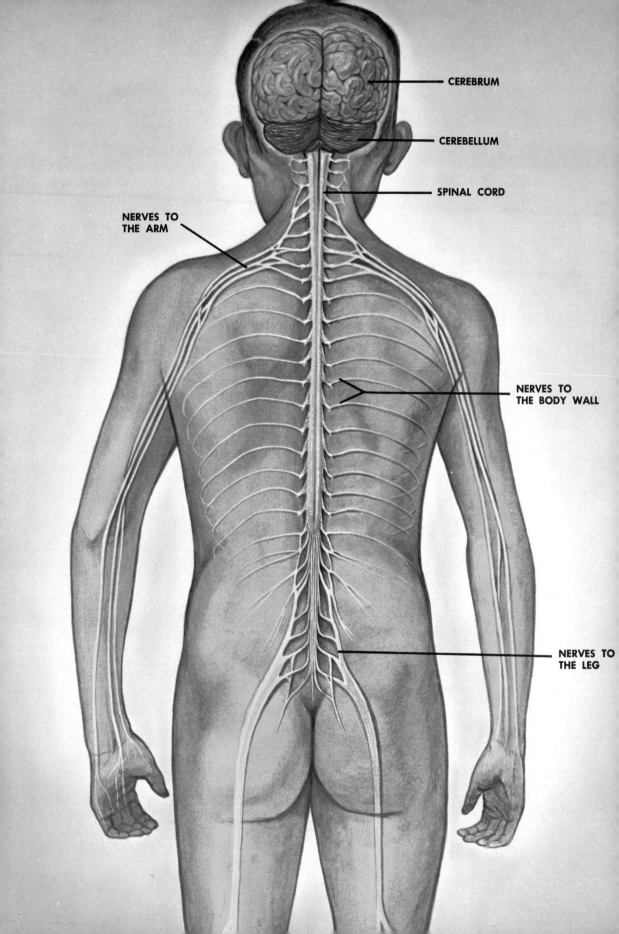

CEREBRUM

CEREBELLUM

SPINAL CORD

NERVES TO
THE ARM

NERVES TO
THE BODY WALL

NERVES TO
THE LEG

The Cerebellum is located just above the neck in the back part of the skull. It is concerned with balance, equilibrium, and the coordination of muscles.

To understand how the cerebellum coordinates the action of the muscles let us notice the movements of the forearm at the elbow. For practical purposes two groups of muscles operate here—one to bend the elbow and the other to straighten it. The muscles that bend the elbow cannot act until the muscles that straighten it relax enough to make this possible. But you do not have to think about relaxing the "opposing muscles" in order to bend the elbow or straighten it. The cerebellum takes care of these details in an automatic manner.

It also keeps the body's muscles ready to act. It does this by maintaining all muscles in a slightly contracted condition (except when a person relaxes completely as in sleep) so that there is no time lost in taking up the slack in a muscle that hangs limp.

The Interbrain (usually called the hypothalamus) is located near the center of the head and just above the pituitary gland. It is surrounded, except on its under surface, by other parts of the brain. The nerve cells contained in the interbrain are grouped to form automatic control centers for several of the body's important functions. Outstanding among these is the control of body temperature.

The interbrain, being located as it is close to the pituitary gland, affects the various functions of this gland and causes changes in those parts of the body ifluenced by the production of pituitary hormones.

The interbrain also serves as a coordination center for the autonomic nervous system—that part of the nervous system that regulates the functions of the body's organs, glands, and vessels.

The interbrain acts in conjunction with certain parts of the cerebrum in providing for the emotions. These are discussed in more detail later in the chapter.

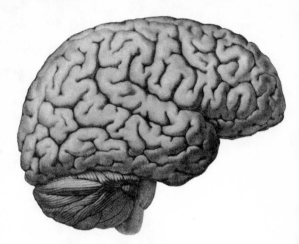

The brain.

The Cerebrum is the largest part of the brain. It occupies the space within the skull from above the eyes, in front, to the very back of the head, just above the cerebellum. It contains billions of nerve cells.

In considering the cerebrum we are most interested in its surface layer, the cortex, which is packed with nerve cells. The cortex is folded into many large "wrinkles" so as to increase its area. This makes the surface of the cerebrum appear something like the surface of a walnut meat.

The cortex of the cerebrum serves as the control board, as it were, for the entire nervous system. Each area of the cortex does a particular work. One part receives the nerve impulses from the various areas of the skin. Another part receives impulses from the eyes; another, from the ears; another, from the organs of smell; and another, from the organs of taste. It is a person's awareness of all these incoming impulses and their significance that constitutes consciousness.

Another part of the cortex of the cerebrum, called the motor area, controls the actions of the body's muscles. The motor area of the right side of the brain controls the muscles on the left side of the body, and the area of the left side of the brain controls the muscles on the right. In most persons, the left side of the brain is more highly developed in its ability to control and coordinate the movement of the muscles, a fact which explains why most people are right-handed.

The motor area of the cortex enables a person to move any muscle of his body just by deciding to do so. Furthermore, he can control his muscles' movements accurately. He can develop skills by moving certain muscles or certain sets of muscles in a specified manner over and over again until a habit is formed. The skills of a musician, of a typist, or of a dentist are developed this way and are under the control of the cortex of the cerebrum.

An area of the cortex of the cerebrum, close by the motor area, provides the patterns of muscle control by which certain muscles are caused to operate in sequence. For instance, the complicated control pattern for walking requires certain muscles to relax while others contract and arranges for the involved muscles to move one after the other in a smooth, predetermined order.

Perhaps the most highly coordinated mechanism for muscle action relates to

Areas of the cerebrum as they are related to the various functions.

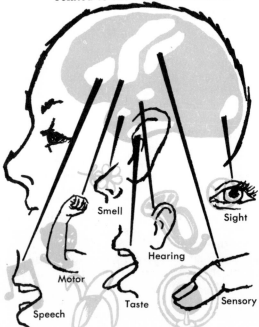

Smell

Sight

Motor

Hearing

Taste

Sensory

Speech

speech. The muscles of the larynx, the tongue, the face, and the jaw, as well as those concerned with breathing, must all be carefully coordinated. And in order for a person to speak intelligently, the "speech center" of his cortex must receive nervous impulses from other areas of the cortex so that what he says carries the meaning he intends.

Although we do not understand exactly how the cortex works, we observe that a record is kept of the thought processes that occur here. This record constitutes memory. Wonderful indeed is that mental faculty that enables a person to recall previous experiences at will and to bring them back into consciousness!

It is also in the cortex of the cerebrum that the higher intellectual functions take place—those that involve judgment, decision, and the recognition of moral values and ethical standards. Here we have many parts of the cortex functioning at the same time in a manner that takes advantage of the memory of previous experiences along with imagination projected into the future.

In order that the various parts of the cortex might function together in these complicated thought processes, many nerve cells serve to connect one part of the cortex with another. Much of the brain substance beneath the cortex is composed of axons which extend from one part of the cortex to another. This deeper tissue in the brain composed mostly of axons is called "white matter," whereras the cortex containing the nerve cell bodies, is called "gray matter."

The Emotions

Earlier in the chapter we learned that the emotions are made possible by the combined activity of the interbrain and the cerebral cortex. Emotions are complex experiences which do not consist of discrete thoughts but rather of attitudes which influence the thoughts. Common examples of emotions are fear, anger, love, and happiness. The nerve patterns for these were built into the nervous system by the Creator for man's protection and happiness.

The emotions influence one's conscious thinking, but they do not need to control it. The cortex of the cerebrum, where conscious thinking takes place, can be used, if a person so desires, to control the other parts of the nervous system. Therefore someone strong in character and mature in attitudes can control his behavior in spite of his emotions.

We have already said that the interbrain serves as a coordinating center for the autonomic nervous system which regulates the functions of the body's internal organs. The nerve cells of the interbrain work quite automatically as they take care of the actions of the heart, the lungs, the stomach, and the other organs. If you had to regulate these organs by conscious thought, you would hardly have time to do anything else. Fortunately, you can leave this to the control centers within the brain. You can forget about your food as soon as you swallow it. From then on it is taken care of by the organs of digestion in ways which best serve the body's needs. And all of these details of digestion, as well as the functions of other internal organs, are cared for by impulses mediated by the nervous system.

Since emotions are activated by the interbrain, the functions of your organs are easily influenced by your emotions.

When you experience the emotion of fear, your interbrain declares an emergency and sends out nervous impulses to the various organs of your body, which modify their functions accordingly. Under the stimulus of fear, the heart beats faster, the blood pressure rises, the amount of blood sugar increases, and your breathing becomes more rapid. These changes make an extra supply of energy food and oxygen available to the muscles. Meanwhile the work of the organs of digestion is retarded so as to give priority to other organs directly concerned with the response to fear. In other words, the emotion of fear conditions your body to run or otherwise protect itself in case of danger, that is, ready for "fight or flight." (See also page 19, this volume.)

Sometimes a person who has not learned to exercise good control over his emotions permits them continued sway for long periods at a time. Thus fear becomes the prolonged emotional state of anxiety. The organs of the body react, as best they can, to a prolonged emotional state just as they do in the case of a short-lived emergency. But when an emotional state continues day after day, the organs suffer the result of an emergency which has no end.

Many forms of sickness begin this way. A person can prevent this kind of sickness by cultivating an attitude of happiness and peace. He can learn to control his emotions in ways that allow his interbrain to function in a normal manner rather than in response to a continuous emotional upheaval.

Injuries to the Nervous System

Now that we understand the basic organization of the nervous system, we can see why people are sometimes handicapped following injuries to a nerve, the spinal cord, or the brain.

When a nerve is cut or torn, as sometimes happens when an arm or leg is mangled or when some part of the body is injured by broken glass or gunshot, the parts of the body previously served by this nerve will be affected. There will be no "feeling" in that portion of the skin. Also, whatever muscles received their nervous impulses through this nerve will now be paralyzed.

In many cases of injury to a nerve, the surgeon succeeds in finding the ends of the injured nerve and stitches them together. This does not restore the function of the nerve until there has been time for the damaged axons to grow past the splice in the nerve and find their way again to the structures with which they normally make connection.

Some severe back injuries damage the spinal cord. This is much more serious than injury to a nerve, for the impulses that would normally go to and from the brain can no longer get past the site of injury in the spinal cord. Therefore the structures supplied by nerves below this level can no longer be controlled by the brain. If the injury to the spinal cord is in the region of the neck, all four extremities (both arms and both legs) may be paralyzed, and we speak of such a handicapped person as a quadriplegic. If the spinal cord injury is below the point at which the nerves to the arms make connections, then the lower extremities are paralyzed, giving rise to the condition called paraplegia. Another serious fact is that, unlike the peripheral nerves, the spinal cord cannot heal in a manner that restores its function.

Injuries to the brain may produce various symptoms, depending upon what part of the brain is involved. Inasmuch as the cortex of the cerebrum serves as sort of a switchboard for the control of all parts of the body, if a portion of the cortex is involved in some kind of injury, those parts of the body which this area previously served will now be difficult or even impossible to control.

Many injuries to the brain come as a result of diseased blood vessels, which either rupture, permitting the escape of blood, or become obstructed by way of a clot of blood. When the blood supply to a certain part of the brain is cut off,

this part of the brain ceases to function just as definitely as though it had been removed by the surgeon.

As explained earlier, the right side of the cerebrum is connected by nerve pathways to the left side of the body and vice versa. The usual "stroke," which a person with hardening of the arteries may have, produces damage to certain parts of the brain. If this damage occurs in the right side of the brain, it is the left side of the body which becomes paralyzed with accompanying impairment of sensations.

Caring for the Nervous System

Even though the nervous system seems more wonderful than other systems of the body, it is still a part of the body and receives its nourishment from the same organs that provide nourishment for all other tissues. It is thus very dependent on all the other systems of the body. The secret of taking good care of your brain, then, is the same as that for maintaining good health in general. When your body is in good condition, your brain will benefit and be able to function well. When you are ill from any cause, your brain suffers accordingly.

Introduction

Of all the organs and systems of the body, the brain and its associated structures in the nervous system are of greatest importance to the normal functioning of the body and to the general welfare of the individual. Reasons for this top-level importance are clear: (1) The activities of all other organs and tissues are controlled by the nervous impulses received from the brain and spinal cord; (2) the brain is the coordinating agency for all nervous activity; and (3) the brain is the seat of consciousness and of all the psychological functions related to consciousness.

When a portion of the nervous system is damaged by disease or injury, a corresponding deficit in function ensues, either in the part of the body normally controlled by the damaged structure or in the related activities of the brain. When demonstrable tissue changes take place in some part of the brain, the spinal cord, or the nerves, we speak of "diseases of the nervous system"—dealt with in this chapter. When the individual's brain functions abnormally but no demonstrable changes occur in the tissues of the nervous system, we speak of "mental illness"— covered in the next chapter, where the neuroses and the psychoses are considered.

Diseases of the Nervous System

PLEASE NOTE: It is urged that the following introductory pages (45-50) be consulted before reading the discussions of the individual diseases which follow. The basic understanding of the causes and manifestations of the nervous disorders thus acquired will enable the reader to place a better evaluation on the particular nervous disease in which he is interested.

Certain diseases of the nervous system pertain particularly to infancy and childhood. These are therefore presented in those chapters which pertain to these age groups. Phenylketonuria is considered in chapter 5, volume 1. Cerebral palsy (Little's disease) and mongolism are described in chapter 6, volume 1. Sydenham's chorea and minimal brain dysfunction syndrome are dealt with in chapter 17, volume 1.

General Considerations. The brain and spinal cord are composed of very fragile tissue. Both are protected by bones, the former by the skull and the latter by bony components of the vertebrae. In addition these organs are surrounded by durable fibrous coverings (the meninges), which provide further protection from injury. Thus, despite their delicate nature, these organs of the central nervous system do well un-

der normal conditions. But once they are attacked by disease, once their supply of blood is curtailed, or once they receive a mechanical impact violent enough to injure their delicate tissues, serious consequences may result. And when a part of the nervous system is damaged other parts of the body, or even the entire body, suffer also.

Common Causes for Disorders of the Nervous System

Many diseases and conditions may involve the nervous system, some affecting only the organs of the nervous system, but others, more general in nature, affecting additional parts of the body. The most common causes of these disorders are listed as follows:

A. *Developmental Defects.* When

Traumata of the Brain

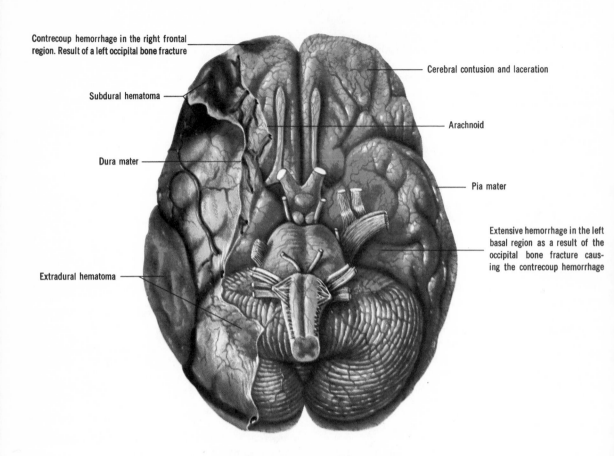

Contrecoup hemorrhage in the right frontal region. Result of a left occipital bone fracture

Cerebral contusion and laceration

Subdural hematoma

Arachnoid

Dura mater

Pia mater

Extensive hemorrhage in the left basal region as a result of the occipital bone fracture causing the contrecoup hemorrhage

Extradural hematoma

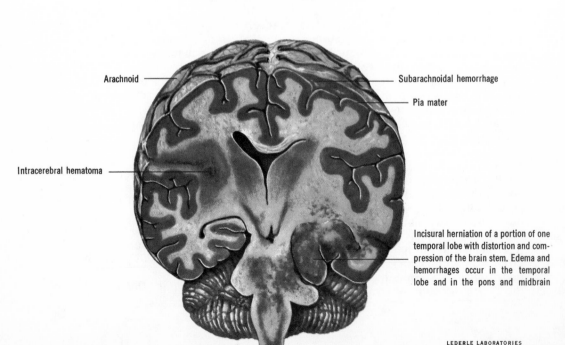

Arachnoid

Subarachnoidal hemorrhage

Pia mater

Intracerebral hematoma

Incisural herniation of a portion of one temporal lobe with distortion and compression of the brain stem. Edema and hemorrhages occur in the temporal lobe and in the pons and midbrain

congenital faults of development affect the nervous system, the results to the individual depend on just what part of the nervous system is affected and on the severity of the defect. Hydrocephalus—an enlargement of the head due to an increase of cerebrospinal fluid within the brain—is an example of developmental defects that may affect the central nervous system.

B. *Infections and Inflammatory Disorders*. These may affect the brain, spinal cord, or nerves just as they affect other tissues of the body. Two examples are encephalitis and meningitis.

C. *Toxic, Metabolic, and Nutritional Disorders*. These are conditions that often affect the entire body as well as the nervous system. Toxins produced by germs (as in tetanus, diphtheria, and botulism), absorption of certain heavy metals (such as lead), or the ingestion of certain chemical agents (such as alcohol) commonly cause damage to the tissues of the nervous system in the brain and other areas. Examples of metabolic disorders which affect the nervous system are phenylketonuria and diabetes. The nervous system is particularly susceptible to deficiencies in the diet, as when the B vitamins are insufficient.

D. *Trauma*. Although the organs of the nervous system are fairly well protected by their bony coverings, falls or car accidents resulting in head or back injury may cause serious damage. In contusion, the delicate brain tissue is damaged by impact or by shearing stresses which pass through its substance, causing varying degrees of disruption of the tissue. Hemorrhage into the brain or spinal cord may cause damage by tearing the tissues or by pressure caused by a blood clot. In some cases of injury the healing process involves the development of extensive scars which may irritate the delicate tissues of the brain so as to cause convulsions. In some injuries nerves are torn as they leave the brain to pass along their course to the structures they serve.

E. *Vascular Disorders*. The blood supply to the brain and spinal cord is very generous—necessarily so because the cells of these active tissues are critically dependent on a continuous supply of oxygen and nutrient materials and on the removal of the by-products of brain metabolism. When the blood vessels of the body become diseased, the brain and spinal cord often suffer more quickly and more seriously than do other organs. Certain symptoms of senility may be the result of a gradual diminution of the blood supply to the brain. When the blood supply to a particular part of the brain or spinal cord is shut off, the resulting symptoms are related to the malfunction of this part. This is the usual background of a "stroke" in which a vessel becomes obstructed.

F. *Tumors*. Tumors of the brain and spinal cord are classed as benign if they do not invade surrounding tissue, or malignant if they do invade surrounding tissue. Even the benign tumors can cause serious symptoms and can threaten the patient's life by pressing against neighboring parts of the nervous system. In many cases of tumor of the brain or of the spinal cord, early surgical removal of the tumor will remedy the situation. Brain surgeons have become very skillful in gaining access to most parts of the nervous system.

Common Symptoms Produced by Nervous Disorders

The human nervous system, consisting of brain, spinal cord, and the many nerves that reach out to all parts of the body, may be compared to a modern communications network. If there is a "break in the lines" at any point, the "territory" normally served by the broken "lines" will no longer be able to exchange messages with the headquarters. That is, if the nerve fibers that control a group of muscles are severed, these muscles will be paralyzed, even though they may be at some distance from the actual site of the injury. Also, if some of the fibers which normally bring sensations from a certain part of the body to the brain are severed, the particular sensations carried by these fibers can no longer reach the brain and thus loss of feeling in that particular part of the body will result. The loss of the ability to detect general sensations that should come from a particular part of the body is called anesthesia.

The important symptoms of nervous disorders are more directly related to the particular part of the nervous system affected than to the specific cause of the disorders. Although a few areas of the brain can be affected without producing specific symptoms, most areas, when involved by disease or injury, cause interference with the sensations, with the control of muscles, or with the coordination of movements.

The common symptoms occurring in connection with nervous disorders are as follows:

A. *Abnormalities of Movement (of Muscle Action).* One of the functions of the nervous system is to control the activities of the muscles throughout the body. When those parts of the brain and spinal cord concerned with muscle activity become diseased or when the nerve connections between the central nervous system and the muscles are affected, the action of the muscles will be altered, and the particular type of the alteration may give a clue to the nature of the disease. The common kinds of abnormality of movement are these:

1. Weakness. Weakness (loss of strength) consists of a reduced power to use the muscles in the normal manner.

2. Paralysis. Paralysis, in contrast to weakness, involves a total inability of a muscle or muscle group to respond to voluntary commands.

3. Spasticity and Rigidity (Stiffness). In conditions of health certain mechanisms cause the larger muscles of the

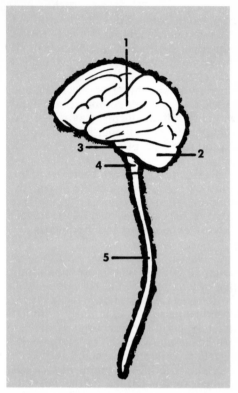

Abnormalities of movement correspond with impairment in specific areas of the brain or nervous system; such as (1) cerebrum; (2) cerebellum; (3) pons; (4) medulla oblongata; (5) spinal cord.

body to remain firm, enabling a person to maintain his posture, for example, without his having to give continuous thought to the movements of his body. When a person desires to use these same muscles in rapid movement, the mechanism otherwise causing them to remain firm is automatically cancelled so that they can now move quickly. In certain diseases of the brain and spinal cord this ability to release the muscles from their contracted state is lost, so that they remain firm even when the person desires to move quickly. Spasticity may be seen in cases of stroke. In spasticity the muscles may still retain their power even though they lack the ability to respond quickly.

4. Involuntary (Uncontrollable) Movements. Certain disorders of the

48

nervous system, such as chorea and athetosis, cause spontaneous, purposeless movements involving certain muscles or muscle groups.

5. Gait Disturbance. Walking is such a complex function that many types of disturbance of the nervous system may interfere with its normal progress. Gait may be altered by weakness, paralysis, spasticity, lack of coordination, disturbed sense of position, and even by hysteria.

6. Tetany. Tetany is a condition in which the muscles become abnormally responsive to stimulation. It occurs in the disease tetanus, in conditions where the amount of calcium in the blood drops to low levels (as in hypoparathyroidism), or in conditions of alkalosis as when a person loses acid from the stomach by excessive vomiting or when a nervous person breathes too deeply with consequent loss of carbon dioxide from the body. Tetany also occurs in certain nervous disorders in which cells within the brain become abnormally responsive to ordinary stimuli.

B. *Disturbances of Speech and Swallowing*. Both of these functions require a high degree of integration and muscle action. Disturbances of speech are particularly significant because they may indicate difficulty not only in the control of the muscles by the brain but in the intellectual processes.

C. *Convulsions*. A convulsion consists of the abrupt occurrence of violent involuntary contractions of muscles, often accompanied by loss of consciousness.

D. *Disturbances of General Sensations*. By general sensations we refer to those that come from the skin, the membranes, and the muscles (pain, temperature, touch, position) as opposed to those which come from the organs of special sense (vision, hearing, equilibrium, taste, and smell).

When a sensation of pain, temperature, or touch is lost, we speak of anesthesia. Also there may be a loss of the sense of position. Oftentimes this loss of sensation is limited to some particular part of the body, and the physician interprets from this clue what part of the nervous system is affected. If irritation of the sensory nerve fibers causes abnormal sensations, such as the feeling of "pins and needles," we then speak of paresthesia. If a normal sensory experience is exaggerated, we speak of hyperesthesia.

E. *Headache*. Headache is perhaps mankind's most common symptom, occurring often in disorders of the nervous system.

F. *Dizziness*. Dizziness is an uncomfortable symptom in which the individual receives a false sense of motion. There are several possible causes of this symptom, some being more mysterious than others.

G. *Impairment of Vision*. Impairment or loss of vision should be taken seriously, and a physician who specializes in diseases of the eyes or of the nervous system should be consulted. Not all impairments of vision relate to the eyes themselves, for the difficulty may be in the nerve fibers that pass between the eyes and the brain or even in the tissues of the brain cortex. Oftentimes defects of vision follow a significant pattern; for example, a restriction in the right side of what is seen by the right eye and in the left side of what is seen by the left eye (bitemporal hemianopsia, as in pituitary tumor). A person may not notice a pattern of sight loss unless he checks the vision of each eye separately.

H. *Unconsciousness*. The term *unconsciousness* is difficult to define, though the difference between the conscious and the unconscious state is easy enough to recognize. Perhaps the closest we can come to a definition of consciousness is to describe it as the normal functioning of a person's mental faculties to the extent that he is aware of his present circumstances and alert to what is going on around him.

Consciousness, in its broad sense, requires the normal functioning of the whole brain. Whatever interferes with a function of the brain interferes, to some extent, with the full experience of consciousness. Placed in the order of increased impairment of consciousness, we may mention such terms as *dullness, lethargy, stupor,* and *coma.* A decrease in awareness of one's surroundings does not necessarily indicate a serious nervous disorder. It may only mean a temporary deficit in the blood supply to the brain, such as occurs in fainting or the presence of toxins produced by germs causing some generalized disease. However, it may indicate a concussion or pressure produced by a tumor. Impairments of consciousness must therefore be evaluated by a physician.

I. *Hallucinations and Delusions.* Hallucinations are false sensory experiences, the individual concerned seeming to hear, see, or smell something when, actually, his eyes, ears, or olfactory organs are not being stimulated in a manner to produce these sensations. Since some hallucinations are the result of abnormal stimulation of the brain areas where these sensations are ordinarily perceived, their occurrence justifies a study of the case by a physician or a specialist in nervous diseases (a neurologist).

Delusions are false beliefs to which an individual adheres in spite of evidence to the contrary. A person with delusions may confuse his identity with that of another, or he may draw conclusions that are false with respect to the information at hand. Delusions are more typical of mental disorders than of nervous disorders, but they may occur in either.

Considerations of the Individual Nervous Disorders

ABSCESS OF THE BRAIN

An abscess of the brain is a localized infectious process with destruction of tissue. It is usually caused by the staphylococcus germ but sometimes by the streptococcus or the pneumococcus. The infection may be introduced at the time of a fracture or by a penetrating wound of the skull, or it may come from some neighboring area, such as from an infection of the inner ear, nasal sinus, or the mastoid cells of the skull. In other cases the infection originates in the lung or the heart and is brought to the brain by way of the bloodstream.

The symptoms of abscess of the brain vary considerably from case to case. In some cases the symptoms are generalized, relating more directly to the infectious process. These include chills, fever, loss of appetite, and a general feeling of illness. Other symptoms are caused by the irritation of the covering membranes (the meninges) and, possibly, of the brain cortex. These include convulsions and stiffness of the neck. Still other symptoms are caused by the disruption or compression of certain nerve fibers as the abscess enlarges. In some cases the only symptoms of an abscess of the brain may be those relating to the nervous system.

Care and Treatment

Abscess of the brain is always a serious condition and carries a mortality rate of up to 50 percent, even with the best of care. It deserves prompt and adequate professional care. The treatment usually includes antibiotics for the infection involved and often surgical drainage of the fluid-filled abscess cavity.

AMYOTROPHIC LATERAL SCLEROSIS

This is a progressive, always fatal disease which affects men more commonly than women and typically occurs above age 40. There is a degeneration of the nerve cells and nerve fibers which supply the muscles of the body, with more and more cells and fibers being involved as the disease progresses. The average length of life after onset is about three years. Annual death rate in the United States from this disease is about one per 100,000 population.

Weakness and atrophy of muscles are the characteristic manifestations. The number of muscles thus involved gradually increases, and various parts of the body may be affected, the most serious development being interference with breathing, swallowing, and chewing. The cause of this disease is not yet known.

Care and Treatment

There is no satisfactory remedy for this illness. The patient should be encouraged to avoid fatigue, but he should remain as active as his condition permits.

ATAXIA

A. *Cerebellar Ataxia*. This is a disease of the cerebellum—that part of the brain located in the back part of the skull. Disease of the cerebellum from any cause may produce the main symptom of ataxia, failure of muscle coordination. There is no loss of muscle power as in paralysis but rather a series of back-and-forth groping movements when any precise action is undertaken. Writing and speaking are seriously handicapped. The symptom of ataxia justifies professional care by a neurologist.

B. *Friedreich's Ataxia*. This hereditary disease is dominant in some families and recessive in others. It usually begins in childhood or youth and is characterized by unsteadiness and tremor. In addition to the lack of coordination of muscle movements, there is a paralysis of certain muscles and a lateral curvature of the spine.

No specific treatment is known. The disease progresses slowly, with death occurring, usually, at about age 20.

CERVICAL RIB

A small percentage of persons develop an extra rib in one or both sides, just above the usual first rib. This extra rib is in the lower part of the neck. Resulting symptoms, when they occur, are caused by a squeezing of nerves and blood vessels leading to the arm and lying between the extra rib and the scalenus anterior muscle. The symptoms are intensified when the arm is used for weight carrying or when it is raised for long periods above the head, as in hanging up clothes or in washing walls. Usually the patient experiences no difficulty until adulthood. The symptoms consist of pain, tingling, numbness, and coolness in the forearm and hand, often on the side of the little finger. The muscles of the hand in this same area may atrophy.

This combination of symptoms is typical of several circumstances which cause damage to the roots of the nerves which supply the arm. Sometimes the symptoms occur when there is no extra rib, being caused by pressure from other structures.

Care and Treatment

When the condition is not severe, the symptoms can be relieved by the avoidance of lifting with the involved arm and by care in supporting it by a pillow during sleep. For an overweight person, reducing often helps. In more severe cases, treatment requires surgery and usually involves the removal of the extra rib.

CHOREA

Two principal diseases carry this name. They differ greatly except that they present the common feature of purposeless, jerking, involuntary movements. Sydenham's chorea (St. Vitus's dance) is a childhood disorder which is considered in chapter 17, volume 1.

Huntington's Chorea. This is a hereditary disease characterized by purposeless, jerking, involuntary movement and by progressive mental deterioration. Symptoms usually appear about age 30 or 40. The purposeless movement and the mental deterioration usually appear at about the same time, but in some cases one group of symptoms precedes the other. The purposeless movements consist of grimacing; lurching; and unsteady, waltzing gait resembling that of drunkenness. As the disease progresses, the muscles become progressively weaker.

The mental symptoms vary from case to case, some patients being very cheerful and others suspicious, spiteful, and destructive. The intellectual faculties gradually deteriorate until the patient often must be cared for in an institution. The disease usually progresses to death in about 10 to 15 years.

Many of the nerve cells throughout the brain and spinal cord show evidences of deterioration. The specific nature of the disease is not understood, but inasmuch as it runs in families as a dominant characteristic, it is advised that persons born into such families deliberately abstain from parenthood so as not to pass this disease on to children.

CONVULSIVE DISORDERS (EPILEPSY)

The cause of convulsions is not fully understood, but they are associated with a functional disturbance of the cortex of the brain which can be demonstrated by the electroencephalogram (tracing of brain waves). Children are more prone to convulsions than adults but may outgrow the tendency. For a discussion of convulsions occurring in infancy and childhood, see chapters 6 and 17, volume 1.

In some instances convulsions may begin in later life. Recurring convulsions are commonly called epilepsy. It is estimated that about two million people in the United States experience these recurring convulsions except as they may control them by the use of medication.

A major (grand mal) convulsion consists typically of the abrupt occurrence of violent, involuntary contractions of the body muscles, usually accompanied by loss of consciousness. The attack is usually of short duration, often followed by temporary confusion, drowsiness, and headache.

The severity of the attacks varies from case to case. In susceptible children diseases with high fever or ordinary breath-holding (such as during a tantrum) may bring on a convulsion. Convulsions may occur in persons with low blood sugar or low blood calcium. They may occur when the blood's reaction becomes more alkaline than normal as in continued deep breathing, persistent vomiting with loss of acid from the body, or from taking too much alkali by mouth. They may occur when a confirmed alcoholic suddenly stops drinking or when a person addicted to barbiturates suddenly discontinues the drug. Conditions that irritate the brain, causing convulsions, include the following: brain tumors, cerebral infections, brain injury, or diseases of the blood vessels supplying the brain.

Convulsions may occur in eclampsia, a serious complication of the latter period of pregnancy. They may also occur in cases of tetanus (lockjaw).

The occurrence of convulsions, especially in an adult who has not been known to have convulsions previously, should be considered a clue to some serious underlying disease. Therefore the services of a physician should be secured promptly. It will then be the physician's responsibility to discover if possible the nature of the underlying condition and arrange suitable treatment. In the meantime, the patient should receive appropriate first-aid care such as is outlined in chapter 23, volume 3.

In less than half the cases of convulsive disorders occurring in adulthood there seems to have been an inherited susceptibility to this ailment. Because this tendency is sometimes inherited, the question is often asked, Should the person who has a convulsive disorder run the risk of passing this tendency on to children, or should he or she deliberately avoid parenthood? The advice given by persons who specialize in treating convulsive disorders is that each case should be studied separately, with all contributing factors being considered. Then, in a given case, if it develops that the hereditary factor is large, the person may be advised to forego becoming a parent.

Another important question in this matter is Can the person with a convulsive disorder live a reasonably normal life? Now that drugs are available which are often able to satisfactorily prevent the recurrence of convulsive seizures, even in cases where there is a tendency for frequent recurrence, the question can be answered in the affirmative. The secret of successful living in such a case is, however, that the person with a convulsive disorder should frankly face the reasonable limitations of his problem and avoid those activities which place him in danger should he have a convulsive seizure unexpectedly. Take the matter of driving an automobile. It would be hazardous not only for the individual but for others who might be involved should an automobile driver experience a convulsive seizure while operating a car. Some states forbid operator's licenses to those who have a history of convulsive seizures. However, most states allow such persons to drive cars provided their condition is so well controlled by medication that they have not had a seizure for a period of a year or so.

Listed below are several agencies which provide helpful information on request to those who have convulsive disorders or to those who are interested in their problems:

The Epilepsy Foundation of America
Suite 406
1828 L Street NW
Washington, DC 20036

Epilepsy Society
3 Arlington Street
Boston, MA 02116

National Epilepsy League
6 N. Michigan Avenue
Chicago, IL 60602

Care and Treatment

The first-aid treatment for a convulsive seizure is described in chapter 23, volume 3. There are now available several effective drugs which act as anticonvulsants and thus reduce the prospect of convulsive seizures.

Each one of these drugs has certain side effects which, of course, are most noticeable when the drug is taken in larger doses. Perhaps the most troublesome side effect is that of drowsiness, which introduces a hazard for driving a car or operating power machinery. By careful trials with the various available drugs and sometimes by using combinations of these drugs, it is usually possible for the physician to work out a maintenance program for his patient that will enable him to live and work quite normally without the fear of a possible convulsive seizure. It is recommended, however, that such patients, even though following an adequate treatment program, should abstain from the use of alcohol and brain stimulants because they increase the tendency to a seizure. They may swim, provided another swimmer trained in lifesaving methods accompanies them.

DELIRIUM

The term *delirium* is used to describe the mental state of a person whose brain cells have been insulted by some unfavorable condition so that he no longer thinks and acts normally. By this definition, there are many causes for delirium. We refer here to those conditions in which a person is said to be "out of his head." Such a patient may be mentally confused, restless, anxious, unable to cooperate. His speech may not be sensible, and his imagination out of control.

The occurrence of delirium depends on several factors, including fever, drugs the patient has received, his general health, his temperament, and the nature of his illness.

Delirium may be caused by any factors which adversely alter the metabolism of the nerve cells in the brain. These include intoxication by alcohol or by other drugs such as atropine, bromides, or barbiturates. Poisoning by lead, by carbon monoxide, or by household or industrial poisons may be the cause. Delirium may occur in severe systemic infections, particularly those associated with high fever. It occurs in diseases which disturb the body's general metabolic processes such as uremia, uncontrolled diabetes, severe loss of fluid, liver disease, heart failure, and pernicious anemia. It occurs in infections involving the brain or its coverings, in head injury, or even in conditions which alter the brain's supply of blood.

Care and Treatment

Because of the many possible causes of delirium, the handling of a patient with this complication hinges on the discovery of the particular cause of his present mental confusion. Once the cause has been identified— whether fever, poisoning, overdose, or metabolic disturbance—efforts should be directed at controlling the problem. For the emergency handling of a person with delirium, see chapter 23, volume 3.

DEMENTIAS

The reason we speak of dementias in the plural is that many basic conditions associated with the brain, usually in older persons, can cause deterioration of the brain. The common feature of dementia, regardless of its cause, is difficulty in all intellectual activities, including defective memory, reduced ability to understand what is taking place in the surroundings, and loss of orientation for time and place. The individual with dementia loses his ability to cope with life's usual activities. In those cases in which generalized destruction of brain cells occurs, the loss of mental faculties is progressive. In about half the cases of dementia, however, the impairment of intellectual function is secondary to some such condition as pernicious anemia, thyroid dysfunction, or the presence of a blood clot pressing against the brain. In such cases, treatment of the underlying condition may bring an improvement in the patient's condition.

One of the most common forms of dementia for which the cause is not known and for which there is no effective treatment is the so-called Alzheimer's dementia. This may begin even earlier than age 65, and it consists of a progressive deterioration of brain cells.

Another condition properly classed as a form of dementia is Korsakoff's psychosis, in which mental deterioration from damage to brain tissue is typically caused by persistent indulgence in alcohol.

Blood vessel disease may cause the deterioration of brain tissue, as with numerous small "strokes," and is responsible for a certain percentage of cases of dementia. Brain tumors, as they develop, may have a similar effect.

Care and Treatment

When symptoms of dementia develop, it is important to arrange for a thorough study of the case in the hope that this may be one that will respond to treatment. For those cases of dementia in which the process of deterioration is progressive, the patient should be gradually relieved of his responsibilities. Preferably, he should remain in a family situation as long as he is capable of cooperation and of performing simple tasks. As the patient becomes less capable and less responsive, it may be advisable to place him in an institution designed for the care of such patients.

ENCEPHALITIS

Encephalitis is a serious condition characterized by an inflammation of the brain tissue. The epidemic type is caused by a virus probably carried from one person to another by the minute droplets of moisture discharged by a sneeze or by way of contact with articles which have been soiled by the discharge from a patient's nose or throat. It may also be spread by insects (see below).

The symptoms of epidemic encephalitis resemble those of influenza, with the addition of signs indicating that the brain and meninges are involved. The patient experiences lethargy (sleepiness) and severe pain in the neck when the head is tilted sharply forward. Symptoms indicating involvement of the brain include disturbance in the action of certain muscles, coarse tremors, purposeless movements, convulsions, delirium, and mental confusion.

Encephalitis has been known in various parts of the world for many years. It typically affects persons between the ages of 20 and 45 years. In recent years special kinds of encephalitis have been recognized, such as the St. Louis type, the eastern type, and the western equine type. Manifestations of these types usually occur in epidemics. In some of these epidemics, the virus may be carried by insects, including mosquitos and ticks.

Forms of encephalitis may also occur as a complication of chicken pox, measles, or mumps; but the seriousness of these cases of encephalitis usually is not as great as that of epidemic encephalitis.

Certain nervous manifestations tend to remain after apparent recovery from the acute phase of epidemic encephalitis. These residual nervous disorders are often grouped under the term *chronic encephalitis.* Some patients have developed, after 20 years or more, a form of parkinsonism. Others develop disorders of the personality, including irritability and asocial types of behavior. Narcolepsy develops in some cases. Some develop various abnormal movements of the muscles such as tics, grimaces, or tremors.

Care and Treatment

Inasmuch as the virus causing a case of epidemic encephalitis may be carried from person to person, great care should be used in disposing of the discharges from the nose and throat of a patient with this disease. Linens and other articles soiled by these discharges must be sterilized or destroyed.

Since encephalitis usually is caused by a virus, there is no specific remedy for this illness. The aim of treatment is to maintain the patient's vitality and to treat the various manifestions in ways that make the patient most comfortable. The patient should be protected from undue noise or excitement.

If the patient has difficulty in swallowing, it is important to make sure that he receives sufficient fluid and that his nutrition is adequate. The physician in charge may find it advisable to provide fluid and nourishment by vein.

FACIAL PARALYSIS (BELL'S PALSY)

In facial paralysis the patient loses control of the muscles of facial expression usually on one side of the face. Although the basic cause often is not known, the paralysis results from a malfunction of the facial nerve. It is impossible for the patient to forcibly close the eye or wrinkle the forehead on the affected side of the face. The mouth droops on the involved side and is

Typical case of facial paralysis.

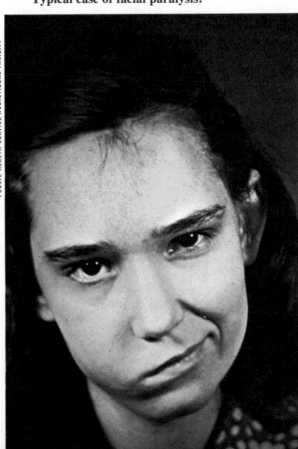

PUBLIC HEALTH SERVICE AUDIOVISUAL FACILITY

drawn to the opposite side when the person smiles.

Facial paralysis affects both men and women of all ages but, most commonly, middle-aged women. The onset is often relatively sudden, frequently after exposure to cold.

In the most common type of facial paralysis (Bell's palsy) there seems to be a reduced supply of blood to the facial nerve as it passes through a narrow, bony canal on its way to the face. In this usual type, improvement may begin within two or three weeks, but complete recovery may be delayed for months.

It is important for the person with facial paralysis to have a thorough neurological examination, for in a small percentage of cases facial paralysis is caused by the presence of a tumor or by some other condition which should have prompt attention, even surgical treatment.

Care and Treatment

For the usual case of facial paralysis (Bell's palsy), most physicians prefer to use corticosteroid medication during the first few days of the illness with the hope that this may relieve any inflammation surrounding the facial nerve that may be causing it to dysfunction. Patients who fail to improve should then be reexamined to determine whether the nerve fibers within the facial nerve are degenerating. If so, some authorities advise exploring the facial nerve by surgical methods to relieve pressure on the nerve.

Because the eye on the affected side does not close securely when the facial nerve is paralyzed, it is important to protect the eye so that its membranes do not become injured or infected. A soothing solution designed for use in the eye should be dropped into the space between the eyelids at least twice a day. A piece of Scotch Tape placed across the affected eyelid serves to keep it closed during sleep. Heat and gentle upward massage to the muscles of the face on the para-

lyzed side will help to prevent their sagging and becoming stretched.

HEAD INJURIES

Accidents are the top-ranking cause of death in the United States for persons under 35 years of age, and injury to the head and brain is the major cause of death in 70 percent of these. For the emergency treatment of head injuries, see chapter 23, volume 3.

The more common types of head injury are these:

A. *Skull Fracture*. Often the actual fracture of the skull is not serious in itself, but concurrent injury of the brain may be. Skull fracture may be complicated by bleeding inside the skull, which can cause damaging pressure against the brain. Also when a fragment of the skull is depressed, the surgeon must relieve the pressure against the brain by elevating that portion of the bone. A compound skull fracture is often complicated by indriven fragments of bone. These may permit the entrance of infection into the damaged tissues of the brain. It is essential to enlist the services of a neurosurgeon in such a case. In some skull fractures, the cerebrospinal fluid, which is watery in appearance, may escape from the nose or from one or both of the ears.

B. *Concussion*. In concussion there has been sufficient damage to the brain to produce some impairment of consciousness. The duration of unconsciousness is a rough measure of the severity of the damage. Often concussion is associated with dizziness, headache, difficulty in concentrating, and a loss of memory for events just preceding the head injury (retroactive amnesia). In minor head injuries the period of unconsciousness seldom lasts more than a few minutes. (In major injuries, unconsciousness may last for several hours or possibly several days.)

C. *Cerebral Contusion and Laceration*. In severe head injuries the surface of the brain may become bruised

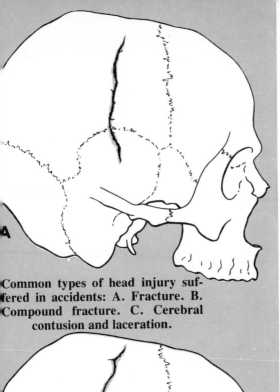

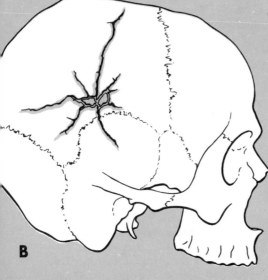

Common types of head injury suffered in accidents: A. Fracture. B. Compound fracture. C. Cerebral contusion and laceration.

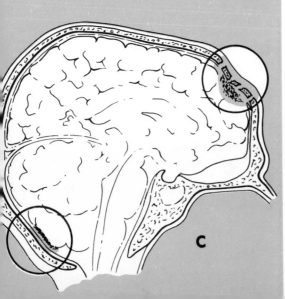

and/or torn. There may be hemorrhage into the brain substance or into the space around the brain. Generally there is swelling of the brain. Confined as the brain is within the bony skull, this swelling poses a hazard. In severe injuries surgical intervention may be necessary in order to control the hemorrhage or to relieve the increased pressure within the skull.

D. *Hemorrhage*. Hemorrhage into the brain substance often occurs in connection with a severe injury in which the brain is damaged. Bleeding into the brain tissue may occur in many locations throughout the area of injury, or there may be a single large accumulation of blood.

In some cases of head injury, associated either with skull fracture or with tearing of the membranes which surround the brain, bleeding will occur and blood will accumulate either within the covering membranes of the brain or between the membranes and the skull. Oftentimes such an accumulation of blood (hematoma) develops slowly. As time passes the clot of blood degenerates; it absorbs fluid and swells, enlarging the hematoma until it produces such pressure against the brain as may endanger the patient's life. This critical complication of hemorrhage inside the skull may develop from several days to even several weeks after the original head injury. The only satisfactory treatment is to remove the hematoma (blood clot) through a surgical opening in the skull.

It is important that a person who has suffered a head injury be observed carefully during his period of recovery. Any impairment of consciousness or speech, or dragging or weakness of a limb, should be reported promptly to the physician. Once the pressure produced by a blood clot becomes great enough to interfere with consciousness, the relief of the pressure must be accomplished quickly if the patient's life is to be saved.

E. *Damage to the Cranial Nerves*.

In some cases of skull fracture, particularly those involving the base of the skull, there may be damage to certain of the cranial nerves at the site where they leave the skull. A nerve commonly damaged is the olfactory nerve, which conveys impulses for the sense of smell. Such damage produces anosmia—a loss of the sense of smell. Other nerves, such as the optic nerve or the auditory nerve, may also be damaged.

Aftereffects of Head Injuries

In many cases of head injury certain symptoms persist which are collectively called the postconcussion sydrome. This group of symptoms, which may continue for some time after the injury, includes headache, dizziness, difficulty in concentrating, and certain alterations in the personality. The severity of the symptoms may not correlate with the severity of the injury. In favorable cases in which the individual receives adequate medical care, the symptoms gradually disappear. In less fortunate cases the persisting symptoms interfere with the patient's return to normal activities.

Another possible complication of severe head injury is the later development of recurring convulsions. These are presumably caused by the irritation of the brain by scar formation. See the item on CONVULSIVE DISORDERS earlier in this chapter, pages 52 and 53.

Care and Treatment

For the first-aid treatment of head injuries, see chapter 23, volume 3. For most cases of head injury and, especially for the severe ones, hospitalization under the care of a physician is necessary.

HERPES ZOSTER (SHINGLES)

Herpes zoster is a painful ailment caused by infection of certain sensory nerve ganglia by the varicella-zoster virus (the same virus that causes chicken pox). Herpes zoster occurs most commonly in older persons. It has been said that in a group of persons 85 years of age, half would have already had an attack of herpes zoster.

The symptoms are localized in an area of skin served by the involved nerve. This occurs on just one side of the body. At the beginning of the attack the individual notices itching, tingling, or burning sensations in the particular area of skin. Within a few days, an eruption characterized by tiny blisterlike lesions develops in the affected area. The area becomes intensely painful.

Any skin area may be affected, but the area most commonly involved is a strip of skin extending from the midline in the back around one side to the midline in the front in the lower part of the chest. The second most common area of involvement is in the region of the head and neck. Serious problems develop when the involved area includes the eye, for there may develop scarring of the cornea of the eye as an aftermath.

For a further discussion of herpes zoster, see chapter 16, volume 3, where this ailment is considered along with other viral diseases and in its relation to chicken pox.

Care and Treatment

Inasmuch as herpes zoster is caused by a virus, there is no specific cure. In caring for such a patient, the aim is to relieve the pain as far as possible by the use of analgesic medications and the application of lotions and powders to the affected skin area. The use of corticosteroid medications has been tried, but the results are not conclusive. When the eye is involved, the care of an eye physician is imperative.

HYDROCEPHALUS

Hydrocephalus is a condition in which the cerebrospinal fluid inside the skull increases in volume. Cerebrospinal fluid is a watery liquid most of which is produced within the internal spaces of the brain (ventricles). It circulates slowly throughout the brain spaces and throughout the space between the exterior of the brain and the membranes which enclose it and the spinal cord. Normally the cerebrospinal fluid is absorbed at the same rate it is produced; but in hydrocephalus there is either an overproduction of cerebrospinal fluid, a reduction of absorption of the same, or, most frequently, a blocking of its normal flow. Thus the amount of fluid gradually increases.

Many cases of hydrocephalus are congenital. In such a case the infant's

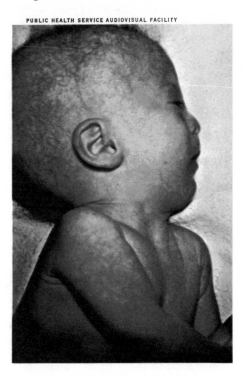

Case of congenital hydrocephalus.

head enlarges, and portions of the brain atrophy because of the larger volume of cerebrospinal fluid. Usually the enlargement of the infant's head is not noticeable until several weeks or months after birth.

In an older person, the skull cannot enlarge to accommodate the larger volume of cerebrospinal fluid. Therefore, increased pressure develops within the skull and this causes damage to the brain.

Care and Treatment

Brain surgeons have developed a method of implanting a plastic tube into the brain in such a manner that it carries away the excess cerebrospinal fluid, allowing it to drain into a vein, a body cavity, or the heart itself. Early treatment is essential.

MENINGITIS

Meningitis consists of an inflammation of the meninges (the covering membranes of the brain and spinal cord). The inflammation may be caused by any one of various disease-producing organisms: bacteria, viruses, fungi, or parasites. Except for the infection of the meninges that develops from a nearby brain abscess or that occurs in contaminated, penetrating head injuries, the infection is usually brought to the meninges from some other part of the body—the middle ear, the nasal cavities and accessory sinuses, the tonsils, the lungs, or the valves of the heart.

We consider here the three general types of meningitis: (A) acute bacterial, (B) aseptic, and (C) subacute.

A. *Acute Bacterial Meningitis (Spotted Fever).* About 80 percent of the cases of acute bacterial meningitis are caused by one or the other of three organisms: the meningococcus, the influenza bacillus, or the pneumococcus. In the description which follows, we select the meningococcic type of acute bacterial meningitis to represent all forms of this illness.

Infection by the meningococcus is spread from person to person by the droplets of moisture violently exhaled at the time of a sneeze or cough. The germs, once taken into the body, establish an infection in the region of the pharynx. While the infection resides there the victim may easily become a carrier of the disease. From the infection in the pharynx, the germs may be carried by the blood to the other parts of the body. It is by this route that the meninges commonly become involved by the meningococcic infection.

59

The disease is endemic in all parts of the world, but from time to time it flares up as an epidemic. Notable epidemics occurred in 1917, 1929, 1936, and 1943. About 45 percent of the cases of meningococcic meningitis occur in children under 15 years of age.

During that phase of the disease in which the infection is being carried by the blood, groups of the germs may congregate in various parts of the skin and membranes, where they cause purple-colored irregular blotches.

Symptoms develop rapidly and may include severe headache, irritability, forceful vomiting, chills with high fever and rapid pulse, convulsions (especially in infants), rigidity of the muscles (especially those of the neck and back), pain on flexing the neck, and delirium progressing to stupor and coma.

Before the availability of modern sulfa and antibiotic medications, the fatality rate for meningococcic meningitis was about 75 percent. With modern methods of treatment the figure has dropped to 10 percent or less.

Care and Treatment

To prevent death or permanent brain damage it is urgent that appropriate treatment be given promptly in this illness. Inasmuch as acute bacterial meningitis may be caused by any one of several germs, the physician's choice of the particular medication will hinge on his knowing just what germ is present. But the identification of the germ in a given case requires laboratory tests which take a few hours. Therefore the treatment program is usually divided into two phases—the initial nonspecific phase and the secondary, definitive phase. In the initial phase, the doctor will prescribe a general antibiotic medication of broad effectiveness so as to keep the infection under control until such time as he knows just what germ is involved in this case. Once this is known, the doctor will then choose the particular antibiotic medication best suited to combat the particular germ. The antibiotic medication should be administered intensively and should continue for at least one week after the patient's fever subsides.

The patient's condition remains serious during the acute phase of this illness. Careful attention must therefore be given to the patient's water balance, kidney function, and the pressure of cerebrospinal fluid within the skull. This requires continuous attention both by the physician and the nurses.

Because the infection by the meningococcus or by the influenza bacillus is easily transmitted from person to person, appropriate precautions should be taken to avoid the spread of the infection from the patient to others. Those who have had close contact with the patient during the early phases of his illness should possibly receive prophylactic treatment with the appropriate antibiotic medication.

B. *Aseptic (Viral) Meningitis.* The cases of meningitis that fall into this category are caused by a virus rather than by one of the bacteria. Such a case usually occurs as a complication of a viral infection that primarily involves some other part of the body such as in measles, chicken pox, rubella, and other virus infections. The symptoms that indicate an involvement of the meninges typically develop five to ten days after the onset of the primary illness. Often in these cases the brain itself is involved (encephalitis) as well as the tissues of the meninges. When it is the meninges that are primarily involved, the symptoms include fever, headache, vomiting, and stiffness of the neck and back. When the brain tissue is also involved, there may be personality changes, impairment of consciousness, seizures, and weakness or paralysis of certain muscles.

The usual course of events in meningitis of this type leads to complete recovery, even though the symptoms in the acute phase of the illness may be alarming.

60

Care and Treatment

There is no specific remedy for this type of meningitis inasmuch as it is caused by a virus. A patient with this illness should receive careful nursing care with attention to the fluid balance within his body and to kidney function. To prevent dehydration, some cases may need to receive fluid by vein.

C. *Subacute Meningitis.* Inflammations of the meninges may occur as a complication of systemic fungal infections, in tuberculosis, and in syphilis. The symptoms are essentially the same as in the acute forms of meningitis, but the illness develops and progresses more slowly. Examinations and laboratory tests must be made to identify the particular fungus or germ which is causing the illness. Only then can the appropriate treatment be arranged.

Care and Treatment

There are specific treatments available for each of the illnesses that fall into this group of subacute inflammations of the meninges. The treatment of the meningitis consists, then, of treatment directed to the primary form of illness. In all cases of suspected meningitis the aid of a physician should be obtained immediately.

MIGRAINE

Migraine is an ailment in which the afflicted person experiences severe headaches in recurring episodes, with the attacks coming at intervals of a few days to as long as a month or more. The headache is often limited to just one side. The attack is usually preceded (15 to 20 minutes prior) by certain unusual sensations, such as the seeing of bright or colored lights, which a person soon learns indicate the onset of another attack. During the attack the patient often suffers severe nausea and vomiting. The attack lasts for several hours, ends spontaneously, and leaves the person rather exhausted.

Migraine headaches may begin at any age, sometimes in childhood, and may continue for many years.

There are many variations in the pattern which migraine attacks may follow in individual cases. The essential mechanism behind the migraine attack is a variation in the control of the blood vessels of the head and neck. In the early part of the attack, these vessels are constricted—so much so as to cause the unusual sensations that occur before the actual pain in the head begins. This constriction of the vessels is followed by a rather sudden expansion, and this is when the pain occurs.

The exact reason for this change in the caliber of the blood vessels of the head and neck is not known, but several trigger factors have been identified. One case may be touched off by one of these factors and another case by an entirely different one. Examples of trigger factors follow: (1) Dietary factors such as the omitting of a meal, unfavorable response to certain foods such as chocolate, indulgence in alcohol, or the withdrawal of caffeine after a person has been accustomed to its use. (2) Hormone factors such as may occur naturally when the balance of hormones in a woman's body changes at the time of menstruation or when birth-control pills are used. (3) Emotional factors. Many persons who suffer from migraine are perfectionists who drive themselves relentlessly toward reaching some goal. Sudden occurrences of stress in such a person's experience may trigger an attack of migraine. (4) Environmental factors such as extremes in temperature, exposure to cigarette smoke, exposure to some offensive perfume, or sudden exposure to a bright light.

Care and Treatment

The first consideration is to try to identify the trigger factor which initiates a person's attack of migraine. Once this is identified, the effort should then be to avoid this particular factor. In those cases where emotional factors play an important role, it may be necessary for the person to change his job or to face up to some

61

family problem that bothers him. It may mean finding some form of enjoyable recreation that provides physical activity to counterbalance the emotional strain under which he finds himself. It may mean a reevaluation of religious philosophy. It may involve radical altering of life-style.

Certain medications have proved effective in selected cases of migraine. Among these are the ergot alkaloids, which have the effect of preventing the blood vessels from expanding. The exact amount of such a drug and the timing of its use is critical to the obtaining of favorable results. The use of such a drug must be under the supervision of a physician, since excessive use may cause serious side effects. Pain-relieving and antidepressant drugs have been used by many persons who suffer from migraine. Their use presents grave danger, however, because the circumstances of recurring attacks of migraine sets the stage for drug dependency which, in the long run, is a worse condition than the migraine itself. Some women whose migraine attacks occur at the time of their menstruation may benefit by the use of a diuretic medicine which causes the elimination of excess fluid from the body. Propranolol (Inderal) is a drug which has recently been approved for use in the treatment of migraine. Early reports indicate that it is quite effective and that it has very few unfavorable side effects. It should be used only under the direction of a physician.

MULTIPLE SCLEROSIS

This slowly-progressive disease involves various parts of the central nervous system and presents numerous symptoms which tend to come and go, only to return again in greater severity. The symptoms usually begin between ages 20 and 40, men and women being affected about equally. In some cases the progression of the disease is so slow that the patient lives out a normal life-span and dies of some other cause. In other cases the disease progresses to a fatal outcome in five to ten years. Early in the course of the disease the patient will appear to be perfectly normal during the periods of remission.

A tremendous amount of research is being carried forward in the hope of discovering the basic cause of multiple sclerosis. The lesions of multiple sclerosis which interrupt the nerve pathways are characterized by a loss of the usual insulating material (myelin) which covers the nerve fibers.

The symptoms vary a great deal from case to case and from time to time in the same case. Some cases exhibit mental symptoms, which may include lack of judgment, inattention, and frequently, unwarranted optimism, but occasionally depression. There is often unstable emotional control. In some cases there are convulsions; in some, abnormal or reduced sensations; and in others, spasticity or weakness in certain parts of the body. Some patients have difficulty in talking. In many cases episodes of double vision or partial blindness occur. Scanning speech is a common symptom, as are also tremors and impaired coordination.

Care and Treatment

As yet no cure is known for multiple sclerosis. Efforts should be made, therefore, to help the patient live as nearly a normal life as possible, consistent with his physical and mental condition. He should use moderation in all he does and avoid fatigue. Physical therapy measures are useful, especially in maintaining function and in preventing deformities of those parts of the body that may be weakened or paralyzed. Intolerance to heat is common. Some medication may be indicated for certain problems.

MYASTHENIA GRAVIS

Myasthenia gravis is a curious disease characterized by the development of muscular weakness that fluctuates from time to time and which especially affects the muscles about the eyes and face. The muscles of swallowing and breathing and those of the limbs are also affected in many cases. The disease may begin at any age but commonly in the second or third decade, beginning earlier in women than in men. The muscles fatigue quickly on use, the first few exertions being nearly normal but the muscle power fading with continued use. The muscles may operate quite normally early in the day, but their strength declines progressively throughout the day.

Some cases progress rapidly to a fatal termination, with death being caused by failure of the respiratory muscles. In others, the patient lives for years.

The immediate cause of myasthenia gravis is an alteration in the chemical activity at the junction between the nerve fibers and the muscle fibers. In a large majority of patients with myasthenia gravis there is some abnormality of the thymus gland or its function. This is consistent with the present understanding that myasthenia gravis is an autoimmune disorder.

Care and Treatment

Patients with myasthenia gravis respond miraculously for a short time following administration of one of the anticholinesterase compounds, such as neostigmine or pyridostigmine bromide. The use of such a drug does not cure the disease or even retard its progress, but it does make life easier for the sufferer. It is administered under a doctor's direction in divided doses throughout the day.

Surgical removal of the thymus gland may be beneficial in those patients in whom a tumor of the thymus is found and in some young persons with a rapidly progressing form of myasthenia gravis. For patients who do not respond adequately either to the use of anticholinesterase drugs or to removal of the thymus gland, steroid medication may be of some help.

MYOTONIA

In myotonia, of which there are several types, the patient experiences difficulty in relaxing the muscles after they have once contracted. Repeated use of the same muscles seems to "warm them up" so that their function becomes virtually normal. Many cases of this unique disorder seem to have hereditary backgrounds.

Some forms of myotonia appear in early life, while others appear later. In some cases the difficulty is aggravated by prolonged rest, by exposure to low temperatures, and by emotional excitement.

Care and Treatment

There is no satisfactory treatment, but in many cases the disease does not shorten life. Many victims of the disease learn to live quite normally in spite of their handicap.

NARCOLEPSY

Narcolepsy is an ailment characterized by (1) the tendency to fall asleep spontaneously, even during the daytime and in spite of adequate sleep at night, (2) the occurrence of unusual dreams, (3) sleep paralysis in which the individual is unable to move his muscles for about the first minute on awakening, and (4) the sudden occurrence of muscle weakness so severe that the patient falls even though he does not lose consciousness. This sudden muscle weakness is called cataplexy and usually comes in response to some emotional experience such as laughter, anger, or fear.

The symptoms develop most commonly during the second decade of life. Narcolepsy is relatively uncommon, but it occurs more frequently in men than in women. It does not interfere with the usual life-span except as it introduces an element of hazard because of the tendency to go to sleep even while otherwise occupied—as while driving a car.

Care and Treatment

Treatment consists of the carefully supervised use of drugs which tend to keep the individual awake.

NEURALGIA

Neuralgia consists of attacks of acute pain in the area supplied by some particular nerve, usually one of the cranial nerves located in the face or neck. In neuralgia, in contrast to neuritis, no demonstrable change occurs in the structure of the nerve involved. Formerly, certain painful conditions such as sciatica were placed under the heading of neuralgia. Now it is recognized that sciatica is usually caused by a compression of one or more nerve roots by the herniation of an intervertebral disk. (See under SPINAL INJURIES in this chapter.) The usual examples of true neuralgia are trigeminal neuralgia and glossopharyngeal neuralgia.

A. *Trigeminal Neuralgia (Tic Douloureux).* The trigeminal nerve is the sensory nerve to the face and consists of three branches, one supplying the skin of the forehead and eye, one supplying the skin of the side of the face between the eye and the mouth, and the third supplying the skin of the side of the jaw, the lower lip, and the chin. One or more of these branches may be involved in trigeminal neuralgia.

Trigeminal neuralgia may occur at any time in adult life but usually begins about age 50. It is somewhat more common in women than in men.

The pain is a lightninglike stab which occurs in paroxysms and usually lasts a moment or two. In the early stages it may not recur for days. If the disease advances, the intervals between paroxysms become shorter. The pain of trigeminal neuralgia is usually so intense that the patient writhes in agony. In most cases there is some activity of the face or mouth which seems to trigger the attack—touching or washing of the face, exposure to cold, talking, eating, or drinking.

Care and Treatment

In treating trigeminal neuralgia, the use of drugs is usually given a good trial before taking recourse to other, more drastic measures. There are now two modern drugs, either one or the other of which is effective for relieving the symptoms of trigeminal neuralgia in about two thirds of cases. The one used most frequently is carbamazepine (Tegretol). In some cases this drug produces such side effects as skin rash, dizziness, ataxia, or damage to the blood-forming tissues of the body. It should be used, of course, only under the supervision of a physician, and he will want to arrange for frequently repeated blood tests and liver-function studies in order to check on the possibility of serious side effects.

Phenytoin is another commonly used drug. It, too, may produce side effects.

Strong pain-killing drugs should be avoided in the treatment of trigeminal neuralgia because, in the long run, they give little lasting relief and because of the great danger of addiction.

Surgical procedures for destroying the sensory portion of the trigeminal nerve have been permanently successful in many cases. It is advised that the patient with trigeminal neuralgia should consult a neurologist—a physician trained in diseases of the nervous system.

B. *Glossopharyngeal Neuralgia.* In this type of neuralgia the patient suffers paroxysms of pain which involve the back of the tongue, one tonsil, one side of the throat, and the middle ear of the same side. The symptom usually makes its first appearance after age 40 and, strangely, affects males more commonly than females. The attack is often brought on by chewing, swallowing, talking, or yawning. The attack of pain is brief, lasting only a few minutes, but being so severe that the patient sometimes faints.

Care and Treatment

As in the care of trigeminal neuralgia, the use of the drug carbamazepine (Tegretol) is the treatment of first choice. The use of this drug must be carefully controlled and monitored by a physician because of the possibility of serious side effects. Here again the use of powerful pain-killing drugs should be avoided because the intensity of symptoms in this ailment readily sets the stage for drug addiction. In cases in which carbamazepine is not effective, surgical interruption of the offending nerve is the alternative treatment.

C. *Causalgia*. Causalgia, though not a typical example of neuralgia, is included here because of the element of excruciating pain. This symptom follows injury to a nerve such as the median nerve in the arm or the sciatic nerve in the hip, thigh, or leg. A persistent burning pain is easily aggravated by almost any stimulus, such as exposure of the involved area to the air, a sudden noise, some startling experience, or mere emotional excitation. It is believed that injury to the sympathetic nerve fibers contained in the injured nerve is responsible for this unusual symptom.

Care and Treatment

In some cases relief has been obtained by surgical severing of the sympathetic nerve filaments which supply this part of the body. The patient should consult a neurologist.

NEURITIS

In neuritis degenerative changes occur in one or more nerves as a result of mechanical damage to the nerve, metabolic disturbance, or toxic insult. When a single nerve is involved we speak of mononeuritis; when more than one or many nerves are involved, we speak of polyneuritis.

Because most of the body's nerves contain various kinds of fibers—some for sensation, some for muscle control, and some for regulating the body's organs—the symptoms appearing in a certain case of neuritis will depend on what kinds of fibers are contained in the injured nerve.

When fibers carrying sensations are injured, the patient may experience sharp pains, burning sensations, sensations of tingling, feeling of "pins and needles," or numbness. When fibers that control muscle action are injured, there will usually be a weakness of the muscles controlled by this nerve and this weakness may progress to complete paralysis.

When the autonomic fibers that control the actions of the body's organs are damaged, there may be an increase in skin temperature in the involved area, sweating, or skin lesions. In other cases there may be paleness and dryness of the skin.

We now mention the three types of neuritis as determined by the three common causes.

A. *Mechanical Damage to the Nerve*. This may occur in connection with penetrating injuries, crushing injuries, or fractures of bones in which nerves are damaged. It may be caused by long-continued pressure against a nerve, as when an intoxicated person sleeps in a chair with his arm over the back. What the patient notices is a distortion of nerve functions such as occurs commonly when a person's leg or arm "goes to sleep" on account of sustained local pressure.

B. *Metabolic Disturbance of the Nerve Tissue*. In these generalized conditions the damage is usually to many nerves, and therefore we speak of polyneuritis. It occurs in conditions in which there is not a sufficient amount of thiamine (vitamin B_1) in the diet. Polyneuritis of this kind develops in such diseases as beriberi and pellagra and in alcoholism. The chronic alcoholic derives much of his energy from calories contained in the alcohol and thus does not eat sufficient food to provide the required nutritional elements, including thiamine. Other metabolic diseases, such as diabetes, may also cause polyneuritis.

C. *Toxic Insults to the Nerves*. Here

65

we include the toxic conditions that result from diseases such as diphtheria, in which neuritis may develop because the toxin from the germs damages certain nerves. Also, there are many chemicals and heavy metals which injure nerve tissue. These include alcohol, carbon tetrachloride, and benzine among the chemicals, and lead, arsenic, mercury, and bismuth among the heavy metals. Persons exposed to these substances in excess are prone to develop symptoms of polyneuritis.

Care and Treatment

Treatment of neuritis consists of discovering and removing the cause of the damage to the nerves. Once the cause is removed, recovery may be prompt in mild cases. In severe cases, however, in which damage to the nerves has been inflicted over a long period, the normal function of the nerve may never be completely restored. A good diet and high intake of vitamins may hasten recovery.

PARKINSONISM (PARALYSIS AGITANS)

Parkinsonism is a chronic, progressive disorder, usually occurring in middle-aged or elderly persons. It is characterized by slowness of movement, rigidity of the muscles, involuntary tremor, and progressive weakness.

The usual case of parkinsonism begins gradually and is without known cause. The rate of progress of the disease will vary from case to case. Usually the patient becomes gradually incapacitated over a period of several years. Parkinsonism occurring earlier in life may be a sequel to encephalitis or some circumstance in which the cells of the brain were deprived of their supply of oxygen for at least five to ten minutes and were thus permanently damaged. Such a circumstance may develop in connection with carbon monoxide poisoning, asphyxia, or head injury.

The victim of parkinsonism presents a characteristic appearance. The muscles of his face become immobile, and blinking of the eyes becomes infrequent so that he appears to stare and seems unable to register his emotions. In advanced cases, saliva may drool from a corner of the mouth. The patient leans forward as he walks, moves with short, shuffling steps, and may break into a run, trying to keep from falling forward. Typically, his arms are flexed at the elbows, and he carries his hands near his abdomen. There may be tremors in various parts of his body, but the most characteristic one involves a repetitive movement by which the tips of the fingers brush past the ball of his thumb—the so-called "pill rolling movement." The tremors are worse when the patient is tired or when he becomes excited, but disappear during sleep.

Although weakness of the muscles develops gradually in parkinsonism, there is a rigidity which interferes with rapid movement of any part of the body. Speech becomes hampered both in volume of sound and in clarity of enunciation. Intellectual capacity is retained quite well until the terminal phase of the disorder.

Care and Treatment

Inasmuch as there is no cure for parkinsonism, the care of a patient with this disorder centers around keeping him active as long as possible, maintaining his morale by cheerful surroundings, and using such drugs as may minimize his tremors and reduce the rigidity of his muscles. Such drugs include some of the anticholinergic medications and certain of the antihistamines.

In about two thirds of cases the symptoms are very materially improved by the use of medication containing levodopa. There is some evidence that the use of levodopa retards the progression of the disease.

In some cases the use of levodopa is accompanied by unpleasant side effects including nausea, vomiting, and, occasionally, transient mental disturbances. The control of such side effects requires cooperation between

the patient and his physician. Variations in the dosage of the levodopa, altering the daily pattern of administering this preparation, using supplementary drugs along with the levodopa, and, especially, using a combination of levodopa and carbidopa will usually reduce the severity of the side effects. Patients treated for long periods of time with levodopa will usually benefit by an occasional period of rest from taking this drug.

PHENYLKETONURIA (PKU)

Phenylketonuria is perhaps the best known of several hereditary metabolic diseases. It strikes about one child in every ten to fifteen thousand and is caused by a lack of an enzyme necessary to the proper synthesis of tyrosine (one of the amino acids). As a result of this metabolic defect, phenylalanine (a precursor of tyrosine) accumulates in the body's tissues and fluids and is excreted by way of the urine. From the standpoint of our present consideration of nervous disorders, the importance of phenylketonuria is that children not treated early in life will display awkward gait, tremors, continuous purposeless movements of the hands, and mental retardation. Epileptic seizures occur in about one fourth of these cases.

The mental deficiency of untreated cases of phenylketonuria develops gradually, beginning soon after birth. If the infant is placed on a special diet at once—a diet which contains only a minimum of phenylalanine—he may not develop mental deficiency or other neurological manifestations.

Prevention and Treatment

The newborn infant who is a candidate for phenylketonuria appears the same as any normal newborn infant. The only way to detect this ailment is to make tests of the urine. Some states require that such a test be made on all newborn infants, this as a means of detecting the occasional one who would benefit by treatment for phenylketonuria and thus be spared the tragedy of becoming mentally deficient. The special diet must be adapted by the physician to the needs of the individul case. The history of a previous child in the family affected by the disease will of course alert the parents and physician.

POSTEROLATERAL SCLEROSIS (COMBINED SYSTEM DISEASE)

Posterolateral sclerosis is a serious involvement of the nervous system associated with pernicious anemia or other macrocytic anemias. A deficiency of vitamin B_{12}, the cause of pernicious anemia, has its effect on the tissues of the nervous system, causing a degeneration of areas of the spinal cord. The degeneration interferes with the normal transmission of both motor and sensory nervous impulses.

Sometimes it is the symptoms of posterolateral sclerosis that first call the physician's attention to the possibility of pernicious anemia in a given case. The first symptoms usually consist of tingling and numbness in the skin of the toes and soles of the feet. Soon the same sensations develop in the fingers. If the disease still goes untreated, the troublesome sensations extend to the legs and, possibly, to the thighs and lower parts of the body. The tingling and numbness of the fingers usually spread to include the hands; but seldom include the arms, particularly the upper arms.

Next is noticed an unsteadiness and stiffness in gait, which may be accompanied by weakness of the muscles of the legs. The patient tends to stumble, especially when walking in the dark. As the weakness progresses, the knees may give way unexpectedly. The hands become clumsy.

In severe cases there is an involvement of the brain, with certain mental symptoms including loss of recent memory, ideas of persecution, and even stupor and coma. Commonly, vision is impaired by a developing blindness at the center of the visual field.

In untreated cases of pernicious anemia the symptoms of posterolateral sclerosis become progressively worse.

Care and Treatment

When treatment is begun early, at least by the time unsteadiness in gait is first noticed, the prospect is good that the symptoms will disappear and, if treatment is continued consistently for the remainder of life, that the victim of this disease can live out a normal life-span. If treatment is long delayed, however, the damage to the tissues of the spinal cord become so serious that normal conditions can probably never be reestablished. Even in such cases, however, treatment may bring a significant improvement.

Since posterolateral sclerosis is part of pernicious anemia, the treatment is one and the same. It consists of the administration, by intramuscular injection, of vitamin B_{12}. A case of pernicious anemia with posterolateral sclerosis should, of course, remain under the continuing supervision of a physician.

SCIATICA

Sciatica is a term used to describe pain in the distribution of the sciatic nerve. This nerve derives its fibers from the spinal cord in the lower part of the back and passes through the buttock and thigh into the leg. The usual cause of sciatic pain is pressure produced by a herniated intervertebral disk. See the discussion of *Herniated Intervertebral Disks* on page 70.

SPINA BIFIDA

In spina bifida a malformation of the vertebral column occurs which, in the more serious cases, may be accompanied by involvement of the spinal cord and the spinal nerves. It usually occurs in the lower part of the back and affects one or more vertebrae.

The least severe cases exhibit no symptoms relating to the nervous system. In the moderately severe cases some of the nerve roots are involved, and the infant may have difficulty in learning to walk and may have a clumsy gait. In the very severe cases there may be a weakness and wasting of the muscles of the legs and feet, in addition to some diminution of the skin sensations in the areas of the buttocks and adjacent portions of the thighs. In these more severe cases there is usually a surface protrusion of the membranes that normally cover the spinal cord, the protrusion appearing in the midline at the lower part of the back.

Care and Treatment

The immediate treatment for cases of spina bifida that have symptoms is reparative surgery. However, surgery will not restore functions of the nervous system already deficient. Furthermore, hydrocephalus sometimes develops as a complication after surgery.

The care of the patient with spina bifida includes a carefully planned program of rehabilitation aimed to make it possible for the child, as he grows up, to live a reasonably normal life.

SPINAL INJURIES

By spinal injuries we refer to those accidents that damage the bony vertebral column and may at the same time injure the spinal cord and/or some of the spinal nerves. The reason spinal injuries may affect the spinal cord or the spinal nerves is the very close anatomical relationship which exists between the vertebral column and the spinal cord with its emerging spinal nerves.

The bony vertebral column consists essentially of the bodies of the vertebrae plus their bony processes which extend to the sides and backward from the vertebral bodies. These bony processes form a complete arch behind each of the vertebral bodies. It is within the spinal canal formed by these arches that the delicate spinal cord (a downward continuation from the brain) is located. The spinal nerves originate from the spinal cord and then pass outward on the right and on the left between the bony processes.

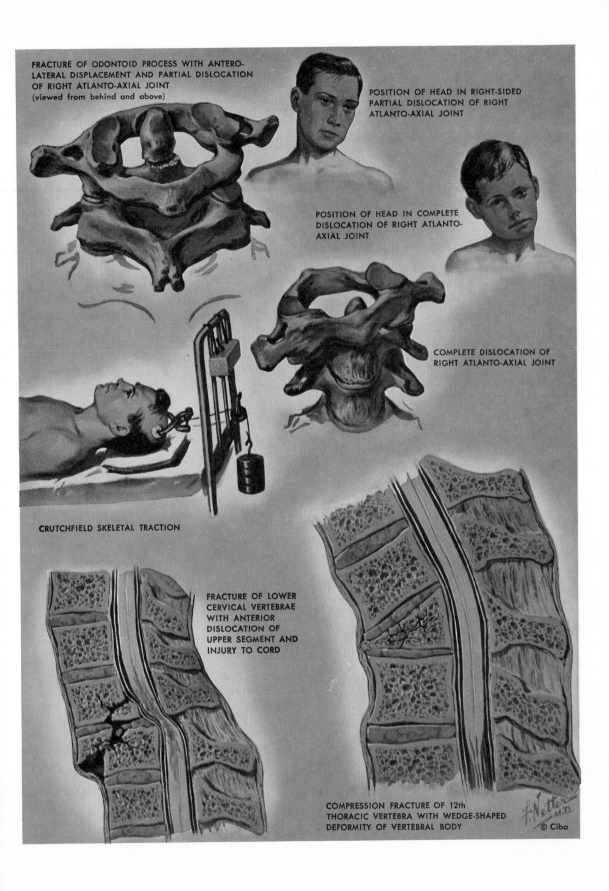

FRACTURE OF ODONTOID PROCESS WITH ANTERO-LATERAL DISPLACEMENT AND PARTIAL DISLOCATION OF RIGHT ATLANTO-AXIAL JOINT
(viewed from behind and above)

POSITION OF HEAD IN RIGHT-SIDED PARTIAL DISLOCATION OF RIGHT ATLANTO-AXIAL JOINT

POSITION OF HEAD IN COMPLETE DISLOCATION OF RIGHT ATLANTO-AXIAL JOINT

COMPLETE DISLOCATION OF RIGHT ATLANTO-AXIAL JOINT

CRUTCHFIELD SKELETAL TRACTION

FRACTURE OF LOWER CERVICAL VERTEBRAE WITH ANTERIOR DISLOCATION OF UPPER SEGMENT AND INJURY TO CORD

COMPRESSION FRACTURE OF 12th THORACIC VERTEBRA WITH WEDGE-SHAPED DEFORMITY OF VERTEBRAL BODY

© Ciba

The greatest danger to the spinal cord occurs when the vertebrae are crushed or sharply bent on one another so that they pinch or crush the spinal cord, or when one vertebra is displaced in its relation to its neighbor so that the spinal cord is sheared. The spinal nerves which emerge between the bony processes of the vertebrae may be compressed or damaged by injuries which bring pressure against them. There are four principal types of spinal injuries as indicated in the following descriptions:

A. *Herniated Intervertebral Disks.* The structure of the bony spinal column, the interposition of intervertebral disks between the vertebrae, and the relation of these structures to the emerging spinal nerves are described in chapter 21, volume 2. It is also mentioned there that certain mechanical stresses and even some elusive forces of pressure can cause the intervertebral disks to deteriorate and "herniate" in such a manner as to bring pressure against an adjacent spinal nerve. These instances of "slipped disk" or "herniated disk" occur most commonly in the lumbar region of the lower back. The second most common site is the lower part of the neck.

The discomfort associated with a herniated disk located in the lower back usually consists of severe aching pain in the buttock and the back and side of the thigh and leg. Often numbness and tingling are felt in the same area. These are the symptoms for which the term *sciatica* is often used because they occur in the areas served by the sciatic nerve. The pain is often aggravated by coughing or sneezing or by straining at stool. It may be made worse by twisting, stooping, or lifting. Certain muscles of the thigh, leg, or foot may become weak. There may or may not be pain in the lower part of the back.

When the damaged intervertebral disk is in the lower part of the neck, the pain involves the shoulder, the arm, the forearm, and the hand, the latter either on the thumb side or on the little finger side. Again there will be numbness and tingling in these areas, with a weakness of certain muscles, particularly the triceps muscle in the back of the arm.

Care and Treatment

Although the symptoms caused by a herniated intervertebral disk result from damage to a nerve, the fundamental problem relates to structures belonging to the skeleton. Therefore the treatment is described in chapter 21, volume 2, where attention is given to methods of relieving the pressure on a nerve caused by a damaged intervertebral disk.

B. *Sprains.* A sprain of the vertebral column involves a stretching of the spinal ligaments which hold the vertebrae in place. Inasmuch as the cervical portion (in the neck) of the vertebral column is most flexible, this is the part most commonly sprained. It is this type of injury, occurring in the neck, that is called whiplash. It occurs as a result of direct violence or excessive muscle pull, as when the head is suddenly thrown backward in an automobile accident.

In a sprain, the vertebrae are usually not displaced; therefore seldom does a sprain injure the spinal cord. Symptoms consist of pain on moving the neck, of local tenderness, and of stiffness.

Care and Treatment

A physician should examine the patient after such a sprain for any actual damage to the bony structures or nerves. Injuries found should be treated accordingly. Otherwise, the aim of treatment is to relieve the patient's discomfort and to promote healing. A treatment program for neck sprain is described in chapter 21, volume 2.

Occasionally a person who has sustained this type of sprain becomes self-centered in his desire for sympathy or compensation. This attitude tends to prolong the symptoms even beyond the time required for the tis-

sues to heal. Most physicians, therefore, advise that these patients return to their normal way of life within a reasonable period of time, encouraging them to ignore their continuing symptoms.

C. *Dislocations.* In a dislocation of the vertebral column an actual displacement of one vertebra in its relation to another takes place. Dislocations are often associated with fractures, torn ligaments, and injuries to the intervertebral disks. Because of the displacement, danger of injury to the spinal cord threatens. Dislocation may be caused by diving into shallow water or by falling on the head, shoulder, or even on one's feet in a standing position. A heavy blow such as causes the vertebral column to bend sharply in any direction may cause a dislocation. Symptoms consist of local pain, tenderness, and a deformity of the bony structures such as can be observed by X ray or by careful digital examination.

Care and Treatment

In any case of dislocation of the vertebrae, great care must be taken in handling the patient lest damage be done to the spinal cord. Even a slight movement of the patient's body might cause the displaced vertebra to compress the spinal cord, with resulting permanent damage.

Immediate care of the case requires the same precautions as when the back is broken. If the patient must be transported, great care should be taken to avoid body or neck movement. For details of the handling of such a patient, see chapter 23, volume 3. Usual hospital treatment for such a patient includes traction of the head so that if parts of the vertebral column shift their location they will do so in the direction of their normal position rather than in a direction that might press on the spinal cord.

D. *Fractures.* Fractures of the vertebrae are somewhat more common in the middle and lower back. Sometimes they consist merely of the compression of a vertebral body without its being displaced. As mentioned above under *Dislocations,* fractures may well be associated with damage to the intervertebral disk or to the ligaments that normally hold the vertebral bodies in place. Fractures are usually the result of a fall with forceful bending, of a direct blow on the back, or of the intense pressure produced by sudden strong muscle action as in a convulsion.

If the fracture involves no displacement of the bony structures so as to endanger the spinal cord or the nerve roots, it is not as serious to the patient's total welfare as a dislocation. Symptoms of a fracture consist of local pain, tenderness, and muscle spasm.

Care and Treatment

Treatment consists, usually, of the use of casts and braces to support the patient's back during the period of healing. For instruction on the first-aid handling of persons with fractures of the vertebral column, see chapter 23, volume 3.

SYPHILIS OF THE NERVOUS SYSTEM

The causes and manifestations of syphilis, which is one of the sexually transmitted diseases, are discussed in chapter 31, volume 2.

Involvement of the nervous system is one of the late manifestations of syphilis, occurring typically in the so-called third stage of the disease. When the disease is treated adequately in its first stage, the infection is stamped out and involvements of the brain and spinal cord are avoided. But in inadequately treated cases, the germs of syphilis remain quiescent in the tissues of the nervous system for many months or even several years after they have entered these tissues. Then, for some unknown reason, they begin to produce damage so disastrous that even intensive treatment may not restore the patient completely to his previous condition.

A person need not remain uncertain

whether he needs treatment for a syphilitic condition. Blood tests for syphilis are now available at any doctor's office, at public clinics, and at public-health headquarters. More than this, it is possible by drawing a portion of the cerebrospinal fluid, to determine whether or not the germs of syphilis have entered the nervous system. If they have, the need for intensive treatment adapted to this complication is most urgent, even though no symptoms of the involvement of the brain or spinal cord have yet appeared.

Syphilis affects the brain and spinal cord in several ways. It may produce a unique type of meningitis, or it may involve, primarily, the blood vessels of these organs. It may produce degenerative changes which seriously affect the intellect or cause a destruction of certain of the nerve pathways. In the present consideration we will discuss the two most important manifestations of syphilis of the nervous system: (A) general paresis and (B) tabes dorsalis.

A. *General Paresis of the Insane.* This is a serious late complication of syphilis, typically developing several years after the individual's first syphilitic infection. It is serious because it destroys the intellect and progressively limits the victim's usual activities, bringing death, on the average, about three years after the first appearance of symptoms. Fortunately, general paresis of the insane is seldom seen now because most cases of syphilis receive treatment in their earlier stages.

The general symptoms of this disorder include headache, ataxia (unsteadiness of gait and station), slurred speech, tremor of the fingers and tongue, and mental deterioration.

A progressive impairment of the individual's efficiency occurs, both in family life and in business. He begins to use poor judgment and is prone to make serious mistakes, such as unnecessarily incurring debt or spending money for things not needed. He suffers a progressive failure in memory and tends to tell untruths. The individual becomes disoriented so that he no longer knows the time of day or the day of the week or month and is confused as to his whereabouts and his identity and the identity of those he contacts. This leads to a dreamlike state. A person with this condition commonly has delusions, imagining himself to be somebody great. The emotions of joy and sorrow may alternate suddenly and without adequate justification. Moral and ethical standards rapidly deteriorate. As the disease continues, the victim becomes apathetic and finally completely demented.

Care and Treatment

Intensive treatment with antibiotic drugs may at least partially arrest the progress of general paresis of the insane; but, inasmuch as the disease involves a degeneration of nerve cells and nerve fibers, treatment cannot be expected to restore the individual completely to his normal state.

B. *Tabes Dorsalis (Locomotor Ataxia).* In this manifestation of syphilis it is primarily the spinal cord and the nerve roots that are affected. Fortunately this disease is much less common now than before adequate treatment for syphilis became available. Tabes dorsalis tends to develop from five to twenty years after the primary syphilitic infection.

In the usual case, the first symptom is an aching pain in the legs, often confused with rheumatism. The pain becomes progressively worse until it is described as lightninglike. These pains come in bouts, usually occurring at least once during each twenty-four hours, the severity usually being more intense at night than during the day. In some cases the patient receives the impression of a tight girdle about his abdomen. In others agonizing pains (so-called tabetic crises) develop in certain organs of the body. These excruciating pains occur most commonly in relation to the stomach. They may last for several days, the pain being either continuous or intermittent. Any attempt to drink or eat causes vomiting. The pain may disappear as suddenly as it began, only to recur at a later time.

Various neuralgias, involving nerves here and there throughout the body, may develop as a part of tabes dorsalis. There may be numbness and a feeling of coldness in various skin areas. Often the patient reports a sensation as though he were walking on cotton. Certain areas of the skin may be less sensitive than normal, approaching a complete loss of sensation. The sense of position suffers greatly in most cases so that the individual becomes unaware of the position of his feet or legs except as he watches them and observes their movements and position. With walking thus made difficult, the victim typically uses a cane and watches each step he takes. When he stands, he stands with feet wide apart to brace himself against falling. He often experiences a loss of muscle tone in his extremities so that they move in a flaillike manner. His strength and energy become progressively diminished. Joint surfaces, such as of the knees, may disintegrate (Charcot's joints).

Care and Treatment

In well-established tabes dorsalis, as well as in general paresis of the insane, the deteriorated nerve fibers cannot be restored even by intensive treatment. Once the damage has been done, repair is impossible. It should be emphasized that any syphilitic infection should be treated intensively promptly after the infection has been acquired.

SYRINGOMYELIA

The person with syringomyelia loses the sensation for pain and temperature in the skin of a certain area of his body, equal on the right and on the left. The area usually involved is that of the arms and upper trunk. Significantly, the sense of touch remains normal even in the areas now insensitive to pain and temperature. The symptom is usually brought to the patient's attention when he observes that he suffers no pain in the involved part of his body from minor injuries or even a burn. Another later evidence of the disease is progressive weakness and atrophy of certain of the small muscles, usually those of the hands.

Syringomyelia is an unusual disease caused by the development of a central cavity within the spinal cord. The first symptoms often appear between ages 10 and 30. The disease is slowly progressive but may remain stationary for several years.

Care and Treatment

Science has found no satisfactory medical treatment for syringomyelia. The patient should be encouraged to remain active as long as feasible. In view of the danger of burns of the skin, now that the natural protective influence of pain and temperature has been lost, appropriate means to prevent injury should be employed. Surgical intervention may slow the course of the disease.

TUMORS

A. *Tumors of the Brain.* There are various kinds of brain tumors. Some grow slowly, others rapidly. All kinds are hazardous because their increase in size brings pressure against the delicate tissues of the brain. Some invade the brain itself, causing destruction of the nerve cells and fibers as they do so. These are classed as malignant tumors (cancer). Others remain within a fibrous capsule and inflict damage by pressure which their growth produces. These are usually classed as benign because they do not invade the surrounding brain tissue. Often they can be safely removed by surgery.

An example of a benign tumor is the meningioma, which develops in the membranes surrounding the brain. An example of a malignant tumor is the astrocytoma, which consists of cancer cells that have developed from cells which normally support the nerve cells of the brain.

Malignant tumors are seldom curable because of their tendency to grow rapidly, to invade the tissues, and to recur after removal. These may be subdivided into primary and secondary tumors. The primary tumors are those that have developed within the brain substance. Secondary malignant tumors are those which have migrated from a malignant tumor in some other part of the body such as the lung or the breast. Small portions of such a tumor are carried by the blood to the brain, where they become secondarily implanted and grow.

Symptoms of tumors of the brain are of two types: (1) those that result from the pressure which the tumor produces, and (2) those caused by the destruction of nerve cells and nerve fibers.

Headache is sometimes the first symptom of a brain tumor. Inasmuch as headache is commonly produced by other causes, this symptom is not diagnostic except as it may persist unnaturally. Unexplained nausea and vomiting are also symptoms which occur commonly in case of brain tumor. In some cases weakness, awkwardness, and/or convulsive seizures develop. In other cases the patient may exhibit drowsiness, changes in personality, strange conduct, and impaired thinking. Vision, hearing, and equilibrium may be involved.

Care and Treatment

The care of a patient with brain tumor should be supervised by a neurologist or a brain surgeon. Three forms of treatment may be applied as the case requires: surgical removal of the tumor, radiation therapy (X-ray treatment), or chemotherapy.

B. *Tumors of the Spinal Cord.* These are much less frequent than tumors of the brain, but are classified in about the same manner. Symptoms depend on the location of the tumor and upon the particular groups of nerve fibers or of nerve cells destroyed or compressed as the tumor grows. There may be weakness of certain muscles and also changes in the sensations relating to certain parts of the skin area—either abnormal sensations or the loss of sensation.

Care and Treatment

Early surgical removal of a tumor of the spinal cord usually offers the best possibility of a favorable result. Even then the outcome will depend upon how much tissue of the spinal cord has already been destroyed. In certain cases of tumor of the spinal cord, radiation therapy is preferable to surgery.

VASCULAR DISORDERS

The brain is particularly vulnerable to any interference with its moment-by-moment supply of blood. Some of the brain cells are so dependent on receiving a continuous flow of oxygen and food materials brought to them by the blood that they suffer permanent damage if deprived for as little as five or ten minutes. Thus problems occur when a blood vessel inside the skull becomes unable to carry its usual quota of blood or when a blood vessel ruptures or when a blood vessel is plugged by a blood clot. The physician speaks of such developments as cerebrovascular accidents or strokes.

Disease of the blood vessels within the skull (cerebrovascular disease) accounts for an astounding amount of disability, especially in the older age group, and, ultimately, for about 10 percent of deaths in the United States.

A description follows of the common types of blood vessel disorders that affect the brain:

A. *Transient Ischemic Attacks (TIAs).* The name of this ailment is quite descriptive of what happens. "Transient" indicates that the symptoms do not last for long—in some cases for only a few seconds; in most cases, for five or ten minutes; never more than twenty-four hours. "Ischemic" means that the problem centers around a lack of blood. In this disease, therefore, a certain part of the brain is suffering because the blood vessel that brings blood is suddenly unable to bring as much blood as this part requires.

And what are the symptoms? They depend on what part of the brain is short on blood. With persons who have repeated attacks, the symptoms may vary from one time to another. The possible symptoms that may occur include these: transient blackout of vision in one eye as though a shade were pulled over the eye, weakness and numbness possibly of one whole side of the body or even of both sides, speechlessness, dizziness, and mental confusion.

The factors that contribute to TIA are the same as those that contribute to a major stroke. We may say, then, that it is a ministroke, the difference being that in the TIA the obstruction to the flow of blood is shortly cleared away, usually before any permanent damage to the brain takes place. We understand further that the occurrence of one or more TIAs is a warning that this person is at high risk as a candidate for a future stroke. If untreated, about one third of persons who have TIAs will sooner or later have a major stroke, about one third will keep on having TIAs without ever having a regular stroke, and about one third will outlive this tendency.

The basic cause in most of these cases is disease within a blood vessel (arteriosclerosis), even one located outside the skull. A small clot tends to form at the site, and from this clot a small fragment breaks away and is carried by the flowing blood until it lodges in one of the smaller vessels that supplies the brain. While the lodged fragment is in place, the individual experiences symptoms. When the lodged fragment is cleared away promptly the incident is properly called a TIA. If the lodged fragment of clot remains where it is or even grows larger because the vessel is diseased at the site of its lodging, a classic stroke supervenes with its enduring symptoms.

Care and Treatment

The aim of treatment is to prevent future TIAs and, ideally, to forestall the occurrence of a major stroke. One immediate treatment consists of administering anticoagulant (blood-thinning or antiplatlet) medication as a means of minimizing the further development of clots within the diseased blood vessels. An angiographic study (picturing the blood vessels by X ray) may need to be made to determine the site of interference with blood flow. On the strength of this information a surgical procedure may be performed to either remove the diseased lining of the affected vessel or arrange an alternate route for the blood to flow around the site of damage.

B. *Stroke*. A stroke is the result of some part of the brain being deprived of its usual supply of blood. The three conditions under which this supply of blood can be interrupted are listed and explained in chapter 9, volume 2. It can be caused by the formation of a blood clot (thrombus) inside one of the vessels that supply the brain. It can be caused by the lodging of a floating fragment of a blood clot (embolus) or, in a minority of cases, it can be caused by a rupture of the wall of an artery in the brain.

A stroke is usually the culmination of unfavorable conditions that have been building up for a long period of time. The actual symptoms occur quite suddenly. In many cases, however, there have been warning circumstances, such as the development of arteriosclerosis and the elevation of the blood pressure. In 50 percent of strokes caused by thrombosis, there have been previous transient ischemic attacks as described in the previous item in this chapter.

The usual outstanding symptom of stroke is the sudden development of paralysis of certain muscles of the body, usually limited to one side. This we speak of as hemiplegia. Often an accompanying loss of sensation (hemianesthesia) occurs in about the same part of the body as that in which the paralysis occurs. There may be the sudden occurrence of difficulty in speaking (aphasia). Also, it is common for the victim of stroke to lose control of the sphincter muscles of the bladder and rectum. There may be headache, vomiting, and altered consciousness.

Prevention and Treatment

Much of the damage which takes place in the brain at the time of a stroke is permanently destructive in nature. That is, when brain cells are destroyed, they are not replaced. Healing may take place, but the healing does not include replacement of the lost brain cells. It is true that a person who survives a stroke may show some improvement in his symptoms so that, even though paralyzed on one side of his body, he may learn to walk again with the aid of a cane. But most of this apparent improvement comes by way of learning to use other nerve circuits and also by a recovery from the tissue swelling at the margins of the brain area of destruction.

In view of the above prognosis, prevention of a stroke should be emphasized rather than treatment after the stroke occurs. Every person should give attention to the following correctable risk factors and thus reduce his susceptibility to stroke: high blood pressure, smoking, overweight, uncontrolled diabetes, a high concentration of cholesterol in the blood, and neglected phlebitis (inflammation of the veins).

With respect to the immediate treatment for the person who has just suffered a stroke, some physicians recommend that for most cases anticoagulant (blood-thinning) medication be used, except in those cases where there is a problem of blood already leaking into the brain or into the spaces which surround it. General supportive nursing care is important, of course. Also, as the patient recovers, it is important for him to be trained in rehabilitation techniques so that he can compensate by using other muscles and other means to perform tasks of which he is possibly capable. Physical therapy and occupational therapy may be helpful. See also item STROKE, APOPLECTIC in chapter 23, volume 3.

C. Cereberal aneurysm and Subarachnoid Hemorrhage. In chapter 9, volume 2, an aneurysm was defined as a weak place in an artery which typically bulges because of the pressure of blood within the artery. Also listed there were the two principal types of aneurysms: (1) congenital and (2) acquired because of arteriosclerosis.

Aneurysms may occur in various parts of the body. Aneurysms of the arteries within the skull rank second in frequency to those of the aorta. Aneurysms may occur at any time of life, with the congenital aneurysms being present even in infancy. Aneurysms within the vicinity of the brain seldom cause symptoms except as they rupture or become so large as to make pressure on nervous structures, such as the cranial nerves.

Middle age is the most common time of life for an aneurysm within the skull to rupture. When such rupture occurs, there develops a sudden violent headache, followed by mental confusion and sometimes loss of consciousness. Blood escaping from the rupture usually finds its way into the cerebrospinal fluid which surrounds the brain, and the presence of blood here causes irritation of the meninges. The evidence of such irritation is severe pain in the neck when the examining physician attempts to bend the patient's head forward. The presence of blood in the space normally occupied by cerebrospinal fluid is designated as subarachnoid hemorrhage.

Care and Treatment

The rupture of a cerebral aneurysm is a serious life-threatening condition. Even though the patient may survive the initial attack of bleeding, the tendency remains, if the aneurysm is not properly treated, for a second episode of bleeding to occur. The accepted treatment for a ruptured cereberal aneurysm consists of two phases: (1) medical and (2) surgical. The immediate medical treatment is designed to reduce the bleeding and allow two or three weeks of time for the patient's condition to stabilize so that surgery, if indicated by diagnostic studies, can then be performed with minimum of risk. The medical treatment consists of cautiously lowering the patient's blood pressure, particularly if it is already high, and of giving such medication as favors the development of blood clotting. The subsequent surgical procedure consists of opening the skull, locating the point from which the bleeding occurred and obliterating the aneurysm.

WERNICKE'S ENCEPHALOPATHY

This ailment occurs typically in chronic alcoholics whose diet has been deficient in the B vitamins. Certain brain cells deteriorate because of the vitamin deficiency. The location of the damaged cells and, therefore, the particular symptoms will vary somewhat from case to case. The usual symptoms include weakness of the eye muscles (causing double vision), ataxia (unsteadiness), neuritis (inflammation of the peripheral nerves), and mental changes such as apathy, disorientation, and forgetfulness. In some cases the patient experiences hallucinations similar to those occurring in delirium tremens.

Care and Treatment

The success of treatment depends upon how early in the course of the disease a nutritious diet, together with mineral and vitamin supplements, especially thiamine (B_1), can be provided. Without treatment, the disease proves fatal. The avoidance of alcohol is also imperative.

Mental Illness: Neuroses and Psychoses

The neuroses and psychoses are conditions in which the brain functions abnormally even though the person suffers from no demonstrable disease in the tissues of his nervous system. This problem stands in contrast to the neurological disorders considered in the preceding chapter, in which the structural pattern of the brain, the spinal cord, or the peripheral nerves has been altered by disease.

The questions logically arise, How can a structurally normal brain function in an abnormal manner? What causes a person to behave strangely even though his tissues are healthy? What sets the stage for a person who has no organic disease to have unfounded fears, to feel depressed, or to have symptoms of disease? Or to imagine things that are not so? What can a person do to keep himself from becoming mentally ill with a neurosis or a psychosis?

Such questions take us into the realm of personality more than into physiology or pathology. The way the individual reacts to the circumstances of his personal experience has more to do with his state of mental health than do germs or viruses or broken bones. To help our understanding of these relationships we will detour for a few paragraphs into a consideration of common frustrating experiences, of the need for adjustments when a person is thwarted, and of the unfortunate consequences when one fails to cope successfully.

Human Reaction to Life's Frustrations

Every person inherits and develops certain incentives to activity. These may be called drives, and they are the inner motivations that force him to play his part in the game of life. One of the outstanding inherited drives is the urge to obtain food. The urge to obtain an education is an acquired drive which, for some persons, entails a great deal of motivating power.

A person's easiest response to his drives is to satisfy them by carrying out the line of activity they suggest. When once a drive has been thus satisfied, the drive itself disappears. However, one's attempts to satisfy his various drives do not always meet with prompt success. Circumstances may be unfavorable. People in some parts of the world have difficulty in satisfying the simple drive to satisfy hunger. The drive to obtain an education may be potentially thwarted by a series of obstacles, some major and some minor.

Three kinds of frustrations may possibly interfere with a person's pursuing his drives to their fulfillment: (1) obstacles in the environment, (2) personal limitations, and (3) conflicts between motives.

1. *Obstacles in the environment.* Many things can occur over which a person has no control. The problem of being late to an appointment because of being caught in a traffic jam is a simple example. The way in which bad weather can interfere with one's vacation plans can be a frustrating experience. Poverty can make it difficult to realize one's urge to be well dressed or to live in a beautiful home. Crop failure can rob the farmer of his cherished hope of buying new equipment. The loss of a finger or a crippling injury to a hand can stifle a young person's drive to be a musician.

2. *Personal limitations.* Being deprived of the chance to realize some fond ambition just because a person lacks the capability is a major disappointment. The girl who wants to be a model but is rejected because she is stockily built knows what it is to be thwarted. The boy whose poor scholarship forces him to abandon his hope of being a scientist is in a serious plight. The handicap of allergy can thwart the person who wants to live in a part of the country where his allergy is aggravated. A wife may desire to experience motherhood, but finds herself unable to conceive. Poor eyesight can deprive a young man of his desire to be an aviator.

3. *Conflicts between motives.* Many human drives are so strong that they impel a person almost mercilessly. The desire for love and companionship is one of these. But a person may have developed some other urge which counters it. What can the person do who has two strong desires, one of which interferes with the other? What can the young man with limited finances do when he wants to marry his sweetheart and at the same time complete the requirements for his doctor's

degree? The young woman who has had a lifelong ambition to travel is similarly frustrated when she finds herself married to a young man whose job requires him to stay where he is. The young physician who wants to be a surgeon and still has a strong desire for country living finds it impossible to practice surgery in a rural community which has no hospital. A person may desire to be healthy and to preserve his personal vitality, but is addicted to cigarettes.

Personalities differ in their ability to cope—in the capacity to adjust to an "impossible" situation. Some people with strongly integrated personalities can ride the waves of difficulties and find ways to live successfully, even so. Others have inherited more fragile personality structures and are caught off guard when life doesn't fulfill their expectations. It is this latter group who are candidates for the neuroses and psychoses described in the present chapter.

But let us notice first the options available to the person whose drives are thwarted. He will be disappointed, yes. But disappointment need not be a permanent attitude. It should be the stimulus which prods the healthy personality into finding a way to solve the dilemma. The goal in solving such a problem need not be to realize one's desire in its original form. Instead, he should strive to live a life of fulfillment, even so, and to find other ways of deriving satisfaction.

In some cases time may remove some of the obstacles that have interfered. But blind persistence in spite of obstacles that won't go away may only bring another thwarting. Repeated frustrations are not only unpleasant, but they also tend to disrupt the personality and make the individual more vulnerable to abnormal behavior.

Compromise is a method of coping that is desirable in many cases. The boy with poor eyesight who is deprived of becoming a pilot may obtain satisfaction by becoming a travel agent. For the wife who finds it impossible to bear

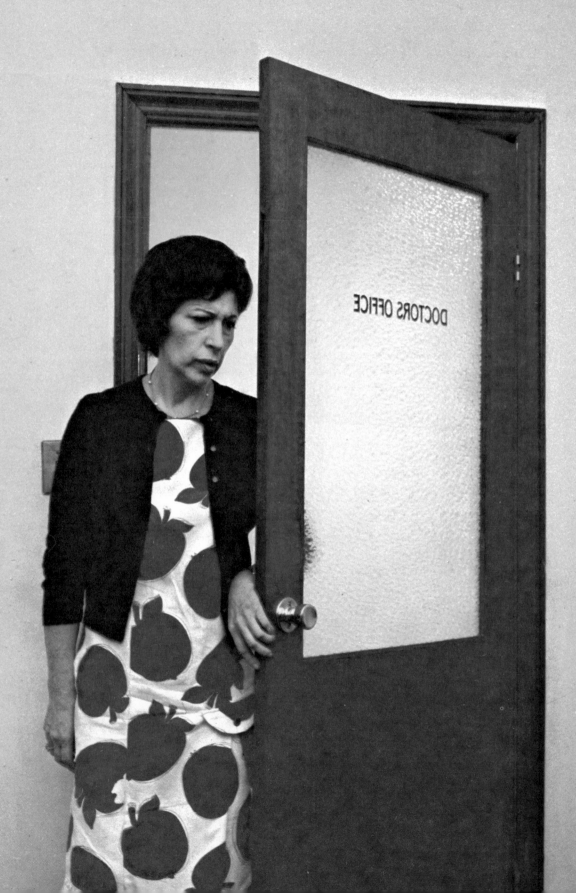

her own child, adopting a child may be the answer.

Substitution is another means of coping. For the person who wanted to be a musician but is now handicapped because of an injury to the hand, becoming an artist with paints or developing skills in public speaking may provide satisfaction.

Help for the Frustrated

A frustrated person needs to have sufficient discernment to evaluate himself and his circumstances correctly. He needs to be able to stand off and objectively observe himself in the stream of events. He needs to make a fair judgment as to the strength of his own personality. He needs to decide whether his goals, now thwarted, have been realistic. He needs to be unbiased in appraising the possible compromises and alternatives. Admittedly, this is too large an order for most persons in the throes of a frustrating experience. They need help from a friend or a professional.

We are dealing here with the very core of the individual's life experience. The person with a well-integrated personality is able to assess the influence of experiences through which he has passed, to judge the significance of the present circumstances, and to readjust appropriately. A person who has religious convictions and who thus sees himself in the perspective of providential interventions has the advantage that confidence in having a Supreme Being on his side provides.

The family physician is in the number one spot for giving help in these cases. If he has known the patient for some time, he can discern the series of events that have brought the patient to his present need. He can appraise the seriousness of the case. His own friendly attitude and impartial advice may be what the patient needs to tide him over this period of discouragement and uncertainty. But if the family physician senses the patient's need of a specialist particularly trained in the care of mental illnesses, he will refer him to a psychiatrist or a psychologist. In some cases the treatment will consist of counseling. In others, the patient will be best served by group therapy where he can hear the experiences of others. In still other cases, the appropriate use of medications will help the patient to adjust to life as it is now.

Neuroses Versus Psychoses

Persons with neuroses are tolerated by their associates even though their thinking and acting may be "different." They are able to think logically and to reason from cause to effect. They are in touch with reality and can usually live somewhat productively.

The psychoses, on the other hand, include several forms of mental derangement, any one of which constitutes "insanity" in the usual meaning of the word. When a person becomes ill with a psychosis, he loses control of his thinking and acting to the extent that his behavior no longer conforms with accepted standards or squares with the realities of his situation in life. His lack of insight makes unsuccessful any effort to persuade him that his thinking is confused and his behavior unacceptable. Reasoning will not change his abnormal patterns.

A. The Neuroses

Ideally a frustrated person adjusts to his disappointments in wholesome ways that permit him to carry on in a satisfying, productive manner. But many people fall short of perfect adjustments and resort, subconsciously, to psychological mechanisms less than ideal. The neuroses fall into this class, for they consist of forms of thinking and of behaving that waste personal resources and interfere in relationships with other people. People with neuroses are not incapacitated, as are those with psychoses; but they pay a high price in inconvenience and unhappiness.

Descriptions of several classic types of neuroses will now follow, along with a statement at the end of the section on

81

treatment generally applicable to all.

ANXIETY

Anxiety is a condition of inordinate fear. It is normal for a person to fear danger. But in anxiety a person recoils from something intangible, he knows not what. Anxiety is an amplification of worry. It is normal for a person to worry about circumstances with which he is familiar but over which he has no control. But in anxiety the person becomes distraught without being able to pinpoint what it is that bothers him. He feels grossly inadequate without knowing what threatens him.

Anxiety produces an emotional upheaval that alters the body's functions. In acute anxiety states the person feels weak, his mouth is dry, his heart beats rapidly, his breathing is fast and shallow, he trembles easily, and perspires excessively. In long-continued (chronic) anxiety states, the patient may experience difficulty in sleeping, heartburn, tiredness, headache, mental stupidity, diarrhea, and frequent urination.

CONVERSION REACTION (HYSTERIA)

In the conversion reaction the individual subconsciously diverts energy pent up as a result of intense anxiety or frustration into some abnormal form of behavior or into some form of supposed illness which tends to protect him from the unbearable situation. The individual is not aware of his having used the hysterical manifestation as a pretext to get himself excused from facing the reality of his problem. This unawareness stands in contrast to malingering, in which the individual deliberately feigns some disability. Nevertheless, the conversion reaction is an unhealthy solution to life's problems. It is a great imitator of many symptoms of disease, such as paralysis, loss of sensation, blindness, loss of memory (amnesia)—either total or for a specific period of time—convulsive seizures, or even loss of consciousness. The physician's skill may be taxed to tell the difference between the conversion reaction and actual disease. The individual's lack of concern for his seemingly serious condition may be a clue.

DEPRESSION

Depression is a state of mind in which the mood has shifted to the melancholy side. Degrees of depression vary all the way from temporary, reactive episodes of being downcast to the serious, incapacitating states of mind which may lead to suicide or which belong in the realm of the psychoses.

Depression is the most common of the mental illnesses. It is estimated that 15 percent or more of persons in the United States suffer from symptoms of depression at some time in their lives.

Crying for insufficient cause is a cardinal evidence of depression. The symptoms include sadness, a sense of hopelessness, loss of usual interest in hobbies or achievements, loss of the ability to experience pleasure, sleep difficulties, loss of energy, decrease in sexual desire, and a feeling of guilt. Depression is often accompanied by certain symptoms relating to the body's functions, such as loss of appetite, constipation, headache, dizziness, and insomnia.

Great progress has been made in recent years in the treatment of depression, especially by the use of medications. One of the unfortunate manifestations of depression is an attitude on the part of the patient that he is unworthy of help. This may make him reluctant to seek medical advice. Those associated with such a person carry a responsibility to arrange for his professional care so that he can benefit by the modern methods of treatment, thus preventing his becoming incapacitated by his depression.

NEURASTHENIA

Neurasthenia is a condition in which the individual feels depleted of energy. The symptoms consist of weakness, exhaustion, fatigue, and an abnormal sensitivity to pain and other sensations that suggest various body and organ ailments. Symptoms often suggest difficulty in the stomach, the intestines, the heart, or the genitourinary organs. Usually the patient suffers a reduced ability to concentrate, irritability, and sleep difficulty.

A person with these symptoms should be given a thorough physical examination to determine whether any organic basis exists for the symptoms. The diagnosis of neurasthenia depends not only on the absence of organic disease but also on evidence that the individual has been experiencing emotional problems and/or has been frustrated in certain of his personal desires.

OBSESSIVE-COMPULSIVE REACTION

An obsession consists of an almost uncontrollable urge to follow the same line of thought over and over. Often the thought is unwelcome, but, try as he may, the individual finds it nearly impossible to banish it from his thinking. An obsession pertains to one's thoughts. A compulsion, by contrast, consists of an unreasonable urge to do something, even though the act is entirely unnecessary and may be unreasonable. A person may become *obsessed* with the thought that he is carrying a germ which could infect other members of his family and even cause their death. As a result he may develop the *compulsion* to wash his hands frequently, particularly at certain times such as before eating, after shaking hands, or at frequent intervals.

A person may develop the obsession that he is changing in appearance, and this fixation may prompt a compulsion that forces him to look in the mirror repeatedly for evidences of such change. A person with an obsession may be constantly troubled by obscene thoughts out of harmony with his standards of conduct. A person may develop the compulsion that he must remove his clothes in a certain routine. This inflexibility may become so troublesome that if anything interferes with the routine, he will have to put his

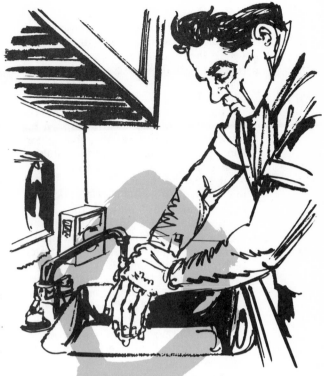

An obsessive fear of germs leading to frequent hand washing can be a part of a psychoneurotic pattern.

clothes on again and start the routine all over. A person with a compulsion may feel that he is forced to touch all power poles as he passes them on the sidewalk.

PHOBIAS

Phobias are unwarranted fears. The afflicted individual panics despite the fact that he consciously knows of no logical reason for him to be afraid. Nevertheless, whenever he comes into the fear-producing circumstance, he seems powerless to restrain his fear. Examples of persons with phobias include the policeman who has become afraid of the dark and the businessman who now climbs ten flights of stairs because he fears riding in a closed elevator. A phobia may involve an unreasonable fear of wide-open spaces, of high places, of needles, of dirt, of germs, of a certain animal, or of cancer. Persons with phobias often go to extreme inconvenience to avoid the thing or condition which they fear. Other than this, their reactions are those of a normal person.

SUICIDE

The person who contemplates self-destruction by suicide is trying, in his own unfortunate way, to solve a personal problem. In his distorted thinking he has found no other way to deal with what seems to him to be a crisis. He feels frustrated and allows his thoughts to center around "ending it all."

The incidence of suicide has been increasing until it has become the ninth-ranking cause of death in the United State. For males age 15 to 34 suicide ranks second as the cause of death, and for females of the same age it ranks third. A condition of depression is the usual prelude to a suicide attempt. However, other factors may contribute, the outstanding one being alcoholism.

Some persons who attempt suicide do not really expect to die. They expect to be rescued from the attempt. Their motive is to attract attention to themselves and to their supposed plight. Others keep secret their plans for self-destruction, and these sincerely expect to succumb. It is this second group that poses the greatest challenge to relatives and to their physicians.

The person who contemplates and/or threatens suicide should be protected until his self-esteem can be restored. Preferably he should be placed in an institution where he can have continuous nursing observation.

TICS

A tic is a habit spasm in which the individual keeps making some unexpected, involuntary, purposeless movement involving a small muscle or a small group of muscles. A tic may consist of a jerking movement, of grunting, throat clearing, or even the pronouncing of a word or a short sentence.

Tics typically make their appearance in childhood and are said to affect at one time or another more than 10 percent of children. Usually these tics disappear within a few days, a few weeks, or at least within a year. In the occasional case, a conspicuous tic will persist into adulthood. A child who becomes self-conscious because of the presence of a tic should have the benefit of consultation with a professional person.

The specific reason why some children develop tics remains a mystery except for the circumstantial evidence that there exists some feeling of personal inferiority.

UNRESOLVED GRIEF

When a person loses something or someone very important or very dear to him, he normally passes through an experience of grief. Normal grief, under the usual circumstances of bereavement or over the loss of an arm or a leg or the loss of control of limbs (as in quadriplegia), does not belong with the neuroses. But when, under such circumstances, the person fails to experience grief or, at the other extreme, continues to grieve for many months after the loss has been sustained, we speak of "unresolved grief," and this is an unhealthy condition.

Normal grief consists of three phases: (1) *Shock* lasting for a few days and consisting of various ways of expressing the intense wish that the loss had not occurred. The grieving person may even try to deny the loss. (2) *Acute mourning* usually lasting for the next three months or a little more. In this phase the grieving person acknowledges the loss but remains unreconciled to it. He experiences waves of intense sad emotions and withdraws from social contacts. (3) *Resolution* or *reorganization* is the final phase in which the grieving person reluctantly accepts the loss and begins to plan his future accordingly. In this phase he resumes and rebuilds his social interests and activities.

It is usually in the second phase that

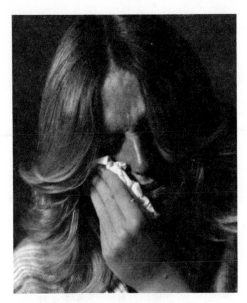

Unresolved grief can be an unhealthy condition.

unhealthy complications of the grieving process occur. In some cases the individual seems unable to express his emotions by crying. In others, he develops symptoms of illness. Some persons become depressed. In still other cases, the stage of acute mourning lingers month after month without giving way to the final stage of resolution.

The person whose grief remains unresolved needs help. It is a mistake for him to try to bypass the sequence of the three stages as listed above. He should be encouraged to express his feelings and to cry when he feels like crying. He needs the presence of a sympathizing friend. And as soon as he has made sufficient progress in expressing his grief, he needs encouragement to resume productive activities—to pull the broken threads together and rebuild his life accordingly.

Treatment of the Neuroses

The person with a neurosis will frequently gain benefit from a series of conversations with his physician or with a psychiatrist. These professionals will help him recognize the relationship between his symptoms and the unsolved problems which lie at their foundation. The patterns of thinking and acting are usually so firmly established, however, that a mere explanation of the cause of the symptoms will not enable the individual to overcome them. He has to have time to reorient his thinking to the extent of accepting his unfavorable circumstances and planning ways of being realistic rather than hiding behind excuses or dodging real issues.

The physician can often aid the patient during this period of reorientation by prescribing one of the modern medications to relieve anxiety or by using one of the antidepressant drugs to help him rise above his periods of depression.

B. The Psychoses

The psychoses include the more serious forms of mental derangement, any one of which constitutes "insanity" in the usual meaning of the word. The person with a psychosis is no longer able to carry his share of responsibility in the family or in the community. He may be irrational and irresponsible. For his own good, he may have to be required to comply with procedures that others consider best.

Fundamental causes of the psychoses are still debated. Most psychiatrists feel that hereditary factors sometimes make one person less able than others to adjust successfully to life's demands and that such an individual's personality may disintegrate under stresses that require greater adjustments than the patient is capable of making. Others, however, believe that the psychoses are caused by some yet undiscovered abnormality of the chemical processes that occur within the nerve cells of the brain.

In some instances persons with a psychosis become difficult to manage. For counsel on how to handle such a person, see chapter 23, volume 3.

DELIRIUM TREMENS

Delirium tremens is a serious, acute, dramatic disorder that affects those

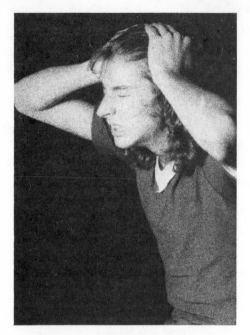

Delirium tremens results from an excessive use of alcohol over a long period.

who have used alcohol excessively for a long time. It occurs when a person, after several days of intoxication, suddenly terminates his use of alcohol. A typical situation would be that of the chronic drinker who, because of accident or infection, is admitted to a hospital. After two or three days, during which he receives no alcohol, he suddenly develops delirium tremens.

The attack is characterized by mental confusion, delusions, vivid and terrorizing hallucinations, tremor, sleeplessness, fever, and profuse perspiration.

In about 80 percent of cases, the episode lasts for three days or less and ends as abruptly as it began. In other cases, the symptoms persist for several days or may be relieved temporarily only to recur as a repeat episode. In the severe cases, the patient may go into shock and may suffer from dehydration because of excessive perspiration. Delirium tremens ends fatally in 5 to 15 percent of cases.

Formerly it was assumed that delirium tremens results from a deficiency of vitamins, as a consequence of the prolonged use of alcohol. It is now recognized, however, that this is a withdrawal complication occurring in a habitual user when alcohol is suddenly withheld.

Care and Treatment

The severe cases of delirium tremens require prompt and precise treatment. Because this ailment may be associated with some other serious condition, search should first be made for the evidence of injury, infection, or inflammation of the pancreas or liver. Such conditions, when present, should be given proper attention. Beyond this, treatment consists of medications that control symptoms, plus the administration of fluids or blood by vein to combat shock and prevent dehydration. It is important that the patient's water balance remain within normal limits. If the patient requires feeding by vein, he should receive supplementary B vitamins as a precaution against such deficiency.

KORSAKOFF'S PSYCHOSIS

Korsakoff's psychosis is characterized by a unique type of memory loss (amnesia). The patient's older, long-established memories are still available, but he is unable to develop new memories of things that happen currently. His other mental processes remain quite normal, so he hesitates to admit that he is out of touch with recent events. He therefore resorts to confabulation, in which he makes up imaginary explanations of what has been recently happening.

Korsakoff's psychosis is caused by damage to those parts of the brain that have to do with memory. When this damage is temporary, as in cases of head injury or subarachnoid hemorrhage, the memory problem may clear up as healing proceeds. But when the damage occurs as a result of alcoholism or some form of encephalitis, the memory loss persists in spite of treatment.

MANIC-DEPRESSIVE DISEASE

This form of psychosis is characterized by an exaggerated mood swing, with only a minor involvement, if any, of the ability to think. Manic-depressive disease tends to occur in attacks, between which the individual is usually normal.

The disturbances of mood may be in either direction, that of mania and elation or that of depression and melancholy. In one attack, mania may predominate; in another, depression. In some patients, the mood in each attack shifts toward mania; in others, toward depression. In still other cases, there may be a shift from mania to depression or vice versa in the same attack.

The first attack of manic-depressive disease typically occurs in young adulthood. It is assumed that heredity plays an important role in setting the stage for the development of this illness. Without adequate treatment, the typical attack of manic-depressive disease may last up to a year or more. With modern methods of treatment, the time is usually shortened.

In the manic phase of the illness, the patient tends to become more and more excited. Tireless overactivities combine with feelings of elation. Judgment and insight are usually poor, and the patient may act in a mischievous manner to the extent of tearing his clothing and engaging in vandalism. Commonly he sings and shouts and even displays occasional delusions of grandeur. He may become easily annoyed with those who try to restrain or control him. He talks a great deal but not on sensible topics.

In the depressed phase the patient is downhearted and fearful and experiences feelings of inadequacy. He sleeps poorly, and all physical activity is accomplished with great effort. He typically develops delusions of self-condemnation in which he believes that he is not worth anything. There may be attempts at suicide. In extreme cases a state of stupor may develop.

Care and Treatment

The treatment of manic-depressive disease consists of four parts: (1) arranging for the professional services of a psychiatrist, (2) placing the patient in suitable surroundings, (3) using medication to hasten recovery from the attack, and (4) influencing the patient by kind conversation to avoid the foolish schemes which he is prone to develop and to look forward to recovery and the resumption of his usual activities.

Lithium carbonate as a medication has been used very effectively in the treatment of manic-depressive disease, beginning in the early 1950s. Because this medication carries the potential of damage to the kidneys, its use should be carefully monitored by the attending physician or psychiatrist.

The patient with manic-depressive disease suffers no essential loss of mentality. He is influenced by his surroundings and conversations to a greater extent than he appears to be. He may even understand quite well that he is ill. Most cases respond favorably to kind treatment in addition to a specific program of medication.

PARANOIA

Paranoia is not a clear-cut condition independent of those just described. It is a type of response seen in persons who may have schizophrenia or manic-depressive illness. Paranoia is characterized by delusions in which the individual attempts to bolster his self-esteem by assuming that people are plotting against him. He craves recognition; but, having failed to obtain the acclaim he desires, he develops false explanations and contends that he has failed in life because of the plottings and jealousies of others.

Paranoia may have its roots in childhood through experiences that deprived the individual of social acceptance. In persons who find life to be disappointing, it is easy for early childhood attitudes of sullenness and hatred to become exaggerated to the extent that a psychosis develops.

Paranoia often leads the patient to imagine himself some great person—a king, a queen, or an inventor. A person with paranoia may become dangerous, with a risk of bodily harm to those he feels are plotting against him.

Care and Treatment

Many patients respond favorably to kindness and sympathy by some person they feel they can trust. Successful treatment of paranoia consists of sympathetic relationships more than of specific therapy.

SCHIZOPHRENIA (DEMENTIA PRAECOX)

Schizophrenia is the most serious of the mental disorders. Although recovery occurs in some cases in response to modern methods of treatment, many cases become progressively incapacitated. Less than 20 percent of the first admissions to public mental hospitals are for schizophrenia, whereas about 60 percent of all who remain permanently in these hospitals are victims of this disease. In schizophrenia the patient loses his ability to distinguish clearly between fantasy and reality. Both his ability to think and his emotional responses become confused.

It is generally assumed that some hereditary predisposition makes certain people susceptible to a breakdown of personality structure once they are subjects to difficult situations. Some persons living perfectly normal lives have traits of personality that resemble, in mild degree, the patient with schizophrenia. Presumably such persons would become ill with this type of mental disorder should they become seriously distressed because of personal problems.

Schizophrenia may develop at any age, but it is less frequent in childhood and after age 50 than it is in young adulthood. The disease often begins insidiously. As the victim begins to withdraw from reality, he appears to others to be preoccupied. His conversations may assume an odd pattern, but the individual experiences no concern even when this aberration is brought to his attention.

As the disease progresses, delusions, hallucinations, and odd mannerisms develop. In his delusions, the patient often hears persons saying unkind things about him. He seems to live in a world apart and may lie staring at himself in the mirror or smiling or laughing to himself. His emotional responses are often inappropriate.

Care and Treatment

Treatment for schizophrenia has been modified a great deal in recent years. The use of drugs particularly adapted for psychotic disorders (antipsychotic drugs) has now largely replaced the previous use of shock therapy. These drugs are not tranquilizers; they are drugs which specifically help to relieve the symptoms of disorganized thinking. The use of psychotherapy and friendly counseling contribute greatly to the success of antipsychotic drug therapy. Although many cases do not recover completely, a large proportion respond enough to be able to live quite normal lives outside the hospital.

SECTION II

The Sensory System

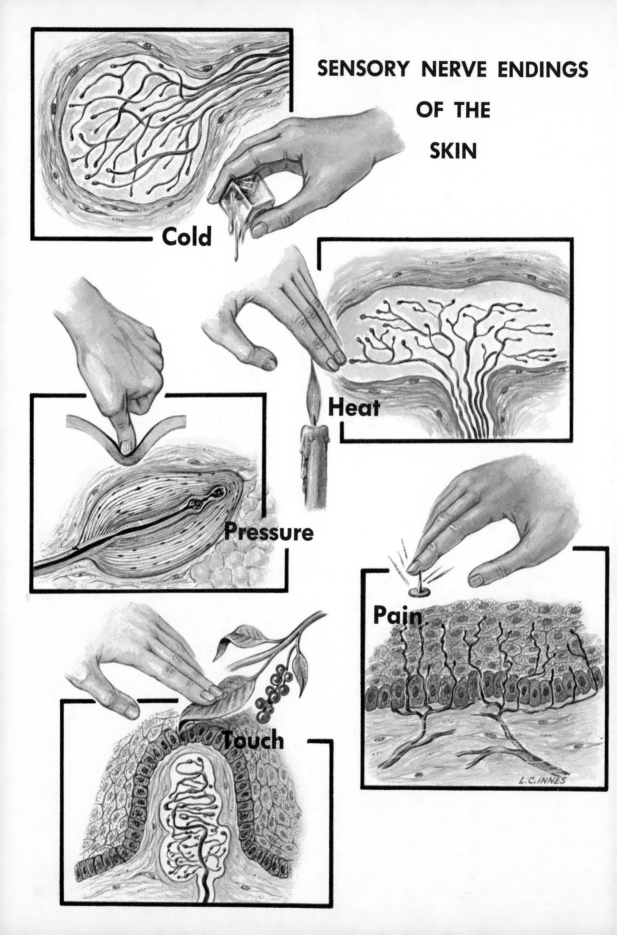

SENSORY NERVE ENDINGS OF THE SKIN

Cold

Heat

Pressure

Pain

Touch

L.C. INNES

The Organs of Sensation

Let us liken the brain to the headquarters station of a large telephone exchange. Here a great deal of equipment is in operation, some automatic and some manually controlled. It is used for several purposes: (1) to relay incoming calls to the persons for whom they are intended, (2) to keep a record of calls made, and (3) to direct the employees of the telephone company in keeping the system operating smoothly.

Similarly the brain receives and sends out many nervous impulses. The incoming ones make the brain aware of surrounding circumstances and events. In response, the various organs and muscles of the body are directed into appropriate activities. Also the brain keeps a record, in the form of memory, of what has taken place. And the brain has a great deal to do in controlling the activities of the body's organs and tissues.

Without the nerves which enter and leave the brain, it would be just as useless as the headquarters station of a telephone exchange if all its lines were severed. The equipment would still be there, but it would be functionless.

Certain nervous impulses come from the eyes, and the brain accepts these as indicating what can be "seen" at the moment. Certain others come from the ears, and these are interpreted in that part of the brain which has to do with hearing. And so with the impulses from the organs of smell, the organs of taste, the organs of equilibrium, and the organs of sensation in the skin and membranes of various parts of the body.

The organs of special sense relay this information to the brain. Thus the brain can think and respond. Consciousness consists simply of the brain's awareness of what is going on in its various parts and in its immediate surroundings.

In the present chapter we will study the organs of special sense. You will be impressed with their marvelous design and their ability to report sensations and happenings to the brain. Each of the organs of special sense is adapted to its work of obtaining one particular kind of information.

The eyes convert the energy of light into nervous impulses which are carried by the optic nerves to the brain. The ears transform the energy of sound waves. The semicircular canals (part of the internal ear) transform the energy of moving fluid into nerve impulses which, when they arrive in the brain, make the body aware of the direction of its movement. The organs of taste and smell are influenced by chemical prop-

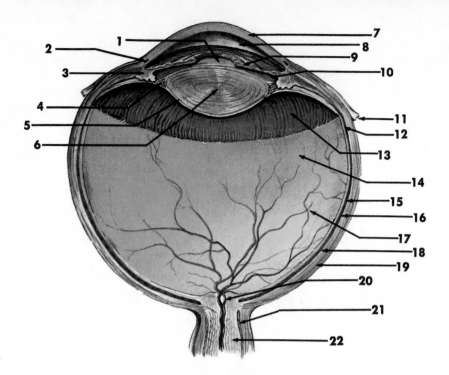

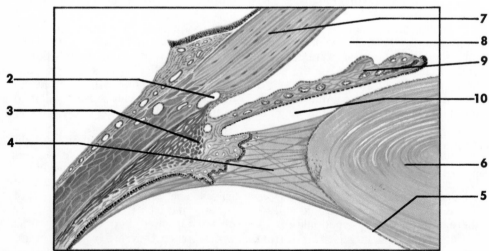

1. Pupil	12. Ora serrata
2. Canal of Schlemm	13. Ciliary processes
3. Ciliary muscle	14. Vitreous body
4. Ciliary zonule	15. Retina
5. Capsule of lens	16. Pigmentary epithelium
6. Lens	17. Retinal arteries and veins
7. Cornea	18. Choroid
8. Anterior chamber	19. Sclera
9. Iris	20. Central artery and vein of retina
10. Posterior chamber	21. Arachnoid
11. Rectus oculi medialis muscle	22. Medullated nerve fibers

Parts of the human eye as seen in a horizontal section.

Microscopic section through ciliary part of eye—low magnification.

erties in food and drink and air. The sense organs located in the skin and other tissues throughout the body transform the energy of pressure, movement, temperature, or mechanical tension into nerve impulses the brain can use.

Vision

Our eyes are considered the most marvelous of the sense organs because they make us aware of various objects all around us, nearby and far away. When we see a tree, we do not have to touch it or climb into its branches in order to know what it is like. We see a friend and can recognize him even though, as yet, he is still at a distance.

With normal vision we reach out "as far as the eye can see" and are thus made aware of events and circumstances around us. Speaking more technically, the eyes—the sense organs for vision—enable us to appreciate the shape, the color, and the movements of the objects and persons around us.

The Structure of the Eye. In order to understand how the eyes permit us to "see," we have to know how an eye is constructed. It is a relatively small organ, and spherical in shape except that its front portion (the transparent cornea) bulges forward just a little. In the average person, the eye is slightly less than one inch (about 2.4 cm.) in diameter. Each eye is located in a bony socket, called an orbit. The orbit is formed in part by the bones that surround the brain, and these are complemented by the bones of the upper part of the face.

In addition to the eye, the orbit contains the muscles which move the eye, the nerves and blood vessels which supply the eye, the tear glands, and a cushion of fat tissue which helps to protect the eye from injury.

In front of the eye are the eyelids, upper and lower, which serve as an opaque screen to shut out light. When the lids separate, the eye is open and the front portion of the eyeball is exposed and light can enter.

The eye is built something like a camera. It has a lens just as a camera has. It has a colored circular curtain called the iris, with an opening at its center, which is placed in front of the lens. Delicate smooth-muscle fibers within the iris control the size of the central opening, letting in more light or less light, just as the diaphragm in a camera controls the amount of light that enters.

In a camera the light is brought to a focus on the light-sensitive film. This produces on the film an image of whatever is in front of the camera. Similarly, the rays of light that enter the eye through its lens are focused on the nervous tissue which lines the back part of the eye. This is called the retina and on it is formed an image of what the person "sees."

The space inside the eye is divided into two chambers. One is in front of the lens, between it and the cornea, and the other is behind the lens, between it and the retina. The front chamber is filled with a clear, watery fluid, the aqueous humor. The chamber behind the lens is filled with a clear, jellylike substance called the vitreous humor.

When observing a person's eye from in front you look right through the transparent cornea and the aqueous humor to see the iris with its opening at the center which we call the pupil. The front surface of the iris appears brown in some eyes and blue or gray in others. The color of the iris, therefore, leads us to say that a person has brown eyes or blue eyes or gray eyes. The reason the pupil appears black is merely that light which passes through it into the eye is absorbed by a layer of black pigment inside. This pigment keeps the light from reflecting from place to place, serving the same purpose as the black paint inside a camera.

The "white of the eye," which surrounds the cornea, is covered by a smooth membrane, the conjunctiva, which folds back on itself to form a lining for the inner surface of the eyelids. Here it appears pink rather than white.

The entire outer layer of the eyeball

93

is firm and tough. It is called the sclera, except at the very front where it bulges forward to form the transparent cornea. The sclera is composed of firm connective tissue. The cornea reminds one of the crystal of a watch. It can be seen best by looking sideways at a person's eye. In a camera the lens is made of glass. It is adjusted by a device which moves the lens forward or backward, just a little, depending on whether the object to be photographed is close or distant. In the eye the lens is composed of a highly specialized tissue flexible enough to allow slight changes in shape. In this case the focusing of the images on the retina is accomplished not by moving the lens forward and backward but by these slight changes as the lens becomes either thinner or thicker. These changes are accomplished by the action of smooth muscle inside the eye.

The Retina. In a camera the sensitive film on which an image has been focused must be "developed" before a person can see the picture. But in the eye there is no such loss of time. A person can "see" the image at the moment it is projected on his retina. The retina consists of highly specialized nervous tissue in direct contact, by nerve fibers that compose the optic nerve, with that portion of the brain which perceives vision. As the accompanying diagram indicates, the image focused on the retina is an inverted (upside-down) image. But the nerve fibers originating in the retina carry their impulses to the brain in such a way that the brain "sees" right side up.

The retina contains many nerve cells which are influenced by the amount of light and by the color of the light to which they are exposed. These cells generate nerve currents; and it is the

The eye and a camera have several features in common.

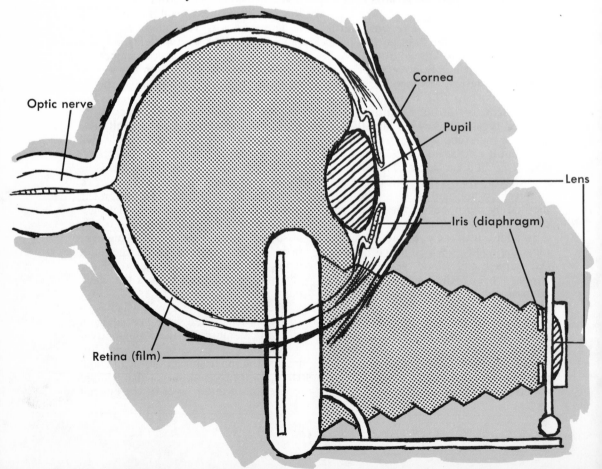

Optic nerve

Cornea

Pupil

Lens

Iris (diaphragm)

Retina (film)

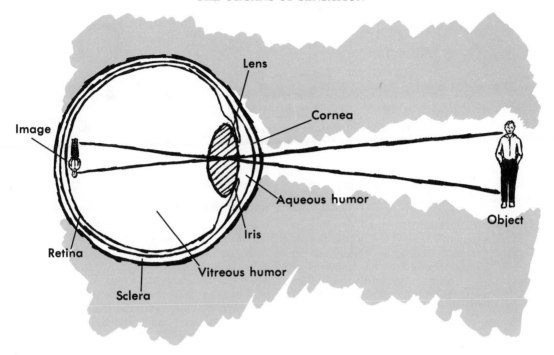

The rays of light cross as they pass through the lens of the eye. On this account the image on the retina is inverted.

nerve currents, not the light itself, that reach the brain.

There are several kinds of cells in the retina but only two capable of being stimulated by the light brought to focus there. These are called rods and cones. There are about seven million cone cells in the retina of each eye. These are most numerous at the central portion of the retina, which receives light from the central part of the field of vision. It is the cones that are responsible for registering the fine detail and the color of the visual image.

There are about 125 million rod cells in the retina of each eye. They permit a person to see even when there is not enough light to cause the cone cells to function. They are most numerous in the parts of the retina other than the central area. The rods are not influenced by the color of what is seen, but they detect motion very readily. The functions of the rods, then, are: (1) to provide "twilight vision" when illumination is faint, (2) to give the "stage setting" for what is seen clearly at the center of the visual field, and (3) to attract attention to anything that moves in the peripheral part of the field of vision.

The Blind Spot. There is a spot in the retina of each eye which is blind—that spot where all the nerve fibers originating in the various parts of the retina pass through the wall of the eye to make up the optic nerve. It is blind because the bundle of nerve fibers occupies the space, leaving no room for rod and cone cells.

The blind spots do not bother a person under ordinary circumstances because the one in the right eye is located to the left of the middle and the one in the left eye, to the right of the middle. That part of the visual image which falls on the blind spot of one eye therefore falls on a light-sensitive spot in the other eye. You can demonstrate the blind spots in your own eyes by examining the accompanying diagram and

X   **O**

To demonstrate the blind spot in your own right eye, close your left eye and focus your right eye on the "X." At the same time move the book closer to you and then farther away. When the image of the "O" disappears (as you see it out of the "corner of your eye") it is because its image is falling on the blind spot. Repeat the experiment with your left eye by closing your right eye and watching the "O" while you make the "X" disappear.

following the directions given just below the large X and O.

Moving the Eyes. Light enters the eye only through its small opening at the center of the iris—the pupil. Therefore, the particular image which falls on the retina depends on what happens to be in front of the eye and on whether the object is situated so that light reflected from it can pass through the pupil. A person's visual field (the area that he can see at any given time) is relatively small when we think of the large area above and below and to the right and to the left of what he is seeing.

A person can control the direction in which he looks, and he exercises this control by two means. First, he can turn his body and his head so as to face any direction he chooses. Second, he can turn his eyes within their orbits so that he can look a little to the right or to the left, up or down, even without moving his body or his head. This movement of his eyes within their orbits is made possible by six small skeletal muscles in each orbit. These fasten to the outer coat of the eye and are thus able to move it in all directions.

Not only do the muscles within the right orbit move the right eye, but they do so in conjunction with the muscles of the left eye so that both eyes can focus on the same object at the same time. This coordinated control of the eye muscles is provided by specialized nerve centers in the brainstem.

The control of these muscles might be likened to the way a driver of a team of horses can turn both horses to the right or left by pulling on the appropriate rein. But the control of the movement of the eyes is much more compli-

cated, for it involves not only movements to the right and left but also up and down and in oblique directions. Furthermore, the axes of the two eyes are not always parallel, for when a person looks at a close object, his eyes must be directed slightly toward each other in order for the object to form images in comparable positions on the retinas of the two eyes. In such a situation the muscles which pull the eyes toward each other must be slightly tighter than those which oppose this action.

The ultimate control of the muscles which move the eyes must come from that part of the brain in which vision is perceived. In other words, the movement of the muscles is modified so as to enable a person to see exactly what he wants to. Of themselves, the muscles have no way of determining just how much they should move the eyes in order to bring the desired object into view. So the control from the brain causes the eyes to move a little to the left or the right as may be necessary.

This same control center influences the muscles that turn the head as well as those that move the eyes, for if the eyes have turned in their orbits as far as possible and still the object is not in view, then the head must turn as well. And the marvel of it is that all of this complicated control of the muscles is carried on without conscious effort. One need not say to himself, "I must tighten a certain muscle in each of my orbits," or, "I must tighten the muscles that turn my head to the right."

Binocular Vision. As we have already mentioned, the control of the muscles that move the eyes is so arranged that, under normal circum-

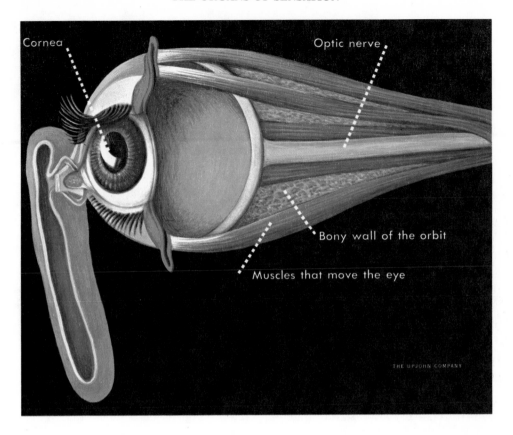

Cornea

Optic nerve

Bony wall of the orbit

Muscles that move the eye

THE UPJOHN COMPANY

stances, both the eyes are directed toward the same object. Thus the visual image registered at any one time by the right eye is almost identical with that registered by the left. Notice that we said *"almost"* identical.

The two eyes are usually a little more than two inches (five cm.) apart, so the object seen is registered by each eye from a *slightly* different viewpoint. The nervous impulses carried from the right eye to the brain are blended with the impulses originating in the left eye. But the brain combines the impulses received from the two eyes into a single perception. In so doing, there is added the extra quality of depth. And this is one of the advantages of our having two eyes—it provides binocular vision on which the perception of depth depends.

In order to appreciate how important is this ability to judge depth and distance, try closing one eye the next time

you reach for some close object. Choose something strange to you, for if you should reach for some familiar object like the toothbrush in the bathroom, the habit of reaching just so far would give you an advantage. With one eye closed you will get the impression that your hand is groping about as you reach for the desired object.

A newborn baby does not have the ability to fuse the visual images of both eyes. In fact, in a very young baby, the two eyes do not always point in the same direction, for the child has not yet become accustomed to interpreting what he sees.

In an occasional case, a child does not learn, on his own, to direct both eyes toward the same object. The difficulty may be that the muscles that move the eyes are not equal in strength. We speak of the condition as "cross-eye" or "walleye," depending upon whether the two eyes are directed toward each other or away from each other.

This condition may also result from a tardy development of the brain centers that fuse the two visual images. As mentioned above, the ability to fuse the two images must be developed as a child learns to understand what he sees.

It is important that a child who is either cross-eyed or walleyed be given corrective treatment before he reaches the age of six. Beyond this age it will be very difficult for him to learn to fuse the two visual images. Even surgery performed to equalize the tensions of the muscles that move the eyes may not help, as he will have already developed the habit of ignoring the vision of one of his eyes. More is said on this subject under the heading "Cross-eye and Walleye" in chapter 17, volume 1.

Adjustment for Near Vision. When a person views a distant object, his eyes are pointing in the same direction, the mechanism that controls the shape of the lens in each eye is relaxed, and the pupil is relatively large so as to admit as much light as possible. But when he looks at a close object, as in reading a book, he must readjust his eyes for closer vision. This is comparable to the adjustment that must be made in an optical instrument, such as a camera or binoculars, when it is focused on a close object.

The adjustment of the eyes for near vision is coordinated by a center in the brain which operates automatically. The three changes that take place are: (1) a slight tightening of the muscles which draw the eyes together so that they are directed toward the same spot at close range; (2) a tensing of the smooth muscles inside the eye, which controls the shape of the lens so that the lens now becomes thicker and brings the rays of entering light to a sharp focus on the retina even though these come from close range; and (3) a reduction in the size of the pupil, as when the aperture of an optical instrument is made smaller, which tends to produce a sharper image on the retina.

In the usual course of events the lens of the eye becomes less pliable year by year so that at about age forty-five its shape does not adjust sufficiently to produce a clear image for close vision. There is no problem regarding distant vision, however. Other factors being favorable, it will be just as clear as ever. But a person forty-five years or older usually begins to hold his newspaper farther and farther from his face. He finds it convenient to wear reading glasses, which consist of optical lenses, that bring the light rays from close objects to a sharp focus on the retina even though the natural lenses are no longer capable of doing it.

Color Blindness. We mentioned earlier the two kinds of receptor nerve cells in the retina—the rods and the cones. It is the cones that enable one to see details clearly and distinguish colors.

There are three kinds of cone cells: those primarily designed to receive respectively the colors blue, green, and red. To register other colors the eye requires cooperative activation of the three kinds of its cone cells.

In some persons' eyes one of the types of cone cells is lacking. Interestingly, this defect is hereditary, usually passed on from mother to son. It is more common in men than in women, occurring in about 4 percent of men and in only about one half of one percent of women.

A person who lacks one of the types of cones in his eyes is said to be colorblind. This term is not entirely correct, however, for he is able to see various colors. His only difficulty is that he cannot distinguish them as easily as a normal person can. The red-green type of color blindness is the most common. A person with this type is particularly handicapped to distinguish traffic signals.

Safeguards for the Eyes. The eyes are such delicate organs and so valuable to the body's welfare and comfort

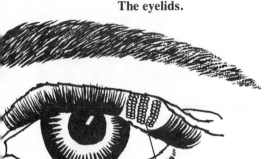

The eyelids.

Tarsal glands

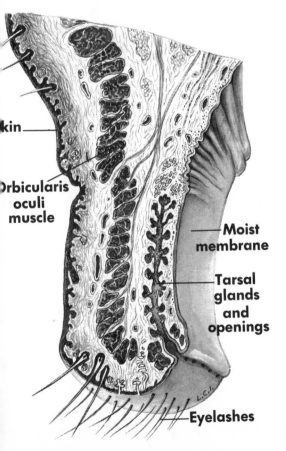

Vertical section of the upper eyelid
(highly magnified view).

kin

Orbicularis
oculi
muscle

Moist
membrane

Tarsal
glands
and
openings

Eyelashes

that the Creator provided extra protection for them. As already mentioned, the eyes are located inside orbits within bony walls. Above, the bones of the forehead overhang the eyes. In the middle is the nose with its bony support. On either side and below are the bones of the face. The eyes are thus protected from mechanical harm from all sides except in front.

The eyelids serve very well to protect the front surface of the eyes from excessive wind, from small particles in the air, and from minor mechanical injury such as could occur from accidental contact with some object. Although made of flexible tissue, the eyelids are firm and tough, and the upper lid is even reinforced by a delicate plate of cartilage. They contain many sensitive nerve endings which cause the lids to cover the eye, reflexly, whenever something threatens its safety.

The eyelashes not only improve a person's appearance but also serve as feelers, causing a person to "blink" in case something like an insect contacts the eyelashes. This reflex control of the eyelids can even be set off by what a person sees, so that when he notices an object approaching his eyes the lids automatically close.

Within the substance of the eyelids are some interesting glands called the tarsal glands. These produce an oily substance which is poured out onto the very edge of the eyelid—that portion which contacts the opposite lid when the eyes are closed. This oily substance serves two purposes: to prevent the tears from running over on the cheek (except when they are produced in excess quantities) and, second, to seal the eyelids so that no air can contact the eye during sleep.

Still another provision ensures the welfare of the eyes—the constant flow of fluid beneath the eyelids, between them and the eye. This fluid is produced continuously by the tear glands, located at the base of the upper eyelid on the side next to the temple. When a person cries, these glands produce large quantities of fluid which over-

99

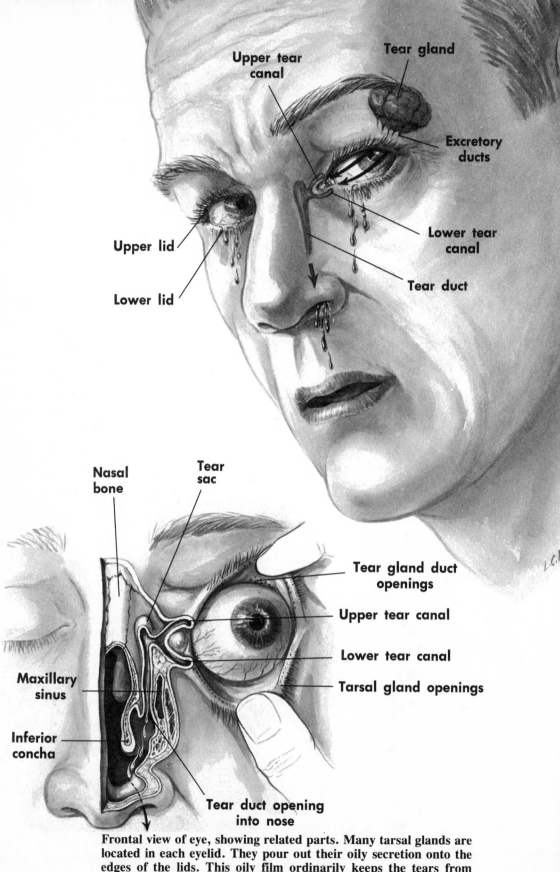

Upper tear canal

Tear gland

Excretory ducts

Upper lid

Lower tear canal

Lower lid

Tear duct

Nasal bone

Tear sac

Tear gland duct openings

Upper tear canal

Lower tear canal

Maxillary sinus

Tarsal gland openings

Inferior concha

Tear duct opening into nose

Frontal view of eye, showing related parts. Many tarsal glands are located in each eyelid. They pour out their oily secretion onto the edges of the lids. This oily film ordinarily keeps the tears from "running over" and also seals the lids closed during sleep.

flows onto the cheeks. But ordinarily they secrete only a small volume of fluid, just enough to keep the front surface of the eyes moist and to wash away any small dust particles that may enter between the lids. This fluid is drained away at the corner of the eye next to the nose. Here two small canals join to form a single duct which carries the fluid into the corresponding nasal cavity.

As the eyelids blink, which they do every few seconds, they spread this fluid evenly over the surface of the eye. This action reminds us of the windshield wipers on a car. The fluid even contains a substance which kills many of the ordinary germs which might enter the space between the eyelids.

Keeping the Eyes Healthy. The eyes are supplied by the same blood that flows through all other organs and tissues of the body. Therefore the eyes are affected favorably or unfavorably by whatever conditions influence a person's general health. Many of the systemic diseases, such as diseases of the arteries, the kidneys, or the endocrine organs, together with various infections, affect the eyes. Severe loss of blood may permanently endanger the eyesight.

Among important substances carried by the blood are the vitamins. The eyes have particular need for at least three of these: A, B$_1$, and C. When the diet is deficient in any one of these vitamins, the person's eyes suffer correspondingly. Deficiency of vitamin A produces "night blindness." Lack of sufficient B$_1$ permits a degeneration of the optic nerve and thus interferes seriously with vision. When vitamin C is inadequate, hemorrhages may occur within the eye.

The eyes are particularly vulnerable to certain poisonous substances, in fact, to a long list of them. We will consider here only three most common ones: ethyl alcohol as contained in alcoholic drinks, tobacco, and wood alcohol (methanol).

Some persons are more susceptible than others to the unfavorable effects of alcohol on the eye. The person thus affected notices a gradual diminution of his vision, with objects appearing foggy.

Tobacco is an even worse offender. The stronger tobaccos used in cigars and pipes also cause a gradual reduction in vision. The use of snuff and chewing tobacco may also cause this damage.

Wood alcohol when taken into the body causes a spectacularly tragic reduction of vision, with a loss of central, acute vision and, in many cases, permanent blindness. Wood alcohol is commonly used as a solvent, and its fumes may be inhaled by workmen using such solvents. Over a period of time, inhaling such fumes can be as damaging as taking wood alcohol by mouth.

Many cases of impaired vision and even blindness are the result of injuries to the eye. The taking of proper precautions could prevent most eye injuries. Children are particularly susceptible on account of the lack of experience, their impulsiveness, their intense activity, and their disregard for caution. A sharp blow received in rough play may damage the eye. Fireworks and firecrackers cause many tragic injuries. Flying rocks, pointed sticks, slingshots, BB guns, scissors, darts, arrows, and other pointed objects damage the eyes of many children.

Adults, too, are susceptible to eye injuries. Industrial hazards include exposure to particles of metal or of stone thrown off by grinding wheels. Sparks from industrial operations may damage the eyes. Workmen in hazardous situations should wear protective goggles, and when the hazard includes exposure to an arc light, one should wear a welder's helmet.

Many of the general infectious diseases involve the eyes in one way or another. Obviously the eyes cannot be protected against these complications except as the individual maintains such a high standard of general health as to avoid these diseases.

101

While we are considering ways of keeping the eyes healthy, we should mention one telltale symptom which when noticed in children should cause parents to arrange for an examination by a qualified physician. We refer to difficulty in reading or to general poor performance in schoolwork. Oftentimes the difficulty can be corrected easily and very satisfactorily by the fitting of glasses.

For other symptoms relating to the eyes, see chapter 8, this volume.

In the schoolroom or wherever reading is done, adequate light is important. Ideally, the source of light should be above and behind the reader. At least it should not be in front of him so that he faces it. Preferably, illumination should be by the "indirect" method.

The fad of wearing tinted glasses has probably been carried to extreme, for the eyes are so constructed that they normally adapt to reasonable changes of light. However, in situations where a person has to face the sun or where reflected light produces a glare, the use of tinted glasses is advisable. Eye specialists strongly warn that a person never look directly at the sun, even though his eyes may be protected by smoked glasses.

The Marvelous Eyes. Now that we come to the end of our discussion on the structure and function of the eyes, it is appropriate that we tarry long enough to express appreciation to the Creator for the marvelous gift of vision.

The fact that the eyes are composed of living tissue and still are able to bring into sharp focus the image of whatever is observed gives us reason to marvel. But we must add to this our appreciation of the advantage of having two eyes, so that objects observed appear to have depth as well as height and breadth.

The registering of the visual image in the cortex of the brain constitutes an additional wonder. Here, what the individual sees not only becomes a part of his immediate processes of thinking but also remains in his memory as a visual image to be recalled later even without the use of his eyes.

The built-in adaptability of the eyes is another remarkable characteristic. They adjust automatically for near vision or for distant vision. They move up and down or to the side. They can follow a moving object as though they were drawn to it by magnetic control. They adapt to varying intensities of light both by changes of the size of the pupil, which controls the amount of light entering the eye, and by changes in the sensitivity of the retina. This latter change enables one to see quite clearly in a poorly illuminated room. In excessive light, adjustment is made so that the image on the retina is not "overexposed."

As is true of many other parts of the body, the eyes are under the control of the will so that a person can look at what he chooses to see. This fact presents everyone with a challenge to determine to look only at things which are beautiful, wholesome, and uplifting.

Hearing

Ask a child what part of his body enables him to hear and he will say, "My ears." Then ask him to point to his ears and he will touch the external features attached to the sides of his head. But the truth is that what we call the ear is only a minor part of the sense organ for hearing.

The Structure of the Ear. The projection on the side of the head called the ear serves as a funnel to direct the sound waves into the ear canal. This canal is a little more than one inch (2.5 cm.) in length and ends at the tympanic membrane (eardrum). It and the feature on the side of the head called the ear constitute the external ear. There are also the middle ear and the inner ear.

The middle ear is an air-filled cavity located just beyond the tympanic membrane. Thus the tympanic membrane has air on both sides and can vibrate freely when sound waves strike its external surface.

The middle ear is connected through the auditory tube (called the eustachian tube) with the back part of the pharynx. It is through the auditory tube that air enters or leaves the middle ear as necessary to keep its pressure equal to the outside air pressure. The auditory tube does not remain open at all times, for its walls are soft and collapse easily. It is when a person swallows or yawns or chews that small bubbles of air enter or leave the middle ear. Usually he can feel or hear the movement of these bubbles of air when his ears "pop."

Often, when one has a "cold in the head," the tissues which line the auditory tube become swollen just as do the tissues of the nasal cavities and pharynx. This may interfere with the passage of air in and out of the middle ear

Drawing of a mechanical model, showing how the energy of sound waves is carried to the inner ear. Notice that the bony ossicles of the middle ear serve as a chain of levers which carry the vibrations from the eardrum (tympanum) to the oval window. Since the inner ear is fluid-filled, the membrane closing the round window must move in a direction opposite to that of the membrane closing the oval window as the fluid pulsates.

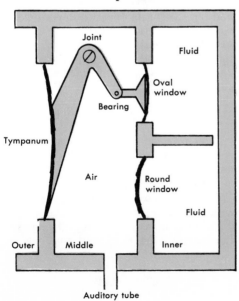

and may thus cause pain because the pressures on the two sides of the tympanic membrane are not equal. Infection sometimes reaches the middle ear by this same route.

At the back part of the middle ear cavity there is an opening into the air cells of the mastoid bone. These are hollow spaces within the bone which serve to reduce its weight. Sometimes an infection which involves the middle ear spreads into the mastoid air cells, causing mastoiditis.

On the farthest wall of the middle ear, opposite the tympanic membrane, are two spaces covered by membranes. The upper one is called the oval window and the lower one, the round window. The chambers behind these membranes are filled with fluid, as will be explained in the description of the inner ear.

Spanning across the roof of the middle ear is a chain of three tiny bones called ossicles. The common names for these bones are hammer, anvil, and stirrup. The handle of the hammer bone fits against the inner surface of the tympanic membrane and the foot-piece of the stirrup bone fits against the membrane which closes the oval window. The anvil lies between them. These bones are set in motion whenever the tympanic membrane vibrates. Because these bones are linked like a series of levers, they transmit the vibrations of the tympanic membrane to the membrane of the oval window and thus set in motion the fluid inside the inner ear. When the membrane closing the oval window is pressed inward, the one closing the round window moves outward.

The inner ear is really a double organ consisting of two parts, the cochlea and the semicircular canals. The cochlea is the essential organ for hearing, and the semicircular canals contain the sensitive nerve structures which register movements of the head and thus mediate the sense of equilibrium. The semicircular canals will be considered under the subhead "Equilibrium" later in this chapter.

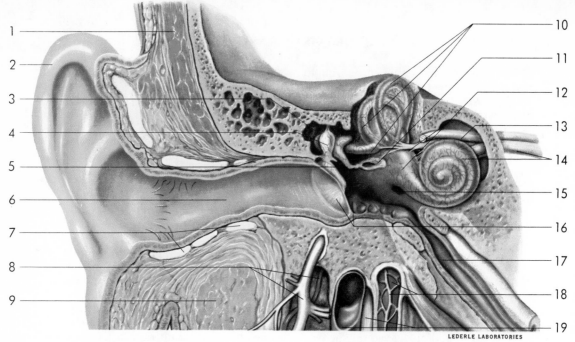

1. Temporal muscle
2. Helix
3. Epitympanic recess
4. Malleus (hammer)
5. Incus (anvil)
6. External acoustic meatus
7. Cartilaginous part of external acoustic meatus
8. Facial nerve and stylomastoid artery
9. Parotid gland
10. Semicircular canals
11. Stapes (stirrup)
12. Vestibule and vestibular nerve
13. Facial nerve
14. Cochlea and cochlear nerve
15. Cochlear (round) window
16. Tympanic membrane and tympanic cavity
17. Auditory (eustachian) tube
18. Internal carotid artery and sympathetic nerve plexus
19. Glossopharyngeal nerve and internal jugular vein

Frontal section showing component parts of the human ear.

The Cochlea. The cochlea fits into a space within the temporal bone shaped like a snail's shell. Three spiral tubes run all the way from the base to the apex of this organ. A tough membrane, the basilar membrane, also runs this same spiral course and helps to separate the fluid-filled tubes from each other. Resting on this basilar membrane are the nerve cells which, when stimulated by vibrations in the fluid, send nerve impulses to that portion of the brain in which hearing is received.

The groups of delicate nerve cells which rest on the basilar membrane constitute what is called the organ of Corti. In one way this is built like a musical instrument, for the cells near its base respond to high-pitched sounds

and those near its apex, to low-pitched sounds. As various parts of the organ of Corti are activated, depending upon the pitch of the sounds that enter the ear, the brain is kept informed so that it can interpret the incoming nerve impulses as music, a human voice, or other sounds, as the case may be.

Advantage of Two Ears. A normal person can hear with either his right or left ear. A person deaf in only one ear can still get along quite well.

The great advantage of having two ears is that the hearer can discern the direction from which a sound comes. Perhaps you have noticed that when you hear an airplane passing overhead, you can know its approximate location in the sky even though you have not yet seen it. This ability to tell from what direction the sound comes often helps you to know where to look in order to spot the plane.

When a particular sound wave reaches your two ears at exactly the same time, your brain interprets the sound as coming either from straight in front, from overhead, or from straight behind, but not from the right or the left. If you turn your head slightly, a sound wave from this same source will reach one ear before it reaches the other. Your brain then interprets this to mean that the source of the sound is now slightly to the right or the left, as far as the new position of your head is concerned. A person deaf in one ear is handicapped in telling the direction from which a sound comes.

Built-in Safeguards. The sensitive part of the ear mechanism is well protected against injury from the outside. The organ of Corti, where the receptor nerve cells are located, is placed deep inside the bones of the skull, where nothing much can happen to it except by skull fracture, by infection, by some degenerative disease, or by a tumor.

The organs of hearing are so delicate and sensitive that loud noises could be damaging were it not for the safeguards which the Creator has arranged. There are two small muscles within the middle ear whose task it is to dampen the heavy vibrations produced by loud noises. One of these (the tensor tympani) tugs against the inner surface of the tympanic membrane (eardrum) to keep it from vibrating too violently. The other muscle (the stapedius) tends to stiffen the attachment of the stirrup bone as it fastens to the membrane which closes the oval window.

These muscles respond reflexly so that whenever violent sound waves enter the ear canal, the muscles contract and dampen the movements of the membranes and tiny bones within the middle ear.

Other reflex mechanisms cause the large muscles of the body to contract when a loud noise is heard. This is the reason you "jump" when you hear a loud blast or the horn of an approaching car.

Keeping the Ears Healthy. Possible injury to the tympamic membrane (eardrum) constitutes one of the first dangers to be avoided in the care of the ears. Doubtless for this very reason this membrane was placed at the inner end of the ear canal. But even this protection may not save it from being injured or punctured if slender or pointed objects are introduced into the canal. To emphasize this danger, someone has humorously said that nothing smaller than a person's elbow should ever be introduced into the ear canal. Bobby pins and pencils are particularly hazardous when used to remove wax from the ear.

It is true that an abnormal accumulation of wax can plug the ear canal and interfere with one's hearing. But the safe way to remove it is to have a doctor wash it out. This washing of the canal will remove the wax without injuring the tympanic membrane.

The tympanic membrane may be injured by a slap of the hand over the external ear or by impact with water when diving with the side of the face downward. In both circumstances, the air contained within the ear canal is suddenly compressed and may cause the tympanic membrane to rupture.

It has been recognized for many years that persistent exposure to loud noises reduces a person's ability to hear. The outstanding example is the factory worker who becomes partially deaf from the din of noisy machinery. Workmen may protect themselves against the damaging effects of these industrial noises by wearing earplugs or sound-insulated earmuffs.

With the advent of jet aircraft, we have another source of loud noise which can be damaging to the ears. Traffic noises have also increased. For the average person the danger is not so much that the noise will deafen him but that it may exceed his nervous tolerance and make him irritable and inefficient.

Another point to observe in keeping one's ears in good condition is to control infections that might involve the ear structures. When a person follows a way of life that promotes good health, all parts of his body, including the organs of special sense, will benefit accordingly.

Equilibrium

In order for the parts of the body to move gracefully and appropriately the brain must receive impulses which indicate the body's position every moment. It must know what parts of the body are being moved and what the body's situation is with respect to the change in rate or the direction of motion. The brain, therefore, receives nervous impulses from muscles and tendons, the joints, the eyes, and the semicircular canals of the inner ear and correlates these into knowledge that indicates the body's present position and the degree and direction of motion.

With such information available, the brain, particularly the cerebellum, modifies its control of the muscles so that when the parts of the body are moved, they move in harmony with existing circumstances. For example, if a person is standing on one foot, it would be senseless for the brain to send out nervous impulses to move the foot until the person's weight is shifted to the other foot. Or, if a person is about to fall backward, it would be disastrous, or at least foolish, for the brain to signal an impulse to step forward.

In the present discussion on equilibrium we are primarily concerned with just those sensations that keep the brain informed on the body's position and degree of motion—the impulses that originate in the semicircular canals.

There are three tiny horseshoe-shaped canals in each side of one's

Diagram showing how the movement of the fluid within a semicircular canal causes the nerve endings to wave and thus to send impulses to the brain indicating that the head is moving.

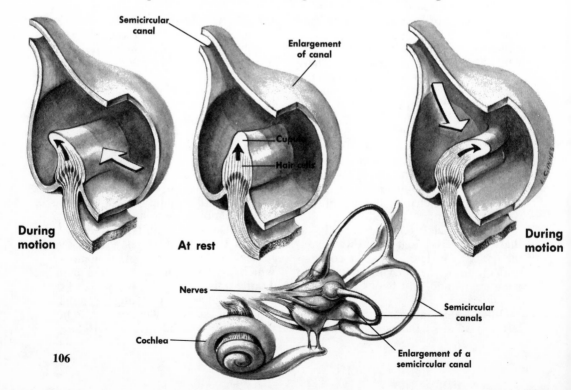

Semicircular canal

Enlargement of canal

Cupula

Hair cells

During motion

At rest

During motion

Nerves

Semicircular canals

Cochlea

Enlargement of a semicircular canal

TONGUE

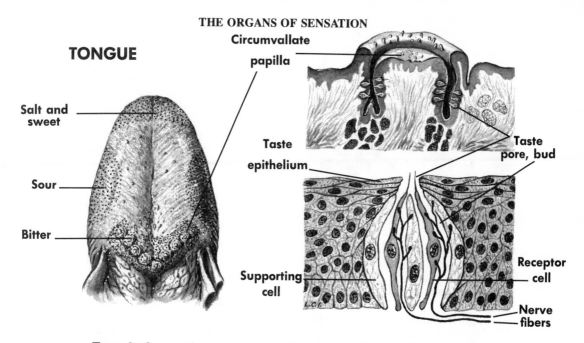

Circumvallate papilla

Salt and sweet

Sour

Bitter

Taste epithelium

Taste pore, bud

Supporting cell

Receptor cell

Nerve fibers

Taste buds are tiny organs served by nerve fibers which twine about specialized cells sensitive to a particular kind of taste. The buds are located in the epithelial layer that covers the tongue and adjacent areas of the mouth, being especially numerous in the walls of the circumvallate papillae.

head, located near the cochlea of the internal ear. Each canal is placed at right angles to the other two. The canals are all filled with fluid, and each has one slight enlargement in which is located a tuft of sensitive nerve cells placed in such a manner that they are stimulated whenever the fluid in the canal moves even slightly across them in either direction.

When a person turns his head, regardless of which direction, the fluid in at least one semicircular canal of each side of his head is caused to move. This motion stimulates the delicate nervous tissue in the bulge of the canal and thus sends impulses to the brain indicating what is taking place.

In some persons the nervous tissue within the semicircular canals is oversensitive. Such individuals are susceptible to motion sickness. Certain diseases may also affect the semicircular canals, making them either more sensitive or less sensitive than normal. These can cause a great deal of discomfort.

Taste

Many persons suppose that the tongue is the organ of taste. This is really not correct, although most of the tiny organs of taste are located on the surfaces of the tongue. These are called "taste buds." They are spherical in shape and microscopic in size, measuring about 0.002 inch (0.05 mm.) in diameter. Particularly numerous along the sides and near the back of the tongue, they are also found in the membranes lining the roof of the mouth and in the pharynx. Each taste bud is located just below the actual surface of the membrane in which it occurs. There is a small opening which permits fluid to enter the taste bud. This carries a sample of whatever substance is being made ready for swallowing. Sensitive cells within the taste bud stimulate nerve fibers which carry nervous impulses back to the brain, indicating the nature of the substance in the mouth.

The taste buds are designed to characterize salt, sour, sweet, and bitter. In

107

general, taste buds which register sweetness are located near the tip of the tongue; those for saltiness, along the sides; those for sourness, a little farther back along the sides of the tongue; and those for bitterness, across the back of the tongue. Even quinine does not taste very bitter until it is moved back to that part of the tongue on which are located the taste buds which respond to bitter tastes.

Smell (Olfactory Sense)

The organ for smell is located in the very roof of the nasal cavities. It registers the nature of substances carried by the air. The reason a person sniffs when he wants to smell distinctly is that the sniffing carries the incoming air currents high into the nasal cavity and thus throws them in contact with the organ of smell.

The sense of smell is very commonly confused with the sense of taste. This happens because many of the foods eaten have an odor as well as a taste. Certain parts of the food are volatile, and these aromas are carried by the air currents up into the nasal cavities while the food is being chewed. Thus, without realizing it, a person tastes and smells his food at the same time.

The reason that food "tastes" so bland when a person has a cold is that the membranes of the nasal cavities are then coated over with mucus and the air currents cannot reach the organ of smell. A slice of apple (if not too sweet) and a slice of raw potato taste about the same when the sense of smell is not functioning.

Sensations of Temperature, Pain, Touch, and Pressure

As we said at the beginning of this chapter, in order for the brain to function effectively, it must be made aware of what is going on both in the individual's surroundings and, also, with respect to his own body. It is in order to complete this provision for informing the brain that the skin, the membranes which line the body's tubes and cavities, the joints, and the muscles are all

well supplied with tiny receptor organs which generate nervous impulses that carry back to the brain information on the momentary conditions of these parts of the body. If one part becomes too hot, temperature receptors in this part send back the information, and the brain directs a move to some cooler place. Similarly, if parts of the body become cold, receptors for cold are stimulated.

Perhaps one of the greatest safety devices the body possesses is the mechanism for detecting pain. The sensation of pain is a danger signal which calls attention to the part of the body in which there is inflammation, or in which the tissues are torn, or in which any other pain-producing circumstance has occurred.

The sense of touch is a help to a person in handling objects, while sense of position allows one to know the exact location of the parts of his body. It becomes highly developed in persons whose movements must be precise and carefully controlled. The musician depends on his sense of touch as well as on his sense of hearing for knowing how to produce the most pleasing sounds on his instrument. The sense of touch is important to the artist as he handles his brushes. It helps the surgeon to know just how firmly to grasp his instruments and how much to stretch the tissues with which he is working. Touch is highly developed in a blind person, who uses this sensation to tell him his whereabouts and even to read.

Some of the delicate receptor organs are placed so deeply in the tissues that they are not stimulated unless the overlying tissues are firmly compressed. These receptors for pressure indicate to the brain how much the tissues are being compressed when a weight is lifted, when a person sits too long in the same position, or when some part of the body is crowded into too small a space.

Some of the receptor organs located in the interior of the body indicate when the tissues in which they are placed are being stretched. Thus, a person becomes aware of bloating or of pressure within his body.

Just as certain taste buds are specifically adapted to receive only sweet tastes, so the receptor organs of which we speak now are also specialized, some being designed to receive only sensations of heat, others of touch, others of pain, others of cold, and still others of pressure. There are certain parts of the skin, as at the tips of the fingers and parts of the face, in which the receptor organs are numerous. In other places, as in the skin of the back, there are relatively few receptors. Nature has been conservative by placing an abundance of receptor organs where needed most and only a few in areas where precise information is not important.

Conclusion

Each of the sense organs is marvelous in its structure and function, and each contributes to the welfare of the rest of the body and to the means by which the brain makes a person aware of his surroundings. In trying to find words to express these relationships in a way that will help readers to appreciate how remarkably every part of the body contributes in enabling the body to function as a unit, one could do no better than to quote the beautiful language of the apostle Paul:

"The body is not one member, but many. If the foot shall say, Because I am not the hand, I am not of the body; is it therefore not of the body? And if the ear shall say, Because I am not the eye, I am not of the body; is it therefore not of the body? If the whole body were an eye, where were the hearing? If the whole were hearing, where were the smelling? But now hath God set the members every one of them in the body, as it hath pleased Him. And if they were all one member, where were the body? But now are they many members, yet but one body. And the eye cannot say unto the hand, I have no need of thee: nor again the head to the feet, I have no need of you. Nay, much more those members of the body, which seem to be more feeble, are necessary: and those members of the body, which we think to be less honorable, upon these we bestow more abundant honor; and our uncomely parts have more abundant comeliness. For our comely parts have no need: but God hath tempered the body together, having given more abundant honor to that part which lacked: that there should be no schism in the body; but that the members should have the same care one for another. And whether one member suffer, all the members suffer with it; or one member be honored, all the members rejoice with it." 1 Corinthians 12:14-26.

Pain

In the previous chapter the sensation of pain was mentioned along with other kinds of sensation that keep the brain informed on what is taking place outside and inside the body. Pain is an especially important sensation because it serves as a warning device to register injury, inflammation, or other kinds of trouble that may occur in various parts of the body. So we here devote an entire chapter to the sensation of pain.

In this chapter we deal with pains as experienced in various parts of the body and indicate the possible illnesses that might cause these pains. The following Outline of the Chapter listing the parts of the body which might be painful will enable the reader to readily find information needed at the moment. Upon finding under a particular listing mention of an illness which may be a possible cause of the pain, he will then turn to the General Index at the back of each volume of *You and Your Health* for the pages describing that illness.

About Pain

Pain is a symptom, not a disease. So when a person suffering pain goes to his doctor he should expect more than

Outline of the Chapter

a prescription for some pain-relieving medicine. He should be patient while the doctor searches for the actual cause of his pain. And, of course, the treatment should be directed toward removing this cause rather than merely stopping the pain.

Some people do not go to the doctor when they experience pain. With the excuse that "it's only a headache," or "it's only an upset stomach," they fall back on some drugstore remedy. Once the pain is thus stifled, they forget that the cause of the pain has not been removed. Thus they court trouble.

You doubtless have had the experience, when taking a hurried drink of water, of having a cramping pain at the center of your chest. It made you so uncomfortable that you waited a moment before taking the next swallow. Then you were careful to drink more slowly and take less water with each swallow. Thus the pain signal helped you to remove the cause of the pain. It made you aware that you had taken too large a gulp of water and by so doing had stretched the tissues of your esophagus.

Even the common headache carries a message which should warn you of possible indiscretions. It usually occurs when you have been nervously tense, when you have driven yourself too hard, or when you have been under emotional strain. The muscles of your neck have become tense, just as the muscles in your leg will tighten up when you sit quietly reading an exciting story. As your neck muscles tighten, they squeeze the blood vessels which bring them their supply of blood. A vicious cycle is established: the tighter the muscles become, the less blood they receive. This interreaction initiates signals of pain from these muscles. At the same time, some of the blood vessels inside the skull participate in this reflex response. In so doing, they stretch the meninges that envelop the brain and cause pain sensations to develop there as well as in the muscles of the neck.

Now you will understand how deep massage of the neck, which tends to relax the muscles and increase the circulation of blood, may be an effective remedy for the common headache. But a persistent headache which lasts day after day may be caused by serious disease. This type of headache should be evaluated by a doctor.

Many times, when one of the body's internal organs becomes inflamed or stretched or deprived of part of its blood supply, the resulting painful sensations seem to come from some area of the body's surface rather than from the organ involved. This displaced sensation is called referred pain. A good example is the pain experienced in a typical case of appendicitis. The discomfort emanates from the wall of the abdomen in the lower right side, not from the appendix itself.

Another example of referred pain is that which involves the chest wall and the left arm in coronary artery disease. The condition which actually sets off the pain is a lack of adequate blood supply in the wall of the heart. The nerve connections are such that the pain which the patient experiences is conveyed by the nerve fibers which serve the chest wall and the left arm.

Some people are more vulnerable to pain than others. A hereditary factor may make some children more stoical than others. More probably, however, it is the example of parents or brothers and sisters. The boy who wants to be like his dad observes that his dad can carry on his usual activities in spite of the discomfort of a smashed finger. So when injured, he too, imitating his father, tries to carry on without complaint.

At first thought we tend to commend such a person's fortitude. Under most circumstances it is good; but some danger lurks also. The person who ignores pain may become so established in this pattern as to neglect it when it signals danger about some serious condition in the body.

On the other extreme, there is a type of pain that originates more in one's mind than in the tissues of his body—

psychogenic pain. From one's memories of painful experiences, an active imagination can construct pseudosensations in the present. But you ask, "Why would a person want to imagine that he is experiencing pain?"

It is not that he wants to imagine pain. Usually the fantasy of pain takes place without any deliberate decision. It typically happens to the person who, without realizing it, has followed a childhood pattern of using pain to attract attention and sympathy. This unconscious recourse to psychogenic pain can exempt a person from experiences that would otherwise be unpleasant. In effect, he accepts pain in preference to trying to live with the tensions that have developed in some of his personal relationships.

When a person experiences the pain that comes from disease or injury in some part of his body, the physician can trace this pain to its source and advise the patient on how he should be treated. But with pain that originates in one's imagination and serves to excuse him from unpleasant realities of life, only the patient himself can bring about a cure. Such a cure requires a change of attitude by which the individual finds greater satisfaction in accomplishing worthwhile things than he does from falling back on the excuse of being an invalid.

Management of Pain

Pain is an uncomfortable experience. It is intended to be. That is the purpose of pain—to motivate the person to remedy whatever is causing the pain.

When a tooth aches, have it repaired or pulled. If you fall and hurt your ankle, find out whether it is broken or merely sprained, and then treat it accordingly. But the ankle may keep on hurting long after the plaster cast is fitted or after the strapping is applied for support. This persisting pain is to remind you that you must be patient until healing is completed.

Pain accompanies appendicitis, and the real remedy is to let the surgeon remove the inflamed appendix. But

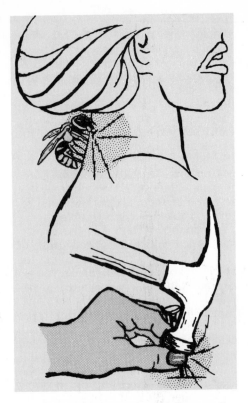

Pain is a sensation intended to motivate the person experiencing it to remedy the cause of the pain.

even while things are being made ready for surgery, the pain persists and the patient suffers. What should be done to make the patient comfortable?

The relieving of pain is one of the major responsibilities of physicians. For a discussion of the available ways to relieve pain, see chapter 55, volume 1, pages 515 to 517.

A. Abdominal Pain

There are many kinds of abdominal discomfort, some serious enough to require consultation with a doctor. The examining physician will want to know the exact nature of the pain in order to make a proper evaluation. When you have pain in the abdomen, try to observe as much as you can about it so that you can answer the doctor's questions. Notice whether it is aching, boring, burning, cutting, dull, gripping, stabbing, sharp, or throbbing. Is it constant, or does it come and go? When was it first noticed, how did it begin—suddenly or gradually? Is it general or located in some particular area? If localized, where is it most noticeable? Has its location changed since it began? If so, from where to where? Has it become more intense or less intense? Has it been relieved or altered by lying down, change of position, or by other activity? Has it been accompanied by other symptoms such as nausea, vomiting, diarrhea, constipation, or gas?

The common conditions that may cause abdominal pain are arranged in alphabetical order as follows:

1. *Allergy to Certain Foods.* Abdominal pain, often associated with nausea and diarrhea, frequently appears soon after one eats a food to which he has allergic sensitivity.

2. *Aneurysm of the Abdominal Aorta.* An enlargement of the aorta in the abdomen, with the threat of rupture, may cause few symptoms until it enlarges suddenly or leaks a little blood or actually bursts. Then the pain is in the mid-abdomen, the mid or lower back, occasionally the groin. This condition constitutes a surgical emergency.

3. *Appendicitis.* The pain of appendicitis usually begins in the middle of the upper abdomen at the level of the umbilicus. It is typically accompanied by nausea and vomiting. The pain may then become more intense and shift to the right side of the lower abdomen. This side becomes tender to touch and pressure, and the abdominal muscle on the right may become firmer than that on the left.

4. *Bladder Disease.* Infection of the urinary bladder (cystitis) causes some pain in the lower part of the abdomen (in the middle) and in the perineum (in front of the anus). This pain is associated with a frequent desire to urinate and a sensation of burning when the urine is passed.

5. *Colic (in Infants).* See chapter 6, volume 1.

6. *Colitis.* This disease consists of an inflammation of the colon (lower bowel). The type and intensity of the abdominal pain varies from case to case and with the type of colitis. In severe cases the patient suffers lower abdominal cramps associated with increased urgency to move the bowels. In milder cases he experiences an aching distress in one or both sides of the abdomen (caused by gaseous distension) which may seem to be aggravated by the wearing of a belt and may seem to be relieved, momentarily, by mild pressure over the aching area or by the passage of flatus.

7. *Diabetes.* Abdominal pain may develop in connection with the acidosis of severe, inadequately-treated diabetes mellitus.

8. *Diverticulitis.* Diverticula (abnormal outpouchings) may develop in the intestine. When these produce symptoms, they are often similar to those occurring in appendicitis.

9. *Enteritis.* This inflammatory condition of the intestine may develop suddenly, accompanied by abdominal pain and tenderness very much as in appendicitis. The disease may follow a more chronic course, with attacks of diarrhea for many months characterized by cramplike, colicky pain in the lower right part of the abdomen.

10. *Epididymitis.* The intense pain which results from an infection of the epididymis is most severe, of course, in the scrotum, but is sometimes radiated to the back in the vicinity of the lowest rib.

11. *Esophagus, Involvements of.* Spasm, ulcer, or tumor of the esopha-

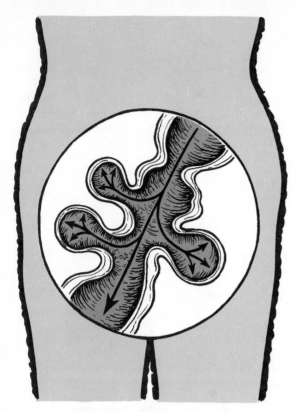

Inflammation of abnormal outpouchings in the intestinal walls is likely to result in an ailment known as diverticulitis.

gus may cause pain just behind the lower end of the breastbone and thus the pain may seem to originate in the upper part of the abdomen.

12. *Fecal Impaction.* In severe constipation the fecal material may become so firmly packed as to produce a hard mass that obstructs the normal movement of intestinal contents. This produces extreme abdominal pain.

13. *Food Poisoning.* Severe pain in the abdomen is one of the common symptoms following the eating of contaminated food, occurring along with nausea, vomiting, diarrhea, and progressive weakness.

14. *Gallbladder Infection (Cholecystitis).* Infection and inflammation of the gallbladder are usually associated with the presence of gallstones. The associated abdominal pain is often present in the midportion of the upper abdomen but more often in the right upper abdomen. The pain may be referred to the region of the right shoulder blade. Nausea and vomiting are often associated.

15. *Gallstones.* Lodgment of gallstones in the bile passages causes a spasm of the walls of these passages with intense pain, producing symptoms as in gallbladder infection.

16. *Gastroenteritis (Acute Infectious Gastroenteritis).* This ailment, which is usually caused by a virus, affects infants and children and is characterized by vomiting, diarrhea, and pain in the abdomen.

17. *Heart Attack.* When a branch of the coronary arteries of the heart becomes seriously narrowed or obstructed, the portion of the heart wall served by this branch is harmed by lack of sufficient oxygen. This series of events, which could be either mild or serious enough to threaten life, is usually accompanied by extreme pain behind the breastbone. Pain may be referred to the left shoulder and arm and also to the upper central part of the abdomen. This occasional occurrence of pain in the upper abdomen at the time of the heart attack may cause confusion as to whether the patient's trouble is within his abdomen or chest.

18. *Heatstroke.* Abdominal pain is often one of the symptoms of this serious illness.

19. *Hemorrhoids.* Severe pain in the anal region is sometimes caused by prolapsed or protruding hemorrhoids.

20. *Intussusception.* This term describes an internal folding (telescoping) of one part of the intestine into the next portion, which, though rare, occurs most commonly in children under five years of age. Cramplike abdominal pain is extreme and comes in paroxysms interspersed with short periods of free-

dom from pain. Prompt surgical treatment is required.

21. *Kidney Disease.* Diseases of the kidney which may produce aching in the back and tenderness in the flank are pyelonephritis (infection of the kidney), glomerulonephritis, tumors of the kidney, and urinary retention.

22. *Kidney Stones.* When a stone formed within the kidney pelvis makes its way through the ureter on its way to the bladder, it may cause a spasm of the ureter, producing excruciating pain. The pain seems to originate in the flank and to radiate across the abdomen into the groin, genitalia, and inner aspect of the thigh. Each episode of pain lasts a few minutes, during which the patient writhes in agony. Nausea, vomiting, sweating chills, and shock are often associated.

23. *Lead Poisoning.* Colicky abdominal pain is usually the symptom that causes a person with lead poisoning to seek medical help. The pain is described as tearing or griping. It occurs intermittently and is usually in the lower abdomen. Associated symptoms are a peculiar taste in the mouth and general weakness.

24. *Liver Disease.* The pain of liver disease is a mild, constant pain just below the rib margin and usually a little to the right of the midline. It occurs in hepatitis, in cirrhosis, and in cases of damage to the liver by certain drugs and poisons. Other symptoms of liver disease must be present to confirm the diagnosis.

25. *Menstruation.* Even the normal occurrence of menstruation causes a certain amount of discomfort. Certain conditions, however, make the occurrence of menstruation more painful than usual. These are discussed in several chapters in *You and Your Health* as indicated in the General Index.

26. *Mesenteric Vessel Occlusion (by*

Thrombosis or Embolism). The mesenteric vessels carry blood to and from the intestines. Their occlusion is a complication of infections in neighboring tissues, of blood vessel disease, or of heart disease. It occurs more commonly in elderly persons. When the onset is sudden, the abdominal pain is usually the first symptom. It is severe, usually generalized throughout the abdomen, and soon accompanied by vomiting. If untreated, the condition moves on within a few hours to dehydration and shock. Surgery provides the only satisfactory treatment.

27. *Obstruction of the Intestine.* Blockage of the intestine may occur in severe hernias, in adhesions after surgery, by pressure from a tumor or invasion by cancer, or by a twist in the intestine. It is a serious, life-threatening condition, usually requiring surgery. Pain in the region around the umbilicus is usually the first symptom. The pain is colicky in nature and occurs intermittently. When the obstruction involves the large intestine, the pain is usually in the lower abdomen.

28. *Ovarian Cyst.* Cysts of various types may develop in the ovaries. When these become large, they may cause an aching pain in the lower abdomen. The pain suddenly intensifies if a cyst becomes twisted at its attachment.

29. *Pancreatitis.* This serious condition involves an inflammation of the tissue of the pancreas. It occurs mostly in users of alcohol or persons having gallstones. The severe pain in the upper central part of the abdomen is accompanied by nausea and vomiting and by local tenderness.

30. *Perinephritic Abscess.* This is a condition in which a collection of pus (an abscess) develops in the tissues surrounding a kidney. The pain in this condition seems to originate in the flank and radiates to the upper part of the abdomen, to the back, and even to the shoulder. The treatment is by surgical

drainage of the abscess, together with the administration of proper antibiotic medication.

31. *Peritonitis*. This consists of an inflammation of the membrane that lines the abdominal cavity and covers its organs. It is always a serious development occurring as an extension of inflammation involving a diseased organ, by perforation of the wall of one of the abdominal organs, by traumatic penetration of the abdominal wall, or as a complication of a systemic infection. In acute peritonitis there is severe, constant abdominal pain and tenderness, often with chills, rising body temperature, and rapid heartbeat.

32. *Pneumonia*. Although a disease involving the lungs, pneumonia may sometimes cause pain in the upper part of the abdomen and thus be confused with disease involving the abdominal organs. It is usually when pneumonia involves an area of the lung next to the diaphragm that abdominal pain occurs.

33. *Pregnancy, Ectopic*. An ectopic pregnancy is one in which the fertilized ovum is implanted in some other location (usually in the oviduct) instead of within the cavity of the uterus. As the embryo grows in this abnormal location it stretches the surrounding tissues to the breaking point. As rupture occurs, it is accompanied by bleeding into the abdominal cavity and by intense lower abdominal pain which is intermittent and does not radiate to other areas. A ruptured ectopic pregnancy constitutes an urgent surgical emergency.

34. *Prostatitis*. Infection of the prostate gland is a common complication of a venereal (gonorrheal) infection. Occasionally it is caused by some other type of infection. It produces some pain in the lower back and, deeply, in front of the anus.

35. *Psychogenic Illness*. Emotional tensions, unsolved personal problems, or fear of cancer may cause functional illnesses in which abdominal pain is a prominent symptom.

36. *Rheumatic Fever*. In children, bouts of diffuse abdominal pain may occur in rheumatic fever.

37. *Salpingitis*. Infection of the oviducts causes cramplike pain in the lower part of the abdomen, usually accompanied by chills and fever, but not by nausea and vomiting.

38. *Spider Bite*. Severe abdominal pain due to muscle spasm occurs typically about 20 minutes after a bite by a black widow spider.

39. *Spleen, Rupture of*. The spleen may be ruptured by a crushing blow as in an automobile accident. Severe pain in the upper abdomen, mostly on the left, develops promptly. The pain is followed quickly by the evidences of internal hemorrhage: abdominal tenderness, abdominal muscle spasm, and shock. A ruptured spleen requires prompt surgical intervention.

40. *Subphrenic Abscess*. In this serious condition an accumulation of pus develops between the liver and the undersurface of the diaphragm. The pain and tenderness are in the upper abdominal area, usually along the lower margin of the ribs. In some cases the pain radiates to the corresponding shoulder. The treatment requires surgical drainage of the abscess, with the administration of an appropriate antibiotic medication.

41. *Tabes Dorsalis*. This disorder, a late complication of untreated syphilis, is characterized by a degeneration of certain of the sensory nerve elements. One of its symptoms is the occurrence of attacks of severe upper abdominal pain ("crises") associated with retching and vomiting.

42. *Ulcer of the Stomach and Duodenum*. Peptic ulcers developing in the stomach (gastric ulcer) or duode-

num (duodenal ulcer) produce typical patterns of abdominal pain. In both types, the pain is relieved by the taking of food or antacids, or by vomiting. In duodenal ulcer, the more common type, the pain is in a small area just below the lower end of the breastbone and may radiate to the back and, sometimes, to the right shoulder. The pain usually begins about an hour after a meal. It is described as gnawing, burning, cramplike, or aching. In gastric ulcer, by contrast, the pain appears when the stomach is empty and may be located a little more to the left than that of duodenal ulcer.

B. Arm Pain

There are many possible causes of pain in the arm, forearm, and fingers. The common ones are now mentioned briefly. For further information on any one of these possible causes, consult the General Index for references to other chapters where these matters are considered in greater detail.

1. *Arthritis*. Several kinds of arthritis affect various parts of the body, including the arms. The racking pain of

Painful deformities are associated with rheumatoid arthritis.

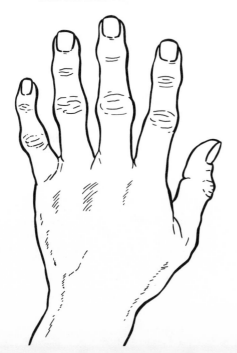

arthritis involves the joints primarily but may be associated with a stiffness which makes it difficult to move the fingers, wrist, elbow, and shoulder.

2. *Buerger's Disease (Thromboangiitis Obliterans)*. This condition affects the legs more commonly than the arms. It involves a partial or complete closure of the lumen of one or more arteries. The resulting pain is caused by a marked reduction in blood supply to the affected part. It occurs most commonly in men in the earlier years of life and, especially, among those who smoke.

3. *Bursitis*. The bursae of the shoulder and of the elbow may become painful as a result of trauma, arthritis, connective tissue disorders, or bacterial infections. The pain of bursitis interferes with the movement of either the shoulder or the elbow as these may be affected.

4. *Carpal Tunnel Syndrome*. This is a condition in which the structures passing into the palm of the hand from the wrist become compressed. The persisting pain that occurs seems to the individual to originate in the fingers, the wrist, and the forearm.

5. *Causalgia*. Causalgia is a form of neuritis characterized by severe, spontaneous, burning pain in the area of a nerve which has been previously damaged.

6. *Heart Disease*. One of the most significant kinds of pain in the arm is that which occurs in the left arm when the blood supply to the heart is curtailed. A severe reflex pain develops in the chest and may include the left arm. This pain occurs in such conditions as ischemic heart disease, angina pectoris, and coronary heart disease.

7. *Neuritis*. Several conditions may cause an inflammation of the nerves within the arms. Among them are arthritis, collagen vascular disease, dia-

117

betes mellitus, and beriberi. The disorder is characterized by pain, weakness, and unusual sensations in the area related to the affected nerve.

8. *Raynaud's Disease*. Raynaud's disease is a benign illness which usually affects the fingers of both hands. In response to cold temperature and emotional stimuli, the fingers change color and become very painful.

9. *Tendonitis*. On occasion the tendons and their sheaths become painful as a result of infection, arthritis, or injury. Tendonitis occurs most commonly in relation to the tendons which pass through the wrist.

C. Back Pain

Pain in the back is a common symptom, because of the many structures that compose the back: the vertebral column, the heavy back muscles with their ligaments and connective tissues, the spinal cord and the meninges that surround it, the spinal nerves, and the blood vessels that supply all these structures. Abnormal conditions in any of these structures may cause pain in the back. Back pain may even occur as a symptom of some systemic disease, as the backaches that appear at the onset of flu or some febrile illness. For more details on the common causes of backache listed below, see the General Index for reference to other chapters where these matters are described.

1. *Cancer of the Vertebrae*. A cancer that originates in the vertebrae is rare. More commonly, cancers originate in other parts (as the breast, thyroid, lungs, prostate, or kidney) and metastasize to the vertebrae. This causes pain because the vertebrae become compressed and transmit pressure to the adjacent nerves. Such pain is described as agonizing and "boring."

2. *Fibromyositis*. This is a condition in which the muscles and the inter-

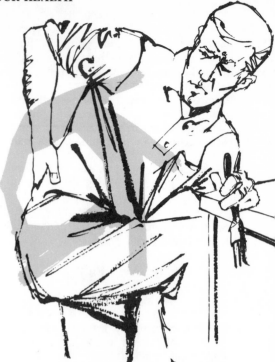

Skeletal abnormalities, as well as systemic ailments, may cause pain in the back.

vening connective tissues of some part of the body become tender and painful when moved, such as stiff neck or lumbago. The onset is often sudden, and the condition may disappear abruptly. The cause is vague. The pain often appears in connection with exposure to cold, infection, trauma, fatigue, postural misfortunes, occupational stresses, or psychic turmoil. Perhaps the best explanation is that a persisting tension of the muscles is followed by a reduction of blood supply to the tissues involved.

3. *Fracture of the Vertebrae*. Fracture of the vertebrae usually results from mechanical violence, but it sometimes occurs in conditions in which the bone structure has become weakened by a loss of inorganic constituents. Fracture causes pain by pressure on the nerves or the spinal cord and meninges, or by tension on the muscles and ligaments.

4. *Meningitis*. Infection of the membranes that cover the spinal cord (the meninges) may cause stiffness of the neck and back, but it is not an outstanding cause of back pain except as a spasm of the back muscles develops.

5. *Menstruation*. Menstruation is commonly accompanied by backache.

6. *Osteoarthritis of the Spine*. Degenerative changes in the vertebrae and in the intervertebral disks are a usual accompaniment of aging and are attributed to unavoidable wear and tear. The changes produce tension in the ligaments and connective tissues about the spinal column and thus cause pain.

7. *Osteomyelitis of the Spine*. Infections involving the vertebrae may cause abscess formation, bone degeneration, and erosion of the surrounding tissues, with possible spreading of the infection to the skin surface. Back pain is caused by involvement of the pain-sensitive periosteum (fibrous covering of the bone) and by irritation of nerve fibers.

8. *Osteoporosis*. Commonly in later life or in connection with debilitating illnesses there occurs in the vertebrae and the pelvic bones a loss of some of the calcium they normally contain. These may collapse, partially, under stress and cause pain because of the displacement of soft tissues.

9. *Pelvic Disease*. Persons with infections of the organs in the lower part of the abdominal cavity (the pelvic organs) often suffer from backache.

10. *Posture, Faulty*. Backache may be caused by faulty posture.

11. *Pregnancy*. Moderate back pain occurs quite commonly in pregnancy. It is probably caused by altered postural stresses.

12. *Prodromal Back Pain*. In many diseases associated with fever and in those in which bacteremia develops, vague back pain is one of the early symptoms.

13. *Protrusion of an Intervertebral Disk*. The cushioning material between adjacent vertebrae (the intervertebral disks) may deteriorate and protrude from between the vertebrae in such a manner as to press on the nerves leaving the spinal cord, thus producing pain. This condition is often described as a slipped disk or a herniated disk. Sometimes one or more of the spinal nerves that compose the sciatic nerve are involved, with the result that the pain seems to come from the thigh and calf of the leg (sciatica). The pain produced by protrusion of an intervertebral disk typically comes in attacks. The condition may also develop in the lower back or the upper back and neck.

14. *Psychogenic Backache*. Back pain of psychogenic origin commonly persists after an actual injury or after an organic illness. This type of pain does not follow the usual pattern of pain associated with actual disease. Efforts at treatment usually intensify rather than remedy it. It may represent the patient's subconscious effort to obtain sympathy or to avoid responsibilities that are unwelcome (see the General Index under "Disease, Functional").

15. *Referred Back Pain*. Many organs when involved with disease become responsible for pain which is "referred" to a particular part of the back. Pain in the upper (thoracic) part of the back can be produced by disease in the peripheral parts of the lungs, by the development of a tumor in the central part of the chest, or by an aneurysm in the thoracic aorta. Disease of the gallbladder or abscess in the vicinity of the liver can cause back pain near the right shoulder. Duodenal ulcer can cause pain in the midportion of the upper back. Irritation in the colon or rectum can cause low back pain. Acute pancreatitis or a weakening aneurysm

of the abdominal part of the aorta can cause agonizing pain in the lower back. Kidney disease commonly causes pain in the flank. Disease of the prostate or of the pelvic organs causes pain in the very low part of the back.

16. *Strain.* Pain in the back sometimes follows the lifting of heavy objects or the attempt to lift an object when the position of the back and legs is unfavorable. It may follow a sudden twisting of the body or making a misstep. Frequently backache results from poor posture, as in obesity, from sitting in a slouched position, or from wearing shoes which have high heels or fit poorly.

17. *Structural Defects.* In some cases a minor congenital defect of the bony structures occurs at the junction of the lumbar and sacral portions of the spine (as in spondylolisthesis). This flaw throws an abnormal load on the ligaments of this region and causes a spasm of the regional muscles, with consequent local pain.

D. Bone Pain

Pain within a bone is usually caused by either infection or tumor. Infection of bone tissue constitutes osteomyelitis, which begins with sudden pain in the affected bone, accompanied by a sharp rise in body temperature. It is painful to move the part of the body in which the affected bone is located, and the patient feels tenderness at that spot. Bone tumors, which also cause pain in the affected bone, may be either benign or malignant. Malignant ones may originate within the involved bone (primary tumors) or may be extensions from tumors which start in some other tissue (metastatic tumors).

E. Chest Pain

Many serious diseases and/or their complications cause pain in the chest, some more serious than others. What

follows will give the reader a basis for judging how serious a given case of chest pain may be. For further information on the conditions that can cause chest pain, consult the General Index for references to other chapters.

1. *Aorta, Pain From.* The aorta is the very large artery that carries blood away from the heart and distributes it to all parts of the body. In the chest it arches to the left, backward, and then downward. Then it passes through an opening in the diaphragm and into the abdomen, where it is designated as the abdominal aorta.

An enlargement of an artery by weakening of its wall is called aneurysm. The usual causes of aortic aneurysm are arteriosclerosis, syphilis, and trauma. Blood flowing within the aorta is under high pressure, and when the wall becomes weakened, a part of the stream may force its way between the layers of the vessel's wall and continue to separate these layers from each other. This is called a dissecting aortic aneurysm.

A dissecting aneurysm of the aorta typically begins in the chest and usually produces excruciating pain which begins suddenly and is extremely severe from the moment it begins. The pain is behind the breastbone and frequently radiates to the back.

2. *Chest, Psychic Pain in.* Some persons experience pain in the chest as a result of concern, fear, or anxiety. The person may be afraid of heart disease or of a heart attack, and yet an examination of his heart reveals no disease. Such pain may occur in connection with the hyperventilation syndrome, in which the individual breathes so rapidly in response to his anxiety that he actually becomes ill from the excessive loss of carbon dioxide from his body.

3. *Chest Wall Pain.* Pain originating in the chest wall may be caused by disease of the nerves, of the muscles, of the bones and cartilages, or of the breasts.

Irritation of the nerves that lie between the ribs may be caused by trauma, by infections or toxic conditions, or by pressure upon the nerves. The pain may be stabbing or burning in nature or may come in paroxysms. Shingles (herpes zoster) is a virus disease that affects one or more nerves, usually on just one side of the body. Osteoarthritis affecting the spine in the region of the chest or a herniated intervertebral disk in this region may cause pain-producing irritation of the corresponding nerve or nerves.

Muscle pain in the chest is caused by the same conditions that cause it in other parts of the body—overuse of muscles unaccustomed to strenuous exercise, or the poorly understood condition of irritation called fibromyositis. Several of the shoulder muscles attach to parts of the chest wall. These, as well as the muscles between the ribs, may be involved. The muscles between the ribs often become strained and painful as a result of persistent cough.

Pleurodynia, a mysterious illness caused by a virus, is characterized by pain in the chest wall.

Bone pain, characteristically intense, aching, and boring, may be caused by a fracture (as a broken rib or a compressed vertebra), by infection of the bone (osteomyelitis), by bone tumors, by pressure against a bone by a tumor originating within the chest, or by an enlarged, pulsating aorta (aneurysm).

The breasts may become painful when fissures develop in the nipples (in the early part of the period of nursing), when the breast tissue becomes inflamed or infected (mastitis), or when cysts or tumors develop within the breast. Perhaps the most severe breast pain is that of mastitis, in which the pain is sharp, cutting, and aching in character and radiates to the armpit and along the inner aspects of the arms and forearms to the little and ring fingers. Also the breasts often become tender just before menstruation. Although pain may occur in connection with a cancerous tumor of the breast, pain is usually a late manifestation in this condition. Unexplained pain in the breast justifies prompt attention by a physician, as does the discovery of a lump in the breast.

4. *Esophagus and Surrounding Tissues, Pain From.* The most common symptom of pain from the esophagus is called heartburn and is caused by an irritation of the membrane lining the esophagus. Hiatus hernia causes pain or a burning sensation behind the lower end of the breastbone.

Tumors, inflammations, or rupture of the esophagus cause chest pains which vary in location, depending on the site of the lesion.

Pain is an important symptom in tumors and inflammations of the tissues which surround the esophagus in the mediastinum.

5. *Heart, Pain From.* Pain originating in the heart is caused when the muscle wall of the heart is deprived of the amount of oxygen it normally requires. When the privation comes gradually, as when the coronary arte-

Angina pectoris is a type of heart pain.

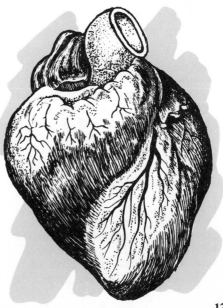

121

ries become gradually involved in arteriosclerosis, the pain comes in attacks brought on by excitement or exertion. This type of heart pain we call angina pectoris.

When the privation comes suddenly, as when a branch of the coronary arteries becomes suddenly occluded, the pain is more severe and prolonged, not being relieved in a few minutes by rest as in the case of angina pectoris. It is this sudden stoppage of blood to a part of the heart's wall that accounts for the serious coronary heart attack. The area of the pain both in angina pectoris and in coronary heart attack is the same. Typically it seems to originate behind the breastbone and then radiate to the upper part of the abdomen and to the left shoulder and down the left arm to the little and ring fingers. There may be variations of this distribution. This pain is described as a tightness, an oppression, and a vicelike gripping.

Inflammation of the pericardium (the membrane that surrounds the heart) may cause pain, but the pain varies from case to case. In some cases it is even similar to that of a coronary heart attack but is influenced more by breathing, coughing, and bodily movements. Typically the pain of pericarditis is over the heart rather than behind the breastbone. Pericarditis may result from various infections as well as from direct injury.

6. *Respiratory Organs, Pain From.* Pain is one of the prominent symptoms of pneumonia. It usually occurs in just one side of the chest and is caused by an involvement of the pleural membranes overlying the area of pneumonia. Such pain is severe and interferes with normal breathing.

Pleurisy is an inflammation of the parietal pleura (the membrane that lines the cavity in which the lungs are located). The pleura is sensitive, and the pain that develops when it is inflamed recurs with each inspiration of air. The patient describes this pain as a catch or stitch. It occurs when disease of the lung involves the pleura, when the pleura becomes inflamed from injury or infection involving the chest wall, when an infection penetrates upward through the diaphragm as from an abscess of the liver, or when infection of tissues in the central portion of the chest (as the esophagus) spreads to the pleura.

Normally no air surrounds the lungs. When, under abnormal circumstances, air accumulates around the lungs, the condition is called pneumothorax. A dull, aching pain with a sense of tightness develops abruptly in the affected side. Breathing becomes difficult because the lung on that side collapses. Pneumothorax occurs in penetrating injuries of the chest wall and in diseases of the lungs in which lung tissue breaks down and permits the air to escape.

A relatively frequent cause of sudden pain in the front, central part of the chest is pulmonary embolism, in which a fragment of blood clot is carried by the blood into the lung and lodges in one of the branches of the pulmonary artery. This pain is accompanied by difficult breathing and a sense of oppression. In the more serious cases where a large branch of the artery is obstructed, the portion of the lung supplied by this branch dies (pulmonary infarction). The fragment of blood clot which causes embolism may come from the veins of the legs, from the veins in the pelvis, or—in certain kinds of heart disease—from the interior of the heart.

Lung abscess may cause chest pain if and when the abscess involves the pleura (the membrane lining the cavity in which the lungs are situated). An abscess can develop in the lung from inhaling some foreign body or from infected materials from the region of the pharynx. The deterioration of a tumor of the lung may cause an abscess. It can develop as a complication of pulmonary embolism, from infection introduced at the time of a penetrating injury to the chest wall, or from an extension of infection from below the diaphragm or from the tissues of the central part of the chest (as the esophagus).

Chest pain is one of the later symptoms of lung cancer.

F. Eye, Ear, Nose, and Throat Pain

Diseases of the eye are considered in chapter 8, this volume, and those of the ear, nose, and throat, in chapter 9. In this chapter we are concerned with pain and therefore include brief mention of conditions that can cause pain in eyes, ears, nose, and throat.

1. *Pain in the Eye.* Any kind of abrasion or scratch affecting the surface of the cornea causes pain. When such an injury to the cornea results in a corneal ulcer, the pain becomes intense. When a foreign body penetrates the eye or even when it lodges next to the conjunctiva (the delicate membrane inside the eyelids) considerable pain is produced.

Persons often use the word *ache* to describe discomfort in the eyes. The eyes may ache after prolonged use, es-

Pain caused by some eye disorders may be corrected by the wearing of glasses.

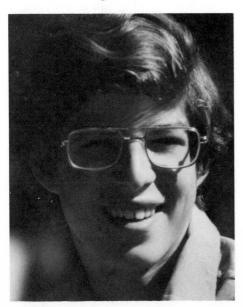

pecially when there is some imbalance of the muscles which move the eyes. There may be this same kind of discomfort associated with uveitis (inflammation of the iris and choroid of the eye). In fact, one's eyes may ache when he becomes extremely fatigued from any cause, even when the eyes are normal.

Glaucoma is associated with discomfort in the eyes, often being a mere ache in the slowly developing type of glaucoma. Intense pain in the eye is associated with acute congestive glaucoma.

Headache may be caused by some disorders of the eyes, especially those which can be corrected by the wearing of glasses.

Discomfort in the eyes is sometimes described as burning or itching. This kind of discomfort is often associated with inflammation of the eyelids or of the conjunctiva. In the allergic reaction of hay fever the membranes of the eyes may burn and itch.

2. *Pain in the Ear.* Pain in the external ear canal may be caused by a break in the skin which lines the canal (as by a scratch with the fingernail), especially when such an injury becomes infected. Intense pain results when a boil develops in the external ear canal. A boil is more painful in this location than in many parts of the body because there is not sufficient room for the tissues to expand as swelling occurs. Injury to the eardrum, as when the side of one's head strikes the water in diving or in rapid descent from a high altitude, causes pain.

The term earache is usually used with reference to an inflammation of the middle ear (otitis media). In this rather common condition the auditory tube often closes, with the result that pressure builds up within the middle ear, causing the eardrum to be stretched.

Pain is often referred to the ear from other nearby areas. Infection of the tongue or of the tonsils may generate the sensation of pain in the ear. Inflammation around a tooth or in the hinge of the jaw (temporomandibular joint) may cause discomfort which seems to focus in the ear.

3. *Pain in the Nose.* Traumatic injury is probably the most common cause of pain in the nose. The development of a boil inside the nostril causes intense discomfort. Sinusitis, an inflammation involving the accessory nasal sinuses, causes pain which seems to originate deep in the face.

4. *Pain in the Throat.* The membranes lining the throat are well supplied with nerves and are therefore sensitive to inflammations of various kinds. Pain in the throat is usually described as sore throat, which consists of discomfort on swallowing and talking. Local irritations of the throat may cause such discomfort. Swallowing very warm drinks or using concentrated mouthwashes may cause such discomfort. Smoking is also a common cause of sore throat. Sore throat usually occurs in the early stages of the common cold and in such infectious diseases as measles, scarlet fever, whooping cough, infectious mononucleosis, and tonsillitis. Vincent's infection is also associated with sore throat. Streptococcal sore throat (strep throat) not only causes a great deal of pain but is a serious infection which requires appropriate treatment in order to avoid dangerous complications.

G. Headache and Head Pain

Headache is a common complaint. It is estimated that 20 million Americans seek help from their doctors on this account each year. And when they do they have two outstanding questions: Is it caused by something serious? and What can I do to get relief?

For two reasons it is important to find the cause of a headache: (1) Some headaches are caused by serious conditions that need to be treated promptly, and (2) The choice of treatment for a certain headache depends on what kind of headache it is.

Indications of "Serious" Headaches:

1. A headache that strikes suddenly and with great severity may be caused by bleeding inside the skull, as from a ruptured aneurysm. A doctor should be consulted at once.

2. A severe headache associated with any of such symptoms as blurring of vision, seizures, clouded consciousness, weakness of muscles, or impairment of sensation may be due to increased pressure inside the skull, as from an expanding blood clot.

3. A headache accompanied by fever and stiffness of the neck may be caused by meningitis, or it may be merely the early sign of flu or some other virus infection. A physician should decide.

4. A series of brief headaches with one or more a day and with increasing frequency or intensity is typical of an enlarging brain tumor.

5. A persisting headache that seems to originate from a particular site, such as an eye or an ear, should be evaluated by a doctor.

Other Types of Headaches:

1. Headaches associated with high blood pressure are uncommon and, when they do occur in this association, are more often related to the treatment than to the high blood pressure itself. Headache does occur spontaneously in some cases of extreme high blood pressure and is then located in the back of the head and is usually most severe at the time of awakening in the morning.

2. Migraine headaches constitute a troublesome affliction in which the symptoms last for several hours with episodes recurring at quite regular intervals of a few days to as long as a month or more. Migraine headaches are considered in chapter 4, volume 3.

3. Posttraumatic headaches are of two types. The first type occurs a few days after the head injury and is the result of an expanding blood clot inside the skull (subdural hematoma). In this case the headache is just one of several symptoms which progress within a

matter of hours and include drowsiness, stupor, and, possibly, partial paralysis. This serious condition requires the immediate attention of a physician.

The second type of posttraumatic headache may linger for even weeks after a serious injury to the head or neck. It is a nagging headache for which there is no immediate remedy. This type of headache eventually disappears spontaneously. The person with posttraumatic headache deserves reassurance and encouragement to resume his normal way of life.

4. The headache of sinusitis is the result of pressure developing within one of the paranasal sinuses when the outlet to the sinus becomes obstructed and fluid accumulates within the sinus. The headache may vary with the time of day and, particularly, with the position of the patient's head. It is often temporarily relieved as the patient raises his head from the pillow on awakening in the morning.

5. Tension headaches occur commonly and typically consist of discomfort in the back of the head and the upper part of the neck. The onset is usually gradual, and it tends to persist with a sensation of pressure that may last continuously, even at night. Tension headaches occur in persons who harbor anxiety and on occasions when the individual is emotionally tense. In women, they often occur just prior to menstruation or during the period of the menopause. Typically, the muscles of the scalp and neck become tight, and it may be that this muscle tension interferes with the circulation of blood both in these tissues and in the vessels that carry blood to and from the brain.

Tension headache is often relieved at least partially by the application of heat or the use of massage to the muscles of the neck. For the long run, attention should be given to the emotional factors that set the stage for this type of headache. Changing one's life-style so as to minimize anxiety may give permanent relief. Recourse to pain-relieving medications carries the risk of drug dependency. This is a poor substitute for

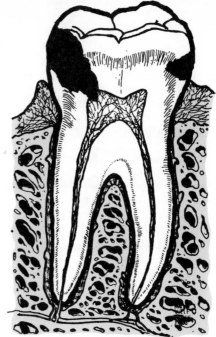

Dental cavities are a common cause of toothache.

removing the basic cause of the pain.

HEAD PAIN

Pain in the head includes several kinds of pain in addition to the symptom of headache described above.

1. Toothache. The various ailments affecting teeth which may cause toothache include dental caries (a cavity in the tooth), pulpitis (in which the central portion of a tooth becomes infected), and periapical abscess (abscessed tooth).

2. Temporomandibular Joint Problems. Difficulties involving the temporomandibular joint (the hinge joint by which the lower jaw is moved) cause pain which seems to originate in the ear. But from that apparent origin it is often referred to the region of the temple, to the neck, or to the angle of the jaw.

3. Trigeminal Neuralgia (Tic Douloureux). In trigeminal neuralgia there are paroxysms of extreme pain on one side of the face.

4. Shingles (Herpes Zoster). Shingles is a virus disease in which the sensory ganglion of some particular nerve becomes involved. Intense pain devel-

ops which seems to originate in the area of skin served by the involved nerve. In about 10 percent of cases the sensory nerve that supplies one side of the face, including the eye, is the one affected.

5. Mastoiditis. Mastoiditis is a complication of middle ear disease (otitis media) in which the internal spaces of the mastoid portion of the temporal bone become infected. There is extreme pain originating in the area just behind the affected ear.

H. Inguinal (Groin) Pain

The inguinal region (groin) is at the lowest part of the abdominal wall at the junction of the abdomen and thigh. In males the scrotum is attached to this part of the body, so we include here pain originating in the scrotum and its contents. Pain relating to the penis is considered in chapter 29, volume 2.

1. Disease of the Epididymis or of the Seminal Vesicle causes pain in the scrotum.

2. Hernia. Hernias developing in the inguinal region may produce pain, even extreme pain, as they cause a tearing of the tissues and, especially, when the hernia becomes strangulated.

3. Prostate, Disease of. Pain from disease of the prostate is often referred to the testes, both right and left.

4. Testis, Disease of. Trauma to the testis as by a sudden blow or by a straddle injury causes extreme pain, which subsides spontaneously unless the tissues have actually been ruptured. Tumor of the testis is also a cause of pain in this organ.

5. Ureteral Disease. Involvement of the ureter, either by infection or by the passage of a stone, causes intense pain which may be referred to the inguinal region.

I. Leg, Hip, and Foot Pain

The so-called lower extremities, which include the hips, legs, and feet, contain many kinds of tissue. They have important functions to perform. They are vulnerable to accidents of many kinds and are therefore the frequent site of pain.

1. *Blood Circulation, Reduction in.* In chapter 9, volume 2, several conditions are described which cause a reduction in the amount of blood which flows to the tissues of the lower extremities. One of the symptoms of reduced blood supply is pain. Conditions that can be responsible are arteriosclerosis, thrombosis, embolism, and thromboangiitis obliterans (Buerger's disease). Reduced blood supply associated with diabetes mellitus may cause areas of gangrene which, of course, are extremely painful.

2. *Bone and Joint Diseases.* The joints of the lower extremities become involved with arthritis just as do the joints in other parts of the body. Infections of bone (osteomyelitis) and bone tumors cause their share of pain in the lower extremities. When the ligaments of the foot become stretched, as in flatfoot, there is pain on weight bearing. A calcaneal spur developing on the bone of the heel causes extreme pain on weight bearing. Bunions cause their share of discomfort.

3. *Injuries.* The lower extremities are susceptible to fractures, sprains, and dislocations. All of these produce pain. However, the pain is a safety device which mandates that time be allowed for the injury to heal.

4. *Muscle Pains.* About 15 percent of children experience "growing pains," with temporary discomfort, especially at night, in the thigh, calf of the leg, and back of the knee. For details see chapter 17, volume 1. Muscle cramps in the leg or the sole of the foot that occur at night are presumably caused by a reflex contraction of the muscles prompted when the foot is allowed to drop forward. Swimmer's leg cramps are caused similarly by reflex contraction of the muscles, occurring

usually when the toes are pointed sharply forward. Claudication is a condition in which painful muscle cramps occur in response to exercise. This develops in persons who have been negligent in the matter of systematic exercise. The pain of claudication occurs when the blood supply to an active muscle is not adequate.

5. *Nerve Involvements.* The various forms of neuritis, including sciatica and causalgia, are painful conditions. In these the actual damage to the nerve may be either in the lower extremity itself or in the vicinity of the spinal column in which the nerves that supply the lower extremity suffer damage. The pain seems to originate in the area of the leg supplied by the nerve, even though the tissues of the leg are otherwise normal.

6. *Toenail and Skin Problems.* A close-fitting shoe or compression by weight bearing may cause such conditions as ingrown toenail, corns, and heavy calluses to become very painful.

7. *Veins, Diseases of.* Varicose veins and thrombophlebitis interfere with the return of blood from the legs and are associated with various degrees of pain.

J. Neck Pain

Pain in the neck comes from several possible causes. Even so, there are certain common characteristics. Pain in the neck is usually increased or aggravated by certain head movements or certain positions of the head. Pain in the neck is usually accompanied by tenderness to the touch and by a certain limitation of motion of the head.

1. *Bone and Joint Disease.* Arthritis affecting the joints of the vertebrae in the neck is a common and distressing cause of neck pain.

2. *Injuries.* Fractures of the vertebrae in the neck are very serious because of the grave danger of compressing the spinal cord. For the handling of a case of serious injury to the neck, see chapter 23, volume 3.

3. *Meningitis.* When the meninges (the membranes that surround the brain and spinal cord) become inflamed, one of the symptoms experienced by the patient is pain in the neck when the head is brought forward.

4. *Stiff Neck (Fibromyositis).* The common form of stiff neck accompanied by severe pain on movement of the head is a poorly understood condition in which certain muscle fibers go into painful spasm.

K. Nerve Pain (Neuritis)

When a nerve becomes inflamed or otherwise irritated extreme pain occurs in the part of the body supplied by this nerve. For the types and manifestations of neuritis, see chapter 4 in this volume.

L. Sexual Pain

Pain in the sexual organs or, more particularly, at the time of attempted sexual intercourse, is typically caused by some inflammation within the sexual organs or the associated urinary organs. In addition, there are some psychological problems by which the sex act becomes repulsive to either a man or a woman, with the result that functional pain develops at the time of attempted intercourse. For a further consideration, see chapters 34, volume 1, and 6 and 30, volume 2.

M. Shoulder Pain

The shoulder is vulnerable to many types of injury. Fracture or dislocation of the structures of the shoulder joint will, of course, cause the patient extreme pain.

Another condition which causes pain in the shoulder and limitation of movements of the arm is bursitis, in which there develops an inflammation of the membranous sac over which tendons glide at the shoulder joint. Bursitis is typically the result of a blow to the shoulder or an injury sustained in falling.

Pain resulting from herniation of an intervertebral disk in the neck region often radiates to the shoulder. Referred pain in the shoulder region may be the result of gallbladder disease.

N. Urinary Pain

Diseases in the organs which produce and transmit urine may cause low back pain or pain either in the bladder or in the abdominal wall in front of the bladder. Pain associated with urination is usually caused by disease of the urethra or of the bladder. It may be caused, however, by disease of the ureter or kidney pelvis, from which the pain is referred to the bladder.

Diseases of the Eye

The eye is the most highly prized of the several sense organs. Even a deaf person says, "My deafness is a handicap, but I am thankful I am not blind."

The proper care of the eyes is so important that a medical speciality has developed concerned only with the care and treatment of problems relating to the eyes—the specialty of opthalmology. Even though the eye is well protected by the bony margins of the orbit in which it is located, it is accessible for examination by the physician and, with the use of modern instruments, its interior can be examined without any discomfort to the patient.

Eye difficulties fall into three age categories: (1) Children and adolescents have eye problems which usually consist of injuries and of difficulties that can be corrected by the wearing of glasses. (2) Middle-aged persons are troubled most with presbyopia, a problem corrected by the wearing of reading glasses. (3) In later life, several sight-threatening conditions need to be recognized early in order to be treated satisfactorily, namely: cataract and glaucoma, hemorrhages in the retina, detachment of the retina, and diseases of the tiny blood vessels within the eye. Many systemic diseases such as diabetes, kidney disease, and high blood pressure also cause damage to the eyes.

The present chapter is divided into two sections: (a) various symptoms that pertain to the eyes, with mention of the disease or diseases in which the symptom may occur; (b) characteristics of and treatments for various eye ailments. The General Index at the back of each volume will be of help in locating the page on which a particular disease is described.

A. Symptoms Pertaining to the Eyes

1. DISCOMFORT IN THE EYES

a. *Smarting and Burning in the Eyes*. This symptom is commonly caused by dryness of the eye membranes, by the irritation of polluted atmosphere (smog), by irritation of the eye membranes associated with allergy (such as hay fever), and in other conditions that may affect the eyelids and conjunctiva. See items 3 and 5 in section B of this chapter.

b. *Itching of Eyelids and Eye Membranes*. This symptom of itching may occur under the same conditions as mentioned for smarting and burning in the previous paragraph. In addition, itching sometimes occurs as a symptom of eye strain, as when a person is doing much reading under unfavorable condi-

129

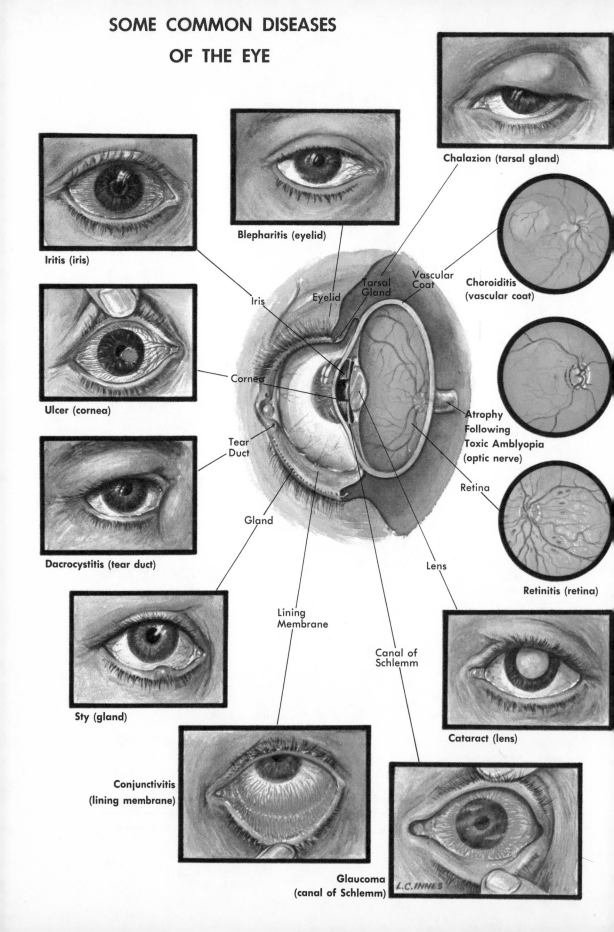

SOME COMMON DISEASES
OF THE EYE

Chalazion (tarsal gland)

Blepharitis (eyelid)

Iritis (iris)

Choroiditis (vascular coat)

Ulcer (cornea)

Dacrocystitis (tear duct)

Atrophy Following Toxic Amblyopia (optic nerve)

Retinitis (retina)

Sty (gland)

Cataract (lens)

Conjunctivitis (lining membrane)

Glaucoma (canal of Schlemm)

Iris

Eyelid

Tarsal Gland

Vascular Coat

Cornea

Tear Duct

Gland

Lining Membrane

Canal of Schlemm

Lens

Retina

L.C. INNES

tions or when refractive errors need to be corrected by the wearing of glasses.

c. *Pain in the Eye.* The most serious conditions which cause pain in the eye are injury, acute glaucoma, and iritis. Injury to the cornea and the presence of a foreign body beneath the upper eyelid cause pain. The pain of sinusitis is sometimes directed to the eye.

d. *Light Intolerance (Photophobia).* This symptom in which discomfort increases with the amount of light entering the eye is typical of inflammations affecting the cornea or the iris. Such conditions are serious and should be evaluated and treated by an eye specialist. See items 4 and 9 in section B of this chapter.

e. *Eye-ache and Headache.* Eyeache may occur under circumstances of general bodily fatigue, regardless of how much the eyes have been used. It may also occur when the muscles which move the eyes are under prolonged strain, as in working at close range or in conditions of increased pressure within the eye as in glaucoma. Headache has many causes, most of which are not related to the eyes. But certain headaches which occur toward the end of the day after the eyes have been used strenuously can be caused by conditions which could be benefited by the wearing of glasses. In any event, persisting headaches should be evaluated by a physician.

2. CHANGE IN APPEARANCE OF THE EYES

a. *Yellow Coloration of the "White of the Eye."* This color change occurs in systemic conditions which produce jaundice by interfering with the normal flow of bile produced in the liver.

b. *Bloodshot Eye; Redeye; Bleeding Into the Eye Membranes.* There sometimes develops a limited area of bright redness in the "white of the eye" area. The cause is a minute hemorrhage into the membrane that covers this forward part of the eye. Such a hemorrhage may occur at any age and without relation to any particular disease. It may appear following sneezing, coughing, or straining at the toilet. Such bleeding usually stops spontaneously within a few minutes. Applying a cold compress to the eye may help to stop the bleeding.

A diffuse redness of the membranes lining the eyelids and covering the front portion of the eye can be caused by anything that irritates these membranes and causes conjunctivitis, such as allergy (e.g., hay fever), foreign body in the membranes, or chemical irritants.

Redness radiating away from the cornea (circumcorneal redness) occurs in the serious conditions in which the cornea or the iris and related internal structures are irritated or damaged, as in corneal ulcer, iritis, and acute glaucoma.

c. *Protruding Eyes.* Some persons' eyes are naturally more prominent than others'. When a certain person's eyes become prominent within a period of a few months, however, disease of the thyroid gland (exophthalmic goiter) should be suspected.

d. *Cross-eye; Walleye (Squint).* In this condition, the individual's right and left eyes are directed in different directions. One eye will be directed to the person or object of attention and the other will either cross or deviate from the first eye's path of sight. This condition is discussed in chapter 17, volume 1.

e. *Differences in Size of Pupils.* This condition is often caused by the inappropriate use of an eye medicine. It may result from an injury to the brain. It may be caused by the development of glaucoma in one eye.

3. ALTERED VISION

a. *Reading Difficulties.* Any condition such as cataract or glaucoma which interferes with the individual's ability to see clearly will, of course, cause difficulties in reading. Such difficulties typically occur also, apart from any disease impairment, two times in life—during childhood and between the ages of 45 and 50. For these a satisfactory remedy is usually available. The reading difficulties of childhood are discussed in chapter 17, volume 1. They may consist of farsightedness or some other refractive error which can be corrected by the wearing of glasses. In the middle-age period the natural lens of the eye becomes stiff, making it difficult for the individual to adjust to near vision. Thus, he begins to hold his newspaper farther and farther from his eyes until finally he no longer can see the print distinctly. The remedy consists in the wearing of reading glasses.

b. *Blurred Vision*. Many problems cause blurred vision, but in all cases this symptom deserves an examination and evaluation by an eye specialist. It may be caused by trouble in the retina of the eye. It may occur in glaucoma, cataract, iritis, and in cases of simple refractive errors which can be corrected by the wearing of glasses.

c. *Partial Blindness*. Certain brain lesions cause a blotting out of vision in certain parts of the visual fields. In such cases it is important to seek professional help promptly because some such conditions are progressive and can be treated most successfully when recognized early. For a detailed discussion of the various types of blindness, see item 1 in section B of this chapter.

d. *Halos Around Lights*. The seeing of halos or rings around lights occurs as one of the symptoms in acute glaucoma.

e. *Spots Before the Eyes*. The seeing of small spots which move leisurely in the visual field of one or both eyes is a common occurrence caused by small opacities floating in the back part of the eye. These become more common as one becomes older or when one is myopic. Spots which seem to blot out certain areas of the vision of one eye occur commonly in beginning cataract or with hemorrhages within the eye which may occur as a complication of high blood pressure or diabetes. The seeing of "sparks" in a certain part of the visual field of one eye often occurs when a part of the vitreous humor becomes separated from the retina. This may be followed by an actual detachment of the retina. (See *Retinal Detachment* under item 11, section B of this chapter.) Some persons who suffer from migraine headaches see moving spots or colored patterns before their eyes for a few minutes before the pain begins.

4. DOUBLE VISION (DIPLOPIA) AND DIZZINESS (VERTIGO)

Double vision occurs when the two eyes "look" at different objects or "see" images of different sizes. In the cross-eye or walleye condition occurring in childhood the two eyes are pointed in different directions, but the child learns quickly to ignore the vision of one eye so that actually such a child is not troubled with double vision. (See chapter 17, volume 1.) Aside from alcoholic intoxication, the usual cause of double vision in an adult is a suddenly developing paralysis of one or more of the muscles that move an eye in the orbit, a condition which allows the two eyes to point in different directions. Such paralysis may occur following trauma, in a case of diabetes, or as a complication of brain hemorrhage or brain tumor.

Double vision is sometimes confused with dizziness because in any one of these conditions, occurring suddenly, the individual does not see clearly, and it may seem to him that his surroundings are moving. For a further consideration of dizziness, see the General Index.

5. DISCHARGE FROM THE EYES

A pussy discharge from the eyes implies a bacterial infection either of the tear duct (dacryocystitis) or of the membranes that line the eyelids and cover the "white of the eye" (conjunctivitis). A watery discharge, consisting mostly of excess tears, occurs commonly when there is chemical irritation, as that produced by polluted atmosphere (smog), in allergic conditions affecting the eyes, in viral infections, as an aftereffect of injuries, and in cases in which the tear duct is obstructed.

6. ALTERATIONS IN LACRIMAL FLUID (TEARS)

As mentioned in the previous item, an excess production of tears occurs when the eye membranes are irritated. The tear glands (lacrimal glands) normally produce fluid continuously so as to keep the eye membranes and the cornea moist. This fluid flows across the front of the eye and is drained away at the corner of the eye next to the nose, where it flows through a tiny duct into the nasal cavity. When tears are produced in such quantities that the tear duct cannot accommodate this volume of fluid, the tears overflow the lower eyelid, and we say that the person may be crying. This occurs in sad emotional states as well as in the conditions mentioned in the previous item. But even with the normal volume of tears being produced, if the tear duct is clogged, the fluid which would normally pass through the duct may overflow onto the face. For additional information on this subject and a consideration of the treatment, see item 13 in section B of this chapter.

B. Specific Eye Ailments

1. BLINDNESS

It is estimated that at least 10 million people in the world are totally blind. But millions of others are partially blind.

What causes blindness? Various diseases, accidents, faulty development before birth, poisonings, or nutritional deficiencies, to name several main causes. Whatever the diagnosed cause, every case of blindness is fundamentally accounted for in one of three ways: (a) There may be some fault in the eye by which its retina does not re-ceive a focused image of what is in front of the eye and therefore cannot generate proper nerve impulses; (b) there may be some interruption of the nerve pathway which originates in the retina and normally would carry impulses to the proper area of the brain; or (c) there may be some fault in the brain by which the visual area of the cortex does not perform the complicated activity by which a perception of vision becomes part of the conscious experience. Examples of each of these follow:

a. *Faults in the Eyes*. Destructive injuries to the eye will, of course, distort or obliterate vision in the affected eye. (See item 8 in this same section of this chapter.) The development of a cataract in which the natural lens of the eye becomes opaque interferes with the passing of light to the retina and thus produces a progressive type of blindness. (See item 2 in this same subdivision of this chapter.) In some cases the retina loses its attachment within the interior of the eye, and portions of this sensitive membrane float within the vitreous humor. Thus the visual image, which normally would be imprinted on the retina, is distorted and partially obliterated. (See item 11 in this same section of this chapter.)

Certain diseases prevail in particular areas of the world that produce various degrees of blindness. One of these is trachoma, prevalent in portions of Africa, the Middle East, and Asia, which affects the lining of the eyelids in such a way as to scar the cornea and thus distort the visual image. (See item 5 of this section of this chapter.) Onchocerciasis, a disease caused by a parasite propagated in the water of natural streams, occurs in tropical Africa and in Central and South America. When in the course of its life cycle this parasite enters the eye, it causes destruction which often results in total blindness. (See chapter 20, volume 3.) Xerophthalmia is a disease caused by deficiency of vitamin A. This deficiency, which occurs in certain parts of the Far East and Central America, causes a softening and even a destruction of the cornea of the eye. (See chapter 12, volume 3.)

b. *Interruption of the Nerve Pathway.* The disease glaucoma (see item 6 in this section) is characterized by an increase in the pressure within the eye. This increased pressure, when allowed to continue, causes destruction of the nerve elements within the retina and the optic nerve, thus causing blindness. One of the tragic complications of diabetes is an involvement of the delicate blood vessels of the retina. Diabetes is said to be responsible for about 10 percent of the new cases of blindness in the United States. (See item 11 in this section of this chapter.)

Degeneration of the nerve elements within the retina and the optic nerve sometimes occurs in longtime users of alcohol and tobacco. The user of these items is particularly susceptible to defects in vision if his diet is deficient in thiamine (a B vitamin). Poisoning by wood alcohol (methanol), whether by accidental drinking of this substance or by inhaling its fumes, introduces the high risk of serious damage to the retina and the optic nerve. Permanent loss of vision sometimes results from arsenic poisoning. Traumatic injury to the optic nerve, such as interrupts some or all of its nerve fibers, causes corresponding blindness of a permanent nature. Meningitis, in which the delicate membranes that surround the optic nerve become infected, may cause permanent damage to this nerve. Tumors within the vicinity of the optic nerve or the other nerve connections involved in transmitting visual impulses often interrupt these nerve pathways and cause corresponding degrees of blindness. (See item 14 in this section of this chapter.)

c. *Fault in the Brain.* A certain part of the cortex of the brain is set apart for dealing with the nerve impulses that come to it from the retinas of the eyes. This so-called visual area of the cortex is connected with other areas of the brain so that the interpretation of vision becomes a part of consciousness. When any circumstance interferes with the function of this visual cortex, the individual will experience a corresponding degree of blindness. The most common disorder affecting the visual area is caused by a curtailment of the blood supply to this part of the cortex. This problem occurs typically in older people whose arteries have become narrowed by the development of arteriosclerosis. The resulting blindness is called cortical blindness because the cortex is no longer able to perform its function in receiving and interpreting the nerve impulses from the eyes.

In certain cases the individual ignores the vision coming from one eye, even though the nerve pathways are still intact. This abnormality occurs particularly in cases of cross-eye or walleye as described in chapter 17, volume 1. It is an instance of so-called amblyopia of disuse. Also, in certain temporary situations (as in some cases of migraine headaches) episodic blindness occurs, total or partial, which lasts for a few minutes.

2. CATARACT

In cataract the lens of the eye becomes progressively opaque. Early in the development of a cataract the patient notices a reduction in the acuteness of vision. As the cataract progresses, his vision continues to fail, until he can perceive only the difference between light and darkness. Frequently cataracts develop at about the same time in both eyes. Of the various types, senile cataract is the most common. It typically develops after the age of 50. Certain systemic diseases predispose to the early development of cataracts, notably diabetes. Sometimes a cataract develops following an injury to the eye. Long-continued exposure of the eyes to high temperatures, as with workers in glass blowing and iron puddling, favors the development of a cataract.

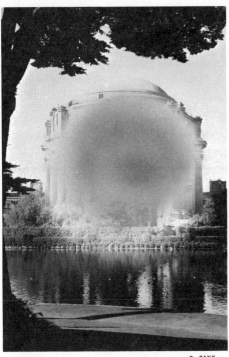

Illustration shows defect in vision experienced by a cataract patient.

Care and Treatment

Everyone should have his eyes examined periodically even though he has no symptoms relating to the eyes. And if a person notices a decline in satisfactory vision, then he should consult an ophthalmologist.

The usual treatment for cataract is surgical removal of the now opaque lens. After recovery from surgery, light can enter the eye in the normal manner, but because no lens is in place, the light rays do not focus on the retina. Therefore all visual images are blurred and appear distorted.

In order to have clear vision, the patient must then be supplied with artificial lenses. These are provided in one of three ways:

a. The wearing of glasses fitted with specially adapted lenses. Such lenses, which appear thicker than usual, provide reasonably good vision in the central visual field, but the lateral range of vision is somewhat limited.

b. The wearing of contact lenses which rest on the front of the eye (beneath the eyelids) and are of proper size to enclose only the cornea. When properly fitted, contact lenses provide satisfactory distant vision. But for reading, such a person must wear conventional glasses in addition to the contact lenses. Contact lenses cause much less magnification and distortion than cataract glasses.

c. The installation of implanted lenses (implants). In this instance, a small, specially prepared plastic lens is inserted into the eye at the time of cataract surgery so that the artificial lens occupies the same part of the eye as was originally occupied by the nat-

Left: How the lens in a normal eye brings light rays to a focus on the retina. Right: How in an eye from which the natural lens has been removed light is focused by an artificial lens worn in front.

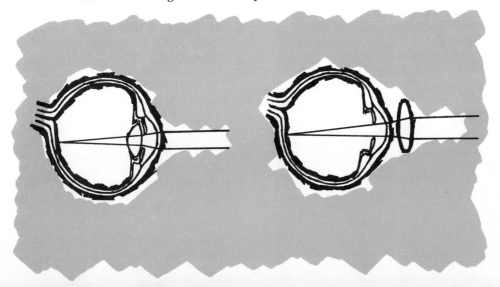

ural lens. Implanted lenses have been used in Europe for several years. Their use in the United States is relatively recent. Certain technical difficulties cause problems in a small percentage of cases in which lens implants are used. The majority of patients with implants are happy with this means of restoring their vision because the implant does not have to be handled and provides the most nearly normal vision.

3. INVOLVEMENTS OF THE CONJUNCTIVA

a. *Conjunctivitis* is an inflammation of the moist membrane that lines the undersurface of the eyelids and covers the "white" part of the eye (up to the circular margin of the cornea). The four principal kinds of conjunctivitis are these:

(1) *Acute Contagious Conjunctivitis (Pinkeye)*. This highly contagious infection of the conjunctiva is easily transmitted from one person to another by fingers or by soiled towels or handkerchiefs. The redness and swelling of the conjunctiva is usually more pronounced on the undersurfaces of the eyelids than over the "white" part of the eye. Early in the disease a watery discharge exudes from between the eyelids. Later the discharge contains more mucus and, in several cases, a mixture of mucus and pus. The patient complains of scratching, burning, and smarting sensations in the affected eyelids. The eyelids tend to stick together during the night.

The infection is caused by any one of several kinds of germs. Both eyes usually become involved. Any age group may be affected, but the disease is most common in children and young adults. Often several persons in the same household or school are affected about the same time. The course of the disease when not treated is 10 to 14 days. There is usually no permanent damage.

Care and Treatment

Take all reasonable precautions to keep the infection from being transmitted to other persons. Wash the hands with soap after each contact with the patient's face. Use paper face towels and handkerchiefs and burn these after use. Bed linen which has come in contact with the patient must be disinfected before it is laundered. Apply a series of compresses wrung out of ice water to the affected eyes for a period of five minutes at least three times a day. Consult a physician. He can prescribe eye drops or ophthalmic ointments to combat the infection.

(2) *Chronic Catarrhal Conjunctivitis*. The symptoms here are about the same as in acute contagious conjunctivitis, only not so severe and usually worse at night. The disease tends to last for weeks and even months. Causes include a carry-over from a neglected case of acute contagious conjunctivitis, irritation from polluted atmosphere, a poor state of general health, insufficient sleep over a long period of time, indulgence in intoxicating drinks, overuse of the eyes, the need for eyeglasses, and chronic inflammation of the tear duct.

Care and Treatment

Correct all conditions that may have contributed to the disease. Follow a general health-building program, including the eating of an adequate diet with sufficient vitamins. Cleanse eyelid margins and lashes at least twice daily with cotton applicators moistened with warm water. Instill antibiotic eyedrops or ointment several times a day as recommended by the physician.

(3) *Gonorrheal Conjunctivitis*. Gonorrheal conjunctivitis is one of the most severe of the infections that involve the eyes, and it can be tragic. It is caused by the same germ that causes sexually transmitted gonorrhea. The germ is carried to the eyes by fingers or towels contaminated by contact with the discharge from a gonorrheal infection. It

can also be acquired by a newborn babe at the time of birth by direct contact with the genital tissues of an infected mother. Without prompt and adequate treatment, gonorrheal conjunctivitis frequently and tragically causes blindness by destruction of the tissues of the eye.

The first symptoms appear from twelve hours to three days after the germs contact the membranes of the eye, and include extreme redness, swelling, and tenseness of the eyelids. A profuse discharge comes from between the eyelids, at first watery and bloody but soon laden with pus. The eye burns and smarts and feels painful. It is tender to touch.

Care and Treatment

From the very first extreme care must be taken to prevent the infection from being carried to the other eye (if only one eye is infected) or to some other person. Any attendant while caring for the patient should wear a surgical gown, face mask, rubber gloves, and protective glasses. All materials used in treating the patient, such as towels and compresses, should be placed at once in a disinfectant solution before being destroyed or laundered. Such a solution can be prepared by dissolving one teaspoonful of Lysol in two quarts (2 liters) of water.

The patient should be placed under the care of a doctor as soon as possible. Preferably, the patient should be treated in a hospital. Methods of treatment now available provide good prospects of recovery with preservation of normal eyesight, *provided* they are employed early in the course of the disease. Antibiotics properly administered usually control the infection promptly. Cold compresses (wrung from ice water) applied to the eyes help to reduce the swelling and congestion of the eyelids and make the patient more comfortable. These can be used continuously at first and then intermittently as inflammation subsides.

(4) *Allergic Conjunctivitis.* This inflammation of the conjunctiva is caused by an allergic reaction rather than by invasion by bacteria. It is usually part of some more general allergic involvement of the body but may be limited to the eyes in case of direct contact between them and an airborne substance that produces allergy. The membranes of the eyes are swollen and red. Itching and extreme production of tears are the usual signs.

Care and Treatment

The fundamental treatment consists of eliminating or avoiding whatever contact is causing the allergic reaction, or of desensitization procedures as for hay fever. In the meantime, the patient can be made somewhat comfortable by the use of a bland eyewash such as Visine Eyedrops or Artificial Tears. Any person who wears contact lenses should avoid wearing these when the conjunctiva is inflamed.

b. *Pterygium.* A pterygium is a wedge-shaped fold of membranous tissue containing small blood vessels which grows from the "white of the eye" onto the cornea. It originates at the inner corner of the eye. It occurs especially in persons routinely exposed to wind and sun. If it is allowed to grow onto the cornea, it interferes with the clarity of vision.

Care and Treatment

The frequent use of eye drops and the wearing of protective eyeglasses can often retard the growth of a pterygium. In cases in which the vision becomes threatened, it may be necessary to remove the pterygium by a minor surgical procedure.

4. CORNEAL INVOLVEMENTS

As mentioned in the previous chapter, the cornea is the transparent, front portion of the eye. It is situated in front of the colored iris and bulges slightly forward like the crystal of a watch. The cornea consists of living cells and transparent intercellular materials. The cells require nourishment just as do other cells throughout the body. The cornea contains no blood vessels, for these would interfere with the direct passage of light rays through the cornea. The cells within the cornea receive their nourishment by the seepage of nutrients from the fluids inside the eye and from the surface tears. The cornea is vulnerable to infections and also to injuries that may cause serious scars. When injuries to the cornea produce scars, the scars, as they heal, interfere with the passage of light and thus distort vision or even cause degrees of blindness.

a. *Keratitis* is a broad term used to denote an inflammation of the cornea by whatever cause. It may develop when the cornea is not kept properly moistened by the fluid produced by the tear glands, when it is injured by scratching or by the penetration of some foreign particle, when it becomes infected either by bacteria or by a virus, when exposed to ultraviolet light (as from the beach, sun lamps, or welding arcs), or when exposed to certain volatile chemicals. The symptoms include severe pain, sensitivity to light, excessive production of tears, redness of the "white of the eyes," and dimness of vision.

Care and Treatment

Mild keratitis caused by exposure to ultraviolet light or to chemicals usually heals spontaneously within hours or at least a few days. In the meantime the individual should wear dark glasses. Anesthetic ointments for the eye should not be used because they will prevent healing, but pain-relieving medications by mouth are often helpful. In cases where the surface layers of epithelial cells have been broken or damaged sufficiently to permit the entrance of bacteria, antimicrobial drops or ointments as prescribed by the physician should be used promptly and continued as long as symptoms persist. Hot and/or cold applications can provide a lot of comfort.

b. *Corneal Ulcer.* A serious possible complication of keratitis is the development of an erosion of tissue (ulcer formation) involving the structures located beyond (deep into) the surface layer of epithelium. Corneal ulcers are of two general types: (1) Those caused by bacteria which have entered through some damaged area of the epithelial layer; and (2) those caused by the herpes simplex virus, Type 1. Dangers associated with a corneal ulcer are these: (1) The ulcer may become so deep that a vision-threatening perforation of the cornea may occur; (2) the infection associated with the ulcer may spread to structures within the eye; and (3) the scar which follows healing of the ulcer may interfere with the passage of light into the eye (more serious when the ulcer is at the center of the cornea).

In corneal ulcer the eye is usually very painful, and the patient avoids all exposure to light. Tears overflow the eyelids. On close observation of the eye, a small grayish-yellow spot may be seen on the cornea. The "white of the eye" appears reddened immediately surrounding the cornea.

Care and Treatment

Corneal ulcer is a serious, sight-threatening condition, and the treatment should be arranged promptly by a specialist in diseases of the eye (an ophthalmologist). He will determine what germ or virus is present and will plan the treatment accordingly. For ulcers caused by bacteria, potent antibiotics are used. For those caused by the herpes simplex virus the eye specialist will often brush away the affected epithelial cells. Following this, medicated eye drops or ointments (containing trifluoridine) are useful.

c. *Xerophthalmia (Keratomalacia).* Xerophthalmia is a condition in which the conjunctiva and the cornea undergo degenerative changes as a result of deprivation of vitamin A. It occurs especially in developing countries where malnourishment is a problem. Otherwise it may occur among confirmed alcoholics or people suffering from an inadequate diet. It is characterized by a loss of the normal luster of the conjunctiva and cornea. The epithelium of the cornea deteriorates; and ulceration, deterioration, and collapse of the eye follow if proper treatment is not initiated early.

Care and Treatment

Intensive doses of vitamin A will arrest the degenerative process if given early in the course of the disease.

d. *Keratoconus*. Keratoconus is a rare inherited condition which first manifests in the 10- to 20-age bracket and which exhibits a progressive weakness of the corneas, allowing them to bulge forward. This alteration in the shape of the cornea changes its refractive properties and thus causes blurred vision.

The circumstance which first calls attention to the condition is the need for frequent changes in the prescription of the glasses being worn. The condition progresses slowly throughout the lifespan. In severe cases a cornea may degenerate, followed by healing which leaves scars.

Care and Treatment

In many cases the wearing of contact lenses serves to aid in the correction of the visual defect. More and more of the moderate to severe cases are now being treated by the delicate surgical procedure of corneal transplantation in which the center of the defective cornea is removed and replaced by a healthy cornea taken from a person who has just died from some unrelated condition.

5. EYELID DISORDERS

a. *Baggy Eyelids (Blepharochalasis)*. Baggy eyelids occur typically in elderly people suffering a loss of elastic fibers in the delicate skin surrounding the

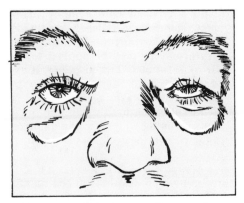

Baggy eyelids is an ailment often suffered by elderly people.

eyes. In some cases the extra folds of skin become so redundant that the individual must raise his eyebrows in order to have a full field of vision. Baggy lower lids may become bothersome not only because of their appearance but because of contact with the lower edge of the frame of glasses.

Care and Treatment

The treatment of baggy eyelid requires a minor plastic-surgery procedure in which a narrow strip of excess skin is removed. The incision is made in a skin fold so that after healing, the scar is not noticeable.

b. *Blepharitis*. Blepharitis consists of an inflammation of the margins of the eyelids. It may be caused by a bacterial (usually staphylococcal) infection of the follicles of the eyelashes, or it may be part of the skin disease seborrheic dermatitis. Frequently both conditions are present, and the eyes are also dry. The symptoms are irritation, burning, itching, and redness of the margins of the eyelids. Occasionally some of the eyelashes fall out, and there may be a shedding of tiny scales in the involved areas.

Care and Treatment

The most effective treatment consists of scrubbing the lid margins for about ten minutes, three times a day, using a small cotton swab moistened

with a small amount of baby sham- poo. Following each such treatment, ophthalmic ointment containing erythromycin may be applied to the areas scrubbed. The instilling of eye drops beneath the eyelids may be helpful. For cases associated with seborrheic dermatitis the physician may recommend the use of a dandruff shampoo on the eyebrows and scalp.

c. *Sty (Hordeolum).* A sty is a minia- ture boil which develops at the margin of the eyelid in connection with the opening of one of the glands contained in the eyelid. It develops commonly in blepharitis, diabetes, or a lowered con- dition of general health.

Care and Treatment

Apply hot compresses, alternating with brief cold, for ten minutes at a time, at least four times a day. This relieves pain and hastens the time when the sty will open on its own. If healing is delayed or if complications threaten, consult a physician, who may find it advisable to surgically open and drain the abscess.

d. *Tarsal Cyst (Chalazion).* A chalazion is a small lump which devel- ops within the eyelid when the outlet to one of the tarsal glands becomes plugged. With the normal outlet now closed, the secretion of the gland accu- mulates, and the size of the mass, com- posed of secretion and tissue debris, in- creases slowly over weeks and months. In contrast to a sty, a tarsal cyst is not caused by an infection but by the sim- ple accumulation of the secretion of a tarsal gland and the body's reaction to it. By the time the little tumor reaches the size of a pea, it causes some disfig- urement of the eyelid and some irrita- tion of the moist membranes of the eye and eyelid.

Care and Treatment

While still small, a tarsal cyst may be treated successfully by applying hot compresses to the affected eyelid two or three times a day, followed

each time by gentle massage. When larger, a tarsal cyst can be drained or opened by a simple surgical proce- dure.

e. *Ectropion.* Ectropion is a rolling outward of the eyelid (one or both) so as to expose part of its lining mem- brane. The exposed membrane is usu- ally swollen and red; and, when the lower lid is involved, there tends to be an overflow of tears. This disorder may be caused by the contraction of scars following face injuries or burns. In el- derly people it may be the simple result of a general relaxation of the tissues. It is a common complication of facial pa- ralysis.

Care and Treatment

In an elderly person, placing the lids in normal position at bedtime and retaining them in place by the use of a bandage or piece of tape may be of help. In troublesome cases a plastic- surgery procedure is indicated in which the tight scar of a previous in- jury is loosened or the margin of the eyelid is shortened.

f. *Entropion.* In entropion there is a rolling inward of the edge of the eyelid and the eyelashes. The rough edges of the eyelids, and especially the lashes, cause irritation of the cornea (keratitis). Keratitis is a serious devel- opment inasmuch as it endangers vi- sion. (See page 138, this volume.)

Entropion often follows burns, injur- ies to the lids, and trachoma in which the formation of scars pulls the tissues out of shape. In the lower eyelid, it may be due to spasm of the muscle. It may follow conjunctivitis.

In certain conditions there may be a few misplaced eyelashes (trichiasis). If these are directed inward, they may ir- ritate the cornea, as described above, even though the eyelid is in normal po- sition.

Care and Treatment

The treatment for these cases re- quires the surgeon to use plastic surgery to reshape the eyelid so that the eyelashes are directed outward. In a case in which a few eyelashes are misplaced, it may be advisable to destroy these lashes and their follicles by the delicate use of electrosurgery in which a tiny wire is inserted into the follicle of the eyelash and a small electric current coagulates the follicle.

g. *Trachoma*. Trachoma is an infectious, highly contagious disease, caused by a minute intracellular parasite, the *Chlamydia trachomatis*. It affects the membranes lining the eyelids and those covering the "white of the eye." It is common in Africa, the Middle East, and Asia. It occurs particularly in districts where poor hygiene and overcrowding prevail. Once it becomes chronic, its principal manifestation is in scarring of the membranes lining the eyelids. These scratch and injure the cornea, with resulting keratitis and the possibility of blindness.

The initial symptoms are redness of the membranes, mild itching, the production of a watery discharge, swelling of the eyelids, and a sensitivity to light.

Care and Treatment

Cold compresses to the eyes help to control the inflammation and thus improve the patient's comfort. The definitive treatment consists of the use of eye ointments containing tetracycline or erythromycin applied three or four times a day for four to six weeks. The use of a tetracycline medication by mouth is sometimes prescribed.

6. GLAUCOMA

A constant production of clear fluid (aqueous humor) goes on inside the front part of the eye. Normally this is drained away as fast as it is produced. In glaucoma, interference with the drainage of this fluid causes increased pressure in the eye.

Glaucoma is the leading cause of blindness in the United States, there being about 60,000 Americans blind on this account. Between one and two million Americans are afflicted with glaucoma, with about one fourth of these unaware of having it. With early detection and proper care, vision can be preserved in 80 to 85 percent of persons with glaucoma.

There are three principal types of glaucoma. In congenital glaucoma (mentioned in chapter 17, volume 1), a faulty development of the eye structures prevents adequate drainage of the fluid produced within the eye. In untreated cases, blindness occurs early. It is estimated that 80 percent of these cases can be recognized by age three months if the evidences of the problem are noticed: (1) extreme photophobia (intolerance of light) and (2) a haze or opacity of the cornea.

The second type is acute (closed-angle) glaucoma, which fortunately accounts for only about 10 to 15 percent of the total cases. In this type the outflow of the fluid in the forward portion of the eye becomes blocked suddenly by a protrusion of the iris, which cuts off access to the canal that normally drains this fluid. Striking symptoms appear, consisting of a sudden blurring of vision with halos around lights, severe pain, and redness in the affected eye. If not treated promptly, this type of glaucoma can cause permanent loss of vision even within a matter of hours. The development of this type of glaucoma therefore constitutes a true emergency demanding prompt surgical intervention.

The third, more common type is chronic (open-angle) glaucoma, which accounts for about 85 percent of all cases. Typically, it develops in persons above 40 years of age, with its onset subtle and unnoticed. Unfortunately, symptoms do not develop until serious damage to the eye has already occurred. For this reason a person above 40 years of age should arrange for routine eye examinations every two or three years. At the time of such examination, the eye specialist will test the pressure within the eye by a simple procedure called tonometry. He will

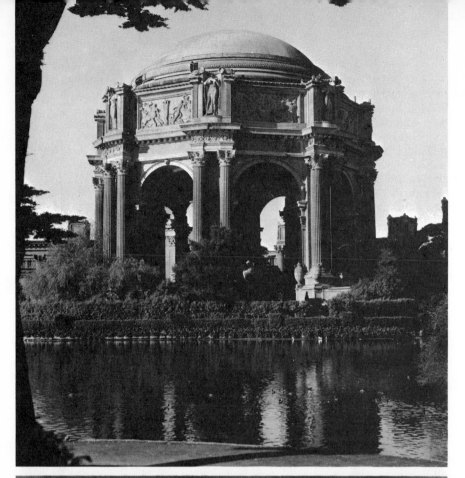

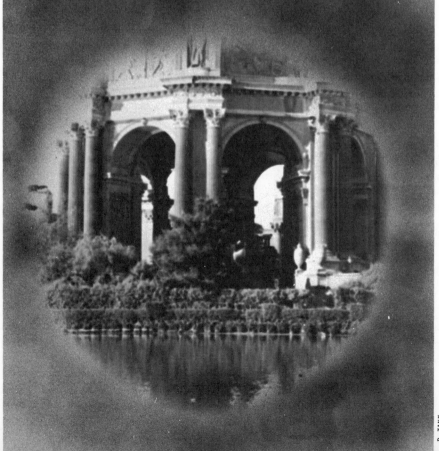

Upper: A scene as viewed by a person with normal vision. Lower: Same scene as viewed by a person with moderately advanced glaucoma.

also use an opthalmoscope to look into the interior of the eye and determine whether there is beginning damage there.

Care and Treatment

Congenital glaucoma must be treated surgically in order to ensure permanent results. The procedure is a delicate eye operation in which an opening is made into the canal which normally drains away the fluid produced in the front portion of the eye.

Acute (closed-angle) glaucoma requires prompt surgical treatment to remove a portion of the peripheral part of the iris so as to permit drainage of the fluid produced in the front portion of the eye.

Many cases of chronic (open-angle) glaucoma can be treated successfully by the use of medication rather than by resort to surgery. This requires the daily use of prescribed eye drops and periodic reporting to the eye specialist. Several effective medications are available. These either decrease the production of fluid within the eye or improve its drainage from the eye.

However, an increasing number of cases of chronic glaucoma are now being treated surgically, especially with the laser. This minimizes the continuing need for daily medication.

7. BURNS OF THE EYES

Burns affecting the eyes fall into two general categories: (a) thermal burns (by heat and intense light) and (b) chemical burns.

a. *Thermal Burns*. (1) Flash burns are caused by the explosive burning of gasoline or some similar volatile substance. Flash burns involve the eyelids rather than the eye proper, for the victim closes his eyes reflexly when the flash occurs. (2) Eye burns caused by actinic light rays injure the eye's cornea. They commonly occur in welders who carelessly neglect to protect their eyes when exposed to the welding arc or in those who ski at high altitudes where the short light rays reflected

from the snow pass easily through the pure atmosphere. The damage to the cornea produces such exquisite pain that the person keeps his eyelids closed for many hours after the burn occurs. (3) Burns from focused sunlight are caused when a person deliberately stares at the sun or when he tries to observe a solar eclipse. The natural lens of the eye focuses the sun's rays to a tiny spot at the center of the retina and actually destroys the retina at this point of central vision. It is a mistake to view the sun even through smoked glass or a photographic negative, for these filter out only the visible rays without impeding the damaging actinic rays.

Care and Treatment

Damage to the eyelids from flash burns is treated the same as burns of the skin in other parts of the body. When destruction of eyelid tissue by a third-degree burn occurs, the healing and repair must be aided by plastic surgery including skin grafts. There is a marked tendency for the scars to contract, causing the eyelids to fit poorly (ectropion).

In damage to the cornea caused by exposure to actinic light rays the treatment usually consists of the use of eye drops to relax the delicate muscle fibers which control the iris, and the use of an antibiotic ointment to prevent infection. Patches are then placed over the eyes to exclude light and keep the eyelids stationary. The patches may remain in place for as long as two days. Eyes thus damaged may remain sensitive to light for many months, requiring the wearing of dark glasses. No treatment exists for damage to the retina caused by focused sunlight, for a small area of the retina is actually destroyed and will not regenerate. There will be a small area of blindness at the center of the visual field for the remainder of life.

b. *Chemical Burns*. The two common types of chemical burns of the eyes involve contact with (1) alkali substances such as anhydrous ammonia or lye and (2) acids. Alkali burns are the most hazardous, for the tissues of the cornea contain no protection against the tissue-destroying effects of alkali. Direct contact with a strong alkali can cause penetration of the cornea within less than one minute. Such damage often results in the loss of the affected eye. Contact with an acid is tolerated better by the tissues of the eye because the cells neutralize the acid more effectively.

Care and Treatment

First-aid treatment for eye burns caused by an alkali must be immediate and vigorous irrigation of the eye with copious amounts of water. The eyelids should be retracted so that the irrigating fluid can wash the entire surface of the eye as well as the lining of the eyelids. The flow of irrigating fluid should be continued for at least 20 minutes.

An alkali burn of the eye is a VERY serious, sight-threatening situation, and the patient should be placed immediately under the care of an eye specialist. Most alkali burns require hospitalization.

For burns resulting from contact with acid, the eye or eyes should be thoroughly irrigated with running water as described in the preceding paragraph. Following this, eyedrops to relax the delicate muscles of the iris should be instilled and an antibiotic ointment placed beneath the eyelids. The affected eye or eyes should then be kept closed by an eye patch for the next day or two. Many acid burns require hospitalization.

8. INJURY TO THE EYE

Most injuries to the eye involve penetration of the eyeball or one of its tissues by some foreign body. When the cornea is involved, symptoms of pain, excessive production of tears, and sensitivity to light call attention to the injury. The seriousness of an injury to the cornea depends on the depth to which the foreign body penetrates and on whether germs were introduced at the time of the injury or can get in later.

Penetrations into the part of the eyeball behind the lens are even more serious than those involving only the cornea, iris, and lens. The seriousness of these deep injuries depends on the size of the object that penetrates and on whether it carried infection into the eye. These deep penetrations may produce severe inflammation which leads to destruction of the delicate light-sensitive tissues.

A sharp blow to the eye, even though nothing penetrates its tissues, may cause the retina to become detached. Unless successfully treated, this detachment produces a partial or complete loss of vision in the involved eye. A blow to the eye may cause hemorrhage into the front part of the eye and may predispose to acute glaucoma. It may also dislocate the lens and require its removal.

Care and Treatment

Injury to the eye justifies immediate care by a physician, preferably a specialist in diseases of the eye. When a small foreign body penetrates the cornea, the procedure for removal is relatively simple. But the danger of corneal ulcer remains even after the removal. Iron and steel foreign bodies in deeper parts of the eye can sometimes be removed by an electromagnet in the hands of a skilled surgeon. Other objects may be removed by small forceps introduced through the original opening.

9. UVEITIS (IRITIS AND CHOROIDITIS)

·Uveitis consists of inflammation of one or more structures belonging to the uveal tract. The uveal tract consists of three principal components: the iris, the ciliary body (the tissue to which the circumference of the iris is attached), and the choroid (the vascular layer of the eyeball located between the retina and the sclera).

There are two principal forms of uveitis: (a) *Iritis (Anterior Uveitis)*, in which the iris is primarily affected; and (b) *Choroiditis (Chorioretinitis; Posterior Uveitis)*, in which the inflammation involves primarily the choroid and secondarily, the retina.

In many cases of uveitis the particular cause remains obscure. In others, uveitis occurs in association with some other disease, such as rheumatoid arthritis, herpes simplex, tuberculosis, toxoplasmosis, or sarcoidosis. It may follow an infection in some other part of the body. It may complicate a disease of the cornea (as corneal ulcer) or be associated with an injury to the eye (either the same, or rarely the opposite eye).

The symptoms of uveitis include throbbing pain in the eye, with the pain radiating to the forehead and temple, blurred vision, sensitivity to light, and an excess production of tears. The "white of the eye" around the cornea appears reddened, and the iris usually appears swollen and dull. The pupil in the affected eye is usually smaller than in the other eye.

The course of the disease varies from case to case. It may clear up in a few weeks or last for several months. Glaucoma and blindness are possible complications.

Care and Treatment

Warm compresses placed over the closed eyelids for two minutes three or four times a day help to relieve the pain. The physician may advise some pain-relieving medication. Dark glasses are worn because of sensitivity to light. The physician will recommend eye drops that have the effect of dilating the pupil. Also he may recommend corticosteroid preparations administered either as eye drops or as medication to be taken by mouth. Attention should be given to any underlying disease which may have predisposed to the uveitis.

10. REFRACTIVE ERRORS

The normal eye is so designed that the entering rays of light are brought to a precise focus on the retina, where the optical image is produced. In some eyes the rays of light are brought to a focus too soon, so that the image on the retina is blurred. This condition is known as myopia, or nearsightedness. In others, the rays have not focused by the time they reach the retina. This is hyperopia, or farsightedness. In still other eyes, the optical system of the eye is slightly distorted so that rays entering in the horizontal plane focus at a distance different from those entering in the vertical plane. This is known as astigmatism.

The fitting of properly designed glasses compensates for the refractive errors of the eye so that all entering rays of light focus clearly on the retina. Such lenses not only provide a clear image but also relieve eyestrain caused by the muscles within the eye as they respond to reflex mechanisms intended to bring the visual image into sharp focus.

The eyes of about 10 percent of young children suffer from refractive errors. Such problems may not be detected until the child starts school and has difficulty in reading. The child himself does not complain of visual difficulties, because he has no basis for knowing whether he is seeing as well as other children. It is advisable, therefore, for a child's eyes to be examined by age four to determine possible need of glasses. See chapter 17, volume 1, for additional information on this matter.

At about age 45 to 50, the natural lenses within a person's eyes lose their elasticity and therefore cannot change shape sufficiently when vision at close range (as in reading) is attempted. We see such a person holding his newspaper farther and farther away from his face. This inability of the eye to adjust for near vision is called presbyopia. Properly fitted reading glasses remedy the situation by causing the incoming light rays to focus on the retina. But the optical strength of a glass lens cannot be varied to accommodate for both near and distant vision. So the person with reading glasses either removes his reading glasses when he looks at a dis-

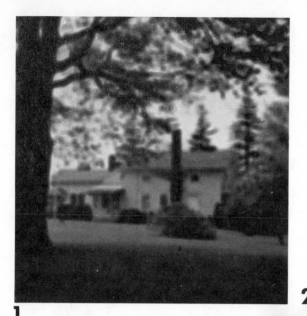

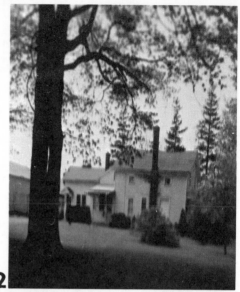

Differing views of the same house as seen (1) by a nearsighted person (blurred); (2) by a person with horizontal astigmatism (blurred, vertical dimensions heightened); (3) by a person with vertical astigmatism (blurred, horizontal dimensions widened).

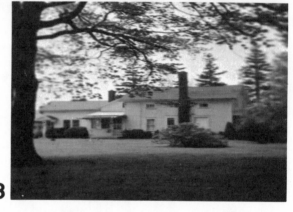

tant object, or he wears double glasses (bifocals)—the lower lens for reading and the upper lens for distant vision.

Contact Lenses. Within recent years a growing number of people prefer to wear contact lenses rather than conventional eyeglasses. A contact lens consists of a small, slightly concave disk of plastic material worn beneath the eyelids to exactly cover the cornea of the eye. This tiny plastic lens can be molded to have the same optical properties as lenses worn in eyeglasses. Most persons who wear contact lenses do so for the sake of appearance, for they are hardly noticeable. In certain eye conditions contact lenses are particularly beneficial. One of these is keratoconus (See under item 4, section B of this chapter), characterized by a tendency for the cornea to bulge forward. Persons who have had cataract surgery also find the wearing of contact lenses preferable to the wearing of conventional eyeglasses, for the contact glasses give them a broader field of vision with less magnification and distortion. Also in some cases of injury to the cornea the wearing of contact lenses is especially beneficial.

Contact lenses have been improved through the years, mostly in the matter of materials better tolerated by the tissues of the eye. Even so, problems of inconvenience persist, in addition to

146

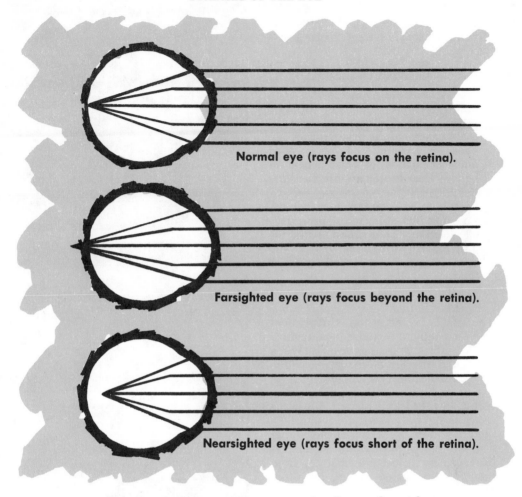

Normal eye (rays focus on the retina).

Farsighted eye (rays focus beyond the retina).

Nearsighted eye (rays focus short of the retina).

In a person needing glasses light rays entering the eye do not focus sharply on the retina, hence the blurring of vision.

the possibility of irritation following many hours of use. An ophthalmologist or optometrist is in a position to advise on whether contact lenses would serve a particular patient's needs better than conventional glasses.

11. INVOLVEMENTS OF THE RETINA

a. *Diabetic Retinopathy.* One of the tragic complications of diabetes mellitus is damage to the blood vessels in the retina of the eye. This condition accounts for about 10 percent of new blindness in the United States each year. Nearly 2 percent of persons with

diabetes are blind on account of this development. The severe damage to the retina typically occurs about twenty years after the onset of diabetes.

The delicate vessels within the retina become weakened, and small hemorrhages occur. Scattered areas of the retina are deprived of their blood supply, and an overgrowth of new blood capillaries develops. The presence of scattered hemorrhages and exudate in the back part of the eye, along with the presence of new capillaries, interferes with the passage of light rays to the retina. The patient experiences a sensation of glare due to the scattering of the light rays, and his visual clarity declines progressively until blindness may result.

Care and Treatment

Considerable progress has been made in the treatment of diabetic retinopathy. For cases recognized early, control of the hemorrhages can often be accomplished by so-called photocoagulation, in which xenon arc light or laser beams are directed into the posterior part of the eye. For patients who have already lost their vision, the highly technical procedure of vitrectomy sometimes allows the now-cloudy substance behind the eye's lens to be replaced by clear fluid.

b. *Other Retinal Vascular Disorders*. The vitality of the retina is dependent upon a continuous and adequate flow of blood through its tiny vessels. When either the arteries or the veins within the retina become obstructed, damage occurs and vision is partially or completely lost. Blocking of the veins of the retina is typically associated with high blood pressure. Blocking of the central artery or one or more of its branches is often caused by the lodgment of a fragment of blood clot from some other part of the body. It may also occur as a complication of arteriosclerosis or inflammatory conditions.

For most such conditions, no effective treatment exists. However, when blindness occurs suddenly in one eye, the patient should be placed promptly under the care of a physician who specializes in diseases of the eye because of the possibility of the other eye becoming similarly involved.

c. *Retinal Detachment*. The retina is the essential part of the organ of vision. It contains specialized nerve cells, some capable of transforming the energy of light into nervous impulses and others designed to convey the nervous impulses by way of the optic nerve to that portion of the cortex of the brain which deals with vision. The retina is

148

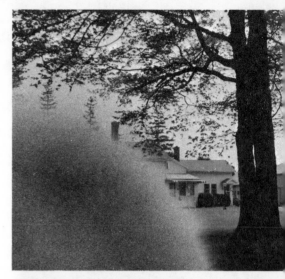
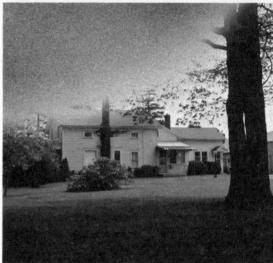
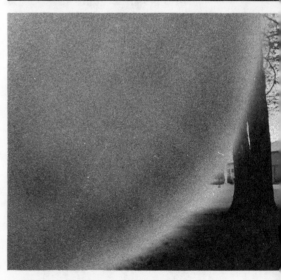

Different ways in which the visual field is partially obscured by a detachment of the retina.

located in the back part of the eye, where it forms the lining layer. Its shape is that of the inner surface of a cup. This back part of the eye is filled with a jellylike substance called vitreous.

The retina is in contact internally with the vitreous and externally with the choroid (vascular) layer of the eye. At the plane of contact between the retina and the choroid a thin pigment layer, dark brown in color, prevents the reflection of light from one part of the retina to another. There is no firm bond between the pigment layer and the retina proper.

Under certain violent conditions, such as a penetrating injury of the eye or a blunt blow to the eye, tears developed in the retina may permit fluid from the vitreous to pass through the new opening and separate a part of the retina from the pigment layer. The separation may progress until large portions of the retina become displaced inward.

In terms of the eye's optical properties, this disturbance would be comparable to deranging the screen on which pictures are being projected in a theater. As the retina becomes detached, the visual image becomes distorted— even to partially or perhaps completely obliterating it.

The first symptoms that a person with detached retina experiences are the "seeing" of floating objects and flashes of light in the affected eye. The vision becomes blurred and, later, as the retina detaches, it is as though a curtain or veil were interposed to obscure part of the visual field.

Care and Treatment

Retinal detachment is a serious condition. Its treatment requires the skill of an ophthalmologist. Fortunately, reattachment of the retina can be accomplished in a high percentage of cases. The methods employed include photocoagulation (attachment by laser beam), cryopexy (attachment by freezing), and surgery.

12. CROSS-EYE AND WALLEYE (SQUINT, STRABISMUS)

These conditions in which the two eyes are not directed at the same object occur in about 2 percent of children. Modern methods make it possible to successfully treat this condition, but for best results it is urgent that treatment be started very early in the child's life. For a detailed discussion of this matter, see chapter 17, volume 1, pages 198 and 199.

13. TEAR DUCT INVOLVEMENT (DACRYOCYSTITIS)

In about 1 percent of newborn infants and occasionally in older children and adults, there develops an obstruction of the tear duct. This causes a pussy discharge at the inner corner of the eye, a redness of the membrane lining the lower eyelid near the inner corner of the eye, and a spilling of tears onto the cheek.

In most infant cases, the condition is caused by a failure of the lower portion of the duct to open at about the time of birth. In a few, there is a fault in development of the tear duct. In older children and adults the obstruction is caused by an injury, by some infection within the nose or sinuses, or, rarely, by a developing tumor. Once the tear duct is stopped up, it tends to become infected.

Care and Treatment

In many infants the tear duct must be probed and, in a few, reconstructive surgery performed.

In older patients the first problem is to control the infection. This is done by the use of antibiotic drugs taken by mouth and application of hot and cold compresses to the inflamed area. Once the infection is controlled, the route for the drainage of tears may have to be reestablished by surgery.

14. MALIGNANT TUMOR (MELANOMA)

Although various tumors can affect the eye or the eyelids or the structures within the orbit, the most serious tumor affecting the eye is the malignant melanoma. As is true in other parts of the body, a melanoma arises from melanocytes (cells which produce the pigment melanin). Melanocytes are numerous in the choroid layer of the eye. The malignant tumor develops when certain of these normal cells undergo malignant transformation.

This tumor in its early stages may be discovered incidentally by the physician when he examines the eyes. Otherwise, a progressive disturbance of vision will alert the patient to a possible problem and prompt him to arrange for an examination of his eye.

Care and Treatment

A malignant melanoma occurring in the eye usually affects one eye only. Such a malignant tumor, if it grows rapidly, threatens to spread to some other part of the body, usually with fatal results (see chapter 11 in this volume).

The procedure for handling a malignant melanoma within the eye is determined by two factors: (1) the size and rate of growth of the tumor and (2) the degree of impairment of vision. When the tumor is small and vision in the affected eye is reasonably good, it is safe to observe it through a series of frequent, periodic examinations to see whether the rate of growth is slow or fast. If it is slow, the removal of the eye can be delayed as long as there is still useful vision. But if the rate of growth is rapid and/or vision is seriously impaired, the affected eye should be removed by surgery.

Diseases of the Ear, Nose, and Throat

Diseases of the ear, the nose, and the throat are traditionally grouped together in the modern specialty of otorhinolaryngology, which pertains to the ear ("oto-"), the nose ("rhino-"), and the larynx ("laryng-"), or voice box. Physicians trained to deal with the diseases of the ear, nose, and throat are properly called otorhinolaryngologists; but more frequently we speak of them as ENT specialists, the ENT standing for ear, nose, and throat. The word *throat,* as commonly used, includes both the pharynx and the larynx. But in *You and Your Health* ailments of the larynx are considered in chapter 13, volume 2, along with other illnesses relating to the respiratory system. In the present chapter the throat is considered to be the pharynx—that region back of the mouth that serves for the passage of food and drink and also forms part of the airway. It is the pharynx that is affected when a person complains of a sore throat.

A. Diseases of the Ear

The structure and functions of the ear are described in chapter 6, this volume. There it is pointed out that the ear has three parts: (1) the external ear, which leads inward to the eardrum (tympanic membrane); (2) the middle ear, an air-filled space spanned by the three bony ossicles; and (3) the inner ear, which consists of the sensitive structures which initiate the nerve impulses for the sensations of both hearing and equilibrium.

The ear is vulnerable to several kinds of disease, as described in the following pages. The associated symptoms may consist of pain and/or of changes or deficiencies in the sensations of hearing and equilibrium. Such symptoms are telltale evidences of difficulty and should cause the person to track down the real cause and receive treatment accordingly.

Common Symptoms Pertaining to the Ears

DEAFNESS
The primary function of the ear is to enable a person to hear sounds. Therefore deafness is the first thing we think of when we consider the ear's ailments. There are several causes of deafness and several manifestations. The following subsection of this chapter (pages 153-156) is devoted to deafness.

DISCHARGE FROM THE EAR
In the normal ear the eardrum

(tympanic membrane) lies at the depth of the external ear canal and serves as a partition between the external ear and the middle ear. Therefore when a discharge of any kind of fluid emanates from the external ear it must come either from the tissues of the external ear canal (as from a ruptured boil) or from the middle ear by passing through an abnormal opening in the eardrum.

In children the usual cause of the "draining ear" (discharge of fluid) is acute otitis media, in which the increasing pressure within the middle ear has caused the eardrum to rupture, allowing the impounded pus to escape to the outside. See chapter 17, volume 1. Discharge from the ear also occurs in cases of chronic otitis media as described in the present chapter, pages 158, 159.

Head injury with skull fracture is sometimes accompanied by a watery or bloody discharge from the ear. A malignant tumor in the vicinity of the ear may cause a foul-smelling discharge to issue from the ear.

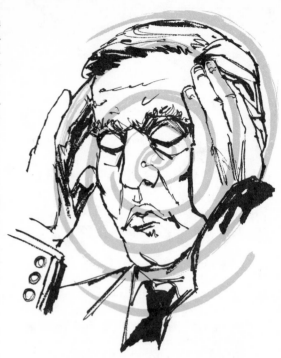

Dizziness is commonly a symptom of disorder in the inner ear.

DIZZINESS (VERTIGO)

Normally it takes three kinds of sensations to keep a person informed on the movements of his body: sensations from his eyes (vision); sensations from his muscles, joints, and tendons; and sensations from the semicircular canals of his internal ear. When a person receives conflicting sensations regarding the movements of his body, as when the semicircular canals register movement and the other sensations indicate no movement, the resulting confusion, with its false impression of movement or unsteadiness, is described as dizziness.

The semicircular canals, being such delicate organs, are easily disturbed by abnormal conditions and may then produce misleading nerve impulses. Also when the nerve which carries impulses from the semicircular canals to the brain is either irritated or compressed, the brain's interpretation of the impulses will be distorted correspondingly.

A common cause of dizziness is an overstimulation of the semicircular canals as in motion sickness (seasickness, car sickness, or air sickness). Reflex stimulation of the canals causing dizziness may occur in excessive use of the eyes, in indigestion, in epilepsy, or in migraine headaches.

In Meniere's disease, a distressing illness of the inner ear, dizziness is a prominent symptom (see pages 161, 162). Dizziness may come from a head injury in which the semicircular canals are damaged. A particular brain tumor known as an acoustic neuroma may cause dizziness by irritating the nerve which carries sensation from the semicircular canals to the brain.

Arteriosclerosis may cause dizziness by limiting the blood to one set of semicircular canals more than to the other. Serious hemorrhage, with loss of considerable blood, as well as anemia, may cause dizziness. Encephalitis caused by mumps may produce dizziness by damage to the semicircular canals. The toxins of some diseases, drugs taken to excess, and allergies sometimes cause dizziness.

EARACHE

Pain in the ear is typically intense and deep-rooted. The soft tissues of the external ear and the middle ear are relatively delicate and are attached firmly to the cartilage or bone which forms their foundation. Limited space makes little allowance for swelling when these tissues become inflamed. The pain, therefore, due to the tension on the nerve endings produced by the swollen tissues, is intense.

One form of earache is caused by an inflammation and swelling of the delicate skin lining the canal of the external ear. It becomes most painful when the infection leads to the formation of a boil. Another cause of earache is pressure on or injury to the eardrum. The problem may arise from severe pressure as in diving or swimming, from sudden changes in the atmospheric pressure as in ascending or descending in an unpressurized airplane, from an actual infection of the eardrum, or as part of an infection of the middle ear (otitis media) as described in chapter 17, volume 1, and in this same chapter, pages 158, 159.

When the tissues of the middle ear are normal, the auditory tube, which extends from the pharynx to the middle ear, permits air to enter or leave the middle ear cavity so as to equalize air pressures. The auditory tube may permit infections to travel from the pharynx into the middle ear, as in cases of the common cold or in pharyngitis. Such infections are a common cause of earache. Blowing the nose too hard sometimes forces infected mucus from the pharynx into the middle ear. When such an infection of the middle ear develops, the walls of the auditory tube may become so swollen that they no longer allow for an exchange of air when the atmospheric pressure changes or for the escape of fluid from the middle ear. When pressure increases within the middle ear, the conduction of sound is dampened. The vic-

tim, therefore, often complains of deafness in the involved ear.

Pressure from infection within the middle ear may force infected fluid into the small spaces within the mastoid bone, thus causing mastoiditis. In such a case, there may be pain on pressure in the area just behind the external ear.

Sometimes pain may seem to emanate from the ear, when the real difficulty is in a tooth, in the tongue or the tonsils, or in the hinge of the jaw (temporomandibular joint). This is an example of referred pain.

NOISE (RINGING IN THE EAR: TINNITUS)

Ear noise is variously described as ringing, roaring, buzzing, pumping, whistling, or clicking. It is a common symptom. Vibratory sounds are typically caused by irritation or inflammation within the middle ear. Clicking sounds may be caused by the contraction of the small muscles associated with the middle ear. Ear noises which synchronize with the heartbeat may be related to nervousness or may be caused by some abnormal condition of the blood vessels in the vicinity of the ear.

High-pitched sounds are usually caused by difficulty within the inner ear (as in Meniere's disease) or by compression of the nerve which conveys hearing impulses to the brain (as by a tumor). The use of certain drugs such as the salicylates and quinine may cause ringing in the ears.

Deafness

To understand deafness and its causes, we must first recall the construction and function of the ear. Being a typical sense organ, the ear helps to make the brain aware of what goes on outside the body. Specifically, the ear is designed to convert the energy of sound into nervous impulses. Sound waves coming to the external ear cause the eardrum to vibrate. The vibrations are carried across the space of the middle ear by a chain of three tiny bones

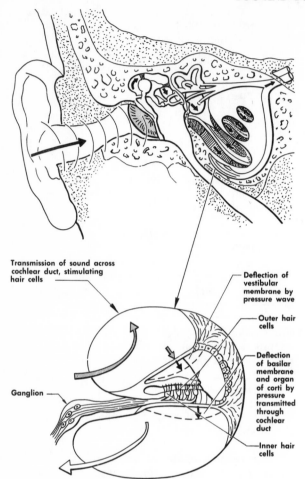

Transmission of sound across cochlear duct, stimulating hair cells

Deflection of vestibular membrane by pressure wave

Outer hair cells

Deflection of basilar membrane and organ of corti by pressure transmitted through cochlear duct

Ganglion

Inner hair cells

(ossicles) which, in turn, agitate the fluid of the inner ear. Delicate nerve cells there generate nervous impulses, which are carried by the auditory nerve to that part of the brain that registers and interprets sounds.

Deafness may involve one or both ears; it may be partial or complete. It consists of two fundamental kinds: (1) conductive deafness, where interference takes place in the passage of the sound waves on their way to the inner ear; and (2) nerve deafness, where interference takes place in the passage of nerve impulses which normally originate in the inner ear and travel to the auditory area of the brain.

CONDUCTIVE DEAFNESS

Conductive deafness stems from sev-

eral possible causes, all of which interfere, in one way or another, with the conduction of sound waves to the inner ear. Mild conductive deafness may be caused by so simple a matter as the accumulation of wax in the external ear canal. A common cause of reduced hearing in children is the presence of excess lymphoid tissue (adenoids) in the back part of the pharynx. Adenoids interfere with the passage of air to and from the middle ear by way of the auditory tube. With such interference, air pressure within the middle ear cavity may be either so high or so low as to interfere with the normal vibrations of the eardrum. A common cause of conductive deafness in young adults is a condition called otosclerosis, in which one of the bony ossicles (the stapes) becomes rigidly attached and therefore not able to vibrate in unison with the sound waves. Chronic otitis media, described later under "Involvements of the Middle Ear" (see pages 158, 159), can damage the delicate structures within the middle ear and thus interfere with the conduction of sound waves. Tumors of the middle ear can have a similar effect.

Care and Treatment

First the cause of conductive deafness must be ascertained, then treatment administered accordingly. Wax in the external ear canal is most safely removed by gentle irrigation with warm water, using a rubber bulb type of syringe. Otherwise it should be removed at the doctor's office. Excess lymphoid tissue in the pharynx ("adenoids") which tends to obstruct the auditory tube can be removed by a minor surgical procedure. The condition of otosclerosis can be treated by a specialist in otorhinolaryngology, who operates on the middle ear with the aid of a specially designed microscope. The procedure is called stapedectomy and involves replacing the bony stapes with a minute prosthetic device. The treatment of chronic otitis media is discussed later in the section on Involvements of the

Middle Ear (see pages 158, 159). Tumors of the middle ear require specialized surgical treatment.

NERVE DEAFNESS

Various conditions can interfere with the passage of nerve currents between the inner ear and the auditory area of the brain—some temporary, others more permanent. When a temporary problem is relieved, the patient's hearing will return to normal or at least improve. In case of a permanent or, perhaps, progressive problem, the defect in hearing remains stationary or even becomes worse.

We will now consider the common causes of nerve deafness:

1. *Advancing Age.* The acuity of an average person's hearing gradually declines with advancing years. This decline is more rapid in some cases than in others. The ability to detect higher-pitched sounds suffers first. As the defect continues, the individual encounters difficulty in recognizing spoken words, even though he still detects the sounds of the speaker's voice.

2. *Congenital Deafness.* Some cases of congenital deafness stem from heredity and some from an unfavorable circumstance occurring prior to birth. Many cases result from the expectant mother's having had rubella (German measles) during the first three months of her pregnancy. For a more complete discussion of congenital deafness, see chapter 17, volume 1.

3. *Drug Damage.* Certain drugs cause damage to the inner ear in a small percentage of those who use them. The salicylates (e.g., aspirin) cause hearing loss and ringing in the ears in a small number of users. In this case, recovery usually follows discontinuance of the drug. Quinine and its synthetic substitutes produce a permanent loss of hearing in some people. Neomycin, one of the antibiotic drugs, causes the greatest damage to the organ of hearing of any of the antibiotic preparations. Strepto-

Decibel Values of Common Noises

	Noise	dB
1.	Traffic at a residential intersection	82
2.	Noise within a city bus	85
3.	Noise of a passing sports car	86
4.	Screams of a child	92
5.	Noise inside a jet airplane on takeoff	94
6.	Noise within a subway car, windows open	95
7.	Power lawnmower at close range	96
8.	Noise of a helicopter motor, close range	104
9.	Sound of a pneumatic hammer, six feet away	108
10.	House party with a four-piece rock band	115

mycin, another antibiotic, may also damage the inner ear, but its damage is focused more on the semicircular canals than on the organs for hearing.

4. *Excessive Noise.* Intense noise, in excess of 95 decibels, damages the delicate nerve cells within the inner ear. The louder the noise and the longer its duration, the greater the potential danger. The ears can recover, somewhat, if the exposure to loud noise has not been too long.

The accompanying chart indicates in decibels the volume of noise which may be encountered in various activities. A person should not be exposed to loud noises, of 95 decibels or more, for more than four hours per day.

Prevention and Treatment

The damage caused to the inner ears by loud noises is permanent. It is important, therefore, for a person to protect himself against such damage. The person who must spend much time in a noisy environment should protect his ears either by earmuff-type protectors or by wearing earplugs. Soft foam-rubber plugs provide the best protection, provided they fit tightly. A plug of cotton is not satisfactory for protecting against loud noises.

For those who have already suffered a hearing loss because of exposure to loud noises, the use of a hearing aid is recommended. Such will not restore a person's hearing to its original condition, but it will be of help.

5. *Meniere's Disease.* Meniere's disease is a condition in which there develops an increase of fluid pressure within the inner ear. This buildup first causes irritation and then gradual destruction of the delicate mechanisms for hearing and equilibrium. It is discussed later in this chapter in the section on Involvements of the Inner Ear, pages 161, 162.

6. *Skull Fracture.* Head injuries that produce a fracture in the temporal bone (in which the inner ear is located) may damage the organ of hearing or sever certain of its nerve connections. In most such cases, the hearing loss is permanent.

7. *Tumor, Pressure by.* A particular kind of brain tumor, called an acoustic neuroma, sometimes develops in the vicinity of the nerve which serves the inner ear. It is slow growing and nonmalignant, but as it grows it brings pressure against the acoustic nerve. The initial symptoms stem from irritation of the nerve and consist of ringing in the ear and dizziness. In untreated cases, these symptoms gradually fade as the progressive pressure on the nerve causes its destruction; but deafness in the corresponding ear and a defect in the mechanism for maintaining body balance results.

Care and Treatment

The acoustic neuroma is a slow-growing, benign tumor and can be successfully removed by a brain surgeon. Recovery is quite satisfactory when the tumor is recognized and treated in its early stages.

8. *Viral Infections.* In an occasional case of herpes zoster (caused by a virus) the nerve which serves the inner ear becomes involved. Among the symptoms in such a case will be hearing loss and dizziness. In most cases hearing will be at least partially restored after the infection subsides.

Involvements of the External Ear

The external ear consists of the feature on the side of the head which we ordinarily call the ear, along with the external ear canal which leads inward for a distance of about one inch (2.5 cm.) to end blindly at the eardrum. Except for accidents in which the external ear is bruised or torn, most of the problems relating to the external ear occur within the external ear canal. This canal is lined with delicate skin within which are tiny glands that produce ear wax (cerumen).

BOIL IN THE EAR

A boil or furuncle in the skin lining the external ear canal is similar to a boil elsewhere except that it is small. Such a boil is usually a complication of external otitis. Extreme pain results because of the limited space within which tissue swelling can occur. Without treatment, such a boil will usually rupture spontaneously within four or five days. The pain subsides promptly once rupture has occurred. Without adequate treatment a tendency persists for boils to recur in the same area.

Care and Treatment

In the early stages of the boil's development, a small pledget of cotton soaked in warm water or warm glycerine can be gently introduced into the ear canal at the site of the boil. Arranging for the patient to lie on a padded hot-water bottle with the af-

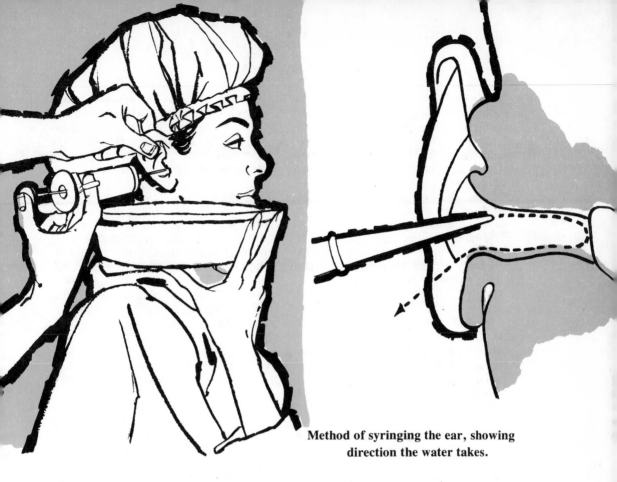

Method of syringing the ear, showing direction the water takes.

fected ear next to the water bottle may give some comfort and help to hasten the readiness of the boil for rupture or lancing. It is preferable to have the boil lanced by a physician, who may choose to place a small wick of gauze, which has been soaked with antibiotic medication, into the incision. Antibiotic medication by mouth is advisable in severe cases, especially if a second boil develops.

EARWAX, IMPACTED

Accumulation of earwax in the external ear canal is a common occurrence. Sometimes the accumulated wax becomes hard and so nearly fills the deeper portion of the ear canal as to cause temporary conductive deafness.

Care and Treatment

It must be remembered that the external ear canal is relatively short and that it ends blindly against the delicate eardrum. In attempting to remove earwax, therefore, beware of damaging the eardrum. Also, the skin lining the external ear canal is delicate, is easily damaged by friction, and is therefore subject to being infected by germs that may be present.

If the earwax is soft, it can be safely removed by gently syringing the ear canal with warm water as indicated in the accompanying illustration. The tip of the syringe must be loosely inserted so as to allow plenty of room for the water to escape.

If the earwax cannot be washed out or if the procedure of syringing causes pain, a physician should be consulted. He has provision for directing a beam of light into the ear canal as he gently removes the earwax with an instrument. In difficult cases, the physician may instill a medication which softens the earwax.

EXTERNAL OTITIS

External otitis consists of an inflammation of the skin lining the external ear canal. It may be caused by damage

157

to the skin such as results from scratches by a fingernail or by the unfortunate use of a blunt instrument to remove earwax. Also, prolonged exposure to water, as in swimming, makes this skin susceptible to inflammation. The skin of the external ear canal is sometimes involved as part of generalized skin ailments as in exzema or seborrheic dermatitis.

External otitis may cause pain which is aggravated by opening the jaw. Usually accompanying swelling may reduce the caliber of the canal.

Care and Treatment

In mild cases, the first portion of the canal may be cleansed by the use of a cotton swab dipped in hydrogen peroxide solution. Great caution must be exercised not to introduce the swab into the deeper portion of the canal lest damage be done to the eardrum. In more severe cases, in which the pain and swelling may be considerable, a physician should be consulted so that he may administer antibiotic medications as indicated.

FOREIGN BODY IN THE EAR CANAL

The problem of a foreign body wedged into the external ear canal is practically limited to children younger than 6 years of age. Such a foreign body may be of any shape and may consist of any material. Its size, of course, is limited to the size of the ear canal. The problem causes discomfort, but the removal of such a foreign body is not so urgent that it must be performed immediately.

Care and Treatment

When the foreign body fits loosely, it may be removed by gently irrigating the ear canal with a stream of warm water provided by a small rubber syringe. For the more difficult cases, the physician may be able to draw the foreign body out by the use of suction apparatus. In still more difficult cases, it may be necessary to give the child a general anesthetic so

that the physician can remove the foreign body by the use of forceps. Being a delicate procedure, it poses danger of injuring the delicate tissues of the ear should the child squirm—hence the general anesthetic.

OTOMYCOSIS

Otomycosis is really a skin disease rather than an ear disease. It is an infection of the skin lining the external ear canal and is caused by a fungus. It is persistent and needs a treatment different from that for fungal infections of the skin in other parts of the body. This infection results in moist crusting of the skin, with a dirty coating on which there may be scattered moldy spots of yellow, green, or black. There is usually a foul smell and more or less itching, stinging, and pain.

Care and Treatment

One treatment consists of cleaning the ear canal gently once a day with small cotton swabs wet with 95 percent alcohol. An alternative consists of irrigating the ear canal with a solution of chloramine-T made by dissolving one tablet of chloramine-T in an ounce (30 ml.) of water. In persistent cases, more effective treatments may be given by a physician specializing in otorhinolaryngology or in dermatology.

Involvements of the Middle Ear

ACUTE OTITIS MEDIA

This is a common affliction of young children. It consists of an inflammation of the tissues within the middle ear and is the common cause of earache. If neglected, it results in rupture of the eardrum, with consequent drainage through the external ear canal. Being primarily a disease of childhood, it is discussed in chapter 17, volume 1.

CHRONIC SUPPURATIVE OTITIS MEDIA

In this condition persisting inflammation of the middle ear causes a progressive destruction of the tissues in this area. It usually follows a case of acute otitis media which has been neglected or improperly treated. Partial destruction of the eardrum allows drainage through the external ear canal of a foul-smelling fluid, which consists of mucus mixed with pus. Perforation of the eardrum and the possible destruction of tissues within the middle ear cavity usually causes a significant decline in hearing in the affected ear.

Care and Treatment

Because of the possibility of serious complications (even that of meningitis) should the infection spread to other tissues, the first emphasis must be on treating the infection, with later attention to the possibility of restoring as much of the function of hearing as possible.

Because the eardrum is perforated, the person with this problem must avoid, by all means, the possibility of water entering the affected ear. He should abstain from swimming and avoid the kind of bathing or showers that would permit water to enter the external ear canal. Home treatment for chronic suppurative otitis media is not usually effective. If the doctor so advises, it is permissible to gently clean the ear canal once or twice a day with a small cotton swab that has been dipped in a mild antiseptic solution in which alcohol rather than water is the solvent. If there develops persistent headache, severe pain on the involved side, or dizziness, the patient should report the symptom promptly to his doctor.

The effective treatment requires a delicate surgical procedure by which all of the infected tissue within the middle ear and the adjacent area of the mastoid bone is removed.

After the infection has been positively eradicated, it is possible for a surgeon trained in surgery of the ear to reconstruct the remaining structures within the middle ear and thus restore some of the function of hearing. The amount of restoration de- **pends, of course, on how much damage was done to the natural ear structures during the course of the infection.**

MASTOIDITIS

Mastoiditis is an inflammation which affects the small spaces in the mastoid bone behind the ear. The condition begins with pain which becomes intense and extends to the whole side of the head. Usually redness and swelling of the skin behind the ear ensues. The area is tender to the touch. Typically the patient suffers fever and weakness.

Mastoiditis develops as a complication of inflammation within the middle ear (otitis media). When neglected, the infection may spread to the meninges—the membranes which envelop the brain—thus causing life-threatening meningitis.

Care and Treatment

The treatment for mastoiditis is the administration of an appropriate antibiotic in generous doses. In severe cases with abscess formation it may be advisable for the surgeon to make an incision behind the ear and clear

Mastoiditis

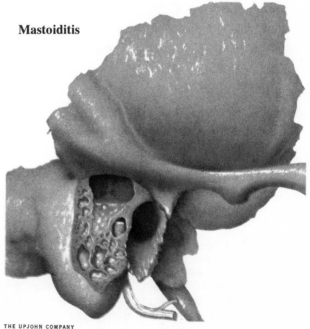

159

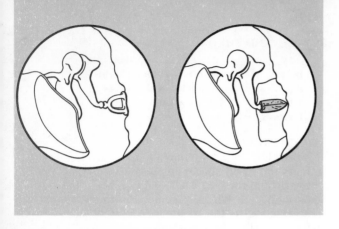

away the affected tissue (mastoidectomy). While time is being allowed for the antibiotic to take effect, the patient may be made more comfortable and the progress of the infection retarded by the placing of an ice bag over the affected area behind the ear.

OTOSCLEROSIS

Otosclerosis is a disease which affects the small bones within the middle ear and the surrounding bone. The footpiece of the stirrup (stapes) becomes fused to the adjacent bone. Because the movements of the stapes are reduced, a progressive loss of hearing results. In many cases there seems to be a hereditary factor which predisposes to this illness.

Care and Treatment

Modern methods of ear surgery can restore hearing, partial or complete, in most cases. The usual operation consists of replacing the stapes with a tiny prosthetic device. The various forms of surgery applicable here are described as stapedectomy, stapes mobilization, or fenestration.

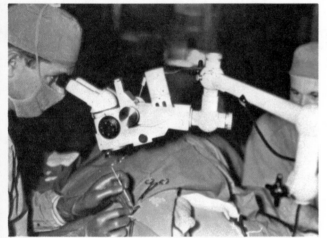

CHAS. PFIZER & CO., INC.

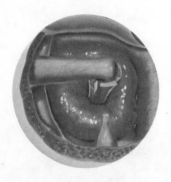

Top: Diagram of positions of normal stapes (left) and prosthesis (right). Center: Restorative surgery for otosclerosis. Bottom: Polyethylene prosthesis resting on a pad of gelfoam over oval window.

Involvements of the Inner Ear

DEGENERATIVE DEAFNESS (NERVE DEAFNESS)

This type of deafness, which occurs typically in the later years of life and involves a gradual degeneration of the sensitive nerve tissues within the inner ear, is discussed earlier in this chapter, pages 155, 156, in the subsection on deafness.

LABYRINTHITIS

The delicate, fluid-filled spaces of the inner ear are designated as the labyrinth. The term labyrinthitis, therefore, refers to an inflammation of the structures within these spaces. The inflammation may be caused by a virus or by pus-producing germs. The source of such a virus inflammation may be difficult to determine, but the germs that

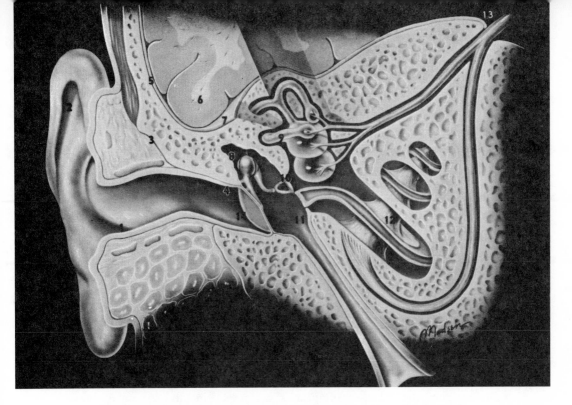

Diagram of the ear showing possible sites of severe lesions: (1) circumscribed furuncle of otitis externa; (2) infection of the cartilage of concha; (3) subperiosteal abscess in case of perforated cortex; (4) sinking of post-superior canal wall, during periosteal inflammation, as seen in acute mastoiditis; (5) epidural cerebral abscess; (6) circumscribed cerebral abscess; (7) subdural abscess; (8) cholesteatoma (pseudo) situated in the attic of middle ear; (9) circumscribed labyrinthitis; (10) fixation of stapes, involving the annular ligament; (11) fistula opening on roof of tympanic orifice of eustachian tube; (12) when these areas are involved, the labyrinth becomes seat of lesion; (13) by pressure on auditory nerve, especially the vestibular branches, symptoms of angle tumor develop; (14) perforated eardrum.

produce the more serious type of labyrinthitis (the pus-producing germs) gain access either from the middle ear (as in otitis media) or as a complication of meningitis. In either event, the inflammation causes profound symptoms: dizziness and/or ringing in the ears, and, in the more serious cases, a loss of the sense of equilibrium and nerve deafness.

Care and Treatment

The virus infections of the labyrinth are typically of short duration and self-limited. There is no specific treatment for these. For the purulent (pus-producing) infections, effective treatment requires the use of antibiotic medications and, in the more serious cases such as are associated with meningitis, surgical removal of the affected tissues. In this latter case the patient will suffer permanent loss of hearing and the sense of equilibrium on the affected side.

MENIERE'S DISEASE (HYDROPS OF THE INNER EAR)

This is a troublesome illness characterized by attacks of extreme dizziness associated with nausea and vomiting. The patient suffers no pain and no fever and shows no evidence of disease of the digestive organs. In addition to the attacks of dizziness, he usually experiences a more or less persistent ringing in the ear accompanied by progressive nerve-type deafness. In many cases only one ear is affected at first, but later both may become involved.

The attack of dizziness associated with nausea and vomiting may last only a few minutes, or it may last several hours. The frequency of attacks varies widely. Meniere's disease affects men somewhat more frequently than women and seldom occurs in persons younger than 40 years of age.

The immediate cause is an increase in fluid pressure within the inner ear. Because the inner ear is concerned with both hearing and equilibrium, both of these functions are affected when the fluid pressure is increased. It is debatable whether the increase in fluid pressure is caused by an excess production of fluid or by a partial failure of the fluid to be reabsorbed.

In some cases Meniere's disease is aggravated or even precipitated by emotional stress. In other cases allergy seems to be the aggravating factor. In still others some metabolic disorder such as hypoglycemia makes the individual susceptible to this disorder.

Some persons experience relief from the symptoms after a few weeks or months. In other cases the symptoms persist for a long time. The usual pattern is that the attacks of dizziness gradually become less frequent and less severe, but the deafness becomes worse.

Care and Treatment

Consultation should be arranged either with a neurologist (specialist in the nervous system) or an otologist (specialist in diseases of the ear). The specialist's first attempt will be to discover the basic cause of the illness. Once the cause is discovered, then removing it should bring about improvement. In extreme cases, recourse may be taken to a delicate surgical procedure in which a bypass

is created to shunt the excess fluid of the inner ear into the fluid-filled space that surrounds the brain.

B. Diseases of the Nose

As explained in chapter 12, volume 2, the nose conditions the air on its way to the lungs. It also contains the receptor organ for the sense of smell. The accessory nasal sinuses which communicate with the nasal cavities provide a certain resonance to the voice.

Disorders of the nose occur rather commonly. They are not usually life-threatening, but they cause considerable discomfort and inconvenience.

ANOSMIA

Anosmia consists of a loss of the sense of smell. The sense organs for smell consist of specialized areas in the membrane in the extreme upper areas of the nasal cavities. Anosmia occurs temporarily in any condition in which the passage of air through the nasal cavities is obstructed. Anosmia occurs in the condition of atrophic rhinitis where the membrane lining the nasal cavities deteriorates. Another cause of anosmia is a skull fracture in which the nerve filaments which carry the nerve impulses from the organ of smell to the brain have been interrupted.

BOIL IN THE NOSE

A boil developing in the nose is very painful and temporarily disfiguring. It consists of a pus-producing type of local infection.

Care and Treatment

A boil in this location should not be lanced but should be treated with warm compresses to hasten the spontaneous discharge of the pus which develops within the boil. Compresses made from gauze (for the exterior of the nose) or from cotton (for the interior of the nose) should be wrung from hot salt water and applied both inside and outside the nostril until softening of the boil occurs and the discharge of pus takes place. Antibi-

otic medication should be given by mouth and, once the boil has ruptured, by the application of an ointment containing an antibiotic.

INJURY TO THE NOSE

Injury to the nose is the most frequent of the facial injuries, because the nose is the most prominent feature of the face. The severity of such injuries varies from case to case, all the way from minor injuries which require no treatment to injuries which cause fractures and displacements of the bony and cartilaginous structures which form the foundation of the nose. In the more severe injuries to the nose there develops swelling of the soft tissues, accumulation of blood in these tissues, and obvious deformity of the nose. When left unattended, the deformities persist, the bones and cartilages heal in abnormal positions, and the partition between the two sides of the nose may be so displaced as to interfere with the normal passage of air through the nasal cavities.

Care and Treatment

The aim in treating a severe injury to the nose is to manipulate the bony and cartilaginous structures which have been displaced, bringing them back into normal relationship, thus restoring the previous shape of the nose. This reshaping of the injured nose can be accomplished immediately after the injury before swelling of the soft tissue has taken place. Otherwise, there must be a delay of three to six days to allow the swelling of the soft tissues to subside before the broken structures can be moved back into their normal position.

The reshaping of the nose is accomplished by pressure from within the nose exerted by the slender handle of an instrument, coupled with external pressure exerted by the fingers of the physician. In many cases it is necessary to administer a general anesthetic in order for this manipulation to be performed. The injured nose is then maintained in normal position by the placing of packing inside the nostrils and by the use of an externl splint of appropriate shape.

NOSEBLEED (EPISTAXIS)

Bleeding from the nose occurs quite commonly in children, in adolescent girls, in elderly persons, and in connection with injury to the nose at any time of life. The blood comes from a rupture of one of the tiny arteries in the soft tissues that line the nose. The usual site of the hemorrhage is at the forward part of the partition that separates the nasal cavities. Conditions that may contribute to nosebleed include the breathing of very dry air, damage to the soft tissue by the removing of crusts from the nose, inflammation of the nasal tissues as in a common cold, high blood pressure, and any one of the systemic disorders exhibiting a tendency to bleeding.

In young, healthy persons nosebleeding is usually not a serious problem, whereas in an elderly or debilitated person it may even be a threat to life. In the usual case, treated promptly, the bleeding stops within a few minutes. In problem cases, however, it may continue for hours, requiring the use of blood transfusions to replace the lost blood and surgical procedures to tie off the blood vessels that bring blood to the bleeding area.

Care and Treatment

For a case of mild bleeding, cut a piece of paper about one and a half inches (3.5 cm.) square. Fold it several times and insert it between the patient's inside upper lip and gum. Instruct him to hold it firmly by tightening his lip against it.

When the bleeding persists in spite of the above procedure, have the patient sit up with his head held forward. Hold a basin below his mouth and nose to catch the blood. Pinch the patient's nose firmly between thumb and finger so that the blood cannot escape from his nostrils. This requires him to breathe through his open mouth. If bleeding continues, the blood now flows backward from the nose into the mouth and flows from the open mouth into the basin. Hold this position for five minutes. In most cases the bleeding will stop within five minutes.

In case the bleeding continues beyond the five-minute period, the cavity of the nose on the side that is bleeding should be gently but firmly packed with a slender ribbon of gauze or soft cloth. It is a good thing to moisten the gauze with hydrogen peroxide before introducing it into the nose. The gauze should be "fed" into the nose, a one-inch (2.5 cm.) loop at a time, using a blunt instrument to push it into place.

For the difficult cases in which nose bleeding persists or recurs frequently, a physician should be consulted or the patient should be taken to a hospital emergency room for treatment.

OBSTRUCTION OF THE NOSE

A common cause of obstruction to the flow of air through the nose is the common cold, which is discussed in chapter 13, volume 2.

Sometimes the turbinate bones in the walls of the nasal cavities become enlarged and obstruct the flow of air through the nose. When they do, a part of them should be surgically removed so that air can get through. The bony partition, or septum, between the nostrils may become crooked and obstruct one or both sides. Relief calls for surgical straightening or partial removal of the deviated bony or cartilaginous septum.

A nasal polyp, a special kind of tumor that usually forms as a result of chronic infection in a nasal sinus, may obstruct a nostril. It also calls for surgical removal. When the lymphoid tissue in the back of the pharynx (adenoids) becomes much enlarged, the victim may be unable to breathe easily through the nose. Under such conditions, the excess lymphoid tissue should be surgically removed.

Children sometimes force a bean, a kernel of corn, or an object of similar size into one of the nostrils. Such can usually be seen by having the child tip his head backward. Inasmuch as the nasal cavities are tall in the vertical direction, it is usually possible to slip a loop of fine wire either above or beneath an obstructing object and gently withdraw it by pulling it forward through the nostril. If this procedure is not successful, a physician should be consulted.

SINUSITIS

Mucous-membrane-lined cavities in the bones of the face and the floor of the skull communicate directly or indirectly with the nasal cavities. These are the accessory nasal sinuses. Their specific locations are described in chapter 12, volume 2.

Whenever excess mucus is produced by the membranes that line the sinuses, it must exit through the openings into

Illustration indicating the positions of the accessory nasal sinuses.

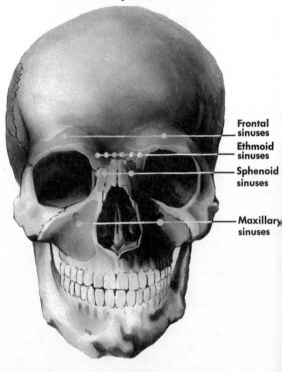

Frontal sinuses

Ethmoid sinuses

Sphenoid sinuses

Maxillary sinuses

COURTESY OF REVIEW AND HERALD PUBLISHING ASSOCIATION

the nasal cavities or else build up pressure inside the sinuses and create discomfort. This problem may occur in a case of allergy or a common cold. If there is no infection, the trouble may correct itself soon; but if pus-producing germs begin to work in the clogged sinuses, inflammation results.

Acute sinusitis causes tenderness of the skin over the affected area, considerable pain, and moderate fever. Chronic sinusitis may produce few or no local symptoms; but, if there is no free drainage for the pus, toxic substances may be absorbed into the circulation, impairing general health and lowering resistance to disease.

Care and Treatment

For acute sinusitis, the cautious breathing of steam, produced in a vessel in which water is boiling, often brings considerable relief. This treatment can be repeated three or four times a day. For an acute case, the use of a nasal spray containing medication to shrink the membrane will give relief. Such a spray is Newphrine (phenylephrine 0.25%) solution. This can be used every three hours but should not be continued for longer than seven days.

Antibiotic medications to combat the infection within the sinuses should be given under a physician's supervision for at least ten days in an acute case and may be used over a period of four to six weeks in the chronic cases. In some chronic cases of sinusitis, even the prolonged use of antibiotic medications does not bring about a cure. In such cases a physician who specializes in otorhinolaryngology should be consulted. He may find it necessary to perform a surgical procedure in which the opening to the involved sinus is enlarged.

Rhinitis

Rhinitis consists of an inflammation of the lining of the nasal cavities. Description of the several types follows:

ACUTE RHINITIS

Acute rhinitis is the most frequently occurring disease of the air passages. The symptoms include a discharge of mucus from the nostrils and a swelling of the membranes that line the nasal cavities. Acute rhinitis is the usual manifestation of the common cold, considered in chapter 13, volume 2.

ALLERGIC RHINITIS (HAY FEVER)

Allergic rhinitis is an inflammation of the membranes lining the nasal cavities that occurs in response to contact with some allergen to which the individual is sensitive. Hay fever is the term applied to the condition when the symptoms

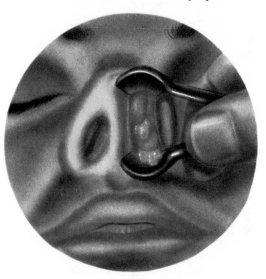

Rhinitis.

occur in certain seasons of the year. It is usually caused by plant pollens from certain grasses, weeds, or trees. Other cases of allergic rhinitis occur throughout the year or at any time of year and are caused by sensitivity to house dust, plant dust, animal danders, and the like, which are borne by the air a person breathes.

This allergic response to an airborne allergen causes the membrane lining of the nose to become congested and swollen. The membrane itches, causing frequent sneezing. The membranes of

165

the eyes usually respond as well. A dry cough commonly occurs.

Care and Treatment

The treatment of allergic rhinitis may be described in four successive steps. If relief is not obtained from the first step, then the second may give relief, and so on to the third and fourth, as may be necessary.

The first step is to avoid contact with the allergen that seems to be responsible for the symptoms. When it is observed that contact with the pollen from a certain kind of grass causes hay fever, staying away from this kind of grass may prevent the attacks. Many hay fever victims obtain relief by remaining in an air-conditioned house during the season in which their symptoms occur.

The second line of attack is the use of antihistamine medications by mouth. Many antihistamine drugs are available without prescription and the individual may need to try several before he finds one that gives satisfactory relief. The hazard in using them is that most of them cause drowsiness. Great caution should therefore be exercised, especially by those who drive cars. The drowsiness may be counteracted, somewhat, by the use of ephedrine, or a similar drug, taken under a doctor's supervision.

The third line of attack would be to try a corticosteroid preparation applied directly to the membrane lining the nose. One such preparation is available as a nasal spray (Turbinaire). Such should be used in small, infrequent doses, preferably under the supervision of a doctor.

The fourth recourse in treating allergic rhinitis is to consult a physician who specializes in allergy, arrange for him to identify the particular substance to which the individual is sensitive, and then arrange for a series of injections to desensitize against this particular substance. For further information on the general subject of allergy, see chapter 14, volume 3.

ATROPHIC RHINITIS (OZENA)

Atrophic rhinitis is a condition in which the membrane lining the nasal cavities deteriorates and develops crust formation, a foul odor, and a tendency to bleed. Loss of the sense of smell (anosmia) usually occurs. The exact cause is vague but presumably repeated infections are responsible.

Care and Treatment

Antibiotic medications in a salvelike combination applied directly to the nasal membranes may be of some help. In some cases, the placing of a small pledget of lamb's wool in each nostril reduces the tendency to crusting and minimizes the drying effect of the air as it passes through the nasal cavities.

VASOMOTOR RHINITIS

Vasomotor rhinitis is a condition in which chronic congestion of the nasal membranes occurs, usually associated with a certain amount of watery discharge from the nose. The condition is not caused by allergy and is not infectious. It occurs quite commonly, almost as commonly as allergic rhinitis. It affects persons of all ages and of both sexes. Persons with this problem seem to be particularly sensitive to such things as cold weather, spicy foods, strong odors, cigarette smoke, oral contraceptives, and even emotional disturbances. Presumably, the disturbance is caused by some imbalance in the autonomic nerve supply of the nasal membranes.

Care and Treatment

No specific cure exists for vasomotor rhinitis. Most persons with this problem have become accustomed to the use of nasal sprays and nose drops. Actually, these remedies do more harm than good, for the tiny blood vessels in the nasal membranes tend to dilate more than ever once the immediate effect of the nose drops has disappeared. Relief is best attained by avoiding the circumstances which seem to aggravate the symptoms.

Smoking, of course, should be avoided, as should contact with others' cigarette smoke.

C. Diseases of the Throat
Sore Throat

A sore throat is caused by inflammation of the mucous membrane that lines the pharynx and is manifested by discomfort in swallowing and talking.

Sore throat may be the result of local irritation of the pharynx, as from drinking irritating or excessively hot fluids, from smoking tobacco, or from using concentrated mouthwashes or antiseptic gargles.

Sore throat is a frequent prelude to the common cold. This acute pharyngitis is caused by an invasion of the pharynx by a virus along with the common types of germs (other than viruses) that invade the tissues once the virus has become established.

A serious form of sore throat is that caused by the streptococcus—so-called "strep throat." Here the tonsils, if still present, become infected, and the lymph nodes at the angles of the jaw become tender. See in this chapter, page 168.

The pharynx may become involved (with consequent sore throat) in a case of Vincent's infection of the mouth and gums. There is actual ulceration of the infected tissues. (See chapter 15, volume 2.)

Sore throat is a part of the initial illness in measles, scarlet fever, and whooping cough. It is an associated symptom in leukemia and infectious mononucleosis.

Tonsillitis and retropharyngeal abscess (see page 168 and this page respectively) cause the pharynx to be extremely sore and painful. The throat becomes sore when involved by such diseases as tuberculosis, syphilis, and cancer. We now describe the kinds of illness that commonly cause sore throat, along with treatment in each case:

ACUTE PHARYNGITIS
Any acute cold or catarrhal condition can affect the pharynx and cause inflammation and soreness. Loss of sleep, breathing stale or smoke-laden air, or almost any deviation from good health habits may bring a sore throat as one of the penalties. On the first day the patient usually feels increasing soreness and discomfort. By the second day his symptoms are usually worse if proper treatment has not been given.

Care and Treatment

If the sore throat is not known to be due to some underlying condition as mentioned above under Sore Throat, proceed as follows:

Gargle every half hour with hot water to which common salt and baking soda have been added, half a level teaspoonful of each to a glass of water.

Apply hot fomentations to the neck for 20 minutes two or three times a day. (See chapter 25, page 445, volume 3, for instruction on the use of fomentations.)

If fever is present, the patient should rest in bed.

Apply a heating compress to the patient's neck at night. (See chapter 25, volume 3, for instructions.)

The diet should consist of liquid or soft foods, and not less than three quarts of liquid should be taken each day.

If the soreness of the throat gets worse, or if it persists more than three days in spite of the above treatments, consult a physician.

RETROPHARYNGEAL ABSCESS
One possible complication of acute pharyngitis is the development of an abscess in the deeper tissues just behind the pharynx. Lymph nodes here function to control the spread of infection in the usual case of pharyngitis. When the infection is severe, these lymph nodes may be overwhelmed, allowing an abscess to form. This causes swelling and tenderness in the back wall of the throat, difficulty in swallowing and breathing, swollen glands in the

neck, and a nasal quality of the voice. In the acute cases there may be chills, fever, and stiffness of the neck.

Care and Treatment

The patient with retropharyngeal abscess should be under the supervision of a physician. The use of antibiotic drugs as prescribed by the physician may bring the infection under control. Once an actual abscess has formed, the pus which it contains must be removed. If the abscess is allowed to rupture on its own, danger threatens that the pus will be drawn into the air passages. Usually, the physician will prefer to drain the abscess by making a surgical incision.

STREPTOCOCCAL SORE THROAT (STREP THROAT)

This severe sore throat is caused by a strain of the hemolytic streptococcus similar to that which causes scarlet fever. In fact, very little difference exists between streptococcal sore throat and scarlet fever as far as the disease processes are concerned, there being in both a serious infection in the tissues of the pharynx. But in scarlet fever the patient experiences in addition, a skin rash caused by the effect of the toxin on the capillaries of the skin.

Streptococcal sore throat occurs both in isolated cases and in epidemics. The epidemics are usually caused by a streptococcal contamination of milk or milk products. Spread of the disease from person to person is usually by the contamination of food and drink with germs from the throat of someone ill with the disease.

The potent toxin produced in the infected tissues of the pharynx makes the patient very weak. The possible complications of streptococcal sore throat include arthritis, persistent infection of the lymph nodes in the neck, middle-ear infection, occasional infection of the lining of the heart (endocarditis), and damage to the kidneys.

Care and Treatment

As with other infections caused by the streptococcus, that of streptococcal sore throat is quite amenable to treatment by antibiotic drugs. Properly selected and administered, these reduce the severity of the illness and shorten its duration.

Nursing care of a patient with streptococcal sore throat should include the usual precautions for preventing the spread of the infection. Discharges from the mouth and nose are laden with the streptococcus germs and should be appropriately destroyed.

In the adult, soreness of the throat may be relieved by using a gargle containing 10 grains of aspirin to half a glass of warm water. In the child, the amount of aspirin in the gargle should be proportionately less.

The painful lymph nodes in the neck are best treated by the use of either hot or cold applications, depending upon which makes the patient more comfortable. Cold can be applied by the use of an ice collar for about 10 minutes out of each half hour. Heat can be applied by the use of fomentations (see chapter 25, volume 3).

It must be made certain that the patient drinks a sufficient quantity of fluid to enable him to produce copious quantities of urine. This forcing of fluids reduces the danger of damage to the kidneys. Remember that the patient is tempted to refuse fluid because his sore throat makes it difficult to swallow. If it is impossible for him to take enough fluid by mouth, a physician's instructions should be obtained relative to administering fluid by vein.

TONSILLITIS AND QUINSY

Tonsillitis consists of an inflammation of the tonsils, organs in the throat located on the right and left opposite the root of the tongue. This is a common disease, especially among children and young people. It is usually caused by the streptococcus germ or, sometimes, by viruses.

In acute tonsillitis the onset is often

accompanied by a chill and aching in the back and limbs. The fever may rise rapidly to as high as 104° F. (40° C.). The patient suffers intense soreness of the throat, with great difficulty in swallowing. The tongue is coated, and the breath is foul. The tonsils are swollen and red, and they may show yellowish or whitish patches on the surface. The neck glands are usually swollen. In some cases the entire throat is bright

Tonsillitis.

red, and there may be a red rash over the chest or the entire body. In such cases the infection is due to germs the same as, or similar to, those which cause scarlet fever.

Quinsy is often associated with tonsillitis. This illness consists of the development of an abscess in the bed of the tonsil or around it. The throat on one or both sides is greatly swollen. The patient suffers much pain and great difficulty in swallowing. The neck glands are swollen, and the victim can hardly open his mouth. Symptoms include high fever and great prostration.

For a discussion of tonsillitis during childhood and a consideration of the pros and cons for removing the tonsils, see chapter 17, volume 1.

Care and Treatment

For tonsillitis use hot or cold applications to the neck, whichever the patient tolerates best. For hot applications, narrow fomentations may be used. (See chapter 25, volume 3, for instruction in the use of fomentations.) Cold is best administered by a padded ice collar (an ice bag shaped to fit around the neck). Apply a heating compress to the neck at night. (See chapter 25, page 450, volume 3, for instructions.)

Use a hot gargle every hour. A suitable solution is prepared by dissolving half a teaspoonful of common salt and half a teaspoonful of baking soda in a glass of very warm water.

The use of antibiotics as arranged by the physician usually brings prompt improvement.

Plenty of water and fruit juices should be taken, preferably hot. A liquid diet should be taken for at least two or three days.

When quinsy develops, it is advisable that the abscess be drained by surgical incision.

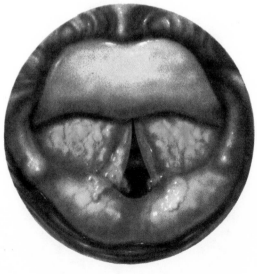

Laryngitis.
(See next page.)

Laryngitis

The larynx often becomes inflamed in association with acute pharyngitis or as part of a respiratory infection. Because the larynx actually belongs to the system of respiratory organs, laryngitis is considered in chapter 13, volume 2.

Cancer

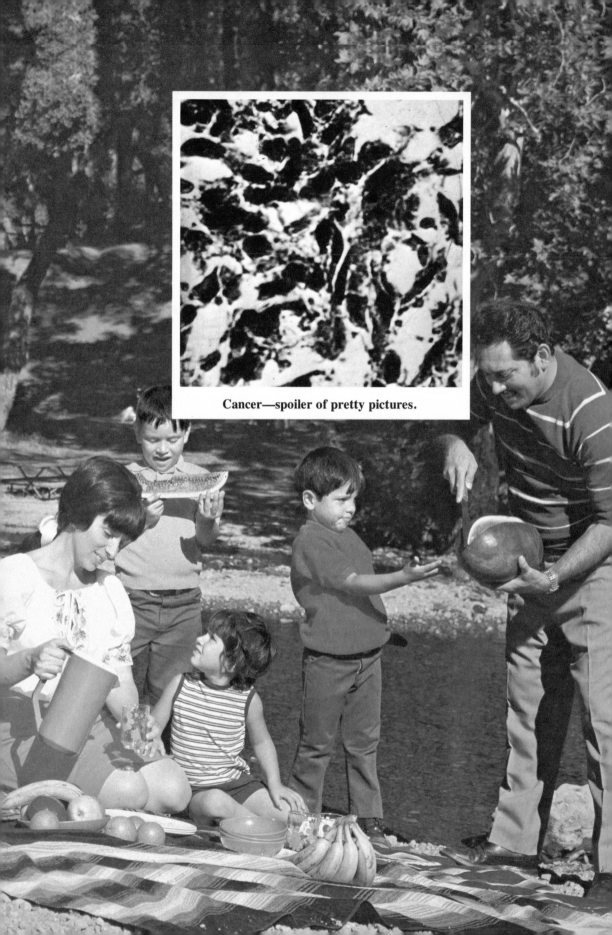

Cancer—spoiler of pretty pictures.

Characteristics of Cancer

Cancer is the second most common cause of death in the United States, being exceeded only by diseases of the heart. In two years cancer kills more Americans than the total number killed in four recent wars: World War I, World War II, the Korean conflict, and the Vietnam engagement. Each year cancer kills about seven times the number of Americans killed in automobile accidents.

For one recent year the estimated number of new cases of cancer in the United States totaled 1,260,000, of which almost one third were cancer of the skin. For this same year deaths from cancer came to an estimated 420,000, a number approximately equal to the population of Atlanta, Georgia. Cancer of the lung accounts for the largest number of cancer deaths among men, and cancer of the breast among women. Present trends indicate, however, that lung cancer will also soon top the list for women.

Cancer is a tragic disease, not only because of the large number of deaths, but because of its high toll of human agony and suffering. The cancer victim who has received the best treatment

that medical science can provide still continues in a state of uncertainty for weeks, and perhaps months. He is haunted by the knowledge that the results of cancer treatment are commonly given in terms of five-year survival rates. He wonders whether he will be alive at the end of five years and, if so, what then?

What Is Cancer?

A cancer is a kind of tumor that threatens life. So to understand the full meaning of the term *cancer* we must first explore the uses of the word *tumor*.

In its broad sense, a tumor means an abnormal enlargement of some part of the body. As usually used, the word refers to a mass of tissue composed of unusual cells that have multiplied more than they normally should, that are not a part of the body's normal design, and that serve no useful purpose. In this sense, the medical scientist prefers the term *neoplasm* (new growth) to the word *tumor*.

In the normal course of its development and growth, the human body maintains precise control over the

173

LEADING CAUSES OF DEATH IN THE UNITED STATES

Rank	Cause of Death	Number of Deaths	Percent of Total Deaths	Rank	Cause of Death	Number of Deaths	Percent of Total Deaths
	All Causes	1,927,788	100.0	8.	Cirrhosis of Liver	30,066	1.6
				9.	Arteriosclerosis	28,940	1.5
1.	Heart Diseases	729,510	37.8	10.	Suicide	27,294	1.4
2.	Cancer	396,922	20.6				
3.	Cerebrovascular			11.	Diseases of Infancy	22,033	1.1
	diseases (Stroke)	175,629	9.1	12.	Homicide	20,432	1.1
4.	Accidents	105,561	5.5	13.	Aortic Aneurysm	14,028	0.8
5.	Pneumonia & Influenza	58,319	3.0	14.	Congenital Anomalies	12,968	0.7
				15.	Pulmonary Infarction	10,941	0.6
6.	Chronic Obstructive						
	Lung Disease	50,488	2.6		Other & Ill-defined	210,606	10.8
7.	Diabetes Mellitus	33,841	1.8				

Source: American Cancer Society, *Ca—A Cancer Journal for Clinicians*, Jan/Feb 1983.

characteristics of the cells that compose its tissues. This control is mediated through the mysterious DNA molecules found in the nucleus of each one of the body's cells (see chapter 5, volume 2). The DNA molecules are "coded" to regulate the growth characteristics and activities of their respective cells, thus enabling them to work in cooperation with other cells.

As the body grows, beginning at conception and continuing to adulthood, the number of cells increases tremendously. This increase is carefully controlled so that only the proper number of each kind of cell is produced. But a developing neoplasm (tumor) is composed of cells which have multiplied irrespective of the body's normal checks and balances.

Tumors are subdivided into two large classes: benign and malignant. In the benign tumors the cells remain isolated from the surrounding tissues and grow within their own capsule. The word *benign* implies that this kind of tumor is harmless. But it does occupy space, and it therefore may cause trouble by exerting pressure on surrounding tissues. A fatty tumor which develops under the skin and which may cause a bump on the body's surface belongs to this benign class.

Malignant tumors are composed of cells so far out of control that they continue to multiply and invade the surrounding tissues. It is such a malignant tumor that is properly called a cancer. As a malignant tumor grows, it sends its processes like tentacles in many directions. As it invades other tissues, it often destroys them, usually by interfering with their supply of blood. Such destruction of the surrounding tissues may cause bleeding and ulceration.

The worst feature of malignant tumors (cancers) is that as their cells multiply and the tumor invades the surrounding tissues, small groups of these wild-growing cells may spread to other parts of the body. The cells may be carried by the bloodstream or the lymphatics, or they may adhere to the lining of body cavities. The new colony of wild cells will establish itself and develop a secondary tumor very much like the original one. The scientist speaks of this process of migration as metastasis. Often the metastatic tumors endanger the patient's life even more than the original tumor.

Most malignant tumors grow for a while at their site of origin before colonies of cells break away and move to some other region. From this observation we understand how important it is to treat a cancer early in the course of its development, before metastasis has taken place.

The specialty of medical science

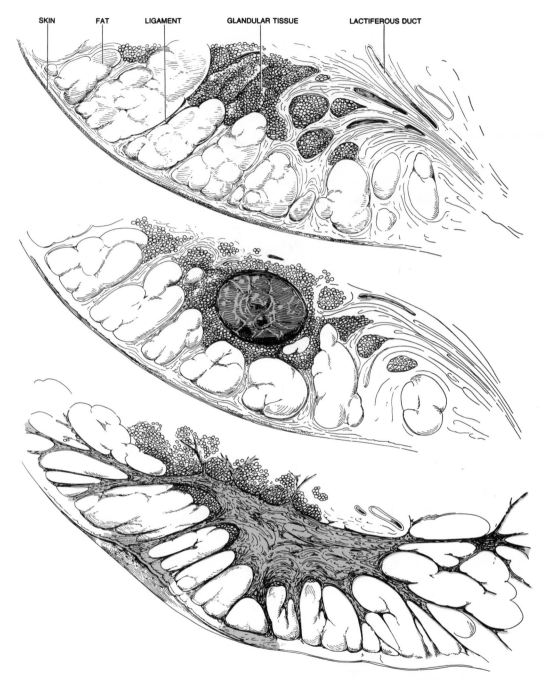

SKIN   FAT   LIGAMENT   GLANDULAR TISSUE   LACTIFEROUS DUCT

GROWTH OF A TUMOR in the breast ordinarily threatens life only when the tumor can spread to distant parts of the body. The normal breast *(top)* is organized into glandular tissue, fat, and other structures. Tumors arise almost exclusively in the glandular tissue. A benign tumor *(middle)* can grow rapidly and become quite large, but it cannot escape the tissue in which it develops. A cancerous tumor *(bottom)* can spread throughout the glandular tissue, can often involve ligaments and skin, and can sometimes penetrate the muscle underlying the breast. In addition cancers can in some cases migrate through the blood or the lymphatic system to establish new colonies of cells in distant, unrelated organs. This is the process known as metastasis.

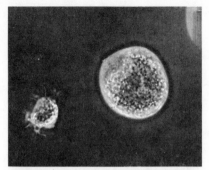

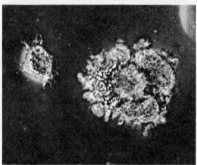

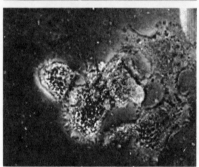

A time-lapse study of the division of a malignant cell, showing four stages of development and growth.

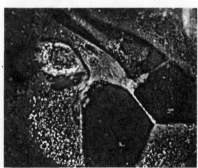

which deals with the identification and treatment of the various forms of cancer is called oncology.

Broad Classification of Cancers

As a cancer develops in some particular part of the body, its cells partake of the nature, more or less, of the normal cells of the tissue in which it originates. For this reason the various kinds of cancer roughly parallel the various kinds of normal tissue in which a malignant tumor may grow. Furthermore, out of a single kind of normal tissue may issue several patterns of abnormal development. Thus it would require several pages to list all the classes and subclasses of cancer that may develop in the human body. For our present purpose we need only to mention the major kinds:

1. *Carcinomas*. The carcinomas compose the largest group of cancers. They are the ones that originate from the epithelial cells that cover the body's surface, line its tubes and cavities, and compose the functioning cells of its glands.

2. *Leukemias*. These develop in the tissues which produce blood cells, such as the bone marrow and the lymph nodes.

3. *Lymphomas*. These cancers develop from the cells of the lymph glands.

4. *Sarcomas*. The sarcomas arise in the body's supporting tissues. Here we have the cancers that develop from fibrous tissue, from bone, from blood vessels, and from muscle tissue.

What Causes Cancer?

Fifty years ago it was assumed that in most cases cancer developed because of some hereditary fault. Instances were cited in which cancer developed in members of a certain family, appearing in one generation after another. Close relatives seemed to be vulnerable to the same kind of cancer.

Now we understand more about what happens in the cells when they undergo transformation to cancer cells. Because of a fault in the body's control mechanism the cells no longer conform to the normal pattern for the particular area of the body in which they reside. Something goes wrong in the chromosomes and genes. Was this change in the control mechanism passed from parent to child as something hereditary? Or did something happen during the present individual's life that damaged the control mechanism within certain of his cells?

In at least 80 percent of cancer cases something in the environment has triggered the changes that cause normal cells to become cancer cells. This understanding of environmental factors is an encouraging development, for it indicates that by removing the cancer-causing conditions in our surroundings, the number of cases of cancer will be reduced.

But heredity does play a part. Some people are inherently more susceptible to the environmental insults that cause cancer than others. Two persons may smoke the same number of cigarettes in a day and inhale just as deeply. One of these may develop lung cancer twenty years later, and the other may not. The woman whose female relatives have had breast cancer carries a three- to five-times greater risk of breast cancer than the woman with no such family history.

Predisposing Factors

By predisposing factors we refer to circumstances and conditions that increase the prospect of the development of cancer. We will group these under four headings: (1) physical agents, (2) chemical agents, (3) biological agents, and (4) circumstances of life and health.

1. *Physical Agents.* Excessive exposure to sunlight is an important predisposing factor to cancers of the skin. The solar keratoses (thickening of epidermal cells) which occur on those portions of the body exposed to the sun are the intermediate stage between normal skin and skin cancer. These occur commonly in farmers and sailors whose activities expose them to the ultraviolet radiation present in sunlight. The effect that sunlight has on the skin depends on the individual's complexion. Darker-skinned persons are not so susceptible, because the pigment in their skin serves to screen the skin's tissues from the effects of the ultraviolet radiation.

Exposure to radiation, as by X ray or by atomic radiation, increases a person's susceptibility to cancer. In the early days of X-ray equipment (around the turn of the century) unsuspecting physicians who worked with such equipment failed to take precautions now professionally routine. According to two scientific studies, physicians of that period who worked with X ray had ten times the incidence of leukemia (cancer of the blood-forming tissues) as did physicians in general.

It has been observed that women patients who receive unusually large doses of radiation therapy for the treatment of cancer of the cervix of the uterus may later develop cancer of the vagina.

It should be explained that modern physicians who deal with X ray know well the hazards and the precautions to be taken in the use of this type of radiation. They sometimes use X ray in the treatment of a malignant tumor. But they always weigh the hazards against the expected benefits and plan procedures accordingly. The usual exposure to X ray—as when X ray is used to reveal the roots of teeth, to show the position of bones in the body, or for other diagnostic studies—is kept well within the tolerance of the body's tissues and therefore does not predispose to cancer.

Long-continued irritation of any certain part of the body may predispose this part to the development of cancer. For example, cancer of the lip occurs quite commonly among pipe smokers. Presumably it is the heat of the pipestem that makes the tissues vulnerable.

Cancer may develop in scars that

177

have been caused by corrosive damage to the skin. The irritating effect of gallstones on the tissues of the gallbladder may make this organ vulnerable. Kidney stones may have a similar effect on the tissues at the outlet of the kidney. The long-continued destructive influence in ulcerative colitis makes the colon more susceptible to the development of cancer.

2. *Chemical Agents.* A great deal of public attention has been focused by the media and otherwise on the possible cancer-causing effects of certain food additives and other chemical substances used in popular drug preparations. Saccharine and cyclamate have taken their turn at being condemned by the government's Food and Drug Administration.

The usual method by which substances are tested to determine any possible carcinogenic properties requires a carefully planned laboratory procedure in which two groups of animals are treated exactly the same, except that one group receives measured and fairly large doses of the substance to be tested. The animals and their progeny are observed over many months. If the treatment group develops cancers and the control group does not, it is declared that the substance being tested is a carcinogen.

This manner of identifying carcinogens has, however, raised questions hard to answer: Would humans react the same as the animals being tested? Would the animals have developed cancer if they had received smaller doses—doses comparable to what a human would ordinarily receive? Do humans possibly have a threshold of tolerance by which small doses do no harm?

According to present policy, the Food and Drug Administration will not approve a substance for human consumption that in a carefully conducted laboratory test has caused cancer in animals. But people may be either more or less sensitive than test animals. The mere fact that the test animals developed cancer does not, of itself, mean that humans would do the same under usual circumstances.

Epidemiological studies of humans (studies of populations) have provided much valuable information regarding the substances that may predispose to cancer. But with most carcinogens a delay period (often as long as 20 years) after exposure must ensue before cancer develops.

Many industrial chemicals are known to predispose to cancer. Coal tar and creosote preparations are used in the laboratory to produce skin cancer in animals. They have a similar effect on industrial workers exposed to these substances. Arsenic preparations, even when taken internally, cause skin cancer in humans. Another industrial hazard is aniline dyes. After continued exposure, workers with aniline dyes are particularly susceptible to cancer of the urinary bladder. It is presumed that the bladder is the vulnerable organ because the offending chemical substances are eliminated by way of the urine. Asbestos is a hazard to those who work with it. Certain industrial solvents and some components used in the manufacture of plastics are carcinogenic.

Persons being given immunosuppressive drugs have higher-than-usual susceptibility to cancer. These are the drugs used to suppress the body's mechanisms which would otherwise cause rejection of a transplanted organ. Susceptibility does not mean, however, that immunosuppressive drugs should not be used. Not all persons, by far, who receive such drugs will develop cancer. Their use is lifesaving for a person who would die were he not to receive the transplant of a healthy organ. The body's immune mechanism is an important part of its ability to resist disease of various kinds. It is understandable that when the immune mechanism is suppressed, the tissues throughout the body are less able than usual to resist the development of cancer.

Those who use alcohol have a higher incidence of cancer of the liver, larynx, and esophagus, than do nondrinkers. The exact influence of alcohol is difficult to determine. For one reason, drinkers nearly always also smoke. Thus, when cancer develops, it is uncertain whether the alcohol or the cigarette smoke is the culprit. Some authorities class alcohol as a cocarcinogen, meaning that its effect is to amplify the influence of other conditions that predispose to cancer. Also, some popular alcoholic beverages contain additives. Is it the alcohol or some additive that does the damage?

Cigarette smoking is now the greatest single cause of cancer, being responsible for one in every four cancer deaths, as of 1982. Smoking is the culprit in about 90 percent of the cases of lung cancer, as well as being implicated as a precipitating cause of cancer in other parts of the body and of other diseases besides cancer. In a recent year lung cancer was the cause of death in 88,000 cases—up threefold from thirty years ago. Lung cancer is the leading cause of cancer deaths among men and the second most frequent cause of deaths among women. The prospect of developing lung cancer is ten times greater for the cigarette smoker than for the nonsmoker, and 40 times greater if he has smoked forty cigarettes a day for twenty years or more.

The smoking of cigarettes increases the incidence of cancer in all the tissues bathed by the smoke stream as well as in some tissues that have no direct contact with the smoke. It is difficult to know just which components of cigarette smoke are responsible for the several effects of smoking on the human body. Presumably it is the tars that increase the susceptibility to lung cancer. The smoke is irritating, however, to all of the tissues with which it has contact: the mouth, the pharynx, the larynx, the trachea, the bronchi, and the delicate air sacs of the lungs. Smoking also increases the risk of cancer of the esophagus, possibly because the saliva swallowed carries with it some of the constituents of tobacco smoke.

Cancer of the urinary bladder is significantly more common among smokers than among nonsmokers. The probable explanation is that certain constituents of tobacco smoke are transferred to the blood and eventually eliminated through the kidneys and the bladder. As the urine accumulates in the bladder, these constituents have a sufficient irritating influence to predispose to cancer of this organ.

3. *Biological Agents.* Much has been written and spoken about viruses as the fundamental cause of cancer—at least certain kinds of cancer: (1) certain kinds of cancer can be induced in animals by inoculating viruses that have been derived from animals that have these kinds of cancer, and (2) the tissues of some human cancer patients contain antibodies which, presumably, were developed to combat a certain kind of virus.

Even so, scientists who specialize in cancer research find no conclusive evidence that infection by viruses is the inciting cause of cancer in humans. Then what is the role of viruses in relation to cancer?

The present understanding is that it takes at least two cancer-producing agents, working side by side, to produce a cancer. The mere presence of a cancer-related virus in a person's body will not, of itself, produce cancer. Under normal conditions the body produces antibodies to combat such a virus. It takes some additional factor which either lowers the body's protective mechanisms or compounds the insult to the body's tissues to trigger the transformation of normal cells to cancer cells.

This recognition of multiple predisposing factors has great practical value. A person cannot avoid the entrance of viruses into his body. But he can avoid many predisposing factors. He can follow a life-style that promotes physical fitness and augments his body's defenses against disease. It is said that our present knowledge is sufficient to enable us, if we will, to avoid more than half the usual risks of cancer.

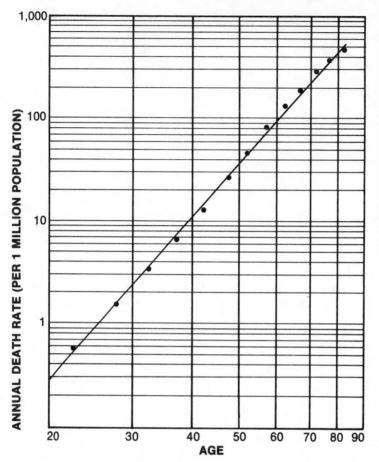

OLD PEOPLE compose the subpopulation that is most conspicuously at risk in the development of cancer. The incidence of almost all forms of cancer increases dramatically with advancing age. Here the U.S. death rate from a representative cancer, that of the large intestine, is plotted against age. It can be seen that the logarithm of the death rate is linearly related to the logarithm of age. The relation can be explained by the hypothesis that several mutations are required to generate a cancer, and that the probability of each mutation is proportional to age. The slope of the line suggests that the number of mutations required is five.

From *Scientific American*, November 1975, p. 67.

4. Circumstances of Life and Health. Certain circumstances of life alter a person's susceptibility to cancer. As examples, note the following:

Age. Two important considerations relate to age: (1) the manifestations of cancer typical of early childhood and (2) the increasing susceptibility to cancer among adults as age increases.

Infectious diseases in former years caused more deaths among children, by far, than did cancer. But now that the infectious diseases are under control, childhood cancer, in ages 1 to 14, causes the most deaths, except for those caused by accidents.

More deaths from childhood cancer occur during the first five years of life than during the next two five-year periods combined. Many cancers affect-

ing young children occur in areas in which the development of the component cells did not reach full maturity. So some of these malignant tumors of early childhood are carry-overs from embryonic life. The organs commonly affected are the blood-producing tissues (with resulting leukemia), the brain and other parts of the nervous system, the eye, the adrenal glands, muscle tissue, bone, and kidney.

The likelihood of cancer increases, year by year, throughout adulthood. Many predisposing factors require an extended time to bring about malignant changes in normal cells. Cancers resulting from exposure to industrial chemicals may occur many years later. The varied damaging effects of tobacco often appear more than 20 years after the individual began to smoke.

CHARACTERISTICS OF CANCER

Cancer Statistics by Site and Sex 1983

The estimates of the incidence of cancer are based upon data from the National Cancer Institute's Surveillance, Epidemiology and End Results (SEER) Program (1973-1979). Nonmelanoma skin cancer and carcinoma in situ have not been included in the statistics. Prepared by Edwin Silverberg, Supervisor, Statistical Information Services, Department of Epidemiology and Statistics, American Cancer Society, New York, New York.

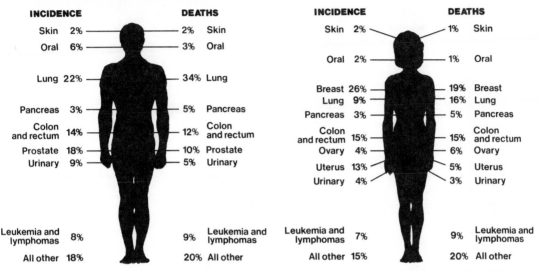

INCIDENCE		DEATHS		INCIDENCE		DEATHS	
Skin	2%	2%	Skin	Skin	2%	1%	Skin
Oral	6%	3%	Oral	Oral	2%	1%	Oral
Lung	22%	34%	Lung	Breast	26%	19%	Breast
				Lung	9%	16%	Lung
Pancreas	3%	5%	Pancreas	Pancreas	3%	5%	Pancreas
Colon and rectum	14%	12%	Colon and rectum	Colon and rectum	15%	15%	Colon and rectum
Prostate	18%	10%	Prostate	Ovary	4%	6%	Ovary
Urinary	9%	5%	Urinary	Uterus	13%	5%	Uterus
				Urinary	4%	3%	Urinary
Leukemia and lymphomas	8%	9%	Leukemia and lymphomas	Leukemia and lymphomas	7%	9%	Leukemia and lymphomas
All other	18%	20%	All other	All other	15%	20%	All other

American Cancer Society, *Ca—A Cancer Journal for Clinicians*, Jan/Feb 1983

Sex. The manifestations of cancer among adult men differ somewhat from those in adult women. The accompanying charts indicate that, for men, lung cancer is not only the most commonly occurring cancer, but also the one that causes the greatest number of deaths. For women, it is breast cancer, as yet, that accounts for the greatest number of cancer cases and the greatest number of deaths.

Marital State. Cancer of the breast is less common among married women than among unmarried. Also, the woman who has her first child before age 25 has a smaller risk of breast cancer than does the woman who has her first child after age 35.

With cancer of the cervix of the uterus, the influence of marriage is in the opposite direction. Women married in their teens or who have their first sexual intercourse while still in their teens have a greater prospect of cancer of the uterine cervix than those married when in their twenties or those who never marry.

Prevention of Cancer

At the present rate, one out of every four people will experience some form of cancer during his lifetime. Only one out of three cancer victims (excluding those with ordinary skin cancer) will survive for five years. No wonder, then, the universal demand that scientists make faster progress in developing a "cure" for cancer.

The concept of this chapter indicates that the problem of cancer is so complex that there will probably never be a single, simple remedy that will serve as a cure for all kinds of cancer. But something more important than merely finding a cure—especially for a disease that will probably leave the patient maimed or handicapped even though his life is spared—consists in applying knowledge already available to prevent cancer in the first place. About 90 percent of the cases of cancer result from predisposing factors in the environment. If, as a nation, we were to apply what we know about avoiding these factors, at least half the usual number of cancer cases could be prevented.

Age-Adjusted Cancer Death Rates* for Selected Sites, Females, United States, 1930-1978

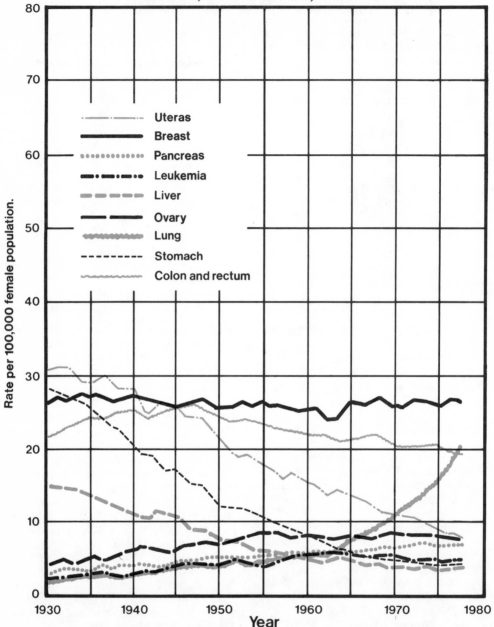

Sources of Data: U.S. National Center for Health Statistics and U.S. Bureau of the Census.
*Adjusted to the age distribution of the 1970 U.S. Census Population.

American Cancer Society, *Ca—A Cancer Journal for Clinicians,* Jan/Feb 1983

A sharp increase in lung cancer among women in recent years and a concomitant decrease in cancer of the colon and rectum show the current incidence of the two about equal. Moreover, the upward trend for lung cancer indicates that it may soon exceed the incidence of breast cancer.

It is a matter of priority. It is natural for a person to assume, "It won't happen to me." It is easy to go merrily on, ignoring the precautions that should be taken. The circumstances that set the stage for cancer are discussed in the previous sections of this chapter. The means of preventing cancer consist simply of avoiding as many of these predisposing factors as possible.

It is true that older persons are more susceptible to cancer than younger people. But an elderly person can be alert to the danger signals, and, realizing that his age places him at greater risk, he can arrange for frequent examinations which make early detection and treatment possible.

Similarly, a woman successfully treated for cancer of one breast should realize the greater risk she faces of having cancer in the other breast, or in some other part of the body, as compared with the person who has never had cancer. Accordingly, she should keep in close contact with her doctor and arrange for whatever periodic examinations he suggests.

The use of cigarettes is now the greatest single predisposing factor to cancer. Smokers are ten times more susceptible to lung cancer than nonsmokers. They are ten times more susceptible to cancer of the larynx. Cancer of the esophagus occurs four times as frequently in smokers as in nonsmokers. Cancer of the pancreas, liver, and bile passages occurs almost three times as frequently among smokers as in nonsmokers. Even cancer of the bladder is twice as common among smokers. As Dr. Brian MacMahon of the Harvard School of Public Health so aptly stated, "No single known measure would lengthen the life or improve the health of the American population more than eliminating cigarette smoking."

The hazard of smoking is compounded in the smoker who also drinks. Not only does alcohol have its own detrimental effect in predisposing to cancer of certain parts of the body, but the risk of cancer in the person who both smokes and drinks is greater than the sum of the risk factors of each of these habits by itself. The risk of cancer for someone who both drinks and smokes heavily is more than fifteen times as great as for the person who neither drinks nor smokes.

Even the food a person eats has its influence. A report made at the 1982 session of the National Academy of Sciences indicates that persons who eat foods that have been smoked or grilled or that have been pickled or salt-cured, have a higher-than-usual predisposition to cancer, especially to that of the esophagus and stomach. Another study indicates that even coffee, used to excess, may contribute to the possibility of cancer of the bladder. Certain food additives, particularly dyes and artificial sweeteners, possibly increase one's susceptibility to cancer.

Early Detection of Cancer

Next best to preventing cancer is being alert for signs of beginning cancer. The type of examination necessary to check for cancer and the frequency of such examinations depend on one's sex and age. The suggestions for such routine examinations are included in chapter 2, volume 2. Under certain circumstances, however, this suggested program for repeated examinations should be modified. It is possible that the signs of beginning cancer will appear between times. It is important, whenever any of the danger signs make their appearance, that the individual's doctor be informed. See the accompanying chart "Cancer Danger Signals."

High-risk persons should have more frequent examinations than those with an average risk. The high-risk category includes smokers, those whose immediate relatives have had some form of cancer, those who have already had one experience with cancer even though the bout may have resulted in a "cure," and those in whom more than one of the usual predisposing factors are present.

If You Have Cancer

When a person learns that he or she

CANCER DANGER SIGNALS

The telltale symptoms listed in the right-hand column suggest the possibility of cancer in the organs named on the left. When the symptoms appear, arrange promptly for an examination by your doctor.

Bladder	Blood in urine; increase in the frequency of urination.
Bone	Local pain and tenderness; unusual thickening on the bone; walking with an unexplained limp.
Blood (leukemia)	Vague symptoms: fever, pallor, bleeding into the tissues.
Breast	Lump or deformity in the breast or nipple.
Cervix	Abnormal bleeding, spotting with blood, or abnormal discharge.
Colon and Rectum	Bleeding by rectum, change in bowel habits.
Esophagus	Difficulty in swallowing.
Kidney (in adult)	Blood in the urine (usually without pain); loss of appetite, fatigue, and loss of weight.
Kidney (in three-year-old or younger)	Firm, painless mass in one side of abdomen.
Larynx	Sudden, unexplained, progressive hoarseness; later, difficult breathing.
Lip	Warty growth; crusting ulcer or fissure (resting on a disk-like, firm area).
Lung	Cough (particularly different from the usual smoker's cough); transient sneezing. Later, blood-spitting.
Mouth and Tongue	An area of roughening; mild burning when eating highly seasoned foods. Later, ulceration.
Skin	A ''pimple'' or small sore fails to heal and gradually enlarges; an old skin lesion now begins to grow; a persistent lesion crusts but bleeds when the crust is removed; an old wart or mole changes size or color.
Stomach	Persistent distress in upper abdomen, loss of appetite, loss of weight.
Uterus	Episodes of vaginal bleeding unrelated to menstruation.

NOTE:
Most cancers are not painful, at least in their early stages. Thousands of cancer victims have lost their lives needlessly because they waited too long before seeing their doctor—thinking that their lesion could not be cancer because it was not painful.

Some cancers do not give a warning signal; they develop ''silently.'' In these the best prospects of cure have passed by the time the symptoms appear. Hence the advice: SEE YOUR PHYSICIAN FOR A PERIODIC CANCER CHECKUP.

has cancer, the first reaction is usually one of consternation or even panic. Previously this person has thought of cancer as a dread disease that picks out people here and there and renders them candidates for unpleasant types of treatment and possibly for invalidism or premature death. "But it can't happen to me," the person thinks.

Even though it is hard for a person to adjust to the reality, it is important that he do something quickly. To delay may make the difference between early treatment and survival, and unnecessary, premature death. Time is of the essence. Cancer moves on relentlessly.

Sometimes doubt intrudes as to whether cancer is really present. But uncertainty and vacillation under such circumstances can be fatal. If any reasonable basis for doubt exists, the patient should ask his doctor to arrange for a second opinion from some other physician. Or perhaps he should arrange for a diagnostic study at a reputable medical center. The cost of such a study is surely justified, inasmuch as life is at stake. But time must not be wasted!

Face the Facts. If you are the one involved and it has been confirmed that you have cancer, share this knowledge with your family members and with your friends. Do not ask for sympathy, but tell them how you feel about it. Confide your fears and ask for their reactions on how you should relate yourself to the uncertainty you face. Sharing your problem helps you to muster the courage to make wise plans and to face the possibility of an unpleasant treatment program.

Plan Realistically. Set yourself the task of becoming well informed about the particular kind of cancer you have. Contact the American Cancer Society, 777 Third Avenue, New York, NY 10017, and ask them to send you information on cancer in general and, particularly, on the kind you have. Request the name, telephone number, and address of the office of the American Cancer Society nearest you.

Discipline yourself to face the prospect that the treatment of your cancer may not be successful. You may recover and you may not. Do not allow your thoughts to dwell too much on the gruesome side of the picture, but think of it and mention it sufficiently so that you gain control of your emotions. Make two plans for your immediate future: one in case the treatment is successful and the other in case it is not. Arrange your personal affairs and your commitments accordingly.

Cooperate in an early, intensive treatment program. The physician who has confirmed your diagnosis of cancer will have a suggestion on the kind of treatment you should have. However, he may not be the one to administer it. Of the several kinds of treatment, some are adapted to one form of cancer and some to others. Some kinds of cancer require a combination of treatment procedures.

Place yourself in the hand of a specialist in whom you have confidence. How do you locate such a specialist? Your family doctor can be of help. Also, you can obtain counsel directly from the American Cancer Society. If you have received a diagnostic study at a reputable medical center, the physician who has been in charge of your case can give you sound advice.

Once your treatment is started, make sure that you cooperate completely. Do not keep secrets from your doctor. Do not deviate from the treatment program without his knowledge and approval. If you feel that you are not tolerating the treatment, talk to him about it.

Beware of nostrums. The problem of cancer lends itself to exploitation by unscrupulous persons who claim to have access to a "cure" for cancer. "Cancer cures" have come and gone for as long as there has been a recognition of cancer. Cancer still persists, but promoted cures have run their courses and disappeared.

It is very tempting to a person with cancer who has just listened to his doctor's explanation of the seriousness of his illness and of its uncertain outcome, to grasp at a straw by listening to the confident promises of some irregular practitioner who reports marvelous results from some "new discovery."

Laetrile, actively promoted in the 1970s, became the most widely known and the most highly acclaimed of all "cancer cures." It was heralded as a "natural remedy" and as "the missing vitamin." Derived from apricot seeds, the active ingredient of laetrile is amygdalin, a chemical which contains 6 percent cyanide by weight. A single 500 mg. dose of laetrile contains enough cyanide to kill a person if the cyanide were released from its chemical combination. Fortunately, most of a dose of laetrile is excreted from the body without being broken into its constituents. However, one eleven-month-old child died of cyanide poisoning after having swallowed about five laetrile tablets taken from her father's supply.

A study of nearly 200 cases of laetrile treatment made by independent analysts failed to reveal a single case in which there was a clear-cut anticancer benefit. The promoters did well financially. Laetrile costs very little to produce, but the tablets sold for more than a dollar each. The documented bank deposits of one promoter totaled $2.5 million within a 27-month period.

Every reputable physician keeps up to date in his understanding of medical progress. He reads medical journals and attends lectures. He has channels of communication by which he can make inquiry of the leading medical authorities on whatever subject he desires. He is therefore in a position to guide his patient in obtaining the best kind of treatment.

The tragedy of irregular cancer cures is that they tempt the cancer patient to neglect the accepted methods of treatment, while, in the meantime, his cancer reaches the dangerous stage in which conventional treatments are no longer effective. Thus, many lives have been unnecessarily sacrificed.

Kinds of Treatment for Cancer

Several forms of treatment for cancer are now available: (1) *surgery,* in which the cancerous lesion and the surrounding tissue are removed; (2) *irradiation therapy,* in which the cancer is penetrated by X rays or other forms of radiation; (3) *chemotherapy,* in which potent drugs are used as medications; and (4) *hormone therapy*, in which hormones or their synthetic counterparts are used as medications to suppress the growth of the cancer. Many medical scientists have looked forward to the development of *immunotherapy,* in which a person could be protected from developing cancer by immunization comparable to what is used to prevent some of the infectious diseases. But immunotherapy for cancer is still in the experimental stage.

The protein interferon has attracted the attention of medical scientists because of its ability to stimulate the immune system. Most of the experimental work thus far has been with animals, and it has yet to be determined whether it may have the capacity to aid in the treatment of cancer in humans.

The examples which follow show how these treatments are used against particular types of cancer.

No uniformly effective treatment for lung cancer exists. But early surgical removal of the affected portion of the lung, sometimes supplemented by irradiation therapy and/or chemotherapy, saves up to about 10 percent of cases.

For cancer of the breast the recent trend is to use surgery conservatively and then follow with irradiation therapy (to kill cancer cells that may remain in the region of the breast) and chemotherapy (to suppress or prevent the growth of cancer cells that may have already migrated to other parts of the body).

With the leukemias (cancer of the blood-forming tissues) chemotherapy, sometimes supplemented by irradiation therapy, gives the best results.

Hormone therapy is especially useful

Age-Adjusted Cancer Death Rates* for Selected Sites, Males, United States, 1930-1978

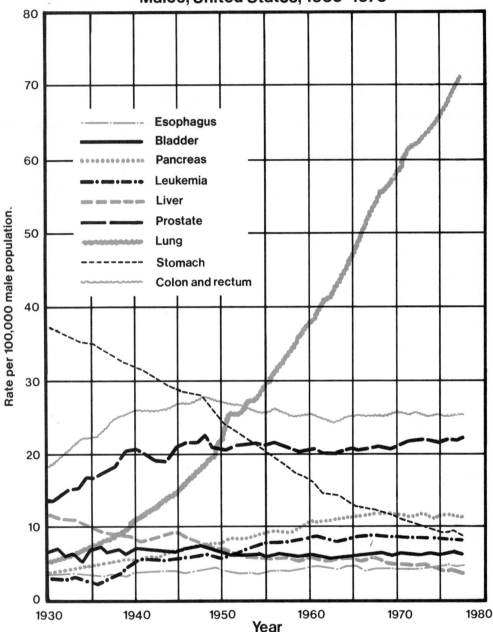

Esophagus
Bladder
Pancreas
Leukemia
Liver
Prostate
Lung
Stomach
Colon and rectum

Rate per 100,000 male population.

Year

Sources of Data: U.S. National Center for Health Statistics and U.S. Bureau of the Census. *Adjusted to the age distribution of the 1970 U.S. Census Population.

American Cancer Society, *Ca—A Cancer Journal for Clinicians,* Jan/Feb 1983

Cancer of the lung has increased sharply during recent years in the United States, currently accounting for more deaths in men than from cancer in any other part of the body.

in treating such cancers as that of the prostate.

With cancer in other locations, choice must be made among the various methods of treatment, with selection of the method or the combination of methods that gives the particular patient the best opportunity for prolonged life.

Progress Report

Education of the public regarding cancer and how to detect it early, coupled with better methods of treatment, are largely responsible for improved survival rates. Take cancer of the cervix of the uterus. Most women now understand that Pap tests performed at regular intervals will indicate whether dangerous changes are taking place in the cervix. Early detection and prompt treatment have reduced the death rate from this kind of cancer to one third of what it was forty years ago.

There has been a substantial improvement in the survival rate in cases of breast cancer, thanks to the custom of monthly self-examination of the breasts and prompt reporting of lumps.

The increasing use of the simple test for hidden blood in the stool has improved the survival rate in cases of cancer of the colon and rectum, because these cases now come to treatment earlier than they used to.

Survival rates have improved for cancers of the bladder, the lining of the uterus, and the prostate. But a long way remains yet to go before cancer is conquered. Future progress depends not only on continued medical research but on the consistent efforts of people to avoid those conditions and personal customs which predispose to cancer and to be continuously on the lookout for the first signs of developing cancer.

Manifestations of Cancer

In this chapter we list, in alphabetical order, the various parts of the body in which cancer may occur and describe its characteristics in these various locations.

BILE DUCTS

The bile ducts may become involved either with cancer within the ducts or with cancer in neighboring structures. The earliest symptom is usually jaundice (manifested by a yellowing of the whites of the eyes and of the skin), an abnormality caused by obstruction to the flow of bile. Surgical treatment of cancer in this location is difficult, partly because of no alternate route for the flow of bile and partly because the cancer is usually advanced before the diagnosis is made.

BLADDER (URINARY BLADDER)

Exposure to certain chemicals such as naphthalenes, aniline dyes, or benzidines predisposes to cancer of the bladder. These substances may be taken into the body by various routes but are eventually eliminated through the urinary system and thus appear in the urine as it is stored in the bladder. Cancer of the bladder often develops as a consequence of cigarette smoking because certain irritating substances in tobacco smoke are eliminated from the body through the urinary system.

The usual earliest sign of cancer of the bladder is blood in the urine (hematuria), often accompanied by pain. Cancer is not the only cause of blood in the urine, but whenever this symptom occurs, it should prompt examination of the urinary system to determine the cause of the bleeding.

Treatment of cancer of the bladder by surgery or by a combination of surgery and irradiation is quite successful when the cancer is detected and treated in its early stages.

BLOOD

The disease leukemia, in which the tissues which form blood cells become involved, is classed as a cancer of the blood-forming tissues. See the discussion of leukemia in chapter 10, volume 2.

BONE

Cancer of the bone may originate within the bone itself, it may have spread to the bone from cancer in adjacent structures, or it may develop secondarily when a colony of cancer cells is carried by the blood from a cancer in some other part of the body (by metastasis). Cancer of the bone typically

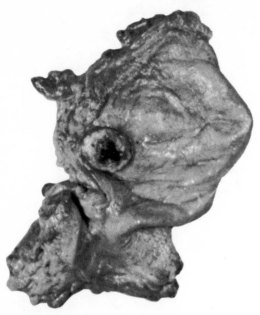

Cancer of the bladder.

causes considerable local pain and also a weakening of the bone so that it fractures easily (pathologic fracture). The treatment of cancer of the bone is difficult and may require radical surgery, irradiation therapy, or chemotherapy.

BRAIN

The largest number of cases of cancer of the brain occur during childhood. Of all cases of childhood cancer, an estimated 19 percent involve the brain and/or other parts of the central nervous system.

Many cancers of the brain are said to be primary because they originate right in the brain substance. Others are classed as secondary or metastatic because a colony of cancer cells has migrated to the brain from a cancer in some other part of the body—most commonly from the lung or the breast.

A cancer developing within the brain is usually in the nature of a tumor that occupies more space than the normal tissue. Inasmuch as the brain is enclosed by the bony skull, a developing brain tumor typically produces abnormal pressure within the skull, which ac-

counts for many of the symptoms of brain cancer. This increased pressure affects everything within the skull, not just the area where the cancer is developing. Therefore, many of the symptoms do not give an accurate clue to the location of the cancer.

The most common symptom of cancer within the skull is headache, mild and intermittent at first, but becoming more severe and persistent. Then nausea and vomiting usually develop, along with drowsiness. The mental changes may include apathy, irritability, depression, and disturbances of consciousness. In about 50 percent of cases convulsive seizures develop at one time or another. A tumor in the area of the pituitary gland (at the base of the brain) usually produces significant disturbances in vision. In another area, toward the back of the brain, a developing tumor will cause disturbances of hearing and of equilibrium.

The patient with symptoms as above should be placed under the care of a physician who specializes in neurology or in brain surgery. Of the several tests and examinations that may be used to determine whether a brain cancer is present, the newer method of brain scan (computed axial tomography) is probably the most useful and accurate. It involves a sophisticated method of examination by X ray.

As with cancers in other locations, so with those of the brain: the earlier the diagnosis and treatment, the better the prospect for the patient's recovery. The specialty of brain surgery has made remarkable progress during recent years, and the lives of many patients with brain cancer can be spared by surgical removal of the involved area of the brain. In some cases, further treatment by irradiation is helpful.

BREAST

The breast is the most common site of cancer in women, there being about 110,000 new cases a year in the United States and more than 37,000 deaths per year (data from the American Cancer Society, 1981).

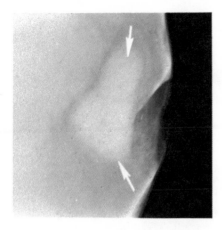

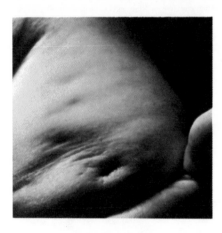

Top: X ray of axillary lymph nodes. A proven case of carcinoma of the breast with axillary metastases. Center: Adenocarcinoma, left breast. Below: Cancer of the breast, late stages of development.

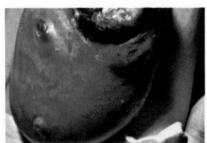

Cancer of the breast is treacherous because it tends to spread early to distant parts of the body. When breast cancer is detected before colonies of cancer cells have migrated to other areas, treatment by surgery and irradiation is quite successful.

Progress during recent years in reducing the mortality rate from cancer of the breast stems largely from early detection and adequate treatment. Women are becoming aware of the tragic outcome of a lump in the breast. By reporting this finding at once to her physician, a woman can receive the benefits of early treatment.

Only about one lump in five discovered in the breast proves to be caused by cancer. But this does not mean that a lump may be safely ignored, for the hazard of delay is so great that any lump discovered in the breast should be reported promptly.

In many instances the physician cannot determine by a simple examination whether a lump in the breast is cancerous or benign. So he removes a small portion of the tissue and arranges for a microscopic examination by a pathologist. If this biopsy specimen proves benign, the surgeon then performs a simple surgery to remove the lump. If, however, the biopsy examination indicates a beginning cancer, the entire breast should be removed, together with any lymph nodes in the axilla (armpit) that seem to have been already affected. This is the so-called modified radical surgical procedure for breast cancer, which spares the muscles located beneath the breast. This procedure may be followed by irradiation. If it appears that the cancer has already spread to other parts of the body by metastasis, the physician will determine the appropriate use of chemotherapy, irradiation, and surgery.

A lump in the breast may develop quickly without attracting particular attention. It may develop between the times of the periodic checkups at the doctor's office. So it is now advocated that women learn the method of self-examination of the breast, as here illus-

191

Breast Self-examination

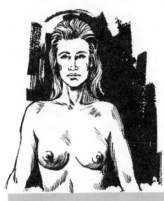

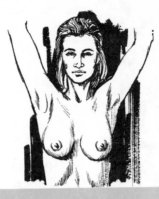

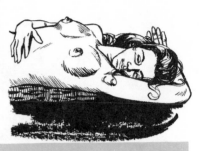

1. Examination of breasts before a mirror for symmetry in size and shape, noting any puckering of skin or retraction of nipple.

2. Arms raised over head, again studying breasts in the mirror for the same signs.

3. Reclining on bed with flat pillow or folded bath towel under shoulder on same side as breast to be examined.

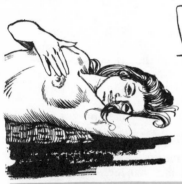

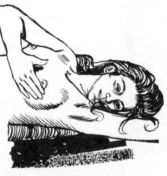

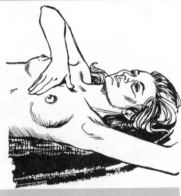

4. To examine inner half of the breast, arm is raised. Beginning at breastbone and working out, inner half of breast is palpated.

5. The area over and around the nipple is carefully palpated with flats of the fingers.

6. Continuing thus to palpate, examination of lower inner half of the breast is completed.

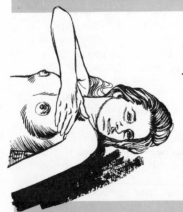

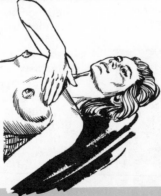

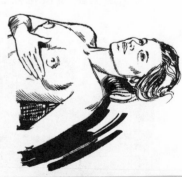

7. With arm down at side, palpation continues with examination of tissues extending to armpits.

8. The upper outer quadrant of the breast is examined with the flat part of the fingers.

9. The lower outer quadrant of the breast is likewise examined in successive stages.

trated, doing it once a month—this in addition to the periodic physical examination by a physician. Of course when a woman discovers a lump, painless though it be, she should report it at once to her doctor. In doing the self-examination she should lie on her back and should use the flat surface of the palm and fingers (not their tips) as she carefully and systematically presses the various parts of each breast against the muscles and ribs which lie beneath.

When a malignant lump in the breast is still small and when it receives adequate treatment promptly (within days rather than months), the prospect of five-year survival is about 85 percent.

In older women, past the menopause, any discharge from the nipple (primarily bloody in nature) is a serious omen and should be reported promptly to the physician. It may be the first indication of a beginning cancer.

CERVIX OF THE UTERUS
See under UTERUS in this chapter, pages 200-202.

COLON AND RECTUM
Cancer in the terminal part of the intestine strikes about 120,000 new victims each year in the United States, and about half of these will eventually die of this disease. Cancer of the colon and rectum seldom develops in persons younger than 40 years of age.

As with cancer in other parts of the body, treatment begun early obtains the best results. Cancer in this location may have been developing for some time before it causes symptoms. The symptoms consist of bleeding from the rectum, changes in bowel habits (which persist more than two weeks), or of persisting discomfort in the abdomen. Many cases of cancer of the colon and rectum are discovered incidentally at the time of a routine physical examination. The means by which the physician can discover this kind of cancer are these: finger examination of the rectum, the use of the sigmoidoscope in examining the terminal portion of the colon, and by testing the stool for the presence of hidden blood.

Cancers in the colon and rectum are relatively uncommon among people in the so-called underdeveloped countries. Dr. Dennis Burkitt, a British surgeon, showed that the diet of primitive peoples contains considerable fiber and very little sugar. It is suggested, therefore, that even healthy persons should include in their diet foods that contain dietary fiber—fruits, vegetables, and whole grain breads and cereals.

Surgical removal of the involved tissues of the colon and/or the rectum is the mainstay of treatment. Some clinics are beginning to use irradiation therapy prior to this type of surgery in the hope of lessening likelihood of spread of tumor cells during the surgery. The use of irradiation therapy following surgery is now frequently recommended.

ESOPHAGUS
Smoking and drinking predispose to cancer of the esophagus, with the risk being the greatest among people who both drink and smoke. Cancer may occur in any part of the esophagus, but it is most common in the mid-portion. It causes difficulty in swallowing. The results of treating this type of cancer have, for the most part, been disappointing. Recently, surgical techniques for approaching the various parts of the esophagus have been perfected, and the survival rate has improved accordingly.

FACE
See under SKIN in this chapter, pages 198, 199.

GALLBLADDER
The presence of gallstones seems to be associated with most cancers of the gallbladder. The symptoms are indigestion, with pain and tenderness in the region of the gallbladder (under the lowest ribs on the upper right part of the abdomen). Jaundice often develops because of an obstruction to the flow of bile. There may be an accumulation of fluid in the abdomen (ascites). Cancer of the gallbladder tends to spread rela-

tively early to the liver. Cancer of the gallbladder is a serious condition and carries a high mortality rate.

HODGKIN'S DISEASE
See chapter 11, volume 2.

KIDNEY
Here we deal with two distinct age groups, infancy and later middle life. The malignant kidney tumor that occurs in infancy (nephroblastoma, often called Wilms's tumor) typically develops before three years of age. The first sign is usually the discovery of a firm, painless mass in one side of the abdomen. Seldom does blood show up in the urine (hematuria), but when it does it conveys an unfavorable import. Fortunately, the disease is usually limited to one kidney. Early removal of the involved kidney, often followed by irradiation therapy, has improved the chances of survival to as much as 50 percent.

The adult type of cancer of the kidney occurs most commonly between the ages of 45 and 60. The warning symptom is the appearance of blood in the urine. This, when it occurs, should be reported promptly to the doctor.

Cancer of the kidney often spreads to other parts of the body—typically to the lungs and certain of the long bones of the skeleton. The primary method of treatment is the surgical removal of the involved kidney.

LARYNX
Cancer of the larynx accounts for about 1 percent of all the cancers diagnosed in the United States. The chances for five-year survival vary all the way from 5 percent for those diagnosed and treated late, to 95 percent for those diagnosed and treated in the very early course of the disease.

Cancer of the larynx occurs most commonly among those who smoke. The damage that smoking does to the larynx is suggested by the typical rough quality of the voice of smokers. Heavy drinking is also listed as a factor which predisposes to cancer of the larynx.

The combination of smoking and drinking is especially harmful in this connection.

When the vocal cords proper are involved in the cancerous transformation, the telltale symptom is unexplained hoarseness. Persisting hoarseness should always signal a need for examination by a physician.

When cancer of the larynx is discovered early and when only one side is involved, partial removal of the larynx may result in a cure. More commonly, the entire larynx has to be removed. Then it becomes necessary for the patient to use one of the methods of artificial speech. Some persons use a mechanical vibrator placed against the skin of the face and then articulate words with their lips and tongue. The newer method, in many ways more satisfactory, consists of swallowing a small amount of air, holding it in the upper part of the esophagus, and then "burping" it gradually as the tongue, cheeks, and lips articulate the words, using the sounds produced by the air escaping from the esophagus. This method of esophageal speech requires training and the development of consid-

Pipe smoking can cause lip cancer.

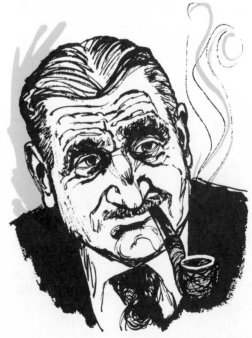

erable skill, but once mastered, it works quite satisfactorily.

LEUKEMIA

Leukemia is considered to be a malignant disease involving the blood-forming tissues. It is therefore discussed in chapter 10 on Blood Diseases, volume 2.

LIP

A sore on the lip which refuses to heal should always arouse suspicion. Cancer of the lower lip usually results from prolonged irritation (as in pipe smoking). When cancer of the lip is treated early, the prospects of cure are given as 90 to 95 percent. The end result in neglected cases can be quite tragic. Treatment is by the surgical removal of the involved area of tissue, with the possible additional use of irradiation therapy, or by radiation only.

LIVER

Cancer of the liver is frequent, but it rarely begins in the organ itself. Cancers from neighboring portions of the stomach, colon, or gallbladder commonly spread to it. Others are transmitted to the liver from more distant parts of the body when colonies of cancer cells are carried by the blood. The symptoms of cancer of the liver vary from case to case. Frequently they include jaundice and the accumulation of fluid in the abdominal cavity (ascites). The liver itself is usually tender to pressure, feels nodular on palpation, and grows steadily in size. The prospect of survival is remote.

LUNG

The number of cases of lung cancer increased alarmingly during recent years. Deaths from this highly malignant disease top the list of all types of cancer in men. Fatalities have also been increasing among women, but at a slower rate. A news item in the *Journal of the American Medical Association* for June 26, 1981, stated, "Lung cancer remains the most lethal cancer for men, is fast becoming that for women, and is expected to account for about 100,000 deaths this year." See chapter 54, volume 1, for a discussion of the relation between smoking and lung cancer.

The mortality rate for lung cancer is so high that less than 20 percent of the stricken victims are alive at the end of five years. Without treatment the survival rate for the usual type of lung cancer is zero. Two reasons account for the high mortality rate. First, cancer of the lung is highly malignant (very prone to spread). Second, it causes no distinctive early symptoms. Cough is often the first sign of lung cancer, but the average smoker has a chronic cough anyway; therefore, the first sign of the cancer usually passes unnoticed. By the time lung cancer is diagnosed, it has usually passed the stage of probable cure.

Surgical removal of the cancerous tissue and chemotherapy are the mainstays for treating lung cancer.

LYMPH NODES (LYMPHOMAS)

Malignancies involving the lymph nodes (lymphomas) are discussed in chapter 11, volume 2.

The lymph nodes are often involved secondarily, as cancers spread from their original locations to other parts of the body. Thus, in connection with cancer of the breast, the lymph nodes of the axilla (armpit) are usually the first ones to give evidence of the spread of this particular cancer.

MELANOMA

The melanoma is a highly malignant form of cancer composed essentially of melanocytes (cells which produce the dark pigment, melanin, found in the deep layers of the skin, the retina of the eye, and elsewhere) which have now taken on the characteristics of cancer cells. In about two thirds of the cases, the melanoma has originated from an apparently harmless mole (nevus). For details of this transformation and a list of the evidences that a mole is becoming malignant, see the item entitled "Melanoma" in chapter 25, volume 2.

Melanomas originate not only in the

skin, but also in certain membranes of the body and in the normally pigmented tissues of the eye. (See chapter 8, this volume.)

Five-year survival rates for patients with melanoma vary from about zero for neglected cases to about 80 percent for cases in which the cancer was completely removed before there had been any migration of tumor cells.

MOLE (PIGMENTED MOLE)

See the item entitled "Melanoma" in chapter 25, volume 2.

MOUTH

See also in this chapter under LIP and TONGUE.

In response to long-continued irritation there may appear one or more irregular, hard, milk-white, dry patches on the membranes lining the mouth, on the tongue, or on the inner aspects of the lips or cheeks. Such a development is called leukoplakia ("white plaque" or "smoker's patch"), and is recognized as a premalignant lesion (capable of transformation to cancer). Cancer of the mouth occurs most commonly in the mouths of smokers, snuff dippers, and tobacco chewers. The use of alcohol and an inadequate diet are also predisposing factors.

A suspicious lesion in the mouth should be examined by biopsy (removal of a small portion for microscopic study) and, if found malignant, treated either by surgical removal or by irradiation.

MULTIPLE MYELOMA

Multiple myeloma is a malignant disease of unknown cause which typically occurs only in persons above 40 years of age and is characterized by tumors in the bone marrow, destructive areas in various bones, anemia, and kidney damage. The bone marrow tumors consist of abnormal plasma cells. The diagnosis is confirmed by the presence of an unusual form of protein (Bence Jones protein) in the urine. The progression of the disease toward a fatal outcome is slow in some cases and

rapid in others. The treatment and care consist of ensuring an adequate intake of fluid, encouraging the patient to exercise as much as his condition permits, judicious use of chemotherapy, and irradiation therapy as indicated to control the local bone marrow tumors.

OVARY

Cancer of the ovary constitutes between 4 and 5 percent of the cancers occurring in women. It is a treacherous kind of cancer, because the early evidences are so insidious that it often becomes far advanced before being recognized and treated. Strangely, but importantly, the symptoms involve the digestive organs more than they do the reproductive organs. In a woman beyond 40 years of age cancer of the ovaries should be suspected if she experiences gastrointestinal symptoms that cannot be explained otherwise. These include bouts of prolonged vomiting, with resulting extreme hunger and thirst. An abnormal mass in the region of the ovary may often be detected by physical examination. Sometimes fluid accumulates in the abdomen (ascites).

The treatment consists of radical pelvic surgery, often supplemented by chemotherapy. The five-year survival rate is about 50 percent.

PANCREAS

Cancer of the pancreas is one of the least favorable forms of cancer, for its five-year survival rate, even after treatment, is less than 1 percent. The incidence of cancer of the pancreas has been increasing during the recent 50 years and now accounts for about 3 percent of all cancers and about 5 percent of all cancer deaths.

The typical symptoms of pain, jaundice, and loss of body weight occur late—so late that in 85 to 90 percent of cases the cancer has already spread to other parts of the body by the time the diagnosis is made. Surgical removal of the pancreas is helpful only when performed early. Chemotherapy and irradiation therapy do not significantly im-

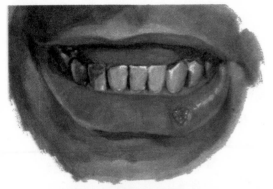

EARLY CARCINOMA OF LIP

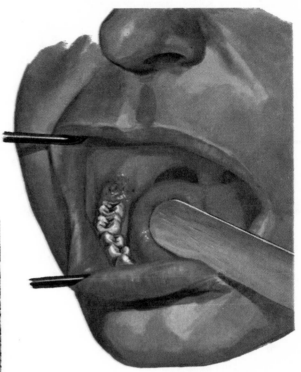

CARCINOMA OF GINGIVA
(RETROMOLAR SPACE)

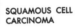

SQUAMOUS CELL
CARCINOMA

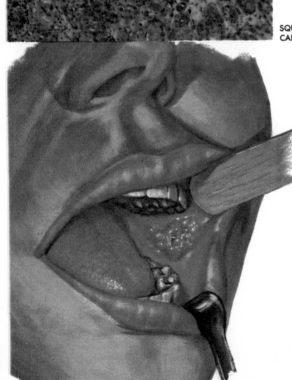

CARCINOMA OF CHEEK

CARCINOMA OF TONGUE
(ON LEUKOPLAKIA)

©CIBA

prove the prospect of survival.

At the time of writing, two well-documented studies have indicated that cancer of the pancreas is significantly more common among coffee drinkers than among those who do not use coffee. Further scientific study of this relationship is in progress. In the meantime, coffee drinkers would be wise to use moderation.

PROSTATE

Cancer of the prostate is discussed in chapter 29, volume 2.

RECTUM

Cancer of the rectum is discussed along with that of the colon, earlier in this chapter, page 193.

SKIN

The highly malignant type of cancer called melanoma is often classed as a cancer of the skin. In this chapter it is listed separately on pages 195, 196.

Chapter 25, "Skin Diseases," volume 2, contains a discussion of changes in the skin which lead to cancer.

Cancer of the skin has been increasing sharply during recent years, particularly in younger people. Present statistics place new cases of cancer of the skin in the United States at an esti-

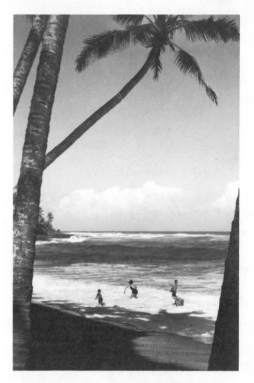

To protect the skin against overexposure at the beach or anywhere, it is wise to use a sunscreen lotion.

Skin cancer occurs commonly on exposed areas, such as the face.

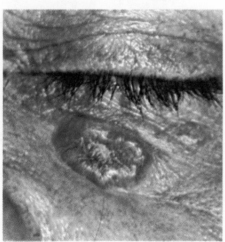

mated 300,000 to 600,000 each year. This increase is caused by the popular customs of wearing fewer and lighter clothes, of exposing large areas of the skin during recreational activities, and of acquiring suntan as an aid to beauty.

Exposure to the sun or to any source of ultraviolet light is the largest single predisposing factor to cancer of the skin. Light-complexioned persons are more susceptible than dark-complexioned to the damaging effects of such exposure.

Fortunately, skin cancer carries the highest rate of successful cure of any form of cancer. More than 90 percent of the ordinary cases of skin cancer (excluding melanoma) are treated successfully, largely because changes in the skin are easily detected. The public is now becoming aware of the possibilities and dangers of developing cancer, and so when a person observes an ulcer of the skin that does not heal or an ulcer developing in an old scar or even a firm mass of tissue in the skin or just beneath it, he usually reports such an observation to his doctor in time for proper treatment to be performed.

Other than being alert to changes in the skin which might indicate a developing cancer, it is wise for all persons, especially those of light complexion, to use sunscreen lotions on exposed areas of the skin when out of doors for any considerable time.

Several forms of treatment are effective for cancer of the skin, the choice in a particular case depending upon the type and duration of the involvement. The several treatments include local freezing, curettage (scraping away the affected areas), electrodesiccation (use of the electric needle), and removal of the affected area by surgery.

Any person treated for skin cancer should observe the treated area afterward and report any unusual develop-

ments to his doctor—this as a means of treating possible recurrences before they have caused greater damage.

STOMACH

Cancer of the stomach is more common in men than in women. The number of deaths from cancer of the stomach has been declining in the United States during recent years, dropping from 25 percent of all cancer deaths in 1930 to 2 percent at the present time.

Some of the early symptoms are loss of appetite, indigestion, and discomfort in the stomach region. Later there may be vomiting of "coffee grounds" material, evidences of blood in the stool, and decline in body weight.

In the early stages, examination by X ray and by the gastroscope gives the most reliable information.

Prompt surgical removal of part or all of the stomach is the only satisfactory treatment. But even with surgical treatment, the five-year survival rate averages only about 25 percent. Cancer of the stomach tends to spread to the liver; and if treatment is delayed until

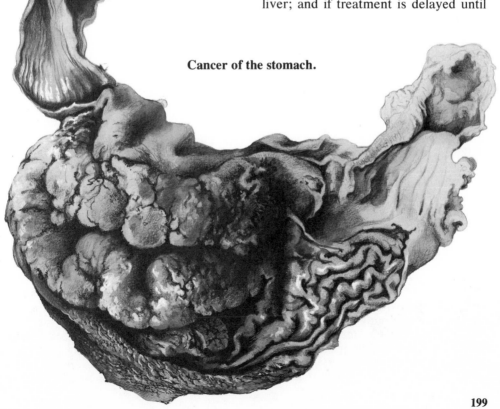

Cancer of the stomach.

after this metastasis has occurred, the outcome is uniformly fatal.

TESTIS

Most tumors developing in the testis are malignant. Therefore any enlarging mass of tissue involving a testis should receive prompt attention by a physician. Untreated cancer of the testis spreads (metastasizes) readily to lymph nodes, lungs, and liver.

The enlarging mass of tissue associated with a developing cancer of the testis is sometimes (not always) associated with pain. Of the several types of cancer of the testis some respond to treatment more favorably than others.

The first step in treatment, regardless of the type of cancer, requires the surgical removal of the involved testis. Microscopic examination of the testis, after removal, will give a clue as to the best form of postoperative treatment. Irradiation of lymph nodes in the pelvic region is often advisable. Newer methods of combination chemotherapy are successful in some types of cancer of the testis.

THYROID

Great variations exist from patient to patient in the characteristics of thyroid disease. It is often difficult to tell the difference between a malignant and a benign condition. Also, some cases of thyroid cancer are more highly malignant than others. Fortunately, cancer of the thyroid is a rare condition.

When a nodule, even though small, can be felt within the substance of the thyroid gland, the advice of a physician should be obtained. Many nodules in the thyroid gland are not cancerous. The nodule of a developing cancer in the thyroid is typically single, firm to the touch, irregular in shape, and somewhat bound to the tissues that surround it.

A physician who specializes in such conditions can make several tests which help to determine whether the condition is malignant. If so, the only satisfactory treatment is the surgical removal of the affected tissue. Conven-

tional irradiation therapy is not effective in treating cancer of the thyroid. In some cases, however, the physician may consider it advisable to use radioactive iodine as a supplement to the surgery.

TONGUE

Cancer of the tongue is a serious disease and causes more deaths than any other cancer within the mouth. The use of tobacco and/or alcohol may cause changes in the surface membrane of the tongue, and this may lead to the development of actual cancer. The tissue transformation often proceeds slowly, and if these precancerous lesions are identified soon enough, discontinuing the use of alcohol and tobacco may cause the lesions to disappear. But when a lesion of the tongue is identified as actual cancer (as when it begins to invade the deeper tissues), it must be treated at once, either by surgery, or by irradiation. Treatment of such a case by surgery requires the removal of the involved half of the tongue, the floor of the mouth on the same side, and also the lymph nodes on the same side of the neck. When performed in the early stages of the cancer, this is a life-saving procedure and it is not as disfiguring or handicapping in the long run as the description makes it sound.

UTERUS

Cancer of the uterus is in third place among cancers that affect women, being exceeded by cancer of the breast and cancer of the colon and rectum. Fortunately, the death rate from cancer of the uterus has declined during recent years, being only one third of what it was forty years ago. The reason for this is that the public is becoming aware of the signs of cancer and of the importance of early detection and treatment. An important contributor to this improvement in the death rate has been the widespread use of the Pap test, by which cancer of the cervix of the uterus (the most common type of uterine cancer) can be detected before it has had time to spread to other tissues.

There are two principal types of cancer of the uterus: (1) cancer of the cervix, the cervix being the outlet to the uterus which projects into the deepest portion of the vagina, and (2) cancer of the endometrium, the endometrium being the tissue which lines the uterus.

1. *Cancer of the Cervix.* An estimated 38,000 new cases of cancer of the cervix occur in the United States each year. The risk factors, one or more of which predispose to the development of cancer of the cervix include (a) early marriage (prior to 18 years of age), (b) multiple pregnancies, and (c) a history of previous disease of the pelvic organs.

The symptoms consist of pain in the pelvic region and bleeding through the vagina other than normal menstruation.

In connection with each routine physical examination of a woman, the physician should obtain a Pap smear, a sample of mucus from the canal of the uterine cervix, to be sent to the laboratory for microscopic examination. The sample of mucus will contain some of the cells normally shed from the membrane lining the cervix. If cancer is present, certain of these cells will show the characteristics of cancer cells. In such instances, the physician will arrange for a sample of tissue to be taken from the cervix for more detailed examination in the laboratory (a biopsy examination). If this confirms the suspicion of a beginning cancer, appropriate treatment must then be arranged.

For a case of beginning cancer of the cervix in which the malignant cells have not yet invaded neighboring tissues, a simple surgical procedure of conization, in which the lining of the canal of the cervix is removed, is the accepted treatment. Following such surgery, Pap smear tests should be performed at frequent intervals to make sure that the cancer has been eradicated.

In a case in which cancer of the cervix has advanced to the stage of invading neighboring tissues, a more radical surgical procedure must be performed,

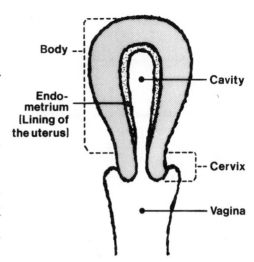

Diagram of the parts of the uterus and their relation to the vagina.

followed by the use of irradiation therapy.

2. *Endometrial Cancer of the Uterus.* An estimated 16,000 new cases of endometrial cancer occur each year in the United States. The risk factors which predispose to endometrial cancer include obesity, infertility (having never been pregnant), age above 50 years, a family history of cancer in other female members, a personal history of having reached the menopause (change of life) at age above 50, and a record of long-term use of estrogen hormone. Of course not all risk factors are present in a given case. The greater the number of risk factors, however, the greater the prospect of this type of cancer developing.

The warning symptom of endometrial cancer is abnormal uterine bleeding through the vagina. When such bleeding occurs after the individual has ceased to menstruate, it is a definite sign of difficulty. When uterine bleeding occurs other than at the menstrual period in a younger woman, it should be considered as a warning of cancer until proven otherwise.

The diagnosis of cancer of the endometrium of the uterus must be confirmed by a microscopic examination of a sample of tissue from the interior of the uterus. The obtaining of such a sample is a minor surgical procedure. The Pap test, so important in the diagnosis of cancer of the cervix of the uterus, does not give conclusive information relative to cancer of the endometrium. Women at high risk of endometrial cancer (those in whom several risk factors are present) should arrange for a pelvic examination each year (especially women older than 50 years). At the time of such an examination the doctor must exercise his judgment as to whether it is advisable for a sample of tissue from the uterine lining to be examined.

Once cancer of the endometrium of the uterus is found to be present, the uterus should be removed by surgery (a hysterectomy). If the cancer has already spread to the lymph nodes in the pelvic area the surgery should be followed by irradiation therapy.

SECTION **IV**

Dietary
Problems

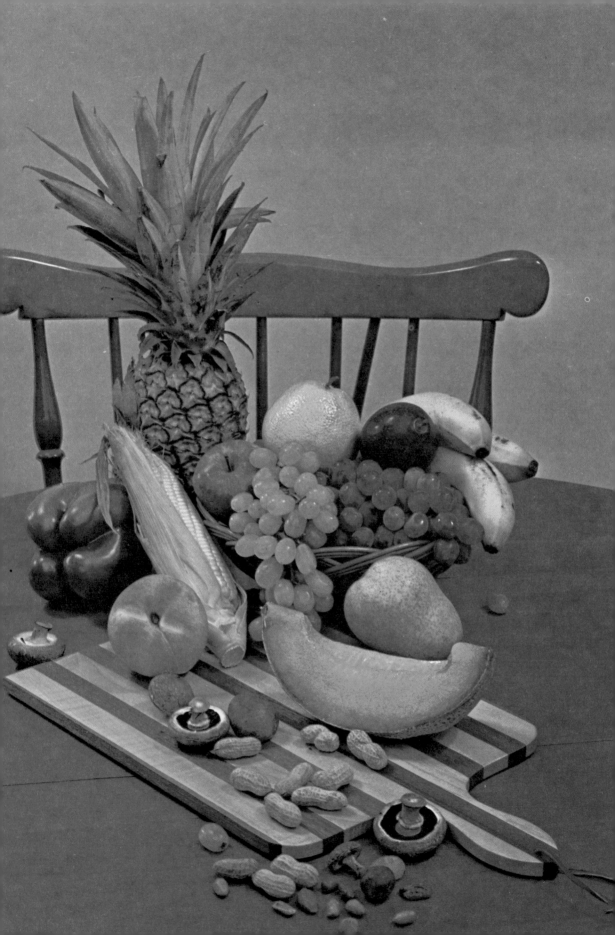

Deficiency Diseases

The deficiency diseases are caused by a shortage in the diet of certain food constituents even when the total amount of food may be adequate.

This chapter is concerned mostly with the body's need for vitamins, minerals, and proteins, and with the consequences when certain of these are in short supply. Consideration is also given to the advisability, and even to the possible hazards, of taking vitamins and minerals as medications or as dietary supplements.

A. Avitaminoses

Illnesses that stem from a shortage of certain vitamins are collectively called the avitaminoses—the prefix *a* indicating "a lack of."

VITAMIN A DEFICIENCY

A mild deficiency of vitamin A tends to produce roughness and dryness of the skin. Another common symptom is night blindness, in which the ability to see in dim light is reduced. A great degree of deficiency causes damage to the epithelial tissues of the body, which then become more susceptible to infection. In later stages, severe infections of the mouth, the genitourinary tract, the respiratory organs, and the eyes may occur. The eye infection often develops into, or in connection with, a se-rious condition called xerophthalmia, which may lead to blindness.

Some evidence suggests that a lack of vitamin A predisposes to cancer. On the other hand, there has been considerable research into the use of retinoids (both natural and synthetic forms of vitamin A) in the treatment of various types of cancer, with promising results.

Adequate amounts of vitamin A are contained in the usual average American diet. This vitamin is especially abundant in such foods as carrots, sweet potatoes, apricots, orange squash, cheese, and milk.

The recommended daily allowance (RDA) for vitamin A varies from about 1500 international units for infants to about 5000 international units for adults. Danger lurks in taking large supplements of vitamin A. It has been demonstrated that doses of 50,000 international units or more per day continued for weeks or months produce such symptoms as loss of appetite, blurred vision, cracking of the skin, headaches, diarrhea, and nausea.

Care and Treatment

Treatment for such conditions as night blindness or other symptoms of mild deficiency of vitamin A consists of the administration of 25,000 international units of vitamin A each day for a period of one or two weeks. In serious deficiencies such as

205

xerophthalmia, the physician may prescribe daily injections of the water-dispersible form of vitamin A in doses up to 100,000 international units continued for a few days, followed by smaller doses by mouth over a period of several weeks.

VITAMIN B DEFICIENCIES

The B group of vitamins includes these: (1) thiamine (vitamin B₁), (2) riboflavin (vitamin B₂), (3) niacin or nicotinic acid, (4) vitamin B₁₂, (5) folic acid, and (6) vitamin B₆ (pyridoxine). We consider the deficiencies of each of these separately.

1. *Thiamine (Vitamin B₁ Deficiency).* The disease beriberi is caused by thiamine deficiency. It is characterized by an inflammation and degeneration of nerve trunks, with resulting disturbances of both motion and sensation. The patient loses his appetite and becomes weak, especially in the legs. The nerves controlling the action of the heart may be affected, and heart failure and sudden death may result.

Beriberi occurs most frequently among people whose diet consists mostly of polished rice, but anybody who lives chiefly on highly refined starchy or sugary foods may get it. It may develop in infants, especially those nursed by mothers who have the disease.

If the disease is not far advanced, correction of diet usually will bring about rapid and complete recovery. If the neuritis has continued until the nerve trunks have degenerated, however, normal motion, sensation, and heart action may never be restored.

Wernicke's encephalopathy is another condition caused by a deficiency of thiamine. It occurs most commonly among heavy users of alcohol. For a further discussion of Wernicke's encephalopathy, see chapter 4 in this volume.

Thiamine deficiency is prevented by a diet which includes whole cereals (unrefined), nuts, milk and milk products, fruits, and vegetables. Meat also contains a moderate amount of thiamine.

Care and Treatment

A severe case of beriberi constitutes a medical emergency. The treatment should start with one injection (into a muscle) of 60 mg. of thiamine. Thereafter for one to two weeks the patient should receive thiamine by mouth in three or four doses per day to make a daily total of 25 mgs. From then on, the dose of thiamine taken by mouth should be reduced to 2.5 mg. per day.

2. *Riboflavin (Vitamin B₂) Deficiency.* Riboflavin deficiency develops gradually, the early evidence being a development of fissures (cracking) at the corners of the mouth and in the lips. The tongue becomes unnaturally smooth and has an unnatural red color. In children, riboflavin deficiency impedes normal growth. Also the eyes are commonly affected, with the cornea becoming opaque in extreme cases.

Prevention of riboflavin deficiency requires plenty of milk in the diet, milk being the outstanding dietary source of riboflavin. This vitamin is also contained, however, in eggs, green vegetables, and meat.

Care and Treatment

Three to 10 mg. of riboflavin should be given by mouth three times each day until the patient shows improvement. Then the dose can be reduced to 1 mg. three times a day until recovery is complete.

3. *Niacin (Nicotinic Acid) Deficiency.* Beginning in the eighteenth century and continuing through the nineteenth, there appeared a disease known as pellagra, characterized by three D's: dermatitis, diarrhea, and dementia. It became prevalent in northern Spain and Italy, and, eventually, in southern United States. It often affected several members of the same family, particularly families whose diet was meager. In 1927 it was discovered that pellagra is the result of a deficiency

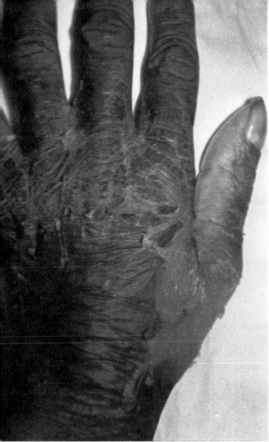

PUBLIC HEALTH SERVICE AUDIOVISUAL FACILITY

Pellagra characteristically causes eruptions on the skin similar in appearance to those caused by burns.

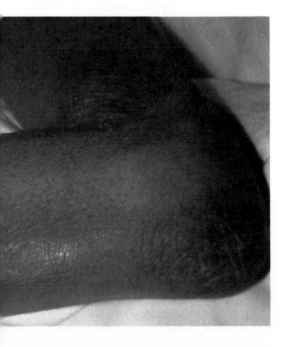

of niacin (nicotinic acid) in the diet.

The skin eruption occurring in pellagra resembles a bad case of sunburn, with considerable cracking, crusting, and scaling. It typically appears on those areas of the skin exposed to sunlight.

The person with pellagra suffers from digestive disturbances and diarrhea. His tongue usually looks abnormally smooth and deep red in color. There may be such nervous symptoms as dizziness, sleeplessness, disturbances of the sense of touch, and weakness. Persons addicted to alcohol seem more susceptible to pellagra than nondrinkers.

Adequate amounts of niacin are available in vegetables, in whole-grain cereals, and in enriched processed cereal products. Meat also contains niacin.

Care and Treatment

The patient with a severe case of pellagra should be treated as an emergency. He should receive niacinamide as a medication taken by mouth two or three times a day in 200 mg. doses. This program of intensive medication should continue for one or two weeks. In the meantime, his diet should include foods high in protein that contain niacin. All use of alcoholic drinks should be forbidden.

4. *Vitamin B$_{12}$ Deficiency.* When the body's tissues do not receive their necessary quota of vitamin B$_{12}$, pernicious anemia (macrocytic anemia) develops. The deficiency is most frequently caused by a failure of the digestive organs to aid in absorbing this vitamin. This condition is explained at greater length, with recommendations for treatment, in chapter 10, volume 2. Also, the effects of this disease on the nervous system are considered in chapter 4, volume 3, under the heading POSTEROLATERAL SCLEROSIS.

5. *Folic Acid Deficiency.* Folic acid, sometimes called folacin, is one of the group of B vitamins. It is an important

and widely distributed vitamin which occurs abundantly in many vegetables. Long-continued cooking of food progressively destroys folic acid.

Deficiency of folic acid occurs commonly among malnourished persons and produces a form of anemia very similar to pernicious anemia. (See the discussion of macrocytic anemias in chapter 10, volume 2.) This form of anemia is most likely to occur under conditions in which the body's requirements for folic acid are greater than usual: in infancy and during pregnancy. Infants who were born prematurely and persons who have had repeated infections of the gastrointestinal organs are particularly susceptible. The condition may be easily confused with that caused by a deficiency of vitamin B_{12}. It is important to avoid such confusion, for the cure of this condition depends specifically on the administration of folic acid.

This type of anemia, when it occurs during pregnancy, occurs during the last three months, at a time when the personal requirements for folic acid are increased because of the rapid growth of the unborn child.

Care and Treatment

The administration of tablets of folic acid, under a physician's direction, usually brings about a dramatic cure.

6. *Pyridoxine (Vitamin B₆) Deficiency.* Pyridoxine is another member of the vitamin B group. Symptoms of this deficiency are particularly serious in infancy and early childhood, when they consist of convulsions. They develop in infants who have received formulas in which the milk or the cereal has been overprocessed, prolonged processing having depleted the vitamin.

Prevention and Treatment

There is an adequate quantity of pyridoxine in human milk, also in cows' milk and in cereals if these latter are not overprocessed.

For the immediate treatment of convulsions due to a deficiency of pyridoxine, an intramuscular injection of pyridoxine gives prompt relief. For infants who seem to be in danger of this deficiency, the physician will arrange for small doses of the vitamin to be added to the diet.

ASCORBIC ACID (VITAMIN C) DEFICIENCY (SCURVY)

Scurvy is caused by a deficiency of vitamin C and is readily cured by taking vitamin C as a medication or by eating foods containing vitamin C. Scurvy is rare in the United States because the usual diet includes fresh fruits and vegetables and because vitamin C has been added as a supplement to many packaged foods.

Going back to the middle of the eighteenth century, scurvy accounted for many deaths, especially among sailors who on their long voyages had no means of preserving fresh foods and thus lived on an impoverished diet. Dr. James Lind, a surgeon in the British Navy, discovered that eating of citrus fruits prevented and cured scurvy. (See also page 482 in volume 2.) Of course it was not known until recent years that the vitamin C in citrus fruits was the healing ingredient.

The symptoms of scurvy include muscular weakness, poor appetite, bleeding and swollen gums, hemorrhages, slow healing of wounds, anemia, and shortness of breath. Even babies may develop scurvy, and when they do they stop gaining weight and appear pale. The slightest bruise of their skin causes a black and blue spot. There may be pain and swelling of the joints.

Prevention and Treatment

For the infant, supplementary orange juice or fortified apple juice or the giving of vitamin drops should begin at about one month of age (see chapter 6, volume 1). For an older child or an adult, adequate amounts of vitamin C are provided by including green vegetables and fruit in the diet. Good sources include citrus fruits, strawberries, cantaloupes, tomatoes, green peppers, and raw cabbage. For the treatment of an actual case of scurvy, administration of ascorbic acid (vitamin C) by mouth in reasonable doses brings prompt improvement.

VITAMIN D DEFICIENCY (RICKETS AND OSTEOMALACIA)

Within the body, vitamin D facilitates the absorption from the intestine of calcium and phosphorus (in the form of phosphate). Calcium and phosphorus are the chief mineral elements in the body's bony framework. Deficiency of vitamin D therefore results in alterations of bone structure. In children, such deficiency causes rickets, a disease characterized by deformities of certain of the bones. Rickets is considered in chapter 17, volume 1. In adults, deficiency of vitamin D causes osteomalacia, a disease characterized by a demineralization of bones.

Osteomalacia is sometimes caused by conditions other than a deficiency of vitamin D in the diet. It may occur in persons whose skin has not been stimulated by sunlight to produce its quota of vitamin D. It may result from faulty absorption of vitamin D from the intestine, or from a kidney ailment which permits the loss of phosphorus from the body.

The outstanding symptoms of osteomalacia are these: (1) pain and tenderness in the bones, especially those of the back, chest, thigh, and feet; (2) muscle weakness, which accounts for a shuffling gait and difficulty in rising from a chair; and (3) bone deformities such as sidewise bowing of the thigh bones, and even incomplete fractures.

Care and Treatment

The immediate treatment of an established case of osteomalacia requires the supervision of a physician. At the beginning of treatment large doses (2000 to 4000 IU) of vitamin D (calciferol) are given by mouth each day for a period of perhaps ten weeks. By that time the daily dosage

of vitamin D can be reduced to between 200 and 400 international units. The patient's diet should include a quart of vitamin D fortified milk per day. It is also desirable for the patient to follow a carefully regulated program of daily sunbaths, inasmuch as some of the vitamin D in one's body is synthesized in the skin in response to the stimulation of ultraviolet light. For the precautions in sunbathing, see chapter 25 in this volume.

VITAMIN E DEFICIENCY

Vitamin E, properly called tocopherol, is known to be a biologic antioxidant. Its chemical structure is such that it is readily oxidized—so readily that it takes priority in the oxidation process over such substances as vitamin A, vitamin C, and certain fats. Thus, when vitamin E occurs in the tissues in association with these other substances, they are free to continue their special functions without their being oxidized until all of the vitamin E has been destroyed.

Symptoms of a deficiency of vitamin E include anemias, fragile red blood cells, and creatine in the urine (indicating breakdown of muscle).

Vitamin E is present in a wide range of foods. It is therefore not probable that a person who receives an adequate diet is in danger of suffering from a deficiency of this vitamin. The deficiency occurs primarily in premature infants on artificial formulas low in E or in adults who have diseases in which fat cannot be digested.

VITAMIN K DEFICIENCY

Vitamin K is the antihemorrhagic vitamin, meaning that it is essential to the complex chemical reactions by which blood clotting occurs. In the absence of vitamin K, bleeding occurs. The common sites for such bleeding are the gastrointestinal tract and the kidneys (causing blood in the urine).

Vitamin K is abundant in dark green leafy vegetables and egg yolk. But less than half of a person's quota of vitamin

209

K is derived from his diet, the larger part being produced by bacterial action in the intestines.

Under usual circumstances a person is in no danger of suffering from a deficiency of vitamin K. The persons most susceptible to such deficiency are these: (1) the newborn infant (especially one born prematurely) until there has been a few days' time during which bacteria within his intestines begin to produce vitamin K; (2) the person continuously taking antibiotic medication, which inhibits intestinal bacteria; (3) the person being fed by vein because he is unable to take food by mouth; and (4) the person taking anticoagulant (blood-thinning) medication.

Prevention and Treatment

An injection of vitamn K given to the mother at the time of childbirth, or a small dose (1-2 mg.) injected intramuscularly into the newborn, serves to prevent hemorrhages in the body of the newborn. For adults in emergency bleeding situations, 10 mg. of vitamin K may be injected intramuscularly. For maintenance in an adult, doses between 5 and 20 mg. of vitamin K may be taken by mouth.

B. Element Deficiencies
Minerals and Trace Elements

The body's tissues contain certain inorganic chemical elements essential to their structure and/or function. These constitute a small part of the body's total weight (a total of six or seven pounds for the average adult), but they are so important that when any one of them is in short supply, the body's functions suffer.

These elements are classically divided into two groups: (1) macronutrient minerals, abundant enough in the body to be readily measured by laboratory methods, and (2) micronutrient minerals (trace elements), which occur in almost infinitesimal amounts but which, nevertheless, are important to the body's economy.

1. *The Macronutrient Minerals,* listed in the order of their decreasing quantity in the body are calcium, phosphorus, potassium, sulfur, sodium, chlorine, and magnesium.

2. *The Micronutrient Minerals (Trace Elements),* of which we have specific knowledge, listed in alphabetical order are chromium, cobalt, copper, fluorine, iodine, iron, manganese, molybdenum, selenium, and zinc.

Functions of the Nutrient Minerals. The minerals in the body perform several functions:

1. The control of water balance.

2. The regulation of acid-base balance.

3. Contributions to the body's structure. Calcium, phosphorus, and fluorine are important constituents of bone and teeth.

4. Contributions to the chemical structure of vitamins, hormones, and enzymes. Cobalt is contained in vitamin B_{12}; iodine is a part of thyroxine; sulfur is a component of thiamine; zinc is essential to the formation of insulin.

5. The catalyzing of certain chemical reactions.

Also, some of the nutrient minerals aid in the transmission of nerve impulses, and some participate in the control of muscle contraction.

Sources of Nutrient Minerals. The nutrient minerals are contained in a wide variety of foods. The person who eats a sensible, average, varied diet is in very little danger of suffering from a deficiency of any of the nutrient minerals (see chapter 53, volume 1, for suggestions on ideal diets).

Deficiencies. Deficiencies, when they occur, are usually the result of some unusual dearth of an element in a person's environment or in his food, or are caused by some systemic disease involving interference with the usual degree of absorption of food elements from the intestine.

C. The Malabsorption Syndrome

The preceding sections of this chapter are concerned with what happens to

SYMPTOMS OF DEFICIENCY

Element in Short Supply	Possible Manifestations of Deficiency
1. Calcium	1. Tetany; neuromuscular irritability; demineralization of bone.
2. Potassium	2. Disturbances of heart action; a form of paralysis.
3. Sodium	3. Edema (water-logged tissues).
4. Magnesium	4. Neuromuscular irritability.
5. Cobalt in vitamin B_{12} (not required in inorganic form)	5. Anemia in children.
6. Copper	6. Anemia in malnourished children.
7. Fluorine	7. Predisposition to osteoporosis and to dental caries.
8. Iodine	8. Endemic goiter; can contribute to cretinism.
9. Iron	9. A form of anemia.
10. Zinc	10. Stunted growth; reduced rate of healing; sexual deficiency.

a person's state of health when certain of the essential vitamins and minerals are in short supply. For the most part it has been assumed that such shortages are brought about by a dearth of constituents (vitamin or mineral) in the food normally eaten. But in certain cases a person's food contains sufficient of the necessary vitamins and minerals, and still he suffers from a deficiency. The problem here is malfunction of the mechanism by which food constituents are transported from the interior of the intestine to the blood. In other words, essential vitamins and minerals are present within the intestine, but they pass on without being absorbed—hence the designation, malabsorption syndrome.

The malabsorption syndrome, its manifestations, and the treatment of these ailments are considered in chapter 17, volume 2.

D. Diet Supplements

A great deal of promotion in the media and otherwise urges people to take supplementary vitamins and minerals on the assumption that a regular diet does not include enough of these. Such promotion is usually prompted by the commercial interests of the manufacturers. As mentioned earlier, an average, wholesome diet contains sufficient of the essential food constituents to provide all the body's needs. Furthermore, many of the packaged foods contain added vitamins and minerals sufficient to replace what may have been lost in the food processing.

In certain forms of disease it is advisable to use vitamin or mineral supplements as medications; and sometimes in special cases, as during infancy, pregnancy, and old age, it becomes expedient to use supplementary vitamins as a safeguard against deficiency. But for the most part, the use of diet supplements is not necessary. Danger of toxicity even threatens in some instances when diet supplements are used to excess.

For a further study of this matter, see chapter 6, volume 1, for a consideration of vitamin supplements for babies; chapter 40, volume 1, for all-purpose vitamins for elderly persons; and chapter 53, volume 1, for a list of the daily vitamin requirements.

Disorders of Regulation

Much modern machinery and equipment is controlled by sensors, thermostats, "black boxes," and computers that do the work that people would otherwise have to do in turning on more power, changing the speed of operations, regulating the flow of water, adjusting temperature, and making calculations. But none of our modern inventions can equal the precision and constancy of the human body's built-in regulatory mechanisms by which chemical processes, enzyme actions, and reflexes respond to the needs of the moment. One of the great marvels of the human body is its ability to regulate its own functions and to adjust to changing circumstances.

Many of the body's checks and controls are discussed in other chapters of this set: water balance in chapter 52, volume 1, control of blood pressure in chapter 7, volume 2, regulation of body temperature in chapter 23, volume 2.

In the present chapter we bring together certain problems of health not adequately considered elsewhere that are caused in whole or in part by disorders of regulatory devices. We deal first with the regulation of food intake, accomplished partly by conscious control and partly by automatic mechanisms. Disorders here account for obesity on one extreme and underweight on the other. Then we consider diabetes mellitus, a disorder involving the body's regulation of the use of energy food. And last we consider gout, in which the regulation of the metabolism of uric acid is at fault; and porphyria, in which the body's metabolism of pigments is disturbed.

A. Hunger

Why does a person want to eat every few hours? Is it from fear of starvation? Hardly. He becomes hungry, that's why. But what is hunger?

Every normal person knows, but who can define it? A sensation that originates in an empty stomach, is how some people define it. But it has been observed that a person whose stomach has been removed by surgery still experiences hunger. Others supposed that the brain contains a "hunger center" which, when stimulated by nerve impulses, as from an empty stomach, would create a desire for food. What we know now for sure, is that there comes a time, a few hours after each meal, when the absorption of food from the intestine is completed. Then the body begins to draw its energy material from stores in the liver and in the fat deposits. It is then that hunger develops.

Of course many conditioning factors may amplify or diminish one's hunger response. Fondness for certain kinds of food, emotional stimulation, fatigue, and social influences may affect the timing or the intensity of a person's hunger.

Satiety is the opposite of hunger. Not merely the absence of hunger, it is a pleasant feeling of satisfaction, the person now desiring a period of quiet relaxation. He is content to wait until he becomes hungry again. Thus there keeps recurring a cycle of hunger followed by satiety, followed by hunger.

Disinterest in eating involves a distortion of the usual hunger-satiety-hunger cycle. This abnormal lack of appetite occurs in many forms of illness. It shows up also as a functional problem in anorexia nervosa, a deep-seated psychological disorder which sometimes troubles teenage girls and young women. See chapter 26, volume 1, for a more complete discussion.

B. Obesity

It has become popular for both men and women to watch their weight. For women the trim figure is considered more attractive, more desirable; for men, the muscular physique.

Credit goes to insurance companies for awakening the general population to the dangers of overweight. Whenever an insured person dies, the company has to pay. The longer an insured person lives, the longer the insurance company has use of the money involved in the insurance agreement, and thus the greater the profit.

A few decades ago the major insurance companies began keeping records of various circumstances relating to clients. They discovered which circumstances of life are associated with early death. One of the main lessons learned is that overweight people tend to die sooner than people of normal weight. The greater a person's weight, the greater his risk of early death.

Estimates of the number of overweight people in the United States vary

---

THESE ARE THE DISEASES THAT CAUSE THE HIGH DEATH RATE AMONG FAT PEOPLE

A figure of 100, if used in the following tabulation, would indicate the usual mortality rate among persons of normal weight. Example: the figure of 383 appearing opposite "diabetes" for overweight males indicates that the incidence of death from diabetes is almost four times as great among men who are overweight as among those of normal weight.

Principal Causes of Mortality of Persons 20 to 74 Percent Overweight

Causes of death	Percent actual of expected deaths	
	Males	Females
Diabetes	383	372
Cirrhosis of the liver	249	147
Appendicitis	293	195
Chronic nephritis	191	212
Cerebral hemorhage	159	162
Liver and gallbladder disease	168	211
All heart disease	142	175

Source: Stare and McWilliams, Living Nutrition, John Wiley & Sons, 1977, p. 90.

---

from 15 million to 40 million.

When an overweight person passes away, his death certificate does not give overweight as the cause. But persons who weigh too much are more susceptible than others to life-destroying diseases. Thus obesity can be named rightly as a contributing cause of death.

The accompanying table showing principal causes of death among overweight people puts diabetes at the head. In the same list are diseases which affect the liver, the kidneys, the blood vessels, and the heart. Being

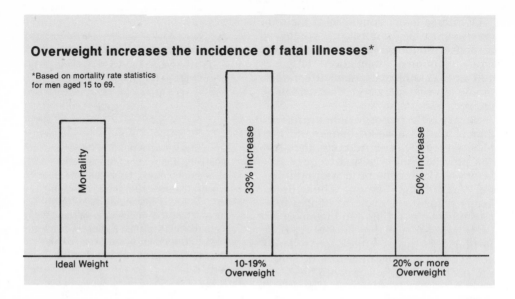

Overweight increases the incidence of fatal illnesses*

*Based on mortality rate statistics for men aged 15 to 69.

Mortality

33% increase

50% increase

Ideal Weight

10-19% Overweight

20% or more Overweight

overweight throws a greater strain on the body's vital organs, making them more susceptible to diseases that cause early death.

What Overweight Does to the Organs

The normal body contains a certain amount of fat in its tissues. It is *excess* fat that causes trouble. Extra fat is deposited in certain parts of the body. An excess layer of fat on the surface of the heart rides as a nonpaying passenger. Obviously it takes more work to move a 200-pound man up a flight of stairs than to move a 150-pound man. This additional activity of the skeletal muscles adds to the workload of the heart.

Overweight interferes with the function of the lungs and with the processes of providing oxygen to the body tissues and of removing carbon dioxide. It requires the blood-forming tissues to build more red blood cells than normally needed. It imposes extra work on the liver.

Why Do People Become Fat?

To say that obesity is caused by overeating is true. But to stop at that is to oversimplify the problem. We must first answer a related question: What causes overeating?

Heredity can properly be blamed for about one fourth of the cases of overweight. In fact, a child born to a father and mother who are both overweight has about a 90 percent chance of being overweight.

But what is it about heredity that may cause a person to be overweight? In many cases the child simply inherits a good appetite.

Approximately another fourth of overweight persons remain fat even when they reduce their intake of food. These are the "easy keepers" in terms of the amount of food they require to maintain their normal body activities. Their digestive organs are more efficient than those of an average person, and a little food seems to go farther in filling their energy requirements. Some of these cases suffer from an abnormality in their endocrine organs. Such persons would do well to consult a medical specialist.

This leaves about half the cases of obesity as victims of a self-inflicted habit of overeating. These are normal individuals who enjoy living. When they see food, they want to eat it; and when they see it in abundance, they eat too much. They have become accustomed to high living standards and are responsive to the social custom of eating with friends. Their thoughts become occupied with the pleasure of eating rather than with the practical aspects of nutrition; therefore, they neglect the counting of calories.

Coupled with this habit of eating too much goes the popular trend toward passive living. Modern mechanization has reduced the need for physical activ-

Having problems with overweight? There's hope. The solution generally lies in control of the appetite. This man lost 181 pounds in one year.

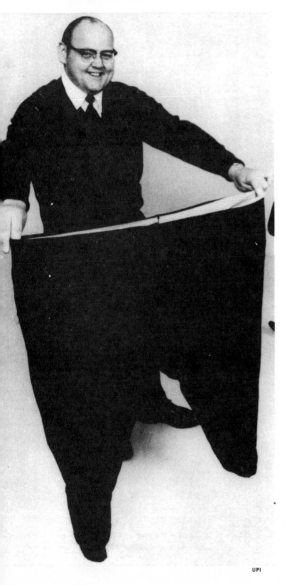

UPI

ity. Even the "workingman" does not use his muscles now as he used to. He rides to and from work. On the job he pushes buttons and moves levers, making machines do the work.

The physical exertion of keeping house has been reduced by modern labor-saving appliances. Housewives today may become just as weary as did their grandmothers, but today's tiredness is more nervous fatigue than physical exhaustion. Who now performs the wearisome tasks of beating rugs, rubbing clothes on a washboard, and obtaining vegetables direct from the garden?

It used to take about 4000 calories per day to provide the energy for an average person's activity. Now, with elevators to take us upstairs and automobiles to carry us to the store, to school, and to work, less than 3000 calories per day can satisfy most people's needs. But the human appetite and the customs of eating remain about the same. It takes only half a slice of bread and a little butter a day beyond a person's food requirements to add a half pound of body weight by the end of the month. This daily addition of sixty-five or seventy calories above one's requirements can account for a weight gain of six pounds during the year and thus of thirty pounds within five years. No wonder that so many people are becoming overweight and that weight often increases as age advances.

Food Tastes Good

We have said that it is one's appetite that tempts him to eat more food than he should. Why is appetite so hard to control? Essentially, people enjoy food. While one eats food that he likes, he receives pleasant sensations from his taste buds. When he stops eating, the pleasant sensations stop. And too often a person allows this enjoyment of food to dictate how long he continues to eat. Thus some people eat until they become uncomfortably "full" rather than stopping when they have had enough. In this way a person can become a slave to his sensation of taste.

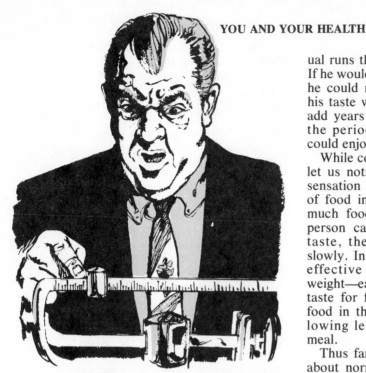

ual runs the risk of shortening his life. If he would reason from cause to effect, he could recognize that by overruling his taste with good judgment he could add years to his life and thus prolong the period of time during which he could enjoy the taste of food.

While considering the factor of taste, let us notice that the pleasure of this sensation depends upon the presence of food in the mouth, not upon how much food is actually swallowed. A person can prolong the pleasures of taste, then, by simply eating more slowly. In fact, this is one of the most effective ways of preventing over-weight—eating so slowly that one's taste for food is satisfied by keeping food in the mouth longer while swallowing less food in the course of a meal.

Thus far we have been saying a lot about normal weight and overweight; but as yet we have not defined normal weight.

What Is Normal Weight?

Originally, weight tables were based on the *average* weight of persons of various stated heights. Naturally, the

Many people begin to hanker for the taste of food within an hour or two after they have had a meal. Without disciplining their desire, they indulge in between-meal snacks, which of course add calories to the day's intake.

By indulging his appetite, an individ-

The percentage of persons who are overweight increases in the older age groups. This means, for the individual, that the older he becomes, the greater is the danger of becoming overweight.

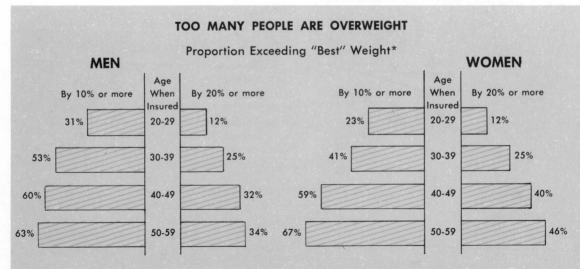

TOO MANY PEOPLE ARE OVERWEIGHT

Proportion Exceeding "Best" Weight*

MEN				WOMEN	
By 10% or more	Age When Insured	By 20% or more	By 10% or more	Age When Insured	By 20% or more
31%	20-29	12%	23%	20-29	12%
53%	30-39	25%	41%	30-39	25%
60%	40-49	32%	59%	40-49	40%
63%	50-59	34%	67%	50-59	46%

*"Best" weight is slight or moderate underweight, ranging from about 5 to 10% below average weight at age 30 to about 10 to 15% below at age 45 or over.

average weight of tall persons is greater than that of short persons. Also, in recognition of the fact that it is easy for weight to increase as a person becomes older, these earlier tables gave several columns with the average weight of persons in different age brackets—from 20 to 24 years, from 25 to 29, from 30 to 39, from 40 to 49, from 50 to 59 and from 60 to 69. By consulting such a table, a person found it easy to excuse adding a few pounds as he became older.

But it is not good for a person to gain weight as he becomes older. To do so throws the greatest work load on the vital organs at a time when they are least able to carry it. With this recognition came the belief that a person's greatest weight should be at the time of life when his body is at its best, and that from then on weight should not increase.

The weight tables now favored by those who have made a careful study of body weight and its relation to health are those built around the average weight of normal persons of the same height and sex at age twenty-five—a standard arrived at on finding that people live longest if they maintain this "desirable" weight. It is at this age that a person has made his physiological adjustments to adulthood and is probably in his prime. It is at this age that the skeletal muscles are best developed and that the vital organs have reached maximum capacity for carrying on their functions. Increase in weight beyond what it was at age twenty-five is therefore a detriment.

It would be foolish to advise everyone, regardless of his type of build, to try to bring his eating habits under such rigid discipline that his weight will conform exactly to a uniform arbitrary figure. Persons of slender build should not weigh as much as persons of broad frame and heavy muscles. Our modern tables, then list the desirable weights in three columns for those of slender build (small frame), for those of average build (medium frame), and for those of stout build (large frame). Furthermore,

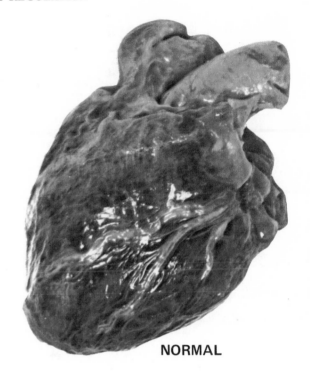

NORMAL

OVERWEIGHT

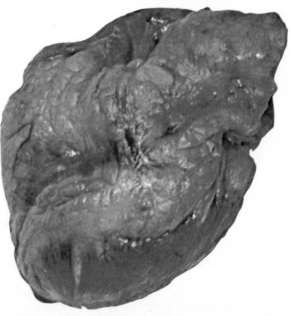

The heart of an overweight person operates under the handicap of a superfluous layer of fat.

217

DESIRABLE WEIGHTS FOR MEN AND WOMEN

According to Height and Frame. Ages 25 and Over.
Height (in Shoes)* Weight in Pounds (in Indoor Clothing)

	Men				Women		
	Small Frame	Medium Frame	Large Frame		Small Frame	Medium Frame	Large Frame
5' 2" .	112-120	118-129	126-141	4'10" .	92- 98	96-107	104-119
3" .	115-123	121-133	129-144	11" .	94-101	98-110	106-122
4" .	118-126	124-136	132-148	5' 0" .	96-104	101-113	109-125
5" .	121-129	127-139	135-152	1" .	99-107	104-116	112-128
6" .	124-133	130-143	138-156	2" .	102-110	107-119	115-131
7" .	128-137	134-147	142-161	3" .	105-113	110-122	118-134
8" .	132-141	138-152	147-166	4" .	108-116	113-126	121-138
9" .	136-145	142-156	151-170	5" .	111-119	116-130	125-142
10" .	140-150	146-160	155-174	6" .	114-123	120-135	129-146
11" .	144-154	150-165	159-179	7" .	118-127	124-139	133-150
6' 0" .	148-158	154-170	164-184	8" .	122-131	128-143	137-154
1" .	152-162	158-175	168-189	9" .	126-135	132-147	141-158
2" .	156-167	162-180	173-194	10" .	130-140	136-151	145-163
3" .	160-171	167-185	178-199	11" .	134-144	140-155	149-168
4" .	164-175	172-190	182-204	6' 0" .	138-148	144-159	153-173

Notice that these measurements of height are with shoes (one-inch heels for men and two-inch heels for women) and the weights are with indoor (lightweight) clothing.

within each of these columns a weight range is listed rather than a single arbitrary figure.

How Many Calories Do You Need?

The energy potential of foods is measured in calories—one calorie being the amount of heat necessary to raise the temperature of a liter (about 1.1 quart) of water one degree Centigrade (1.8 degrees Fahrenheit). The number of calories a person needs each day, to be derived from the food he eats, depends upon at least three things: (1) his size and "desirable" or ideal weight, (2) his physical activity, and (3) the individual factors that determine how efficiently his food is used (metabolism). A person has very little control over the third factor. It depends on heredity, on the structure and functional pattern of his digestive organs, and upon the physiological balance among his endocrine glands.

With respect to the factor of physical activity, the amount of calories necessary to provide the energy for exercise may vary, even from hour to hour. For example, when an average-sized person is resting quietly, he uses up only about sixty or seventy calories per hour. When he is using his muscles in strenuous work, he may use as many as 200 to 300 calories per hour for many hours at a time. Under extremes of all-out exertion, he may use calories at the astonishing rate of 1000 or more per hour for a few minutes at a time.

To answer the question, How many calories do I need? see the table on the next page listing caloric allowances for men and for women in the three adult age groups. The allowances as listed are for persons whose daily expenditure of energy (daily activity) is moderate. The allowance may be shifted up or down for persons of maximum or minimum activity.

Recommendation for the Number of Calories Per Day

	Age	Calories per Day
Men	19-22	3000
	23-50	2700
	50+	2400
Women	19-22	2100
	23-50	2000
	50+	1800

Source: National Research Council recommendation as revised, 1973.

Reducing by Limitation of Food

The nutritional principle involved in reducing body weight is very simple: Merely cut down the daily number of calories taken in until it is less than the number necessary to provide the daily energy requirements. The difference is then made up from the fat contained in the body tissues. So if you eat less food than required to maintain usual activities, the reserve supply of fat is correspondingly reduced.

But limiting the amount of food eaten is not the only way to reduce the extra fat in your tissues. Consider a moment how you maintain the balance in your bank account. You write checks, day by day, to pay bills. These are charged against your checking account. Also, you make deposits, which become credit entries. Now if you wish to reduce the credit balance, you can do it in two ways: (1) decrease the amount of your deposits or (2) increase withdrawals by writing more or larger checks.

Similarly, in reducing the amount of fat in body tissues, you can either decrease the amount of food intake (com-

parable to reducing the amount of money deposited in the bank) or you can increase the number of calories used each day to provide the energy for physical activity (equivalent to writing larger checks).

Here we will consider both possibilities—first, limiting the diet, and later, increasing exercise as a means of reducing the "fat account."

A pound of body fat can supply about 3500 calories when it is used as a source of energy. Therefore, if each day's diet contains 500 calories less than the day's energy requirement, it will take seven days to lose one pound of weight. When a person follows such a program for ten weeks, he will have lost ten pounds of body weight. Simple, isn't it?

In principle, yes; but in practice, no—too many factors complicate the process. For example, it is hard to be accurate in counting calories. Second, activities vary from day to day, and thus the number of calories consumed per day is not always the same. Then, the element of human frailty enters. A person may break over occasionally and eat an extra slice of bread or a piece of candy. Being invited out to dinner carries the strong temptation to forget about calories "just this once."

One reason a person may become discouraged when he places himself on a restricted diet is that the bathroom scales may not register any loss of weight the first day. Fact is, they may not show any results for several days—in some cases for as long as three weeks. Why? Because a person's weight, as measured by scales, consists of more than fat and bone and muscle. It includes the weight of the water in his body. Weight can vary two or three pounds either way, depending on the amount of water that happens to be in the tissues at a given time.

So do not worry when it seems that several days pass and you weigh just the same. Simply persist in following your limited diet, and the scales will finally reflect the improvement. Then you will be gratified to find that you are

SOME FAVORITE FOODS WITH HIGH CALORIE COUNT

Approximate Number of Calories

3 four-inch griddle cakes	225
1 seven-inch waffle	200
1 tablespoon butter	100
1 tablespoon maple syrup	60
1 tablespoon of jam	55
1 slice of wheat toast	65
$^1/_7$ of a nine-inch apple pie	350
$^1/_7$ of a nine-inch lemon meringue pie	300
$^1/_2$ cup of ice cream	130
$^1/_{16}$ of a nine-inch chocolate layer cake	235
10 roasted peanuts	50
10 large potato chips	100
5 cashew nuts	55
1 chocolate almond bar	200
1 glass of ginger ale	85
1 serving of chocolate malted milk (8 ounces)	500

Persons who are reducing should partake of these sparingly

bottle? Not exactly, but to control weight a person must balance the number of calories contained in his food with the number of calories that his body needs for its usual activities.

The danger in following a reducing diet not carefully planned is that it may not contain sufficient protein, vitamins, and minerals. The difference between a normal diet and a reducing diet is not merely smaller servings. The reducing diet should contain as great a quantity of protein, vitamins, and minerals as does a normal diet. The essential difference, then, between an average diet and a reducing diet is less fat and carbohydrate in the latter. It is not desirable to eliminate all foods containing fat, however, because some fat is important to the body's nutritional needs.

We now present a reducing diet. First we list the daily food pattern, indicating what foods and how much of each may be eaten within the day to provide the necessary nutrients and still limit the calories to 1200. Then follows a sample menu for each of the day's three meals. And last we give lists of approved foods from which the items in the menus may be chosen.

1200-Calorie Reducing Diet Daily Food Pattern

3   cups nonfat milk or buttermilk
1   egg 3 or 4 times a week
1   serving citrus fruit or tomato juice
2   servings fresh fruit or fruit canned without sugar
$^2/_3$ cup raw vegetable salad
2   servings cooked or raw vegetables, one yellow or green
1   small potato
3   slices whole-grain bread; or substitute 1 slice with $^1/_2$ cup whole-grain cereal; or use 1 rounded tablespoon 100 percent wheat germ instead of $^1/_2$ slice bread
2 or 3 servings low-calorie protein foods
1   tablespoon fat

Sample Day's Menu
Breakfast

2   servings fruit, one citrus (see the

on schedule after all. For this reason some counselors advocate that people on a reducing diet should weigh only once a week rather than once a day.

While speaking of bathroom scales for checking one's weight, we should mention that the weighing should always be done at the same time of day and with the same amount of clothing on. The ideal time is just after rising in the morning, before any food or drink has been taken. The weight table appearing in this chapter specifies that "indoor clothing" be worn at the time of weighing. It may be more convenient, however, when weighing in the early morning, to wear night clothing. If you do this, make a correction of about three pounds less in the weights listed in the weight table.

Can Calories Be Counted?

Can calories be counted like pills in a

list which follows for portion size)

1/2 cup whole-grain cereal or 1 slice bread

1 egg poached or boiled

1 cup nonfat milk (may be incorporated into hot drink)

1 teaspoon margarine or 2 teaspoons half-and-half

Dinner

1 generous serving protein food (see list under *Group II* below)

1 cup buttermilk or nonfat milk

1 medium-sized baked potato

2/3 cup mixed green vegetables or sliced tomato

1 serving vegetable from *Group I* or *II* (see list below)

1 serving simple dessert, usually fruit (if desired)

1 slice whole-grain bread

1 1/2 teaspoons margarine or oil

Supper or Lunch

1 1/2 servings fruit chosen from list, or vegetable soup

1 cup nonfat milk or buttermilk

1/2 cup low-fat cottage cheese or other low-calorie protein food

1 slice whole-grain bread

1 teaspoon margarine or oil

Fruits and Approved Portion Sizes

1 apple 2 inches in diameter

1/3 cup apple juice

1/2 cup applesauce

3 medium-sized apricots

4 dried apricot halves

1/2 medium-sized banana

2/3 cup blueberries

3/4 cup other berries

1/4 cantaloupe* 6 inches in diameter

10 large or 15 small cherries

2 dates

2 medium-sized fresh figs

1/2 cup canned fruit

1/2 small grapefruit*

1/2 cup grapefruit* juice

12 grapes

1/4 cup grape juice

1 piece (one sixth) honeydew melon 6 inches in diameter

1/2 medium-sized mango

1 small-sized orange*

1/2 scant cup orange* juice

1 medium-sized peach

1 small or 1/2 large-sized pear

1/2 cup or 1 slice pineapple

1/3 cup pineapple juice

2 medium-sized dried prunes

1/4 cup prune juice

2 tablespoons raisins

Rhubarb as desired

1 large tangerine*

1 slice watermelon 1 1/2 x 10 inches

Vegetables
Group I

3/4 cup of any:

Asparagus
Beetgreens
Broccoli
Cabbage
Celery
Cucumbers
Endive
Lettuce
Mustard greens
Radishes
Sauerkraut
Spinach
Summer squash
Swiss chard
Tomatoes
Mushrooms

*Asterisk indicates high vitamin C content. At least one of these should be chosen daily.

Group II

1/2 cup of any:

Eggplant
Green beans
Kohlrabi
Banana squash
Turnips
Artichoke (1 small)
Beets
Carrots
Onions
Rutabagas
Brussels sprouts

Indicated amounts of any:

3 scant tablespoons corn

1/4 cup green peas

2 tablespoons lima beans

221

$^1/_4$ cup parsnips
$^1/_3$ cup salsify

Protein Foods

2 vegetable steaks of about 1$^1/_2$ ounces each or other equivalent low-calorie meat alternate
$^1/_2$ cup ground gluten
$^1/_2$ cup low-fat cottage cheese
$^1/_2$ cup cooked beans
2 ounces cheddar cheese

Diet Pills

Since weight control has become popular, many preparations have been marketed with the claim that they will remove one's desire for food or that they will suppress the appetite or that they will provide the necessary nutritional elements in a compact, low-calorie package. Enough years have now passed since the introduction of such preparations to evaluate their effectiveness scientifically.

Dr. Walter Modell, Director of Clinical Pharmacology at Cornell University Medical College, published such an evaluation in the *Journal of the American Medical Association*. He noted that the one drug (dinitrophenol) formerly used quite successfully for weight reduction, eventually proved to have toxic effects and had to be abandoned. Dr. Modell observed that "no similar drug is currently used."

Crash Programs for Reducing

Many spas and health culture salons offer programs claiming to take off several pounds per week. The more spectacular of these include the use of steam baths, starvation diets, and moderate to vigorous exercise. The number of pounds lost can be demonstrated, day by day, on the scales. Some of these programs require the use of purges, massage, and mechanical exercising devices such as shaking belts and slimming machines.

The rapid weight loss in such programs is accounted for, however, not by reduction of body fat, but by the quick elimination of water through perspiration or by the cathartic action of the medicines used. A person's normal water balance will be quickly restored, once he discontinues the regimen. Promoters of these programs hope that the prompt weight loss as measured by the scales will encourage their patrons to continue the program until the starvation diet and the program of exercise has brought about an actual reduction in body weight.

Passive exercise such as massage and manipulation actually accomplish no more than "busy work" to keep the individual's attention distracted during the time his food intake is being curtailed. Active exercise where the individual uses his own muscles is beneficial. The crash programs, however, do not allow enough time for the individual to build up his tolerance for the amount of active exercise that would ensure permanent results.

In the late 1970s a so-called "liquid protein diet" gained some popularity as a means of rapid weight reduction. The diet consisted almost entirely of protein or a mixture of protein and carbohydrate and contained such a small number of calories that the program was described as "protein-supplemented fasting." It truly made possible the loss of many pounds of weight in a matter of a few weeks, but an alarming number of mysterious deaths occurrred among those who followed this program. The deaths ocurred suddenly, possibly related to a chemical imbalance (low potassium), and the physicians caring for these patients could find no other cause but that of malfunction of the heart.

The Value of Exercise

The subject of exercise is considered in chapter 52, volume 1. We are mentioning it here again as part of a reasonable program of weight reduction. In order for exercise to be effective as a means of losing weight, it must be carried out systematically. The weekend game of golf is not enough.

As indicated in the accompanying table, the more strenuous the exercise, the greater the consumption of calories. Consider the strenuous activity of

THE NUMBER OF CALORIES PER HOUR CONSUMED BY COMMON EXERCISES

Walking moderately (3 miles per hour)	270
Walking fast (4 miles per hour)	350
Bicycling slowly (5 miles per hour)	250
Bicycling fast (10 miles per hour	450
Riding horseback	150-600
Playing golf (average)	300
Rowing (strenuously)	1,200
Swimming	300-650
Climbing	700-900
Skating fast	300-700

These are the rates at which you may expect exercise to use up the extra calories contained in your diet.

testines. The most desirable program, of course, for losing body weight is to limit the intake of food to the same amount as previously taken so that the exercise will consume some of the calories that otherwise would be stored as fat. Thus the exercise will constitute an additional factor in the program of weight reduction.

Another important consideration is that active exercise changes the nature of the body tissues by increasing the volume of muscle. For example, a certain man began a systematic program of daily exercise as a means of restoring his physical fitness. After he had continued a few weeks, a friend remarked, "You've lost weight."

The man who had been exercising replied, "Not by the scales. I've just shifted weight from my face and neck to other parts of my body." With the development of his muscles had come a reduction in the amount of fat. Even though he weighed the same as before, his weight now consisted of more muscle and less fat.

Hints for Success

In following a program of weight reduction it is *you* who must determine whether you will succeed. Even though the doctor places you on a rigid program, it is your degree of cooperation that will determine whether you lose the amount of weight that you should. The following suggestions are designed to help you maintain enthusiasm and thus ensure satisfactory results.

chopping wood. If the calories in a person's diet were maintained at a constant level, chopping wood for half an hour per day for one year would bring about a reduction of twenty-six pounds in body weight. Exercises less strenuous would of course cause a reduction of correspondingly fewer pounds.

In order for a person to engage safely in a program of vigorous exercise, he should build up gradually. In case of any question as to his fitness or the ability of his heart to tolerate additional activity, he should check with his family doctor before launching such a program.

Many persons contend that exercise increases appetite. This is true, but consider the plus factors as well as the minus factors. At the same time that exercise increases a person's appetite it also increases the activity of the various organs of his body, thus using up more calories and hastening elimination of wastes from the kidneys and in-

1. Keep a diary just for information relating to your program of weight loss. Make a brief notation each day regarding your diet program. If you have broken over by eating a snack or eating some rich dessert beyond your limit of calories, admit this lapse in your diary. Also, for each day, make a note on the exercise you have taken. At least once a week make an entry indicating how much you weigh.

2. Discipline yourself to forget foods you cannot have. Learn to enjoy the taste of simple foods. Eat slowly so that the taste of food lingers longer in

FOUR WAYS OF JUDGING THE EFFECTIVENESS OF EXERCISE
IN TERMS OF CALORIES CONSUMED

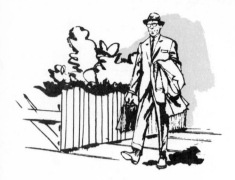 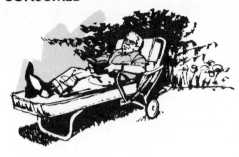

Walking is better than sitting because muscles are brought into play.

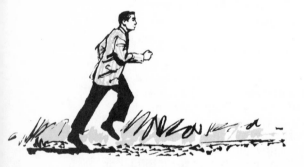 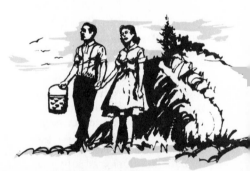

Playing tennis is better than typing because larger muscles are used.

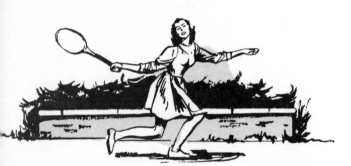 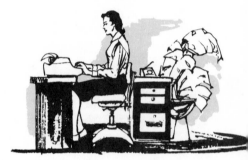

Running is better than walking because the muscles are used faster.

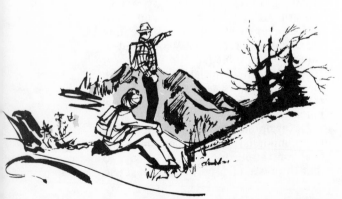 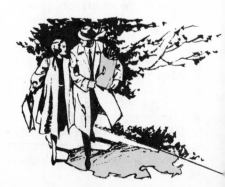

Hikes are better than short walks because the muscles are used longer.

your mouth and in your memory.

3. Don't expect results too soon. If your weight remains constant for a week or two or if you even gain a pound as measured by the scales, recognize that these variations may be caused by temporary changes in the water balance within your body. It is the long-range results that count.

4. Tell your friends about how much better you feel as you begin to lose a few pounds of weight. This not only helps to focus your attention on the benefits of reduced weight but pledges you, in the eyes of your friends, to continue your program of weight reduction until you have reached your goal.

C. Diabetes Mellitus

When a person uses the term *diabetes* without qualification, he refers to diabetes mellitus, a serious metabolic disorder characterized by defects in the body's use of carbohydrates. It may be caused by a deficiency in insulin production by the pancreas or else by an inability of the body cells to use the insulin available. The other kind of diabetes—diabetes insipidus—quite a different disease and relatively rare—is discussed in chapter 2, volume 3.

Diabetes mellitus, once established, persists throughout the life of the individual and often produces serious, life-threatening complications, and thus reduces life expectancy. An estimated ten million Americans (almost 5 percent of the population) have diabetes of some degree. Among diabetics, blindness occurs twenty-five times as frequently as among nondiabetics; kidney disease occurs seventeen times more frequently; gangrene of the tissues is fifty times more prevalent among diabetics; and heart disease occurs twice as often among diabetics as among nondiabetics. Although diabetes, as such, is not curable, the modern treatment programs, when faithfully followed, can relieve the patient of the symptoms of his disease and can reduce the prospect of his developing tragic complications. We may say, then, that even those who develop diabetes in early life may, by a rigid program of treatment, live comfortably and productively for several decades.

Role of Insulin

Insulin is a hormone produced by the beta cells in the islets of Langerhans in the pancreas. See chapter 1, volume 3. Insulin is carried by the blood as it flows to all parts of the body. The cells throughout the body use glucose (blood sugar) as their fuel. They have receptors on their surface to which insulin becomes attached. This binding of the hormone insulin through a complicated series of events within the cells, enables the cells to use the glucose circulating in the blood by converting it into energy or storing it as fat. The process by which insulin controls the body's use of glucose is rather complicated. Any defect in this process, however, either in the pancreas where insulin is produced or at the site of attachment to the cells throughout the body, interferes with the body's use of fuel to produce energy. The two major types of diabetes mellitus are caused by interference with this process in two different ways.

The Two Types of Diabetes Mellitus. There are certain times of life during which diabetes mellitus is especially prone to develop. For children, the occurrence of new cases is highest among 5- and 6-year-olds and again among those between 11 and 13 years of age. For adults, most cases of diabetes mellitus begin after 40 years of age. The particular manifestations of the diabetes that begins in childhood differ from those of the type which begins later in life. The two types are designated as (1) insulin-dependent diabetes (juvenile-onset diabetes) and (2) non-insulin-dependent (maturity-onset diabetes). The insulin-dependent type is by far the more serious of the two and, fortunately, accounts for only about 10 percent of the total number of cases of diabetes mellitus. The first type—the

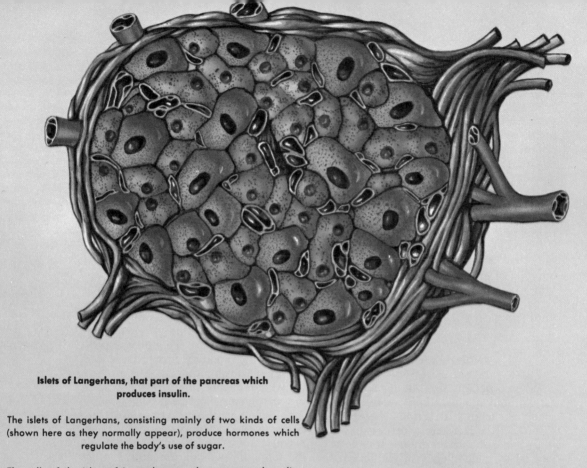

Islets of Langerhans, that part of the pancreas which produces insulin.

The islets of Langerhans, consisting mainly of two kinds of cells (shown here as they normally appear), produce hormones which regulate the body's use of sugar.

The cells of the islets of Langerhans as they appear when diseased and no longer able to perform their essential function.

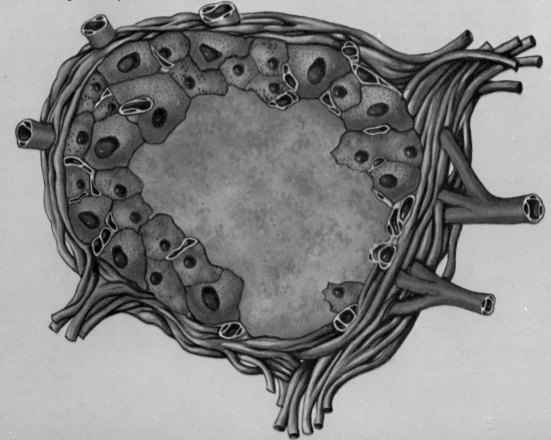

type that begins in childhood—is not limited to childhood. Beginning in childhood, it continues throughout life.

The fundamental cause of insulin-dependent diabetes is a reduction in the production of insulin by the beta cells of the islets of Langerhans in the pancreas. The symptoms of this type are relieved by the use of injections of insulin. (See chapter 17, volume 1, for additional information on this type of diabetes.)

In the non-insulin-dependent type of diabetes that occurs in later life, the body has an adequate supply of insulin, but a defect has developed in the mechanism by which insulin enables the cells to make use of glucose. Therefore in this type, the administration of insulin is not always necessary.

Causes. For many years it has been recognized that children of diabetic parents have a greater-than-usual prospect of developing diabetes. A hereditary factor causes some people to be more susceptible than others. For insulin-dependent diabetes (the type that begins in childhood) evidence shows that the actual damage to the beta cells in the pancreas may be caused by the invasion of one of several types of viruses. Perhaps some persons inherit a susceptibility to the damage which such viruses can cause, whereas others have a natural resistance to such damage.

The fundamental cause of non-insulin-dependent diabetes (maturity-onset diabetes) seems to be an overburdening of the body's energy-producing mechanisms. It is significant that obese persons are particularly susceptible to non-insulin-dependent diabetes.

Risk Factors. In view of the information given above, it is possible to list the following risk factors by which certain persons are predisposed to diabetes: (1) family members who have diabetes, (2) obesity, (3) older age. Diabetes is two and a half times more probable in persons whose relatives have had diabetes. The fact that 85 percent of diabetic patients were at some time overweight speaks for itself. As for age, four out of five diabetics are over 45 years of age.

Symptoms the Patient Notices. When diabetes begins during childhood, the symptoms include excess production of urine, excessive thirst, a desire to void at night, bedwetting, an increase in appetite in spite of a loss of body weight, weakness, and itching of the skin. For cases which begin during adulthood, the symptoms are excessive production of urine, increased thirst, weakness, and itching of the skin.

What the Physician Finds. When a physician examines a person with diabetes, he finds sugar in the urine, a higher-than-normal concentration of glucose in the blood, and evidence (revealed by a glucose tolerance test) that the individual is not using up his blood sugar as quickly, following a meal, as in a normal case. These all indicate that the body is unable to use glucose in a normal manner. In other words, glucose accumulates in the blood and is eliminated by way of the urine instead of being used in the body for production of energy.

Complications. The great tragedy of diabetes of either type is the unpredictable prospect of serious complications. These do not arise in all cases. They are most likely to happen in cases of long standing and in cases where carelessness occurs in the program of care and treatment.

Something about diabetes favors the development of arteriosclerosis (hardening of the arteries); narrowing of the blood capillaries; the development of new capillaries, particularly in the eye; and degenerative changes in the nervous system. In a person who happens to be otherwise susceptible to arteriosclerosis, the occurrence of diabetes hastens and intensifies this development. Diabetes compounds the effect of smoking as it relates to arteriosclerosis. Definitely, the diabetic should not smoke.

The diabetic is particularly susceptible to coronary heart disease with its possibility of heart attack, to foot problems resulting from poor circulation in the feet, to kidney disease with the prospect of uremia because of the constriction of the blood capillaries in the kidney and destruction of the glomeruli (kidney filters). He is also susceptible to proliferative retinopathy with its prospect of blindness because of the abnormal development of blood capillaries in the back part of the eye and to various kinds of nervous ailments because of the degeneration of nervous tissue.

Also, a diabetic faces the ever-present danger of loss of consciousness. Two situations representing opposite conditions may cause unconsciousness. The first develops gradually, when the glucose in the blood reaches high levels and is not offset by an adequate amount of insulin. This condition is called *diabetic coma* (ketoacidosis, hyperosmolarity, lactic acidosis, etc.). The second situation that can cause unconsciousness may develop quite suddenly when, for some reason, the supply of glucose in the patient's blood and tissues reaches such a low level that the cells of his body run out of energy. This second condition is called *hypoglycemic coma*. It may develop when the diabetic patient has taken a larger dose of insulin (or a similar medication taken by mouth) than he presently requires. For the emergency treatment of these two conditions see chapter 23, volume 3, in the section on "unconsciousness."

Care and Treatment

It is because of the lurking danger of coma that a diabetic patient is advised to carry a wallet card or wear a bracelet stating that he is a diabetic, and that if he is found to be acting strangely or if he becomes unconscious, a doctor or an ambulance should be called. The card should give the following information: pa-

tient's name, address, and telephone number; a statement that he has diabetes; and his physician's name, address, and telephone number.

Careful regulation of diet is essential in the control of diabetes. Many cases, particularly those that develop during adulthood, can be handled satisfactorily without the use of insulin or other medications, provided the patient follows a proper dietary program. A suitable diet for a diabetic is relatively normal, except that it contains very little of the rapidly absorbed carbohydrates, is low in fat to protect against arteriosclerosis, and high in fiber to slow absorption. The special feature is that all portions must be carefully measured so that the patient eats neither too much nor too little. The various food elements must be carefully regulated. It is important that the diabetic patient avoid becoming or remaining overweight. It is when a diabetic patient becomes careless in following his diet that he encounters difficulty.

Particularly in the insulin-dependent type of diabetes, the use of insulin or one of the hypoglycemic agents becomes a vital part of the treatment. Insulin administered by hypodermic is the reliable means of controlling the level of the patient's blood sugar. Great advances have been made in the preparation of insulin, and the physician may choose among various products as he adapts the treatment to the particular needs of his patient. The so-called hypoglycemic agents are insulin enhancers and can be taken by mouth. They should be used only after careful consideration by the physician in charge of the case.

Once diabetes has been diagnosed, it is good for the patient to spend several days in the hospital for education on how to control his illness. Here he learns how to regulate his diet, how to test his urine for sugar, and how to take his insulin or insulin substitute, if such is necessary. His opportunity to enjoy good health thereafter depends on his being consistent in following his treatment program. Periodic checkups are necessary as a means of measuring his progress and of modifying the treatment program to fit changes in his condition.

A diabetic should give special attention to the care of his feet. It is estimated that one half of all diabetics will experience at least one major complication affecting the feet during their lifetime. These problems are the result of poor circulation of blood as well as of involvement of the nerves. Gangrene may develop in the foot or leg. In neglected cases, amputation of a limb may become necessary to save the patient's life. Many such complications could be avoided by appropriate foot care, such as daily inspection, management of corns and ulcers, surgical treatment of ingrown toenails, and consistent use of well-fitting shoes.

Certain circumstances require special attention. Pregnancy is one of these. In the event of surgery, the diabetic's condition must be carefully monitored. When an infection develops in the skin or in any other part of the body, the diabetic should have appropriate special care.

The person with diabetes should regulate his physical exercise almost as carefully as he regulates his diet. It is good for him to have some physical exercise every day. But excessive exercise changes his requirements for food.

D. Hypoglycemia (Low Blood Sugar)

Hypoglycemia is the condition in which the amount of glucose (blood sugar) drops below the level of 50 mg. per 100 ml. of blood. Hypoglycemia is not a separate disease as such, for it may stem from any one of several causes.

The symptoms of hypoglycemia may follow two patterns, which can occur separately or in combination. First, certain symptoms relate to the nervous system and result from the brain's be-

ing deprived of sufficient glucose (energy food) to maintain the normal activity of its cells. These symptoms may include mental confusion and anxiety, hallucinations, aimless activity, convulsions, and even coma.

Second, certain symptoms result from the body's automatic attempt to compensate for the lack of blood sugar by producing an emergency supply of epinephrine. These include sweating, pallor, chilliness, trembling, hunger, weakness, and palpitation.

The Causes of Hypoglycemia:

1. Hypoglycemia may result from an overdose of insulin. Insulin has the effect of accelerating the body's use of blood sugar. An overdose of insulin, therefore, reduces the amount of sugar in the blood. Hypoglycemia may also follow the excessive use of hypoglycemic agents.

2. Failure to eat the usual amount of food after taking insulin may cause hypoglycemia. In a diabetic patient, the amount of insulin must be balanced against the amount of food the patient is expected to eat in order to maintain the normal level of blood sugar. When the patient does not eat this necessary amount of food after taking insulin, the effect is comparable to that of an overdose of insulin, with the result that blood sugar is reduced.

3. Hypoglycemia may result from excessive exercise. If the body's sources for replenishing the available supply of blood sugar thus used are not momentarily adequate, hypoglycemia will result. A person with diabetes mellitus is particularly susceptible in this instance.

4. Hypoglycemia may result from an overproduction of insulin within the body, as in a particular type of tumor of the pancreas in which the insulin-producing tissue becomes overactive.

5. It may develop in cases of liver disease in which the blood sugar is not stored or released by the liver in a normal manner.

6. Hypoglycemia may occur in connection with diseases of certain endo-

crine organs, as the adrenals and pituitary.

Care and Treatment

The treatment of an acute attack of hypoglycemia will vary, depending on whether the patient is in a hospital or is given emergency treatment elsewhere and on whether he is able to swallow or has already lost consciousness. In a hospital intravenous glucose is given. Elsewhere the administration of glucagon by injection will usually produce a rapid elevation of the blood sugar level. Glucagon is a hormone normally produced in the pancreas which has the effect of counterbalancing the influence of insulin. The giving of glucagon may need to be followed by the intravenous injection of glucose to replenish the body's supply. Subsequent treatment is determined by the results of laboratory tests indicating the level of the patient's blood sugar.

When the patient is not in the hospital but is still able to swallow, he should be given any sort of sweetened drink, such as orange juice, or its equivalent in candy or sugar. The symptoms of the immediate attack should improve within fifteen minutes. Then he should eat bread or other food containing starch and protein to provide the necessary source from which his tissues can produce additional glucose. When the patient is not able to swallow, intravenous therapy is given. Prompt effort should be made to secure the services of a physician or to take the patient to the emergency room of a hospital.

For cases in which the cause of hypoglycemia may be organic disease of the pancreas or liver, a physician should study the case in order to determine the exact cause and to arrange the treatment accordingly. Surgery or other definitive treatment may need to be carried out promptly.

For cases of functional hypoglycemia, when no actual disease of the liver or pancreas exists, an alteration in the patient's diet may correct the tendency to hypoglycemia. In such cases, the body's control mechanism may have become unusually sensitive to the taking of carbohydrate food so that insulin is produced in excessive amounts. A helpful procedure is to adopt a diet low in refined carbohydrates (sugar and white-flour products), moderate in protein, low in fat, and high in fresh fruits and vegetables and unrefined grain rich in fiber—thus enabling the individual to derive the necessary number of calories for his energy needs without overstimulating his own production of insulin.

E. Gout

Gout is a systemic disease characterized by an inherited fault in the way the body metabolizes uric acid. Uric aid is one of the by-products of the digestion of food. In most persons, uric acid is readily eliminated by the kidneys. But in a person with a tendency to gout, the uric acid is not eliminated as quickly as it should be, and the body's fluids and tissues contain more than is normal. Such an excess of uric acid in the body's fluids (hyperuricemia) occurs in 5 to 10 percent of American men above the age of 30, but in only about one tenth as many women. Many persons with hyperuricemia have no symptoms and do not know that they have this condition. But in a minority of this group (about three persons per thousand population), one or the other of four possible complications develop:

1. *Acute gouty arthritis* occurs in attacks which come unannounced and, if untreated, will run a course of one or two weeks each. This problem is discussed in chapter 21, volume 2.

2. *Tophaceous gout* is a chronic condition in which hard masses of uric acid crystals, called tophi, make their appearance in various tissues of the body. One of the favorite sites for a tophus is the lobe of the ear. Commonly, tophi are situated in the vicinity of joints.

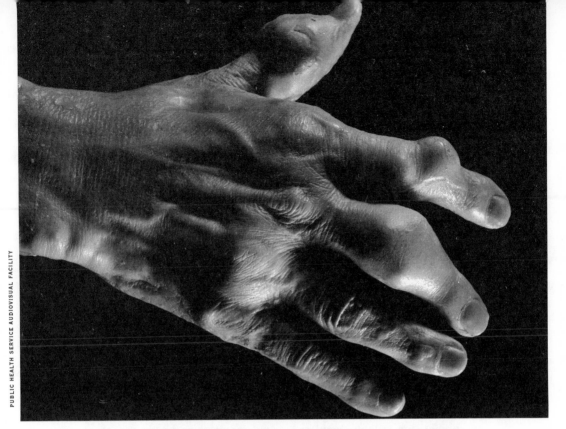

The hand of a person suffering from gout, one form of arthritis. Lumps in knuckles are caused by excess of uric acid leading to formation of urate crystals around the joints. See diagram below.

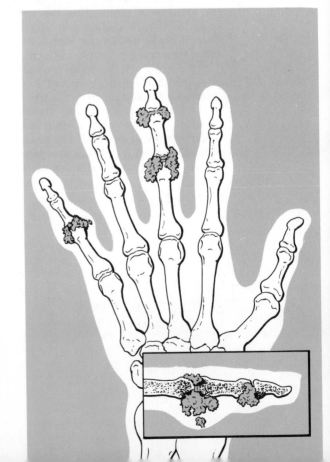

The body's tissues react to these tophi as to foreign bodies, with a resulting mild but persistent inflammation. When untreated, a certain destruction develops in the tissues adjacent to a tophus, which may involve the bones and surrounding soft tissues.

3. *Kidney Stones*. Gout is not the only condition in which stones develop within the pelvis of the kidney, but the development of kidney stones is frequent in persons with hyperuricemia. Kidney stones are discussed in chapter 27, volume 2.

4. *Gouty kidney disease*. There appears to be a two-way relationship between gout and degenerative disease of the kidney. About one third of the cases of hyperuricemia seem to be aggravated by or possibly even caused by inefficiency of the kidneys to eliminate uric acid from the body as readily as it should be. On the other hand, the mere

condition of hyperuricemia seems to have a damaging effect on the kidneys. In some cases kidney disease seems to contribute to gout; in others, gout contributes to kidney disease.

Care and Treatment

Many persons who have high levels of uric acid in their body fluids and tissues are not aware of this until one of the complications of gout develops. A difference of opinion exists among specialists on the use of medications to lower the level of uric acid in the body fluids in cases which show no symptoms of gout. At any rate, the person who knows that he has hyperuricemia should do what he can to reduce his intake of uric acid in food and what is reasonable to hasten and facilitate the elimination of uric acid from his body. Meat and animal fat (such as butter) should be kept to the minimum in his diet. If the patient is overweight, his weight should certainly be brought within normal limits. Such a person should drink up to three quarts of water per day to aid the kidneys in eliminating the uric acid. He should abstain consistently from alcoholic drinks, for such indulgence may bring on another attack.

The person who has developed any one of the complications of gout should be under the care of a physician. Within recent years several medicines have been successfully used in the treatment of gout. The choice of medicines for a given case depends on the specific manifestations of the disease and on the stage of the disease during which the treatment is begun. Medicines particularly useful include probenecid (Benemid), sulfinpyrazone, and allopurinol. When used selectively and discriminatingly, under a physician's direction, medicines can make the difference between invalidism and a life essentially free from disability and deformity.

F. Disorders in Pigment Metabolism

The outstanding example here is the disease porphyria, in which there is a disturbance of the metabolic process by which the body uses the chemical substance known as porphyrin to help build its hemoglobin and some of its other pigments and enzymes. Heredity is blamed for most cases of porphyria. There are various forms of the disease, all resulting in an excess of porphyrin compounds in the urine.

In some forms of this disease there is a sensitivity of the skin to sunlight or to artificial ultraviolet light, with resulting skin lesions and abnormal pigmentation. In one form the patient shows symptoms of abdominal pain, vomiting, and constipation, together with paralysis of certain of the muscles. Acute attacks are usually brought on by the use of alcohol, by certain drugs, or by infections.

The treatment consists largely of avoiding alcohol and drugs and of protecting the skin from sunlight.

SECTION V

Allergies and Infections

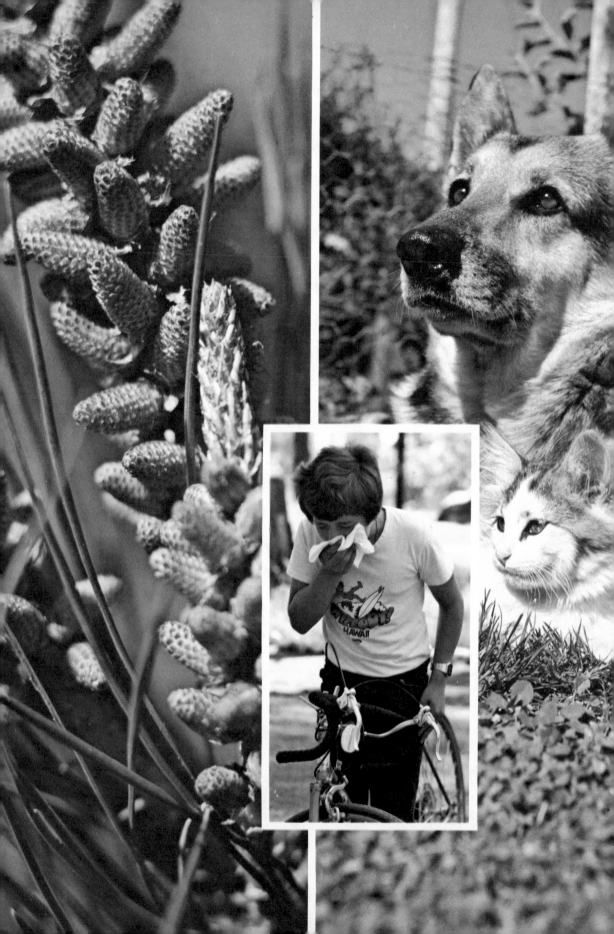

Allergic Manifestations

It is not intended that this chapter will add significantly to our list of diseases. It is expected, rather, that it will improve the reader's understanding of the causes of some of the diseases described in other parts of the book.

In the broad sense, allergy is the body's response to the presence of some aggravating agent called an allergen. Individuals react differently in their responses to allergens; therefore some people are said to be more allergic than others.

It used to be assumed that all allergens were protein substances, and it was common to speak of "protein sensitivity," by which was meant that a given protein substance would cause certain tissues to react abnormally. It is now understood that some allergens are carbohydrates, and at least a few are chemically related to the fats. Regardless of their chemical nature, all allergens have one thing in common— they stimulate a sensitive individual to react by producing antibodies.

The mechanism by which tissues react unfavorably to the presence of an allergen is bound up with the body's intricate chemical processes, such as enzyme reactions, and is even related to the processes by which immunity is developed. Becoming immune to a certain germ whose products have served as an allergen is one form of response which could be thought of as allergy but is best termed immunity. When the antibodies which a certain allergen produces are fixed to a group of the body's cells rather than remaining free in the bloodstream, then these cells on which the antibodies are located may be unfavorably affected when exposed to this specific allergen.

Kinds of Allergens

1. Some allergens enter the body by being inhaled. These include pollens; dusts; vapors, such as tobacco smoke; emanations from epithelium, such as dandruff; and strong odors, such as perfumes.

2. Certain foods provoke an allergic response in persons who may be sensitive. These include wheat, milk, chocolate, eggs, strawberries, nuts, pork, and fish.

3. Some persons become sensitive to drugs or biological agents. These substances, then, can serve as allergens.

4. Certain germs may function as allergens so that the symptoms produced when these germs invade a person's tissues are the direct result of the allergic response and are not caused, primarily,

by tissue injury through direct contact with the germs.

5. Some allergens cause the allergic response through a mere contact with the skin or the mucous membranes of a sensitive person. These include products from plants such as poison oak and poison ivy, and certain dyes, metals, plastics, furs, leathers, rubber products, cosmetics, and chemicals such as insecticides.

6. Even physical agents such as heat, cold, light, and pressure occasionally awaken a response similar to an allergy. Many a sufferer from hay fever has noticed that he begins to sneeze when he steps into bright sunlight. This can be either a triggering of the allergy or a vasomotor response due to sensitive membranes and thus not a true allergy.

Preventing the Allergic Response

In general, the allergic response may be prevented or its symptoms modified in four ways:

A. *Avoiding the Allergen*. The simplest way to prevent the allergic response is to prevent the allergens to which a person is sensitive from entering his body. Sufferers from hay fever can often prevent their attacks by staying indoors during the time of year when the plants bloom that produce the pollens to which they are sensitive. If these plants are limited to a certain locality, the sufferers can avoid symptoms by staying away from this locality. Allergy to a drug can be avoided by not using the drug. Allergy to some specific food may be handled by excluding this food from the diet. Persons sensitive to a particular dust may benefit by wearing a filtering mask. Airconditioning systems with good filters often bring relief to victims of hay fever and asthma.

B. *Desensitization*. Just as it is possible to make a person immune to snake venom by injecting gradually increasing doses of this venom into his tissues, so it is possible to build up a person's tolerance to some allergens by a carefully controlled program of administering gradually increasing doses of this allergen. Physicians can obtain preparations of the usual allergens from medical supply houses and can inject these into a sensitive patient, beginning with very small doses and building up gradually week by week, until the patient's tolerance has improved to the point where he will no longer develop symptoms when exposed to the allergen. This method has proved quite successful in bringing relief to many patients suffering from hay fever and to some suffering from types of asthma which result in large part from allergy. It may be necessary to administer doses of these preparations at regular intervals the year round in order to maintain the individual's tolerance to the offending substance.

C. *The Use of Antihistamines*. In most cases of allergy, histamine is one of the chemicals which the body's tissues liberate in response to the presence of an allergen. An antihistamine drug, which counteracts histamine, may relieve the allergic response in such cases. There are many varieties of antihistamine drugs, and it happens that one kind will benefit some allergic persons and another kind, others. It may be necessary to use the trial-and-error method to determine which form of antihistamine will bring the greatest benefit in a particular case. Some hay fever sufferers derive enough benefit from the use of antihistamines that they prefer using them to obtaining relief by the more time-consuming desensitization method.

Some hazard is involved in the use of antihistamine drugs, because in some cases these have the side effect of making a person sleepy. It is dangerous, therefore, for the person taking such drugs to drive a car lest his reactions have been slowed to the extent that his driving is unsafe.

D. *The Use of Hormones*. In cases of extremely serious allergic reactions,

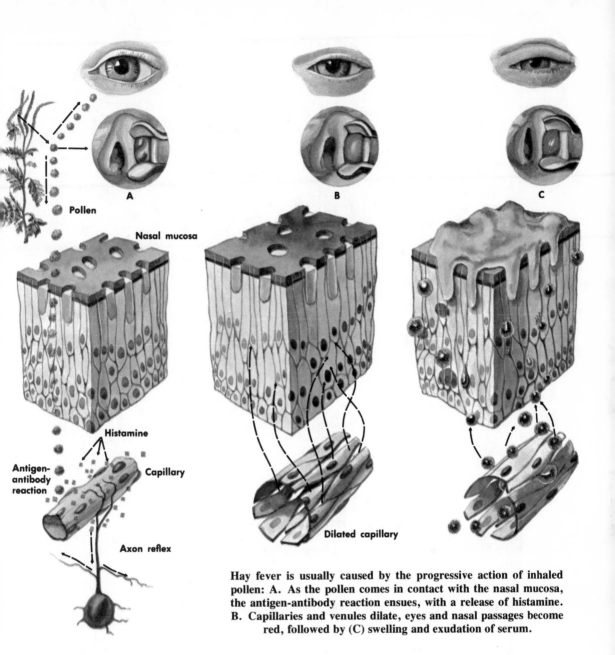

Pollen

Nasal mucosa

Histamine

Antigen-antibody reaction

Capillary

Axon reflex

Dilated capillary

Hay fever is usually caused by the progressive action of inhaled pollen: **A.** As the pollen comes in contact with the nasal mucosa, the antigen-antibody reaction ensues, with a release of histamine. **B.** Capillaries and venules dilate, eyes and nasal passages become red, followed by (C) swelling and exudation of serum.

the appropriate use of steroid preparations derived from the cortex of the adrenal gland may provide some benefit. These powerful medicinal agents should be used only under the direct supervision of a physician.

ALLERGIC RHINITIS (HAY FEVER)

The symptoms of this illness depend typically upon an allergic response to an offending protein substance breathed in by way of the inspired air.

The symptoms of this illness are described in chapter 9, this volume.

ATOPIC DERMATITIS (ECZEMA)

Atopic dermatitis, in most cases, is an allergic manifestation affecting the skin, causing itching, burning, and redness. The symptoms vary from person to person. Atopic dermatitis is likely to occur during three age periods—infancy, childhood, and adulthood. It may appear for the first time in any one of these. A comprehensive consideration of atopic dermatitis appears in chapter 17, volume 1.

ASTHMA

At least half the cases of asthma seem to be caused or aggravated by allergy. Asthma is discussed in chapter 17, volume 1. Emergency treatment for an acute attack of asthma is described in chapter 23, volume 3.

URTICARIA (HIVES; ANGIONEUROTIC EDEMA)

This is a skin malady which typically occurs in response to some offending allergen. It may affect the membranes lining the air passages and thus, in extreme cases, endanger a person's life. More information and suggestions for treatment are provided in chapter 25, volume 2.

SERUM SICKNESS

Serum sickness is an allergic reaction triggered by the injection of a serum of animal origin (usually horse serum). Certain antitoxins, valuable in the treatment of specific infections, have been formed in animal serum. The acute allergic reaction typically occurs in persons who have had a previous injection of this same kind of serum and have had sufficient time to become sensitive to it.

Sensitization *can* occur 10 to 14 days after the *first* exposure. It is because of the possibility of serum sickness that physicians prefer to use human anti-serum preparations, when available, rather than the type produced in animals.

Symptoms of serum sickness begin with a skin eruption which may appear like urticaria (hives). There is fever, enlargement of the lymph nodes, pain in the joints, nausea, and abdominal pain.

Emergency treatment for serum sickness requires the use of small intravenous injections of a 1:1000 solution of epinephrine. Depending upon the patient's condition, the injection may need to be repeated two or three times at intervals of a few minutes.

DRUG ALLERGY

An allergic reaction may occur in sensitive individuals after the taking of certain drugs. Hundreds of drugs at one time or another have provoked an allergic response in sensitive persons. Certain drugs are more common offenders than others, the notable ones among the modern drugs being the sulfonamides and antibiotics.

The development of a skin rash is the usual manifestation of a drug allergy. Fever and symptoms of shock may occur in the more extreme cases. Discontinuance of the offending drug is the obvious method of treatment. The symptoms usually disappear within a few days after the drug is discontinued. (See the item on "Drug Eruptions" in chapter 25, volume 2.)

ANAPHYLACTIC SHOCK

In some persons an allergic reaction to an insect sting or to a drug such as penicillin is so sudden and so intense as to be designated as shock (anaphylactic shock). The beginning symptom is usually a skin reaction as in urticaria (hives). The membranes of the air passages swell, and the condition progresses rapidly to collapse. Further details and instructions for the emergency treatment of anaphylactic shock are found in chapter 23, volume 3.

Infections

The invasion of the human body by infectious agents, germs, and viruses is a major cause of diseases and disabilities. Not all diseases are caused by infectious agents, however. Some are caused by injuries, deficiencies, faults in the body's control systems, poisonings, degenerative processes in the tissues, or unhappy or unfortunate states of mind. Many diseases have multiple causes. But we are concerned in this chapter and in the five following chapters with certain of the health problems for which various kinds of germs are responsible.

The word *infection* refers to the entrance into the body's tissues of disease-producing organisms. These may enter by many routes. A break in the skin caused by a wound, a scratch, or an animal bite allows them to enter the tissues underneath the skin. Puncture by a sharp object or by a nail, or penetration of the skin by an insect bite may introduce germs. The membrane surrounding the eye can be easily penetrated by germs brought there by dirty fingers or a contaminated handkerchief. Membranes of the nose or throat are susceptible to penetration by organisms carried by small particles of dust or droplets of moisture. Infections involving the lungs may be caused by germs and viruses emitted by a sick person when he sneezes or coughs.

Contaminated food or liquid carries germs into the digestive organs. In sexually transmitted infections, the agents are transferred from one person to the other by contact with the delicate skin or membrane of the sex organs.

The Body's Defense Against Infectious Agents

The human body has an efficient, built-in defense mechanism designed to combat invasion by disease-producing organisms. Phagocyte cells in the tissues and in the circulating blood are capable of engulfing or even destroying many types of germs. Invasion by germs and viruses stimulates the production of specific antibodies custom-built to combat the particular agents that have invaded. After a particular infection subsides, the antibodies produced to combat this infection may become permanently available for action in case this same kind of organism should enter the body another time. The details of the body's mechanisms of defense are explained in simple terms in chapter 5, volume 2.

When infection occurs there develops a conflict between the aggressive action of invading organisms and the resisting action of the body's defenses. Certain factors tend to swing the outcome of the conflict in either a favorable or an unfavorable direction. The

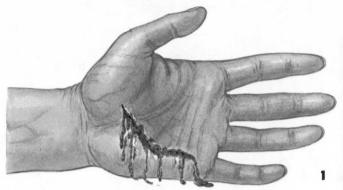

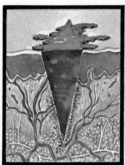

**One route by which disease-producing organisms
enter the body is by a wound.**

number of invaders is one factor. When in large numbers, they tend to overwhelm the body's defenses. Some are more deadly than others.

A person's relative susceptibility is another variable in this conflict. The person who has once recovered from rubella has antibodies within his tissues which can protect him for the remainder of life from an illness caused by this particular virus. But the person whose tissues do not contain antibodies for this certain virus may become an easy victim once the virus enters his body.

The efficiency of a person's defense system may change from time to time. When fatigued or in poor health, a person is more susceptible to infections than when vigorous. A person suffering from an illness is more vulnerable to the threat of some unrelated infection than a person in good health.

Local Infections

In many infections, especially those in which the organisms enter through a break in the skin or at some particular site, the body's defense mechanisms are able to limit the spread of the infection so that it remains in just this one part of the body. Then we speak of the infection as a local infection. This prevention of spreading is accomplished by the invasion into the infected area of phagocyte cells which "close ranks" to wall off the zone of infected tissue. This maneuver occurs, for example, in

the area surrounding a boil, a boil being a good example of a local infection. The same walling off process occurs in miniature in the immediate area of a pimple. This area of compacted cells tends to prevent the spread of the germs into surrounding healthy areas. It is because of the danger of breaking down this barrier zone that a boil or even a pimple should not be squeezed, lest the organisms still alive in the infected area be forced into healthy tissue beyond.

When the germs producing a local infection are sufficiently virulent, the tissue at the focus of the infection may actually be destroyed. This destruction occurs at the center of a boil. The fluidlike material at the center of such an area is called pus and consists of tissue debris, dead germs, some active germs, and cells belonging to the defense system. As the boil ruptures or is lanced it is pus that escapes through the new opening.

When an area of active local infection develops in some internal part of the body, the destruction of tissue may result in the formation of a fluid-filled cavity that we call an abscess. The fluid within an abscess is pus, just as at the center of a boil. Once an abscess develops, it is desirable for the pus to be evacuated. Abscesses developing in internal organs require surgical treatment, sometimes with the insertion of a tube to permit continuous drainage of

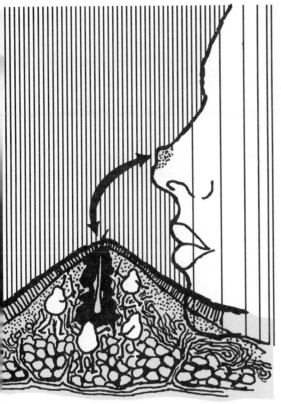

White blood cells, operating as "police" cells, engulf and destroy many types of germs.

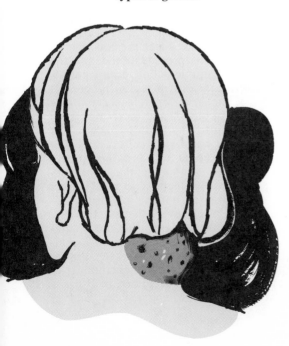

the pus while the infection persists. Obviously, danger of contamination and of spread of the infection threatens when an abscess is being treated.

General Infections

In the battle between invading germs and viruses and the body's defenses, the possibility remains that the invaders will overwhelm the defense mechanisms or that some of the invading germs will slip past the barriers that the body provides for their containment. The lymphatic system with its lymph vessels and lymph nodes is designed to prevent the spread of infections and to keep the infection from entering the circulating blood. The lymph nodes serve as filters for the lymph so that this fluid, together with any organisms or foreign material that it may carry, must run the gauntlet of the defense cells located within the lymph nodes. Even so, germs occasionally enter the circulating blood and are carried by it to the various parts of the body. This circumstance is called bacteremia, the word meaning bacteria or germs in the blood.

In a healthy person, mild degrees of bacteremia do not last long, for even the circulating blood must pass through organs such as the spleen and liver in which are phagocytic cells belonging to the body's defense system. Mild degrees of bacteremia occur frequently when local infections in some part of the body are being treated. A tonsillectomy, extraction of a tooth, surgical drainage of an abscess, a surgical procedure involving the urinary organs—such procedures often allow some germs to enter the circulating blood. Because of this possibility, surgeons often administer antibiotic medications to a patient before he undergoes surgery, so as to destroy germs that may happen to enter the circulating blood.

The principal risk attending bacteremia is the possibility that germs being carried by the blood may establish themselves in the tissues which line the heart, thus causing the serious condition of endocarditis.

The term *septicemia* is used to de-

241

scribe the condition in which germs or toxins are present in the blood.

In some of the infectious diseases described in the following five chapters, the germs which cause the disease are carried by the blood in the early stages of the illness. This is the means by which such general infections extend to all parts of the body.

Infectious and Contagious Diseases

An infectious disease is one caused by the entrance of germs or viruses into the body. By this broad definition, many of the diseases considered in earlier chapters qualify as infectious diseases. The reason they are described there rather than in the five chapters which follow is that they affect organs or organ systems with which these earlier chapters deal. There remain some diseases, however, in which the invading organisms cause infections general in nature. They may affect many organs or just certain ones at random, at times one organ and at other times a different one.

Malaria is an infectious disease, occurring as it does only when the malar-

The common cold is spread from one person to another by viruses.

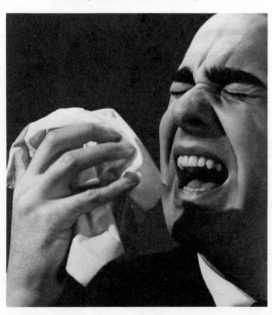

ial parasites enter the body. Measles (rubeola) is also an infectious disease, caused not by a parasite, but by a virus. Arteriosclerosis, by contrast, is not an infectious disease, because it is not caused by the entrance of organisms into the body. It is one of the degenerative diseases.

We sometimes use the term contagious disease. A contagious disease is caused by some germ or virus which may be transferred from one person to another so as to cause the same disease in the second person. Not all infectious diseases are contagious because not all of them are "catching" in the sense that the organisms can transfer from a sick person to cause a well person to become sick with the same disease. Syphilis is a contagious disease. Sometimes we speak of the contagious diseases as communicable diseases.

Physiological Responses to Systemic Infections

The human body responds in many ways to an infectious disease. Some of its responses are for the purpose of combating the infection. Others are mere evidences of the damage the infection is causing within the body's tissues and organs. Fever is a uniform accompaniment of any serious infection, but, as far as we know, it does not contribute to the control of the infection.

The responses which the body makes to an infection provide an index to the severity of the infection. In a vigorous individual, enormous numbers of phagocytic cells are released into the circulating blood, and these may even migrate into the tissue spaces. The number of phagocytic cells revealed by the blood count (a laboratory procedure) gives some indication of the severity of the infection. In most cases, the greater the number of phagocytic cells, the more severe the infection.

Fever (an increase in the body temperature) occurs quite commonly in infections and infectious diseases. But fever also occurs in other conditions: in crushing injuries, in cancer, in diseases of the blood-forming tissues, and in stroke. Therefore it cannot be assumed that the presence of infectious agents is the direct cause of fever. As explained in chapter 23, volume 2, the body temperature is controlled automatically by intricate mechanisms within the nervous system. Our best explanation of fever is that some by-product of tissue destruction is carried by the blood to those centers in the brain that regulate body temperature and that this substance, whatever it may be, changes the setting of the body's "thermostat."

The human body does not tolerate excessive increases in its temperature. Therefore, in cases in which fever becomes excessive, it is advisable to use treatments that reduce fever. For methods of reducing fever by the use of hydrotherapy see the section on "Rubs and Sponges" and on the "Graduated Tub Bath" in chapter 25, volume 3.

In cases of severe, rapidly progressing infection, the serious complication of toxic shock (septic shock) may develop. This condition requires energetic treatment directed both to controling the infection and to maintaining the vital functions of the patient.

Delirium becomes a symptom in many cases of systemic infection.

The Outcome of Infections

In the battle that takes place between the invaders and the body's defense mechanisms, the outcome depends upon which of the conflicting forces prevails. When the body's defenses prove inadequate, the illness may be prolonged indefinitely or may become so serious as to take the patient's life. When the defense mechanisms prove adequate, the invaders are killed and healing takes place.

Many infectious diseases are said to be self-limited. By this it is meant that the body's defenses eventually win out as they bring the infection under control within a few days or, at most, a few weeks.

Some cases of infection, without treatment, end fatally; some continue as a prolonged illness; and some end quite promptly because the body's defenses overcome the invading organisms. We now raise the questions, What is the purpose of treatment? and What may treatment accomplish?

How Treatment Helps

Treatment, properly administered, may save the life of a patient who, otherwise, might succumb to an infection or an infectious disease. Even in those illnesses that would be self-limited, proper treatment can shorten the course of the illness. Treatment may also make the patient more comfortable during the time the infection persists.

Our next question is, What are the principles upon which treatment is based?

There are two principles. The first is to reinforce and augment the patient's defense mechanisms by which his body resists and counteracts the presence and effects of the germs and viruses which have invaded. The second is to combat the invaders more directly by introducing into the patient's body certain chemical agents that are destruc-

Local application of disinfectant kills germs and controls infection.

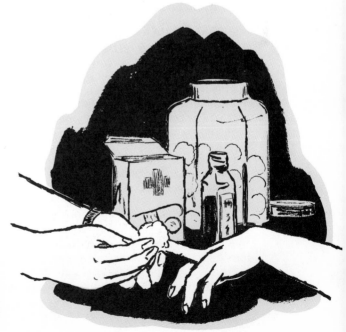

tive to the organisms. We will now consider the applications of each of these principles.

Stimulating the Patient's Defenses. Once a person becomes ill with an infection or an infectious disease, his body's defenses begin to operate as best they can. The efficiency of these defenses is determined by the patient's inherent vitality. When fatigued or otherwise run-down, his defense mechanisms do not operate well. When in a good state of general health, his defense mechanisms cope with the challenge of invading germs and viruses.

So, in aiding a person to combat an existing infection, we aim to improve and conserve his inherent vitality. Even though he may be inclined otherwise, we urge him to conserve his strength by remaining in bed. We provide simple, easily digested food. We arrange for him to obtain adequate sleep and to avoid undue excitement. In addition, we employ certain procedures of physical therapy which have the effect of stimulating his defense mechanisms. These are described in chapter 25, volume 3.

The choice among the physical therapy procedures depends somewhat upon the patient's present degree of vitality. If reasonably good, the procedures in which contrasting temperatures of heat and cold are applied to the skin surface have the effect of increasing the flow of blood through his tissues and of increasing the production of phagocyte cells. When applying such procedures, there must be consistent effort to keep the patient from becoming chilled, for shivering would require an unnecessary expenditure of his energy and thus reduce his vitality.

Using Antibiotics. The many types of germs and viruses mentioned in the five chapters that follow produce various kinds of illness. Certain germs are killed by one type of antibiotic medication, whereas others respond to a different chemical preparation. In order to use antibiotic medications properly,

therefore, it must be determined first what type of organism is involved. The testing process often requires laboratory procedures in which the patient's body fluids are examined or cultured so as to identify the germs causing his problem. While waiting for the laboratory report, it may be advisable to administer a broad-spectrum antibiotic— one capable of destroying more than one kind of organism. But best results, in a case of severe infection, are obtained from the use of a medication particularly effective against a single agent.

The use of the modern antibiotic medications is complicated by the fact that many strains of germs have become resistant to certain antibiotics. Additional antibiotic medications are being developed in an attempt to control even those infections in which the organisms have become resistant to the older medications.

It should be mentioned that the use of antibiotic medications in the treatment of infections and infectious diseases may not necessarily improve the patient's own mechanisms of defense or immunity.

One of the marvels of the defense mechanisms which our bodies possess is their ability to produce surplus antibodies which remain on call, so to speak, in case this same kind of germ or virus should enter the body at some future time. Thus a person may become immune to a certain infection once his body has combatted it successfully. Such immunity may last for several months or even for a lifetime. The program of artificial immunization, urgently recommended for all infants and children, and for certain adults (see chapter 6, volume 1), consists of stimulating a person's defense mechanisms to produce antibodies without his having to experience the actual illness which a certain organism causes.

Maintaining the Body's Defenses

We commonly speak of curing an infection, or perhaps we say that a certain form of treatment provides a cure for a particular illness. Actually, however, the conquest of a disease depends upon what goes on within the patient's tissues. The doctor does not cure a disease. Medication does not cure a disease. The battle for the control of disease is waged within the patient's own body. Medications may kill infectious agents and physical therapy may stimulate the body's defense reactions, but the healing process involves a miracle which takes place within the tissues.

Many types of infectious agents are constantly present on the surface of the skin, in the membranes of the nose and throat, and in the intestinal tract, just awaiting an opportunity to invade and produce damage. The reason a healthy person remains healthy is that his body's defenses are in good condition. Once his vitality wanes and his resistance to disease declines, he becomes more vulnerable to infections of one kind or another.

One secret of good health is to maintain one's vitality at the highest possible level. The principles on which this can be accomplished are mentioned in the earlier chapters of this set of books. Maintaining a high level of vitality requires adequate sleep, wholesome nutrition, consistent and systematic physical exercise, abstinence from debilitating indulgences, and the maintenance of an optimistic and peaceful state of mind. It is far better to avoid disease in the first place than to treat it once it becomes established.

Maintaining a high level of vitality protects against infections just as maintaining a healthy bank balance ensures against financial problems.

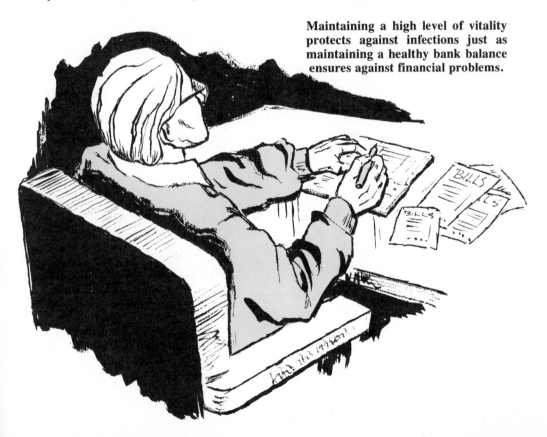

Viral Diseases

Viruses are tiny particles which exist inside of living plant or animal cells, most of them too small to be seen through the light microscope. More than 600 different viruses from animals and humans have been isolated. Some seem to be harmless, but many are the causes of serious diseases. The core of a virus contains a form of nucleic acid, either DNA or RNA, but not both. The fact that they contain only one type of nucleic acid distinguishes them from bacteria and other disease-producing agents. Viruses lack other cellular constituents necessary to self-existence. They may therefore be considered as minute parasites, for a virus depends on the cell within which it lives for its metabolic needs.

Great progress has already been made toward the prevention of certain virus-induced diseases by means of vaccination. Smallpox, a worldwide scourge of previous centuries, has now been eradicated. Effective immunization against yellow fever, poliomyelitis, measles, rubella (German measles), and mumps is now available and only needs to be used more generally. Immunization is available and practicable in selected instances for influenza, hepatitis B, and rabies.

The means of treating virus-induced diseases, once the illness is established, poses a continuing problem.

Viruses are not killed by the antibiotic medications so useful in the treatment of diseases caused by bacteria. But progress is being made in the development and testing of two types of medications: (1) synthetic drugs such as amantadine, vidarabine, and acyclovir; and (2) agents such as the interferons, which are produced by lymphocyte cells. The synthetic drug acyclovir (Zovirax) was approved in 1982 for use in the United States. It is applied as a topical ointment in the treatment of the initial attack of genital herpes simplex. It does not cure the disease, but it hastens the healing of the ulcers that develop in the initial attack of this illness. It is hoped that other antiviral medications will soon become practical for the routine treatment of viral infections.

This chapter consists of a listing in alphabetical order, with discussions, of the various common viral diseases. Several of these diseases are designated by more than one name. Therefore, if the reader has difficulty in locating here the particular disease in which he is interested, he should consult the General Index at the back of this volume.

CAT-SCRATCH DISEASE

This mild, noncontagious illness affects children more commonly than adults and usually follows a scratch or bite inflicted by a kitten. Occasionally scratches by animals other than cats, or even a puncturing thorn, have been the means of introducing the causative agent, probably a virus, into the body.

In the usual case a scabbed ulcer of the skin develops at the site where the scratch occurred. This may disappear at the end of two or three weeks. In the meantime an enlargement of the lymph nodes has usually developed in the affected part of the body—axilla, groin, or neck. General symptoms of loss of appetite, weakness, and nausea may also develop. In an occasional severe case, an affected lymph node breaks down to form an abscess.

Care and Treatment

Recovery usually occurs spontaneously within a few weeks. There is no specific remedy. Good nursing care to make the patient comfortable is usually all that is required.

CHICKEN POX (VARICELLA)

This very contagious disease, occurring in all parts of the world, is caused by a virus and appears most commonly in children under eight years of age. It is characterized by general symptoms of mild illness and by a skin rash consisting of lesions which pass through a sequence of four stages.

The illness usually begins ten to sixteen days after contact with someone who has chicken pox. At the onset the patient usually suffers a slight fever, a feeling of chilliness, aching in the back and extremities, and vomiting. The older the patient, the more serious the symptoms are likely to be. The skin rash makes its appearance about one day after the symptoms begin. The skin lesions appear in "crops," which usually develop first on the scalp and face and eventually become most numerous on the chest and upper back.

The skin lesions pass through four distinct stages. First is the small macule—an area of mild redness. Second, the macules develop into red papules, slightly elevated and resembling fleabites and mosquito bites.

PUBLIC HEALTH SERVICE AUDIOVISUAL FACILITY; LOMA LINDA UNIVERSITY SCHOOL OF MEDICINE

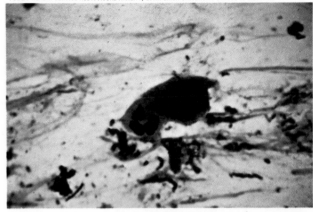

A

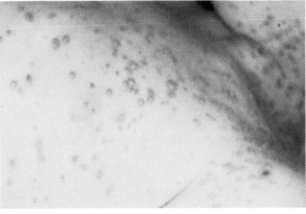

B

A. Greatly enlarged view of multi-nucleated giant cell as affected by chicken pox virus. B. Red papules on the skin. C. Small crusted blister.

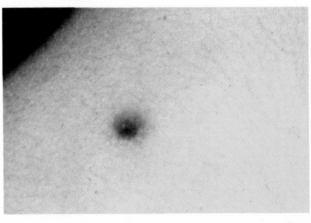

C

247

Third, the papules become small vesicles (water blisters), each surrounded by a tiny red zone. Fourth, if the vesicles do not become infected by ordinary germs, there develop crusts that soon break away, leaving no permanent scars.

With the skin lesions developing in crops, there may be present at one time on any given area red spots of different sizes, blisters, and scabs. The recovery from chicken pox is usually uneventful and rapid, once the skin rash disappears. In occasional cases, complications occur involving various organs of the body. The most common complication is that the itching skin lesions become infected by ordinary germs.

The virus which causes chicken pox is the same virus that also causes shingles (herpes zoster). For a discussion of this disease, see under SHINGLES in this same chapter, page 260.

Although chicken pox is highly contagious, it is not considered serious. Children of school age who have chicken pox should be kept home until the skin lesions have developed crusts and have become brown in color. If there happens to be another child in the family who is not in good health and who has not had chicken pox, it is best to keep such a child away from the patient in the hope that the frail child will not catch the disease.

As yet no satisfactory way exists of preventing chicken pox by vaccination.

Care and Treatment

The itching of the skin is the most troublesome symptom during the usual course of chicken pox. This may be relieved somewhat by sponging the affected areas with a strong solution of baking soda. Calamine lotion may also help to relieve the itching.

It is important to guard against infecting the skin lesions. The patient's fingernails should be clipped short and kept clean, and his hands should be washed at frequent intervals. If an infection develops in skin lesions which have been scratched, the physician's attention should be called to this complication. He may find it advisable to use antibiotics for the control of such an infection.

As the lesions progress to the crusting stage, gentle application of olive oil to the skin surface will have a soothing effect.

COLD, THE COMMON

The common cold, caused by any one of a number of different viruses, is considered in chapter 13, volume 2.

COLORADO TICK FEVER

Colorado tick fever is a tick-transmitted disease which occurs in Colorado and other western states and, possibly, in western Canada. The illness occurs most commonly in spring and summer. It may affect persons of any age.

The symptoms occur three to six days after the patient has been bitten by an infected tick. They appear suddenly and consist of headache, muscle aches, sensitivity to light, and a rapidly rising body temperature (fever). The symptoms disappear suddenly after about two days, only to recur three days later, with the body temperature this time usually rising a little higher than at first. The symptoms of the second episode disappear in about three days, but the patient remains weak for several weeks thereafter.

Eventual recovery is usually complete, and the recovered person then remains immune to the disease.

Care and Treatment

There is no specific treatment. Nursing care consists of making the patient comfortable.

DENGUE (BREAKBONE FEVER)

This epidemic disease which occurs in tropical areas is caused by a virus usually transmitted by the *Aedes aegypti* mosquito. The disease is not common in the United States, but one case did occur in Brownsville, Texas, in 1980 after a 35-year period in which there had been no such cases in the continental United States.

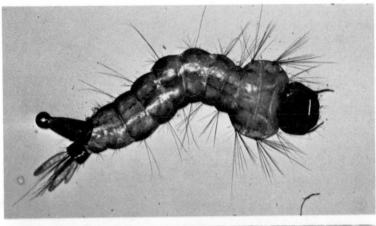

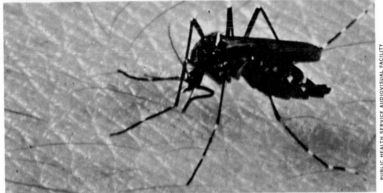

The *Aedes aegypti* mosquito, larval and adult forms, usual transmitter of dengue (breakbone fever).

The symptoms appear after an incubation period of five to eight days. Symptoms appear suddenly, the fever rising rapidly, in severe cases as high as 106° F. (41° C.). The face becomes flushed, and there may be marked soreness in the eyeballs. The throat is sore, and the patient suffers pains in the head, lower back, and joints. The victim is usually nervous, and sleep is often disturbed. Prostration may be great.

About the third or fourth day the temperature usually drops to normal, only to recur after an interval of about three days. The second wave of illness is usually less severe and shorter than the first. A skin eruption usually appears at about the time of the second series of symptoms. The eruption be-

gins on the hands and feet and spreads to the arms, legs, and body. The skin eruption soon fades. Convalescence is usually slow, but the disease is self-limited and the acute symptoms do not last long.

Care and Treatment

There is no specific remedy for dengue. Deaths from the disease are almost unknown. Good nursing is the most important part of the care of the patient. The patient should be kept in bed and should be given abundant water to drink.

When the patient's body temperature rises as high as 104° F. (40. C.), it may be reduced by the use of cool enemas, tepid sponges, or alcohol rubs. Placing an ice bag on the pa-

249

tient's forehead may help relieve his headache.

ENCEPHALITIS
Encephalitis is a serious involvement of the brain caused by a virus. It may affect children (see chapter 17, volume 1, or adults (see chapter 4, volume 3).

EXANTHEM SUBITUM (ROSEOLA INFANTUM)
This viral disease of early childhood is considered in chapter 17, volume 1.

GASTROENTERITIS (ACUTE INFECTIOUS GASTROENTERITIS)
This disease, usually caused by a virus, is one of the serious diseases that may affect infants (see chapter 6, volume 1); it may affect children (see chapter 17, volume 1); and it sometimes occurs in adulthood (see chapter 17, volume 2).

GERMAN MEASLES
See RUBELLA in this chapter, page 258.

HEPATITIS
Hepatitis is considered in chapter 19, volume 2.

HERPANGINA
This illness is described in chapter 17, volume 1.

HERPES SIMPLEX
Although this disease is caused by a virus, its principal manifestation is in the skin. It is therefore considered in chapter 25, volume 2.

INFLUENZA (FLU)
Influenza is a contagious disease of short duration caused by either A, B, or C type of influenza virus. The disease is transmitted from person to person by droplet infection, a susceptible person inhaling virus-laden droplets released by a sneeze or otherwise from a person who harbors this virus. The incubation period is between one and three days.

The symptoms consist of a sense of

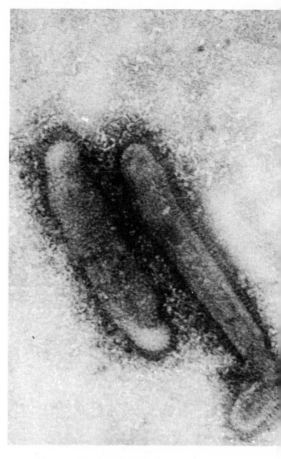

Photograph of influenza virus (Imai strain) showing magnification of 166,400 times.

chilliness, followed by fever, general weakness, various aches and pains, including headache and pain in the muscles, loss of appetite, and inflammation of the membranes of the nose and pharynx.

Once the vitality of the membranes of the nose and pharynx has been weakened by the influenza virus, it is common for bacteria (not viruses) always present in the mouth and pharynx to invade the tissues and produce complications such as sinusitis, ear infection, and bacterial pneumonia. The most serious of these is bacterial pneumonia.

Except for the development of complications, influenza is self-limited and usually lasts no more than a week. The patient usually remains somewhat weak for several days after the other symptoms have disappeared.

Prevention. Polyvalent influenza vaccine is available for the protection of persons particularly susceptible to this type of infection. The U.S. Public Health Service recommends that high-risk persons should receive an injection of such a vaccine every autumn. High-risk persons include those with chronic heart disease, chronic pulmonary disease, diabetes, and persons older than 65 years. The manufacturers of the polyvalent vaccine alter its composition year by year, so as to combat the particular type of virus expected to be prevalent during that year. The protection provided by influenza vaccine does not protect against other types of respiratory infection.

Care and Treatmenet

For the uncomplicated case of influenza the care consists simply of making the patient as comfortable as possible. When secondary infections or complications develop or threaten, it is urgent to arrange for the services of a physician.

Rest in bed for the duration of the symptoms helps the patient to conserve his strength and hasten his recovery. As symptoms subside, return to activity should be gradual. An ice bag applied intermittently to the forehead helps to relieve headache. For cough, steam inhalation three times a day is helpful. A simple diet, including much fruit juice and other liquids, is indicated as long as symptoms persist.

The drug amantadine hydrochloride has given some promise of combating the influenza viruses and of hastening recovery from such infection. As yet, the results of the use of this drug have not confirmed the original high hopes.

MEASLES (RUBEOLA)

Measles (rubeola) is a distinct disease and must not be confused with

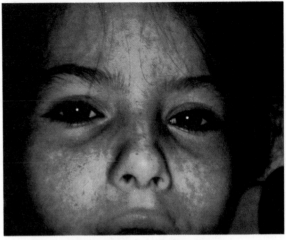

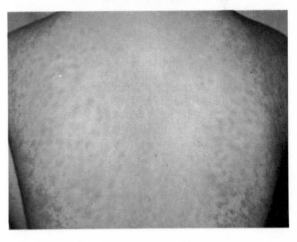

The pink spots of measles appear first on the head, spreading next to the trunk and limbs.

rubella (German measles). These are separate diseases, even though both are contagious and both present a skin rash as a characteristic of the illness.

Measles is a contagious, viral disease, easily transmitted from person to person in the early stage before symptoms become full-blown. The virus is conveyed by invisible droplets of moisture discharged from the mouth or nose of a person becoming ill with this disease. The incubation period is between seven and fourteen days.

The earliest symptoms are similar to those of the common cold, with the addition that the individiual is sensitive to bright light. Fever develops and gradually rises day by day in a sawtooth pattern. There is usually a hoarse, dry cough, with pain and soreness in the chest.

Three to five days after the first symptoms appear, there develops a skin rash which consists of well-defined pink spots, first seen behind the ears, on the neck, on the scalp, or on the forehead. Later the rash appears on the trunk and limbs. These pink spots tend to become darker as time passes, becoming almost purple before they disappear. As these spots increase in number, they tend to run together to form irregular blotches. Even in the cases in which the rash is profuse, small patches of natural-appearing skin may be seen among the blotches. Often the rash on the face begins to fade before it is fully developed on the legs. White lesions (Koplik's spots) develop on the inner surfaces of the cheeks.

The severity of measles varies a great deal from case to case. In severe cases the patient may suffer high fever, delirium, cracked tongue, rapid pulse, and even unconsciousness.

A possible complication of measles is encephalitis, caused by the invasion of the measles virus into the brain. Other complications may result from a lowered resistance to other germs. The hazard of measles is really not in the disease itself, for, without complications, recovery is quite prompt. The serious complications include pneumonia, middle ear infection, damage to the heart, and exacerbation of latent tuberculosis.

Prevention. In the early 1960s a vaccine to keep susceptible persons from developing measles became available. It was partially successful but did not immunize all persons who received the vaccine. This early vaccine was superseded in 1967 by a different, more effective type.

Vaccination for measles is now routinely included in the immunization program recommended for infants and children. (See schedule in chapter 6,

volume 1.) The resulting reduction in the number of cases of measles has been most gratifying. However, the disease has not disappeared, and it is predicted that it will not disappear in the United States until at least 90 percent of susceptible persons are immunized. Health authorities are urging cooperation in their campaign for stamping out measles in this country.

Care and Treatment

The care of a patient with measles is directed primarily toward the prevention of complications. Secondarily it is intended to make the patient as comfortable as possible during his illness.

The patient should remain quietly in bed until after the skin rash disappears. Then he should be protected for at least two more weeks from sudden changes of temperature or from other conditions that might make him susceptible to infections. During the illness, the patient's eyes should not be exposed to strong light. It is not necessary that the room be completely darkened, but only that the light be subdued.

Increasing the humidity of the room or arranging for steam inhalations may reduce the patient's tendency to cough. The diet should be simple and easily digestible and should include an abundant intake of fluid.

Itching of the skin may be at least partially relieved by the application of phenolated calamine lotion applied to the skin several times a day. This medication is available at most drug counters.

Antibacterial drugs are indicated only as a means of preventing or controlling certain of the complications that may develop. The physician's judgment will indicate when these are needed.

MENINGITIS

For a discussion of the types of meningitis that may be caused by a virus, see chapter 4, volume 3.

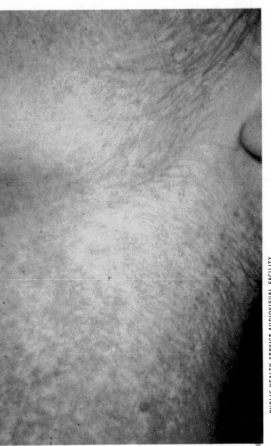

PUBLIC HEALTH SERVICE AUDIOVISUAL FACILITY

A symptom of mononucleosis is enlargement of the lymph nodes.

MOLLUSCUM CONTAGIOSUM

Molluscum contagiosum is a contagious viral disease of worldwide distribution which affects only humans and occurs most commonly in children, especially boys. It produces small papules in the skin. It is transmitted person-to-person among those who have close relationships, as among wrestlers, persons using the same swimming pool, or people living under the same roof.

The incubation period varies from two weeks to two months. The individual skin lesions heal without scarring in about two months, but additional lesions develop over a period of six months to three years until a spontaneous recovery occurs.

The skin lesions are waxy, pearly-white papules with depressed centers which may grow to a diameter of one-fourth inch (6 mm.). The lesions rupture easily.

Care and Treatment

There is no specific cure. When the lesions are gently ruptured, they then heal without scar formation. Secondary infections, when they occur, should be treated as under other circumstances.

MONONUCLEOSIS (INFECTIOUS MONONUCLEOSIS)

Mononucleosis, also called infectious mononucleosis, and formerly called glandular fever, is an acute, viral, infectious disease which continues for a variable period between one week and three months. It occurs worldwide and commonly affects those between the ages of 15 and 30 years. The specific cause is an infection by the Epstein-Barr virus, one of the herpes viruses.

Usually the disease occurs sporadically, but occasionally it spreads as an epidemic where young people have close association, as in schools. The disease is probably transmitted from person to person by way of contaminated oral secretions.

After an incubation period of between 30 and 60 days, fever and enlargement of the lymph nodes are the outstanding characteristics. Sore throat, weakness, muscle pains, and loss of appetite are accompanying symptoms. The spleen and liver frequently become enlarged. One of the serious complications of the disease is caused by rupture of an enlarged spleen. Precise diagnosis requires a laboratory examination of the blood.

Care and Treatment

Bed rest and good nursing care are the mainstays of treatment for mononucleosis. The disease is spontaneously self-limited, but the recovering patient may lack endurance for several weeks.

253

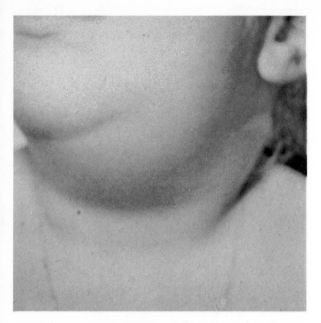

The chief characteristic of mumps is
a swelling of the salivary glands.

MUMPS (PAROTITIS)

Mumps is a contagious, viral disease
characterized by enlargement of one or
more of the salivary glands. The usual
case occurring during childhood ends
in spontaneous, complete recovery
within a few days. In persons older
than 12 years of age the illness is more
serious and may cause complications.

Symptoms—chilliness, headache,
lack of appetite, and moderate fever—
begin within two to four weeks after
contact with a person who has the disease. Within a few hours after the first
symptoms appear, one or more of the
salivary glands become painful. It is
usually the parotid gland, situated just
in front of and below the ear that is primarily affected. Pain in the involved
gland is induced by external pressure
on the area, by swallowing, or, particularly, by taking sour substances into
the mouth. The swelling of the involved
salivary gland or glands usually lasts
from three to six days.

The most common serious complication of mumps is an involvement of the
sex glands, either of the testes
(orchitis) or of the ovaries.

In about 25 percent of the cases of
mumps among older boys and men, at
least one of the testes is affected. The
affected testis becomes swollen and
very painful. In some cases the organ
later atrophies, thus being rendered in-
capable of producing male sex cells;
but unless both testes are thus involved, a man is still capable of father-
hood. Even when one or both testes atrophy, the male sex hormones are
produced in normal fashion. The comparable involvement of the ovaries in
women is not so common or so serious
as is the involvement of the testes in
men.

About 10 percent of all cases of
mumps develop some degree of encephalitis, with severe headaches,
drowsiness, and vomiting. Usually this
complication clears up spontaneously.

Another occasional complication of
mumps is pancreatitis, in which severe
nausea, vomiting, and abdominal pain
develop. Even with this unpleasant and
rather serious development, spontaneous recovery usually ensues within a
week.

Prevention. A mumps vaccine is
available for purposes of immunization.

Care and Treatment

No specific treatment for mumps
exists. Unless complications develop,
it is considered to be one of the less
harmful contagious diseases. A child
with mumps should be kept at home
and out of school until all swelling of
his salivary glands has disappeared.
Effort should be made to keep him
away from other children or from
grown people who have not had this
disease. Persons older than 12 years
who have mumps should remain in
bed until their fever has disappeared.
The nursing care for mumps may be
summarized as follows:

The patient should be protected
against chilling throughout the period
of his illness. This precaution is especially important for patients above 12
years of age. Swollen salivary glands

may be less painful if either a hot-water bottle or an ice bag is placed over the swollen area for a few minutes out of each hour. The choice of heat or cold depends upon which makes the patient more comfortable. The patient should receive a light diet of food easily swallowed. The patient is made more comfortable by rinsing the mouth every two or three hours with a warm salt solution (one level teaspoonful to a pint of water).

All cases of mumps in which complications develop should be under the supervision of a physician. In cases in which the testes become involved, the patient should be kept at absolute bed rest and the scrotum should be supported by a large tuft of cotton or by an adhesive-tape bridge placed between the thighs so as to support the weight of the swollen scrotum. The periodic application of an ice bag to the scrotum may provide some relief. When the pancreas becomes involved, it is usually advisable to feed the patient by vein rather than by mouth. This treatment, of course, must be administered in a hospital.

PLEURODYNIA (EPIDEMIC MYALGIA)

Pleurodynia is an uncommon, acute, viral disease which has occurred in various parts of the world and which may affect persons in any of the age groups. Its principal symptom is paroxysmal, severe chest pain over the lower ribs or breastbone. The pain, when it occurs, is made worse by deep breathing, coughing, or body movement. The pain is described as knifelike, smothering, or stabbing. Pleurodynia is caused by viruses which usually enter the body through the mouth in contaminated food or water. Other symptoms typical of a viral infection are also present. The duration of the illness varies from case to case and averages about one week. The illness is usually self-limited and recovery is complete. Possible complications include viral infections of other organs such as the heart, the liver, or the testes.

Care and Treatment

There is no specific cure for this ailment. Nursing care is directed toward making the patient comfortable.

PNEUMONIA

Viral pneumonia is one of the diseases of the respiratory organs, described in chapter 13, volume 2.

POLIOMYELITIS (POLIO)

Thanks to the development of poliomyelitis vaccines and their widespread use, beginning in 1955, poliomyelitis has the potential to become a conquered disease. In spite of the availability and efficacy of poliomyelitis vaccine, there occurred in 1979 a rather serious outbreak of poliomyelitis in an area of the United States in which families were opposed to the use of vaccine in any form. This outbreak proved that the poliomyelitis virus is still circulating in the United States, even though very few cases of the disease now occur.

Older persons of the present generation seem to have forgotten and younger members of this generation never knew of the horrors and tragedies of poliomyelitis prior to 1955, when the vaccines became available. In those days every parent shuddered at the mention of poliomyelitis, lest his own child might be stricken with this disease and die or be permanently crippled. The tragedy of our present situation is that only about 60 percent of young children have been immunized against this dangerous disease. Just because the disease is not now prevalent, it has become easy to assume that danger no longer lurks.

Poliomyelitis is an acute infection caused by a virus which most commonly (80 to 90 percent of cases) produces a mild illness lasting one to three days, but which sometimes produces a major illness resulting in serious damage to certain of the nerve cells controlling the muscles of the body and which therefore often produces paralysis of the corresponding muscles. In those serious cases, slightly more than 50

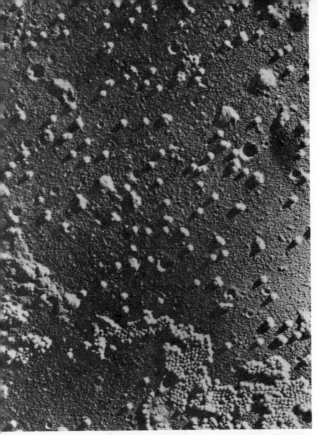

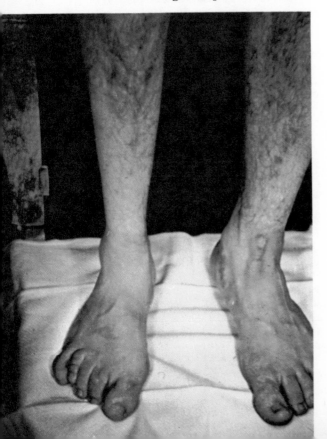

Above: A photomicrograph of one type of polio virus, enlarged 77,000 times actual size. Below: Atrophy of leg from polio.

percent recover without permanent paralysis of the muscles; about 25 percent have minor muscle weaknesses for the remainder of life; and the remainder (slightly less than 25 percent) carry severe disability for life because of permanent paralysis of important muscles. In these severe cases the greatest danger lies in possible failure of the breathing mechanism. It is for these that the use of the mechanical respirators (iron lungs) may be lifesaving.

Prevention. The more recently developed type of vaccine (live attenuated vaccine) is administered by mouth and is so effective in preventing poliomyelitis that no reason now exists for anyone having this dread disease.

Care and Treatment

There is no specific treatment for poliomyelitis once a person becomes ill. For the minor type of poliomyelitis, the treatment consists of bed rest for several days, an adequate intake of fluid, and good nursing care. For the major type of poliomyelitis with involvement of the central nervous system, there must be absolute rest in bed. The patient must be under the care of a physician, and it may be necessary for the patient to be hospitalized in order to receive care for the complications that may develop. Fomentations (Kenny packs) applied to arms or legs in which the muscles have become weak help to relieve the painful muscle spasms. For cases in which the muscles of breathing have become weak, the use of the iron lung provides a means of artificial respiration.

RABIES (HYDROPHOBIA)

Rabies is a serious disease which typically follows the bite of an infected animal and ends fatally if not treated. It is caused by a virus capable of invading the brain of many mammals, especially the carnivores. Once the virus enters the body through a break in the skin, it travels by way of the nerves to the brain and then to the salivary glands so that the saliva of an animal or person ill

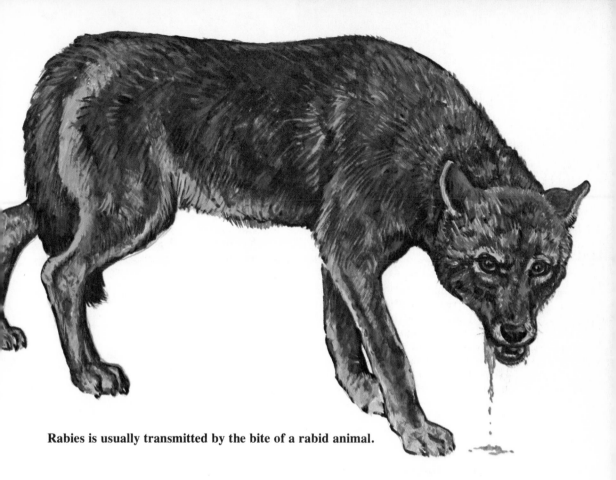

Rabies is usually transmitted by the bite of a rabid animal.

with this disease becomes contaminated and can carry the virus to another animal or person.

The disease occurs quite commonly among wild animals such as skunks, bats, foxes, raccoons, and coyotes. In some other countries in which rabies in dogs is not well controlled by immunization, the domestic dog is a common agent for infecting man.

Although skunks, domestic cats, foxes, and other animals have all been responsible for transmitting rabies to humans, in recent years the bat seems to be among the animals most frequently involved. This new development may be due to the fact that the bat does not always manifest the typical foaming at the mouth and the wildness exhibited by other animals.

Because of the involvement of the brain, an animal with rabies sometimes behaves in a furious manner, and because of its own discomfort bites other animals or humans, even without provocation. The wound caused by the

bite becomes infected because the animal's saliva is laden with the virus. The infection may be transmitted even though the animal does not bite, if circumstances permit the infected saliva to come in contact with an open wound or a break in the skin or mucous membrane of the susceptible animal or person.

In the human, symptoms of the disease may develop any time between ten days and one year after exposure. The average is thirty to fifty days. The period is shorter when the wound through which the virus enters is in the region of the neck, face, or head. Once the symptoms of the disease begin, the infection invariably progresses to a fatal outcome. It is therefore imperative that treatment be given as soon as possible after exposure to the virus. If early and adequate treatment is given, the symptoms will not develop.

The symptoms in man start with mental depression, fever, and a growing restlessness which progresses to a

257

stage of excitement. As the salivary glands become involved, there is excessive production of saliva accompanied by painful spasms of the muscles of the larynx and pharynx. These spasms are triggered by minor activities such as the attempt to take a drink of water. It is in fear of causing another of the painful spasms that the patient now refuses to drink. Death occurs within about five days after the symptoms begin.

Care and Treatment

Treatment of the person who has been exposed to rabies, either by the bite of a possibly rabid animal or by contact with the animal's saliva which may have permitted the virus to enter the tissues through some break in the skin or membranes, consists of two phases: (1) local treatment of the wound and (2) systemic treatment to provide immunization by the use of the newly developed human-diploid-cell rabies vaccine.

In the meantime, attention should be given to the condition of the animal which inflicted the bite. If the bite was by a wild skunk, fox, coyote, raccoon, or bat, it must be assumed that the animal was rabid and that the person bitten must therefore have the systemic treatment. If the animal was a domestic dog or cat, the animal should be confined and observed for ten days to determine whether or not it becomes ill. If it becomes ill, it should be killed and its brain examined by a specialist to determine whether rabies was present. Rodents and rabbits so rarely carry rabies that it is not necessary to suspect them of transmitting this disease.

The local treatment of the wound requires a thorough cleansing with large amounts of soap and water. After such treatment, it is recommended that the wound be left open, without suturing.

The systemic treatment consists of several intramuscular injections of the human-diploid-cell rabies vaccine given over a period of twenty-eight days, each injection consisting of 1 ml. of the vaccine. At the time the first injection of vaccine is administered, the patient should also receive one dose of rabies immune globulin (10 IU per kg. of body weight), half of which is injected into the tissues around the wound and the remaining half injected intramuscularly.

The decision regarding the use of the antirabies vaccine must rest with the physician who cares for the person who has been exposed. The general rule is that the series of vaccine injections should be started immediately under any one of three conditions: (1) when it is known that the biting animal has rabies; (2) when the animal is not available for examination but rabies is known to have been prevalent in the area; and (3) when the bite was inflicted by one of the wild animals mentioned above commonly known to be carriers of rabies.

When the bite was inflicted by a domestic dog or cat which was then kept in confinement for ten days and has proven to be healthy at the end of this ten-day period, the series of intramuscular injections of the vaccine may then be safely discontinued.

RUBELLA (GERMAN MEASLES)

Rubella is a mild, contagious disease caused by a virus. The symptoms, which usually begin between seven and fourteen days after exposure, vary a great deal from case to case. The first symptoms may be a cold, with cough and sore throat; or there may be headache, a feeling of general illness, aching of the muscles with fever, and an enlargement of the lymph nodes, especially those behind the ears. A skin rash usually appears within 24 hours of the first symptoms. It consists of a faint blotchy redness of the skin. It usually appears first on the face and neck and spreads rapidly to the trunk and extremities, sometimes leaving one area before it appears at the next. The red areas fade under mild pressure. The rash usually lasts two or three days.

Persons of all ages, above six months

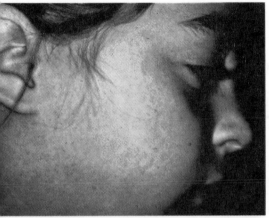

The rash of rubella appears on the face and neck first, spreading then to the trunk and extremities.

of age, may be susceptible to rubella. It is especially common among young adults. The virus is transmitted from one person to another by personal contact and seems to enter the body through the membranes of the respiratory passages.

Rubella is usually a mild disease and rarely causes complications. The tragedy of this disease, however, is that it may interfere with the development of an unborn child when an expectant mother becomes ill with this disease, especially during the first three months of her pregnancy. About one third of the children born to mothers who have had rubella during the first three months of pregnancy have some kind of congenital defect. The possible de-

fects include abnormalities of the heart, eyes, ears, brain, and bones. Such a child may be mentally retarded, or it may be deaf.

Vaccination for rubella is now the accepted procedure for preventing the disease. It is part of the schedule for immunization of children as advocated in chapter 6, volume 1. But in spite of the recommendation that all children should be vaccinated, many grow up without this protection. And some who do receive it lose their immunity sometime following vaccination.

The body's reaction to this vaccination is essentially the same as to a regular illness with rubella. Therefore, if a young woman happens to be vaccinated for rubella at the time she is or becomes pregnant, she runs about the same risk of having a deformed child as does the expectant mother who has had this disease during the early part of her pregnancy. Thus, a girl should not wait until she arrives at young adulthood before she is vaccinated for rubella.

Many authorities now recommend that all girls should be vaccinated for rubella at about age 10. This recommendation applies to those who have been vaccinated in infancy as well as to those who have never been vaccinated. By being vaccinated at age 10, the vaccination will serve as a "booster" for those who have been vaccinated in infancy and as a means of present immunization for those who have never been vaccinated. The immunity conferred by vaccination at age 10 should carry over into young adulthood, and thus prevent the danger of damage to an unborn child.

Care and Treatment

There is no specific treatment for rubella once the illness develops. The care of the patient consists of making him as comfortable as possible. The usual symptoms are mild, and the illness is self-limited. The patient should be kept at home and isolated from other persons until after the skin rash has completely disappeared. In cases associated with fever, the patient should be kept in bed until the temperature becomes normal.

When the lymph nodes at the back of the neck become particularly painful, an icebag applied over the area for a few minutes out of each hour may give considerable relief.

In the case of an expectant mother who has just been exposed to rubella, a physician should be consulted at once.

SANDFLY FEVER (PHLEBOTOMUS FEVER; PAPPATACI FEVER)

Sandfly fever is a self-limited, viral, relatively mild disease that occurs in Europe, in the Middle East, in parts of Africa, in central Asia, in southern China, and, occasionally, in Central America and Brazil. It is transmitted by the bites of infected sandflies, flies so small that they can penetrate ordinary window screens.

The onset of the symptoms is sudden, with moderately high fever, severe headache, dizziness, general itching, and pain behind the eyes. The symptoms persist for three or four days.

Prevention. The prevention of this disease centers around the irradication of sandflies, which hide in weeds and shrubbery during the day and lay their

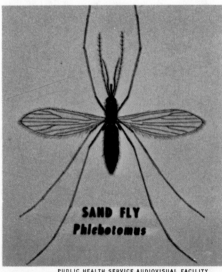

SAND FLY
Phlebotomus

eggs in dark, damp places. Using insect repellents on the exposed skin, sleeping under fine mesh bed nets, and the wearing of close-woven clothing helps to avoid being bitten by the sandflies.

Care and Treatment

No curative remedy exists for sandfly fever. Rubbing alcohol or an alcohol-based lotion applied to the skin areas affected may help to relieve the discomfort.

SHINGLES (HERPES ZOSTER)

Shingles (herpes zoster) is caused by the varicella-zoster virus, which is the virus that causes chicken pox. It is supposed that when a person has chicken pox (varicella), usually during his childhood, he builds up an immunity to this particular virus. This immunity keeps him from having another attack of chicken pox even though he may come in contact with a person who has this illness. Even so, the virus remains latent in his body's tissues for the remainder of life. When at some later time, usually after age 50, this person's general vitality wanes or some circumstance of poor health causes his immune system to weaken, the latent virus may again become active in causing illness. This time, however, the virus affects one or two of the sensory nerve ganglia and the associated nerve trunk or trunks. This manifestation is called shingles (herpes zoster).

Shingles affects a certain limited area of the skin and underlying tissues on only one side. It may affect an area of the upper body (55 percent of cases), of the neck and arms (20 percent), of the lower body and legs (25 percent), or of the upper part of the face (10 percent). The affected area becomes extremely painful and develops a vesicular rash.

The skin eruption is limited quite sharply to the area supplied by one or two nerves. When the upper body is affected, the skin eruption extends like a band from the midline of the back around to the midline in front.

Extreme pain in the affected skin area may begin as much as two or three

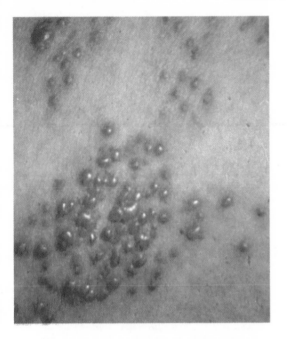

Shingles. Note typical mini-blisters.

days before the skin eruption appears. The pain is variously described as burning, stabbing, itching, or aching. The skin eruption begins with pink maculo-papules which develop into fluid-filled vesicles that may rupture and then heal by the formation of crusts. The crusts often persist for two more weeks. Permanent scars often remain. The pain typically disappears or lessens at about the time the crusts fall away. In some persons, especially in people more than 60, the pain in the area continues for several weeks or even months after the skin has healed (postherpetic neuralgia).

Care and Treatment

Shingles is a self-limited disease which runs its course regardless of what remedies are used. There is no specific cure. In the usual uncomplicated case the duration is two to four weeks. Treatment consists of making the patient as comfortable as possible by the use of moist compresses on the affected skin and by the use of aspirin or other pain-killing medicine that the doctor may prescribe. Moist com-presses may be applied for half an hour as many as four times a day. Between times the skin area should be gently dried and a soothing powder sprinkled over the affected skin. In cases in which the skin lesions become infected with ordinary germs, the doctor may prescribe an appropriate antibiotic to control the infection. Some physicians use corticosteroid in the treatment of shingles, but it is questionable whether this actually shortens the course of the disease.

Special care is required in those cases in which the opthalmic division of the trigeminal nerve in the face is involved. The tissues of the eye become affected in such a case, and it is imperative that a physician, preferably an eye specialist, give detailed directions for the patient's care.

SMALLPOX (VARIOLA)

The description of smallpox can now be phrased in the past tense, for smallpox is a conquered disease, worldwide.

Smallpox was an acute, highly communicable, virus disease, characterized by suddenly developing symptoms of severe illness and a progressive skin rash followed, after recovery, by blemished and pitted skin.

Prior to the widespread use of vaccination, smallpox was very common, usually contracted during childhood. Thousands of people died in the severe epidemics, and those who recovered were usually disfigured for life by scars left from the skin lesions.

A consistent worldwide cooperation in the program of vaccination to prevent smallpox has resulted in the eradication of this disease. The last case of epidemic smallpox occurred on October 26, 1977, in Somalia. The World Health Organization has maintained close scrutiny since that date, to make sure that no other cases of smallpox appear. Investigations have been made of all rumors regarding cases of smallpox, only to find the supposed cases were those of other diseases such as chicken pox. The eradication of smallpox repre-

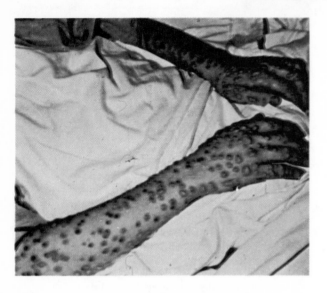

Smallpox in the vesicle stage.

sents a great victory for the world's health-promoting organizations and sets an example of what may be accomplished in controlling contagious diseases if the general population will only cooperate completely in programs of immunization.

YELLOW FEVER (YELLOW JACK)

Yellow fever is a frequently fatal, epidemic, viral disease, transmitted by the bite of the *Aedes aegypti* mosquito or one of several closely related species. In the past there have been widespread epidemics in the eastern and southern parts of the United States. The disease is more or less prevalent in some other parts of the world, chiefly in tropical areas. The disease is still endemic in South America and in sub-Sahara Africa. Travelers in these areas are advised to be immunized before entering.

The illness begins about three to six days after a person is bitten by an infected mosquito. The onset is abrupt, with a rapid rise in temperature to 103° F. (39.4° C.) or more. A person may feel perfectly well, and then within a few hours he may be critically ill. The face is flushed and swollen, and the eyes are bloodshot. All the typical symptoms of an acute infection are present.

Vomiting, first of mucus and then of bile, appears early. The kidneys are affected, and a large amount of albumin can be found in the urine by the third or fourth day. The fever remains high for a few days, being a little higher in the evenings than in the mornings; then it declines steadily. A characteristic finding is a marked slowing of the pulse while fever is still present.

With the decline of fever, improvement in the acute symptoms occurs; but the victim may become increasingly toxic along with the appearance of the most characteristic features of yellow fever—jaundice and hemorrhages. The whites of the eyes first become yellow, and the jaundice (yellow color) can soon be observed over the whole body. The gums swell and bleed. Then bleeding from the bowels and the stomach occurs, characterized by bloody stools and vomitus appearing like coffee grounds. Frequently there are hemorrhages under the skin showing up as black-and-blue spots. Liver damage may be extreme.

Severe yellow fever may be fatal. If the victim survives for as long as nine days, he will probably get well. The first evidence of probable survival is a fall of the temperature to near normal. Until this happens, however, even a moderately severe attack must be considered dangerous, because a sudden turn for the worse often occurs.

Prevention. The Center for Disease Control recommends the administration of 17D yellow fever vaccine to persons who will be traveling in the areas where yellow fever still exists. Some nations require a certificate of vaccination for travelers who have recently passed through a country where yellow fever still occurs. It is assumed that a person will be immune to the disease beginning ten days after vaccination. A booster vaccination is required after ten years. Vaccination for yellow fever should not be administered to a pregnant woman.

When caring for a patient ill with yellow fever, everybody in the neighborhood of the sick person should take as much care as possible to avoid being bitten by mosquitoes, since the disease is not transmitted in any other way than by mosquito bites. All possible measures should be taken to destroy mosquitoes and keep them from breeding. For safety, no standing water should be allowed anywhere near the house. Experience has shown that the thorough and repeated use of mosquito-killing spray in houses in a neighborhood in which there is a case of yellow fever is a valuable procedure.

Care and Treatment

Anyone ill with yellow fever should be under a physician's care and preferably placed in a hospital. No specific remedy exists for this disease, but good nursing care is important, and the physician may prescribe suitable remedies to help make the patient comfortable. The patient should be kept at absolute rest in bed. It is very important that he receive abundant fluid, and this may require administration of fluid by vein, particularly if the patient is losing fluid from his body by vomiting or diarrhea.

Rickettsial and Chlamydial Diseases

A. Rickettsial Diseases

The rickettsial diseases are caused by "germs" called *Rickettsieae*. They are intermediate in size between viruses and bacteria. Like viruses, they require a living cell in which to grow. Structurally, they are much like bacteria. They contain both kinds of nucleic acid (RNA and DNA). They are susceptible to some of the same antibacterial drugs used for the control of bacterial diseases.

The rickettsial diseases are grouped into three categories: (1) the spotted fevers, (2) the typhus fevers, and (3) Q fever. The rickettsial organisms are usually harbored and maintained in the bodies of animals and are transmitted to humans by insects or contaminated dust (for Q fever). In the case of epidemic typhus, the rickettsial organism *(Rickettsia prowazekii)* is harbored in the human body and is transmitted from one person to another by lice. In a few recent cases of epidemic typhus occurring in the United States, evidence indicates that the organisms were first harbored in the bodies of flying squirrels.

SPOTTED FEVERS
1. *Rocky Mountain Spotted Fever.*

This disease was at first supposed to be limited to the Rocky Mountain area but is now known to occur throughout most of the United States, as well as in Canada, Mexico, Columbia, and Brazil. In recent years, more than half of the cases occurring in the United States involved persons living in the Southeastern part of the country. The rickettsial organism responsible for this disease is introduced into the body by the bite of an infected tick.

The illness comes on suddenly three to eight days after a tick bite. The patient suffers chills, sweats, fever, headache, eye discomfort from bright light, pain in the skeletal tissues, sore throat, and vomiting. The breathing and heartbeat become rapid. A skin rash usually appears between the third and fifth days of the illness, beginning on the ankles and wrists, and spreading to the legs, arms, and trunk. At its onset, the rash consists of small rose-colored spots that blanch under pressure. In some cases there is an associated obstruction of the tiny blood vessels in the skin, which accounts for bluish to purplish blotches which in severe cases give rise to local areas of skin destruction. In some severe cases nervous symptoms occur, consisting of sleeplessness, restlessness, delirium, and possibly stupor or coma.

Without specific treatment, the disease runs its course in about three weeks. In fatal cases, death may occur about two weeks after the onset. Formerly, mortality rates for this disease were alarmingly high. Now that effective drugs are available, the mortality rate is as low as 3 percent, the deaths usually occurring in those who receive the treatment late in the course of the disease.

A vaccine is now available which produces immunity to Rocky Mountain spotted fever. Immunization by this means is recommended for those who live in areas where the disease is prevalent.

Care and Treatment

Selected antibiotic medications are very effective in treating this disease when given early—at the time the skin rash appears. The medications of choice are chloramphenicol and tetracycline. These must be administered under the direction of a physician. Nursing care is directed toward making the patient comfortable and conserving his strength.

2. *Rickettsialpox.* This is a mild, nonfatal, self-limited disease transmitted from mice to humans by mites. About twenty days after the mite has penetrated the skin, a single initial skin lesion develops at the site of penetration. This initial lesion becomes red and elevated, spreads to about half an inch in diameter, and eventually develops a blister at the center. A few days later the patient suddenly experiences chilly sensations, sweats, headache, loss of appetite, pains in the muscles, and fever which remits each morning. These symptoms continue for about a week. A generalized skin rash, similar to that of chicken pox, usually develops either during the period of fever or immediately thereafter. This rash continues for about a week.

Care and Treatment
This disease is mild compared with

Rocky Mountain spotted fever, described in the previous item. However, the treatment for the two diseases is the same.

TYPHUS GROUP

1. *Epidemic Typhus Fever (Louse Typhus).* Epidemic typhus is one of the "five great pestilences" that caused the loss of millions of lives before these diseases were brought under control by modern medical science, the other four being smallpox, yellow fever, plague, and cholera. During World War I epidemic typhus became rampant in Russia and Eastern Poland, numbering an estimated 30,000,000 cases. There were 3,000,000 deaths. Because of the advances made in the treatment and prevention of such diseases, epidemic typhus is now of minor importance in the United States and many other coun-

Skin rash characteristic of Rocky Mountain spotted fever.

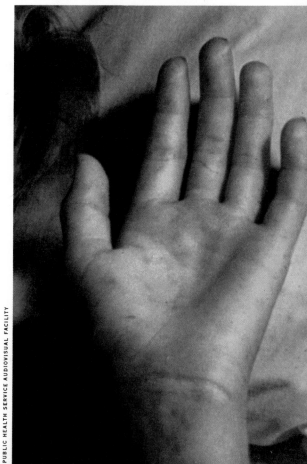

PUBLIC HEALTH SERVICE AUDIOVISUAL FACILITY

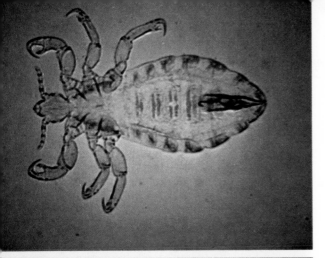

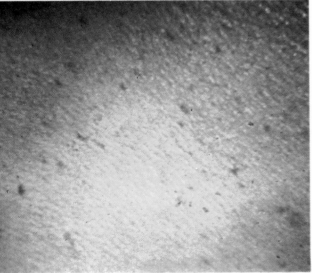

Epidemic typhus fever, characterized by pink spots on the skin, is
caused by organisms transmitted by
body lice.

tries. We must not be complacent,
however, for the rickettsia which
caused this disease is still present in the
world. The near control of this disease
depends upon maintaining proper standards of sanitation and on the availability and use of the insecticides and
medications required for prevention
and treatment.

Epidemic typhus is transmitted from
person to person by the body louse,
called the *Pediculus corporis* or
Pediculus humanus. Spread of the lice
from the body or clothing of one person
to those of others is favored by close
contact and lack of personal

cleanliness, especially in cold weather
when warm clothing is worn. Extermination of body lice is the secret of success in preventing typhus fever.
Dusting powders developed especially
for this purpose have proved very effective.

Shortly before the appearance of
typical symptoms, the typhus victim
may seem to have a common cold. The
onset of symptoms is sudden, with
chills, high fever, headache, general
pains, prostration, nausea, vomiting,
constipation or diarrhea, with possible
delirium or stupor developing early.
About the fifth day small pink spots appear on the skin of the neck, chest, abdomen, and limbs. They change to red,
then to purple, and finally to a brownish color. In nearly all cases there is
marked bronchitis with cough and excess sputum. The pulse is rapid, but the
blood pressure is low. The disease is
most serious among elderly people. In
untreated cases, the mortality ranges
from 10 to 50 percent.

*Prevention of Epidemic Typhus Fe-
ver.* The most effective means of preventing epidemic typhus fever in an
area where the disease is prevalent is
by the use of DDT or lindane powders
or their equivalent to eradicate lice.
Also, a vaccine is available which will
prevent or at least greatly reduce the
severity of this disease.

Care and Treatment

**The preferred antibiotic drugs for
the treatment of epidemic typhus fever are chloramphenicol and tetracycline, which must be administered
under the supervision of a physician.
When these drugs are administered
early in the course of the disease, the
symptoms disappear within about 48
hours. The nursing care consists of
making the patient comfortable, of
making sure that he receives sufficient fluid, and, very important,
eradicating lice from the patient's
body and clothing. The clothing
should be sterilized, preferably by
heat. Great precaution should be
taken in attending the patient lest the**

germs be spread to another individual. These precautions are especially important because the germs which cause this disease may remain viable in dried louse feces such as may contaminate the patient's skin or clothing.

2. *Murine Typhus (Endemic Typhus).* This is a mild type of typhus fever caused by a rickettsial organism harbored by rats and mice and transmitted to humans by the bite of the rat flea *(Xenopsylla cheopis).* While this disease is seldom fatal, the control problem is difficult. It is virtually impossible to exterminate the fleas that carry it. They do not stay on the body or in the clothing, or always in the house of the patient; and no way exists to fumigate the outdoors. Rat extermination, however, is a valuable control measure.

The incubation period for murine typhus is between eight and sixteen days. The symptoms begin with a shaking chill accompanied by headache. The patient's body temperature rises rapidly, and in untreated cases the fever and related symptoms last for about twelve days. Most patients develop a suddenly appearing, generalized, dull-red, macular skin rash. The rash usually appears about five days after the onset of the fever and lasts for about six days.

Care and Treatment

The antibiotic medications preferred in the treatment of murine typhus are the same as those used for epidemic typhus: chloramphenicol and tetracycline, which must be administered under the supervision of a physician. In the meantime, consistent efforts must be used to eliminate rats and mice from the living quarters and to exterminate fleas as far as possible.

3. *Scrub Typhus.* The rickettsial organism that causes scrub typhus can be transmitted by numerous species of mites. The mites pick up or transmit the organism only in its larval or blood-sucking stage, but they can carry it in their bodies until it matures and then pass it to the next generation of mites through their eggs. It is possible that rodents may act as reservoirs of infection.

In a typical case, a painless papule appears first, usually on some part of the body ordinarily covered by clothing. It enlarges and becomes dark in the center, eventually forming an ulcer less than half an inch (1.2 cm.) in diameter which leaves a scar when it heals. The lymph nodes in its vicinity swell and become tender.

As the disease develops, the patient suffers a gradually rising fever, which eventually becomes high; but the pulse rate is much slower than might be expected. In many cases, but not all, a body rash appears about the fifth day, spreads widely, and lasts from one to ten days. The spleen is enlarged and tender. At the height of the disease severe headache behind the eyes, loss of appetite, vomiting, muscular twitching, difficult breathing, cough, deep prostration, and delirium may be present. Without specific treatment, up to 20 percent of the victims die, the mortality differing widely in different localities.

Prevention. No vaccine is available for the prevention of scrub typhus. The only effective prevention consists of using chemical substances to exterminate mites (such as dibutyl phthalate or benzyl benzoate), applying these to the clothing and the skin.

Care and Treatment

The same antibiotic medications used for the other forms of typhus are effective for scrub typhus (chloramphenicol and tetracycline). These must be administered under the supervision of a physician. Fortunately, scrub typhus is more amenable to these medications than the other rickettsial diseases. These drugs administered at any time in the course of the disease bring about improvement within twenty-four to thirty-six hours.

Q FEVER

Q fever is a nonfatal, self-limited disease that occurs worldwide, except in Scandinavia. It differs from other diseases caused by rickettsias in that it exhibits no skin rash and is transmitted by the inhalation of contaminated dust rather than by the bites of insects.

Q fever occurs among people who have close contact with cattle, sheep, or goats. Inasmuch as this disease is contracted by the inhaling of contaminated dust, it is the lungs that are primarily involved with the development of a condition described as atypical pneumonia.

An abrupt onset of symptoms usually occurs, with high fever, headache, pain behind the eyes, and pain in the chest. Complications are rare, but in occasional cases the liver or the heart becomes involved by the infection. The symptoms last for one or two weeks.

Prevention. An available vaccine is recommended for persons at high risk of this disease, people such as dairy workers, slaughterhouse workers, wool sorters, and tanners.

Care and Treatment

If untreated, this disease will run its course in about two weeks. However, the drugs of choice (tetracycline and chloramphenicol) when properly administered early in the course of the illness will cause prompt recovery. Rest in bed, easily digested food, and cool sponges to reduce the patient's fever are the principal features of patient care.

B. Chlamydial Diseases

The *Chlamydia* are disease-producing organisms more closely related to bacteria than to viruses. The diseases they cause are not transmitted to humans by insects (as is usually the case with the rickettsial diseases), but occur, rather, by close contact between persons or by close association with birds. Fortunately, these organisms are susceptible to certain of the antibiotic medications.

LYMPHOGRANULOMA VENEREUM

This is a sexually transmitted infection caused by a strain of *Chlamydia trachomatis*. It is discussed in chapter 31, volume 2.

NONGONOCOCCAL URETHRITIS

About half the cases of nongonococcal urethritis in men (see chapter 29, volume 2, and chapter 31, volume 2) are caused by *Chlamydia trachomatis*. The sexual partner of a man with this ailment usually has these organisms in her uterine cervix; but the organism does not seem to cause urethritis in the female.

PSITTACOSIS (ORNITHOSIS; PARROT FEVER)

This disease is caused by the *Chlamydia psittaci*. Infection with this organism may affect parrots, parakeets, pigeons, finches, chickens, pheasants, and turkeys. Usually a bird which harbors this infection shows few, if any, signs of illness. The organisms which cause this disease are present in the bird's nasal secretions, feathers, and excreta.

Humans most susceptible to this disease are those who have close contact

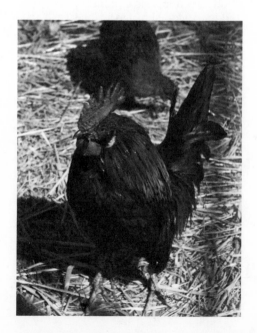

with the birds mentioned above. Pet shop employees, pigeon fanciers, and poultry raisers are at risk. The organisms enter the human body by being inhaled. The lungs are the organs primarily affected, and the usual manifestation is an atypical form of pneumonia.

The incubation period is seven to fourteen days. The severity of the disease varies from case to case, from a mild illness similar to influenza to a severe type of pneumonia. When the disease is mild, recovery occurs in about ten days. In more severe illnesses, the fever may continue for three weeks or longer. In untreated cases, the mortality rate is about 20 percent. When antibiotic drugs are used to control the infection, the mortality rate is less than 5 percent.

Care and Treatment

The antibiotic drugs effective in the treatment of psittacosis are tetracycline and chloramphenicol, tetracycline being preferred. Improvement in the patient's condition usually occurs within two to three days after the antibiotic medication is started. This medication should be continued for seven to ten days after the symptoms improve, this as a means of avoiding relapse.

The patient should be kept in bed while the symptoms persist. In the severe cases, oxygen inhalation, as in other forms of pneumonia, may be indicated. Fomentations to the patient's chest, morning and evening, will help to preserve his vitality and stimulate his resistance to the infection. See chapter 25, volume 3, for the method of giving fomentations.

TRACHOMA

Trachoma is an infection of the conjunctiva of the eye caused by a strain of *Chlamydia trachomatis*. Trachoma is discussed in chapter 8, volume 3.

Bacterial Diseases

Bacteria are one-celled microorganisms which contain both kinds of nucleic acid (DNA and RNA) and are capable of active reproduction. Bacteria are widely distributed in nature, and many of them perform useful functions, such as drawing nitrogen from the air for the use of growing plants and aiding in the decomposition of organic matter. Many harmless bacteria inhabit the intestinal tract of humans and even aid in certain chemical processes there.

Certain bacteria are properly classed with other types of "germs" and are capable of producing disease once they enter the tissues of the human body. In *You and Your Health* many of the diseases caused by bacteria are considered in chapters concerned with the body's organs and systems. In this present chapter we bring together the descriptions of bacteria-caused diseases not mentioned elsewhere in these volumes. The reader is advised to use the General Index at the back of each volume to locate the chapter and page where any particular disease in which he may be interested is described.

ACTINOMYCOSIS (LUMPY JAW)

The rod-shaped organism *(Actinomyces israelii)* responsible for this disease resides commonly in the mouths of persons habitually careless in matters of mouth cleanliness. It may be harbored in the tonsils or in decayed teeth. Also it may be present within the intestine. It usually causes no trouble until a break occurs in the tissues, as when a tooth is extracted, or the patient suffers an injury to the face or jaw, or a break occurs in the membrane lining the intestine. Infection typically occurs after oral trauma or dental procedures that bruise the tissue or cause anaerobic conditions. The disease is characterized by local inflammation of tissues and the formation of sinuses (hollow spaces).

There are four possible manifestations of this disease: (1) The most frequent consists of abscesses and draining sinuses within the neck. (2) In some cases the organisms are carried by air currents into the lungs, where they cause a condition resembling pulmonary tuberculosis. The chest wall may become involved, and there may be sinuses which open through the skin. (3) When the intestine is affected, there may be partial intestinal obstruction, together with draining sinuses and fistulas in the abdominal wall. (4) In a few cases the infection becomes generalized to involve other organs of the body.

Care and Treatment

The drugs of choice are penicillin or one of the tetracycline drugs.

These must be continued for several weeks after the patient appears to have overcome the infection. It is often necessary to use surgical procedures to aid in the eradication of the fistulas and sinuses.

ANTHRAX (MALIGNANT PUSTULE; WOOLSORTER'S DISEASE)

Anthrax is a disease of animals which may be transmitted to humans. The germs of anthrax *(Bacillus anthracis)* occur commonly as spores (the latent form), which adhere to the skin or hair of animals and may remain potentially dangerous for a long time. Humans at risk of this disease are those who handle animals, their hides, or their hair. The spores usually enter through a break in the skin. In a small number of cases the spores are inhaled into the lungs. In another small group of cases the spores are introduced into the body by eating contaminated meat.

The disease which results when the spores are taken into the lungs or into the organs of digestion is more serious and progresses more rapidly than that in which the spores enter through a break in the skin. Even in the latter, the mortality rate for untreated cases is about 20 percent.

In a typical case of anthrax involving

Typical case of anthrax.

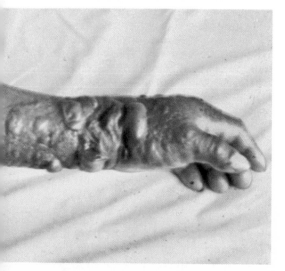

the skin, a small, red, slightly-raised spot appears at the spot where the spores entered. The lesion increases rapidly in size to form a flattened blister which becomes a dark-colored ulcer around which the tissue is swollen. The patient may experience itching but very little pain. It is usually this dark-colored ulcer surrounded by swollen tissue that attracts attention to the infection.

Prevention. Human involvement with anthrax can be prevented by a vaccine, strongly recommended for persons at high risk in the animal industry.

Care and Treatment

Anthrax occurring in humans responds well to several of the antibiotic medications. When the infection enters through the skin, the patient should receive about two million units of penicillin twice each day for seven days. For the more serious cases, in which the lungs are involved, much larger doses of penicillin are recommended.

BRUCELLOSIS (UNDULENT FEVER)

Brucellosis is a disease which primarily affects animals, especially cattle, sheep, pigs, and goats. Pregnant animals are especially susceptible. The causative organisms are present in the milk, the excretions, and the flesh of infected animals. The disease is readily transmitted from animal to animal and from animals to humans but, rarely, if ever, from human to human.

In former years, the disease was most commonly transmitted to humans by raw dairy products from infected cows or goats. Now that milk is pasteurized, the persons at greatest risk are those who have contact with animals and those concerned with the processing of meat. The germs enter the human body through wounds in the skin, by being inhaled with contaminated dust, by being swallowed in contaminated meat or dairy products, or by penetration into the delicate membranes around the eyes.

The incubation period for human brucellosis averages about two weeks, but may be as short as five days or as long as thirty-five days. The symptoms, manifestations, and duration of the illness vary from case to case. Typically the patient experiences chills and fever, headache, muscle pains, and a rise in body temperature each evening. The intermittent fever continues for one to five weeks. Then, in mild cases, after a period of apparent improvement lasting a week or two, sequences of symptoms may recur one or more times.

Prevention. Elimination of infected animals from dairy herds has gone a long way toward protecting humans from this disease. Also, pasteurization of dairy products has been a great help. Those who handle animals or carcasses likely to be infected should wear rubber gloves and should carefully protect any break in the skin.

Care and Treatment

Most cases of brucellosis respond well to antibiotic medication, tetracycline being the preferred drug. It is given by mouth in doses of 0.5 gms. at four-hour intervals (four doses per day) for three weeks.

Bed rest throughout the acute phase of the illness is advised. Tepid sponge baths and alcohol rubs are usually effective for the control of high fever. The patient should be encouraged to drink adequate water and fruit juice. He should have an easily digested and adequately nourishing diet. Attention should be given to maintaining the patient's courage and optimism. Complications, if and when they develop, should be treated as recommended by the physician.

CHOLERA

Historically, cholera has been one of the five major pestilences of the world, having caused millions of deaths, particularly in India, Southeast Asia, and China. The most recent pandemic of cholera occurred between 1961 and 1975, originating in the Celebes and spreading to Korea, Africa, and southern Europe.

The germs of cholera, after having been swallowed, take up their residence in the upper part of the small intestine. While residing there, they produce a toxin that causes an extremely severe diarrhea—so severe that the patient's life is endangered because of the sudden loss of fluid and essential chemicals.

The organism that causes cholera (*Vibrio cholerae*) lives only in human beings. The excretions of a person ill with cholera are loaded with these organisms. They are transmitted to another human only by contamination of liquid or food which the susceptible person swallows. It is evident therefore, that the continuing incidence of cholera depends upon conditions of poor sanitation. Cholera is usually spread by contaminated drinking water, but contaminated food is also an important means of transmitting the disease.

The incubation period for cholera is brief—from six to forty-eight hours. The symptoms begin abruptly with the onset of watery, painless diarrhea. The diarrhea is so excessive that a quart (1 liter) of body fluid may be lost within an hour. Effortless vomiting is often associated with the diarrhea, this problem complicating the loss of fluid from the patient's body. This rapid loss of fluid soon leads to profound shock. There may be severe muscle cramps due to the loss of essential chemicals from the body. When untreated, the illness runs a course of between one day and one week, with a mortality of about 50 percent when the loss of fluid is excessive.

With adequate treatment by prompt and continuous replacement of body fluid and essential chemicals, complete recovery is the rule. The reason for the tragically high death rates in underprivileged countries when pandemics of cholera occur is that the available supplies of fluid and essential chemicals suitable for intravenous injection are soon exhausted. Also, in such countries, many persons do not have access to medical care.

Prevention. A standard commercial vaccine is available which provides protection from cholera for a period of four to six months. For persons living in areas where cholera may occur, the standard method of vaccination requires two doses of the vaccine (0.5 ml.) given one month apart. For travelers passing through an area where cholera may occur, a single dose of the vaccine given prior to travel is recommended.

Care and Treatment

The mainstay of the treatment of cholera consists of vigilant nursing care and the continuous replacement of body fluids and essential chemicals. These are preferably administered by intravenous injection at a rate which approximates the loss of body fluid and chemicals by way of diarrhea and vomiting. The essential chemicals which must be contained in the fluid are salts of sodium, potassium, and carbonate. The intravenous injection of fluid may be supplemented by fluid taken by mouth.

The patient with cholera should be kept in bed and should be protected from becoming chilled. If necessary, his body temperature should be maintained by the use of a hot-water bottle and/or fomentations. As the patient becomes able, he may receive strained vegetable broths and strained cereal gruels.

It is very important to prevent this infection from being transmitted to other persons. The patient's bowel discharges should be boiled or otherwise sterilized before being discarded. His bedding and clothing should be disinfected before being laundered. All foods and beverages in the vicinity should be protected from flies and other insects. All persons who may have been exposed to this infection should receive a course of cholera vaccine. Those who attend the patient should take precise pre-cautions to avoid being infected or being the means of transmitting the infection to others. See chapter 24, this volume, for details.

DIPHTHERIA

In years past, diphtheria was a dread disease, often occurring in epidemics and causing thousands of deaths. Even after surviving the illness, many persons suffered permanent handicaps from damage to the heart or the kidneys, or from paralysis of certain of the muscles.

Since 1923 there has been available a toxoid which, when administered to a susceptible person, stimulates the development of immunity and thus keeps him from acquiring the disease. Immunization with the toxoid has reduced the incidence of diphtheria, but some parents have become careless in arranging for their children to be properly immunized. So diphtheria is still with

Appearance of throat in diphtheria.

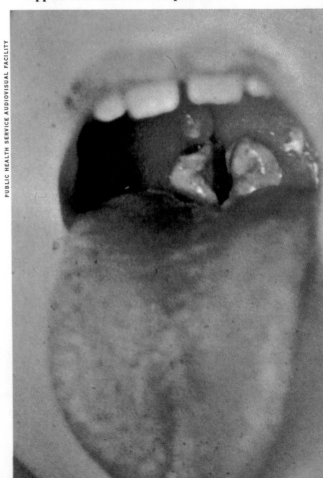

PUBLIC HEALTH SERVICE AUDIOVISUAL FACILITY

us, and it is still a lethal disease. The number of cases that occur in the United States each year runs between 200 and 400, and the mortality rate varies from 6 to 14 percent.

Diphtheria is a highly contagious disease caused by the diphtheria bacillus, Corynebacterium diphtheriae. Children between the ages of 1 and 10 are especially susceptible, but the disease also attacks older persons. The bacillus does not survive long when not in contact with human tissues. The germs are usually carried by infected secretions from the nose or throat of a person who harbors these germs. They are introduced into the body of the susceptible person by the inhalation of contaminated droplets of moisture, by contact with contaminated fingers or a soiled handkerchief or towel, or by the use of contaminated food or milk. The incubation period is short, being one to five days.

Usually the bacillus invades the membranes of the upper air passages (pharynx, larynx, and trachea). There serious damage results from a unique structure called a pseudomembrane, which develops and coats over the infected areas. The pseudomembrane becomes thick and constitutes the first threat to the patient's life because, as it loosens from the underlying tissues, it may obstruct the passage of air and cause death by asphixiation. In serious cases where the passageway through the larynx is obstructed, life is sometimes saved by the surgical procedure known as tracheotomy, in which an opening from the outside into the trachea is made in the lower part of the neck.

Once the diphtheria bacillus is entrenched in the upper air passages, it produces a very potent toxin which circulates throughout the body by way of the blood. Except for the danger of asphixiation as mentioned above, it is the effect of this toxin that accounts mostly for deaths from diphtheria. It damages the heart, the kidneys, and the nerves, damage to the heart or the kidneys causing most of the deaths. The nerve damage may cause paralysis of muscles, more commonly in the area of the throat and face but occasionally in other parts of the body also. In many recent cases in the United States there has been a skin lesion in which the diphtheria bacilli have invaded a preexisting wound causing a deep, "punched-out" ulcer, which may vary in size up to one or two inches (2.5 to 5 cm.). This manifestation occurs typically among older indigent and alcoholic patients who live under conditions of poor hygiene.

The symptoms in the usual early case of diphtheria (pharyngeal diphtheria) include a mild sore throat, an elevation of body temperature, difficulty in breathing and swallowing, and the beginning evidences of damage by the toxin produced by the diphtheria germ. The circulation of this toxin through the body causes severe prostration. In some cases there is a tremendous enlargement of the lymph nodes in the neck.

Prevention. In addition to the immunization of young children by the use of diphtheria toxoid, a booster injection of toxoid should be administered at ten-year intervals. Cases of diphtheria that now occur in the United States usually involve those who have not been immunized or who have neglected to have their booster immunizations.

Care and Treatment

One of the classic successes in the development of specific methods of treatment was the preparation in 1890 of an effective antitoxin which, when administered early enough during the course of diphtheria illness, will prevent the usual complications of this disease. The administration of antitoxin does not kill the bacteria which cause this disease, but it does neutralize the toxin which these bacteria produce. The present-day physician in charge of a case of diphtheria will not only administer the antitoxin but will also use an antibiotic preparation such as penicillin in order to kill the diphtheria germs.

The patient with diphtheria should be kept absolutely quiet in bed for at least two weeks—longer if complications have developed. During the acute phase of the illness the patient's breathing must be constantly monitored to safeguard against obstruction by the pseudomembrane that develops in the air passages. Because of the patient's difficulty in swallowing, it may be necessary to administer fluid and nourishment by intravenous injection.

Pain, caused by swollen lymph nodes in the neck, may be somewhat relieved by applying an ice collar for fifteen minutes out of the hour. Mouth and throat irrigations with warm salt solution (1 tsp. of salt to a pint of water) may relieve some of the discomfort of the sore throat.

Because of the possibility of damage to the heart, the diphtheria patient should be very deliberate about resuming his normal activities following the acute phase of the illness. The recovering patient should not be permitted to mingle with people until after two successive laboratory examinations have indicated that the diphtheria germs are no longer present in his tissues.

Because diphtheria is highly contagious, the nursing procedures should include all precautions to prevent transmission of the germs to other people. See chapter 24, this volume, for details.

LEPROSY (HANSEN'S DISEASE)

Leprosy, sometimes called Hansen's disease, is a chronic infectious disease caused by a germ which resembles the germ of tuberculosis. Leprosy occurs most commonly in tropical countries. An estimated 10 to 20 million persons are affected with leprosy worldwide. In the United States, a recent increase in the number of cases has brought the total to about 200 newly recognized cases per year, a statistic attributed to immigration from countries where leprosy is common.

The germs are believed to gain en-

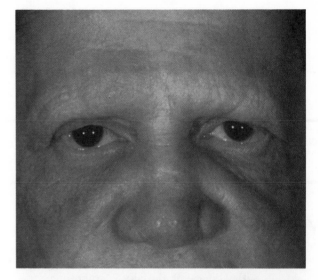

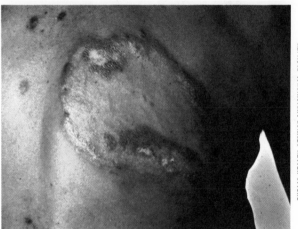

PUBLIC HEALTH SERVICE AUDIOVISUAL FACILITY

In the lepromatous variety of leprosy, loss of eyebrows constitutes an early symptom, and in the tuberculoid, spots on the skin.

trance to the body through the membrane lining the nose or through breaks in the skin. Biting insects may possibly introduce the germs into the skin, and there may be other modes of infection.

The incubation period for leprosy is two to five years or longer. The disease has a gradual onset. The usual first evidence is an area of skin that lacks sensitivity to temperature, pain, and touch. Other early symptoms are nosebleed, headache, and fever.

There are two fairly well defined varieties of leprosy: (1) the lepromatous, in which the patient manifests no resistance to the disease and (2) the tuberculoid, in which he shows considerable biological resistance.

The lepromatous variety is characterized by the formation of nodules and diffuse infiltration of the skin. The nodules, frequently most abundant on the face, soon alter the appearance of the victim. They cause the beard and the eyebrows to drop out and the cheeks, brows, and ears to have an irregular, swollen appearance. These nodules tend to break down and ulcerate, sometimes destroying the ears and at other times the nose; sometimes laying bare the bones of the skull; sometimes attacking the eyes; and sometimes making large openings through the cheek into the mouth. The senses of smell and taste are usually lost. The nodules may also appear on the extremities, from which the flesh may fall away, leaving bones exposed. The lymph nodes become enlarged. The peripheral nerves are usually affected, with the patient suffering pain in some area of the body followed by the loss of sensation. The nerves that activate certain muscles may be destroyed, with a resulting loss of function so that the individual may be unable to move the forearm or to walk.

The tuberculoid variety is less severe. It progresses slowly. It may consist principally of discolored and insensitive skin areas. Even in this variety, the damage to nerves may be considerable.

Prevention. While the danger of contagion is not great, all persons not infected should avoid body contact with a leper. They should not handle objects that he has handled, should not wear clothing that he has worn, and should not eat food that he has touched or that has been exposed to flies or other insects that might have been in contact with him. Special care should be exercised to avoid contact with the body discharges from a person with leprosy, especially discharges from the nose.

Care and Treatment

Effective drugs are now available for the treatment of leprosy. However, use of these drugs must be continued for long periods (at least five years). The initial treatment for a case of leprosy is best conducted in a clinic or an institution in which the program can be supervised by a physician specialized in the treatment of this disease. After spending a few months in such a clinic or institution, it is feasible for the patient to return to his family, with his continuing treatment program being supervised by a physician. The sulfone drugs, of which dapsone is most commonly used, are preferred. Rifampin, a semi-synthetic antibiotic drug, is also effective in such cases, its disadvantage being that it is expensive.

Persons with mild infections of leprosy do much better when they keep active than when they resort to bed rest. Patients with leprosy should have a nutritious diet, should be aided in maintaining personal hygiene, and should be encouraged to be optimistic.

NOCARDIOSIS

Nocardiosis is a condition caused by one or more subtypes of bacteria closely related to that which causes actinomycosis. When these organisms are introduced into the skin, as when a skin injury is contaminated by infected soil, the organisms cause damage similar to that in actinomycosis or maduromycosis. This form of the disease is becoming more common in the southern areas of the United States. However, the disease in its various forms is worldwide in occurrence.

When these bacteria are inhaled, they may cause severe lung disease, the early symptoms of which often resemble those of pulmonary tuberculosis. Cough and the raising of pussy sputum are the chief symptoms, but the infection can cause larger areas of consolidation, also cavities in the lungs;

and the disease may spread to the ribs and burrow through the chest wall.

Any part of the body may be attacked, but involvement of the brain and its coverings is the most serious development.

Nocardiosis affecting the lungs or other parts of the body is a serious condition. Before the sulfonamides became available for treatment, three fourths of the patients with this serious type of the disease died at the end of an illness of about six months. The administering of sulfonamides has greatly reduced the mortality rate.

Care and Treatment

Many patients with the primary cutaneous type of nocardiosis recover spontaneously without treatment. In the more serious form of the illness, which affects one or more of the internal organs, the administration of sulfonamides is the only effective treatment and may be lifesaving.

PLAGUE (BUBONIC PLAGUE)

Plague is one of the five great pestilences that, historically, have afflicted mankind. Now that effective antibiotic medication is available, the hazard of plague has been greatly reduced. However, the disease still exists in wild rodents in many parts of the world, even in western United States. Australia is the only continent free from this disease. It is still prevalent in South America, Africa, and parts of Asia. A few cases in humans occur each year in the United States.

Plague is caused by a specific organism called *Yersinia pestis*.

Although the organism which causes plague is carried in the bodies of many wild rodents, it is the domestic rat that most often transmits the disease to humans. The organisms are usually carried from the rat to the human by the bite of a flea.

The incubation period for plague is from a few hours to ten days. A typical case begins suddenly with a high fever, great weakness, chills, severe headache, and pains in the back and limbs.

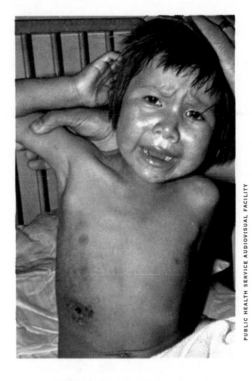

In bubonic plague, buboes usually appear in armpits the second day.

There may be vomiting and diarrhea. The organisms move through the lymph channels, and the lymph nodes become infected. Those in the groin, under the arms, and in the neck become enlarged and tender and are called buboes. Abscesses may form in the buboes, and these may break through the skin.

In the serious cases, the organisms find their way beyond the lymph nodes and enter the blood, spreading then to all parts of the body.

A serious complication occurs when the lungs become involved. The pneumonia thus developed is serious and, in untreated cases, is almost uniformly fatal. This type of pneumonia (pneumonic plague) can be transmitted from person to person by bacteria-laden droplets discharged from the patient's mouth and nose as he coughs, sneezes, or speaks forcibly.

Prevention. A vaccine is available for immunizing persons at high risk of plague, especially those involved in the care of patients with this disease. Protection for the general population consists of the eradication of rats and fleas.

Care and Treatment

Prompt administration of the appropriate antibiotic medication is a very effective treatment for plague. Streptomycin given in doses of one gram by intramuscular injection twice a day for ten days is the usual program.

The patient with plague should be isolated from all unnecessary contacts with other humans. Full precaution should be taken to avoid the spread of the infection. For details of this type of patient care, see chapter 24, this volume.

The patient should be kept in bed, and his diet should consist of easily digested foods such as soups and broths. He should be urged to drink as much fluid as possible so as to keep his kidneys active. High fever may be reduced by the use of cool sponges, alcohol rubs, and cool enemas. Ice bags applied intermittently over the painful buboes may give some relief to the pain.

RAT-BITE FEVER

Rat-bite fever is an uncommon infection transmitted to humans by the bite of a rodent—usually a wild rat. The infection may be caused either by a bacillus (*Streptobacillus moniliformis*) or by a spirochete (*Spirillum minor*). The illness is quite the same regardless of which organism causes the infection, and the treatment is also the same. The incubation period is usually less than ten days for the infection with the streptobacillus and more than ten days for that caused by the spirochete.

The infection caused by the streptobacillus produces symptoms similar to those of a virus infection. Joint pains commonly occur, and these may persist for a few months in untreated cases. In most cases a macular rash develops on the skin of the extremities, involving even the

palms and soles. Infection of the lining of the heart (endocarditis) is the most serious complication. The mortality rate is about 10 percent for untreated cases.

Rat-bite fever caused by a spirochete is mentioned on pages 292, 293, volume 3.

Care and Treatment

Most cases respond well to intramuscular injections of procaine penicillin G, 600,000 units given twice each day, for seven to ten days. Larger doses are used for severe cases or for those which develop endocarditis.

SCARLET FEVER (SCARLATINA)

Scarlet fever is one of the manifestations of an infection by beta-hemolytic streptococci. This is the same kind of infection that causes streptococcal sore throat (strep throat) as described in chapter 9, this volume. In both diseases the patient suffers a serious infection of the tissues of the pharynx. In fact, about the only difference between streptococcal sore throat and scarlet fever, as far as the disease processes are concerned, is a skin rash in scarlet fever caused by the toxin's effect on the capillaries of the skin. Formerly, scarlet fever was a common ailment, but since the advent of antibiotic medications the incidence has declined sharply.

Scarlet fever is an acute infectious disease in which the symptoms appear from one to ten days after contact with a carrier or with a case during the communicable stage of the disease. In the usual case, the disease lasts for about three weeks after symptoms first appear. The illness is characterized by fever, extremely sore throat, vomiting, headache, a coated tongue, and a skin rash which makes its appearance about two days after the onset of other symptoms.

The principal site of infection in scarlet fever is the soft tissues of the pharynx. It is here that the toxins are produced that may cause serious damage in various organs of the body.

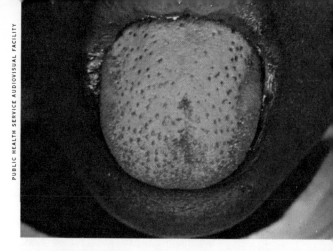

PUBLIC HEALTH SERVICE AUDIOVISUAL FACILITY

Germs of scarlet fever are carried from person to person by the air or by the small droplets of moisture emitted through a person's nose or mouth. A person with this infection may transmit it to others, beginning about a day before his symptoms appear and extending as long as a month or more after recovery. Certain persons become carriers of the infection even though they have never been ill with the disease.

The skin rash of scarlet fever appears first on the upper chest and back, later on the lower back, upper extremities, abdomen, and lower extremities. Often the rash does not appear on the face, but the face is flushed, with a pale area around the mouth. Typically, the tiny elevations of the skin rest on a background of redness which fades on pressure. The tiny elevations are about the size of goose pimples, and these remain after the red color of the skin has become pale. In most cases numerous tiny blisters develop. As the rash fades, the skin begins to peel, with large sections of skin becoming loose, particularly on the palms and soles.

Typically in scarlet fever the lymph nodes of the neck become greatly enlarged. Occasionally abscesses develop in these nodes. Complications which may occur in untreated young children include sinusitis, middle ear infection, mastoiditis, and impetigo. Other possible serious complications include damage to the heart and damage to the kidneys.

Prevention. In children who have been exposed to scarlet fever and in whom it is desirable to prevent the disease because they are not vigorous, the prompt administration of penicillin may keep the disease from developing.

A coated tongue and a skin rash help to identify scarlet fever.

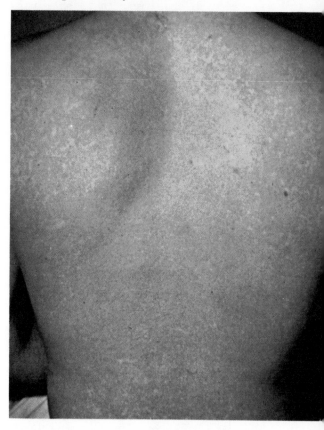

Care and Treatment

If no serious complications develops, scarlet fever runs its course in two or three weeks. The danger of complications is grave, however, and therefore it is important that an appropriate antibiotic be administered, for this has the effect of hastening recovery and, more important, of preventing the serious complications. Penicillin is the medication of choice, injected into the muscle or given orally. It may be given in one large injection of benzathine penicillin G (600,000 to 900,000 units for small children or 1.2 million units for older children and adults), or by a ten-day program of oral penicillin in which 200,000 to 400,000 units are taken by mouth four times a day. It is important when the ten-day oral program is followed that the medication be taken four times a day for the complete ten-day period, even though it appears that the patient has become well in the meantime.

Nursing care for the scarlet fever patient should provide rest in bed, adequate fluids, and an easily digested, nourishing diet. For excessively high fever, tepid sponge baths or alcohol rubs may be helpful. Continuous heating compresses to the neck are helpful in allaying the discomfort of severe sore throat. See chapter 25, volume 3, for details. Cleanliness of the mouth may be promoted by using a salt-water mouth rinse (one level teaspoonful of salt to a pint of water). At the time scaling of the skin occurs, it is helpful to rub the skin with olive oil.

It is recommended that the recovering patient remain in bed a few days even after symtpoms disappear and that he be slow in returning to full activity—this as a means of minimizing the danger that may have been done to the tissues of his heart or kidneys.

SHIGELLOSIS (BACILLARY DYSENTERY)

Shigellosis is a disease of the bowel caused by germs belonging to the *Shigella* group of bacilli. It is characterized by frequent stools (up to 100 or more a day) which contain mucus, blood, and pus. The patient suffers abdominal cramps, a general feeling of illness, and fever. The disease occurs in all parts of the world, particularly in the tropics.

Shigellosis occurs frequently where families live in overcrowded quarters where the sanitation is not satisfactory. It affects young children more commonly than older people. It is a contagious disease, the responsible germs being carried from person to person, usually by food which has lacked re-

frigeration and which has been contaminated by contact with germ-laden soil or with flies that have carried the germs from human excrement.

The symptoms begin within one to four days after the germs have been taken into the patient's mouth, the onset often being sudden, particularly with children. They include fever, loss of appetite, drowsiness, a desire to vomit, abdominal pain, and the frequent passage of stools which soon contain mucus, blood, and pus.

In the case of a young child, the greatest danger to life is caused by the loss of fluid from the body (dehydration). Also, as the illness persists, the lack of nutrition becomes serious.

Prevention. The general principles for preventing the spread of shigellosis require adequate sanitation, the safeguarding of food supplies (refrigeration and avoiding contamination), effective disposal of sewage, and proper methods to exterminate flies and to keep even an occasional fly from entering the house.

Care and Treatment

Healthy adults who develop shigellosis will usually overcome their fever, even though untreated, in about four days. The diarrhea and abdominal cramps usually continue for a few days longer.

The primary consideration in treating this illness is to restore the fluid and the essential chemicals lost from the body by way of the extreme diarrhea. Such replacement is particularly imperative when dealing with children, especially infants, and with frail patients. The restoration of the fluid and essential chemicals is best performed in a hospital by the use of intravenous injection.

Appropriate antibiotic medication shortens the duration of the illness. The preferred antibiotic medication is ampicillin administered over a period of five days.

The problem of nutrition becomes a major concern in the case of an infant with shigellosis. As soon as the

vomiting and diarrhea have ceased, the infant can be given nourishing liquids by mouth at hourly intervals. As recovery progresses, the usual formula can be added to these liquids.

STAPHYLOCOCCAL INFECTIONS

Staphylococcus aureus germs are typically involved in infections of the skin such as boils, in infections that produce abscesses, in some kinds of pneumonia, and in septicemia (bloodstream infection). Treatment of such infections is sometimes difficult because certain strains of the staphylococcus (the so-called resistant strains) do not respond well to the common antibiotic drugs.

Staphylococcal infections are most serious in the very young and the very old and in those whose resistance has been reduced by illness. The danger of staphylococcal infections is greatest in newborn infants, nursing mothers, persons ill with influenza, those with such chronic lung diseases as emphysema, those with long-standing skin disorders, persons recovering from surgery, and persons with extensive burns.

Staphylococcal germs (shown here highly magnified).

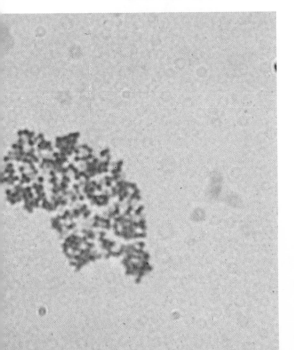

Prevention. Because some staphylococcal infections are life-threatening, and because their treatment is difficult, emphasis is placed on preventing them in preference to treating them after they occur. Particularly in hospitals, both in nurseries and in the facilities for surgery, great care is used to avoid the transfer of staphylococcal germs to someone who may be susceptible. Precautions involve the use of all possible methods of preventing contamination.

In the hospital nursery sterile gowns and masks are worn by those who take care of the infants. The hands of the attendants must be washed with soap and rinsed with disinfectant solution. Any infant with an infection is isolated to prevent spread of the infection to others. Any materials or body discharges that may possibly carry staphylococcal germs are handled strictly in accordance with hospital techniques. Similarly in the handling of surgical patients, all precautions are taken to prevent the entrance of staphylococcal germs into the tissues of susceptible patients.

When a patient with such an infection is cared for at home, the patient should be isolated from other persons who may be susceptible. His bedding, personal linen, and all body excretions must be handled in a manner to prevent contamination.

Care and Treatment

Many of the older antibiotic preparations may not be effective in combating a staphylococcal infection. Several of the newer antibiotics are quite useful. The physician in charge of a case will use his judgment in selecting the antibiotic most effective against the type of staphylococcal germ involved.

An abscess that develops in the course of an infection must be surgically drained. The patient should receive an adequate amount of easily digested food during each twenty-four-hour period. High fever is best controlled by the use of tepid sponge baths or by alcohol rubs.

281

TETANUS (LOCKJAW)

Tetanus is a life-threatening disease in which a potent toxin is produced when spores of the *Clostridium tetani* are introduced into human tissues on the occasion of some penetrating injury. Because of the general use of preventive immunization, the actual disease is now rare in the industrialized nations. Cases in the United States number only 100 to 150 cases annually. But worldwide, tetanus accounts for an estimated 1,000,000 deaths per year, almost half of which involve newborn infants.

The germ that causes tetanus grows only in the absence of oxygen. The spores of this germ are abundant in gar-

Puncture wounds give tetanus germs access to the body.

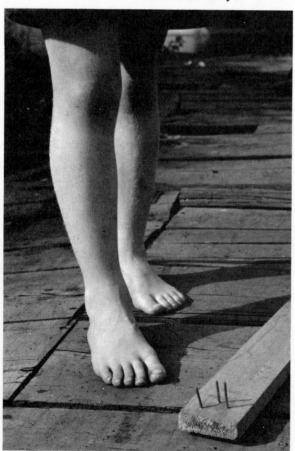

BLACK STAR

den and barnyard soil, in the dust along the roadside and in playgrounds, and especially in soil or dust mixed with horse manure. When spores find their way into a deep wound, particularly a puncture wound where they have no access to the air, they grow and produce their toxin. It is the toxin which gives rise to the serious symptoms characteristic of this disease.

Symptoms usually appear within five to ten days after the injury. The original wound may have begun to heal by this time. There develops a stiffness of the muscles of the face, noted when the patient attempts to open or close his mouth. The victim becomes restless and worried. The stiffness spreads to other muscles of his body. His face becomes contorted, and he responds so sensitively to slight noises or any sudden contact with his skin that all the muscles of his body may suddenly contract. Pain becomes intense, and he suffers high fever with sweating, exhaustion, and retention of urine.

For patients who survive, the severe symptoms, including the muscle spasms, persist for about a week and then gradually diminish during the next several weeks. In the United States, the mortality rate for tetanus cases varies between 50 and 60 percent. Because of the seriousness of this disease, once it develops, it is urgently recommended that parents consistently arrange for their infants and children to be protected by the administration of tetanus toxoid, beginning at two months of age, continuing at intervals through childhood, and repeated every ten years thereafter, as advised in chapter 6, volume 1, and chapter 2, volume 2.

Procedure for the Person Who Sustains a Penetrating Injury. The person who sustains a penetrating injury, as by stepping on a nail, or by sustaining a deep wound possibly contaminated by dust or street dirt, should receive treatment at once. There is danger in delay, for if time is allowed for the toxin to be produced and circulated throughout the body, then no way exists of preventing the suffering which the symptoms produce or of avoiding the risk of a fatal outcome.

A physician should clean the wound thoroughly, even by making a larger opening as necessary to remove all fragments of tissue that have been damaged. He should inquire about the patient's history of immunization. If the patient has previously completed the immunization schedule for tetanus but has not had a booster injection of toxoid within the preceding five years, he should then receive such a booster injection. If the patient is uncertain about his immunization history or if he has never been immunized for tetanus, he should then promptly receive an injection of tetanus immune globulin which confers protection for a few days.

Care and Treatment

Once a person actually experiences the symptoms of tetanus, his care becomes extremely critical. If possible, he should be placed in the intensive care unit of a hospital where he can receive continuous nursing care under the supervision of a physician. He must be protected from all disturbing influences, for noises and other distractions may cause his muscles to go into serious spasm. In many cases it becomes necessary to provide artificial assistance for the patient's respiration. Medications may be necessary to reduce the strength of his muscle contractions. The patient will need careful professional supervision for a period of several weeks.

TUBERCULOSIS

Tuberculosis was near the top of the list of dread diseases in the previous century. It was called the white plague. It struck down persons of all ages, but especially young adults in the prime of life. It was easily transmitted from person to person, and once the disease entered a person's body death usually followed within a matter of months. In the 1870s, approximately one out of every five deaths was caused by tuberculosis. In 1900 tuberculosis was still responsible for 10 percent of all deaths in this country.

Back in the 1870s a better method of treating this disease prompted a glimmer of hope. The method was discovered almost by accident by Edward Trudeau, a young physician who had himself contracted the disease as he cared for his brother during the last few weeks of the brother's life.

Expecting that his own illness would soon run its usual, fatal course, young Trudeau made an unusual decision. He reasoned that if he were going to die, he might as well die happy. Earlier in his life he had spent a few weeks on a hunting trip in the woods of the Adirondacks in upstate New York. Now he determined to return to Paul Smith's hunting camp and enjoy outdoor life while he lasted. But instead of

An X ray of the chest reveals possible presence of tuberculosis.

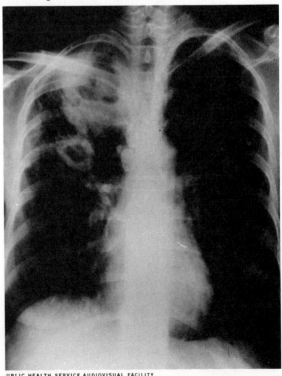

dying, Trudeau lived on and even improved. He had not followed the traditional pattern for the treatment of tuberculosis. Why should he? And as he improved he became interested in helping other persons who had tuberculosis. And this led to the development, beginning in 1885, of the Adirondack Cottage Sanitarium for the treatment of tuberculosis.

Trudeau's method of treatment was simple. It is well summarized by the acronym for which he became famous—PAMSETGAAF. The letters of this word stand for Pure Air, Maximum Sunshine, Equitable Temperature, Good Accommodations, and Abundant Food. Even in cold weather, Trudeau's patients were wrapped in blankets and placed outdoors for a while each day. This kind of treatment was aimed to build up the body's resistance to the disease. The improvement that many patients made under this regimen was proof in itself that tuberculosis is essentially a systemic infection and that there occurs within the body a virtual warfare between the germs that cause the disease and the body's defense mechanisms.

A very decided decline in the number of cases of tuberculosis and in the number of deaths from this disease dates back to the beginning use of certain medications which specifically control the *Mycobacterium tuberculosis,* the germ that causes this disease. But even though tuberculosis is now treatable, curable, and preventable, it is still causing about 30,000 new cases each year in the United States and about 3000 deaths.

How does a person become infected with tuberculosis? Usually by inhaling what someone else has exhaled. For the common type of tuberculosis caused by the *Mycobacterium tuberculosis,* humans provide the essential reservoir of the infection, meaning that the disease is transmitted from one human to another. And the means of transmission is by tiny droplets of moisture expelled from a person's mouth or nose when he coughs, sneezes, or speaks.

These tiny droplets float easily in the air, and when inhaled by another person, they carry the germs into this second person's organ of breathing—usually right into his lungs.

Still another organism, *Mycobacterium bovis,* is responsible for tuberculosis in cattle, a type which may be transmitted to the human by the drinking of contaminated milk. The careful management of dairy herds and pasteurization of milk has virtually eliminated this kind of tuberculosis in the United States and Western Europe. However, it is still common in certain other parts of the world.

The Primary Infection. When a person inhales aerosol particles contaminated by the germs of tuberculosis, they are carried into his lungs and into the delicate air sacs. Here the germs multiply, and many find their way into the lymph nodes near the center of the

The tubercle bacillus multiplies rapidly in a dark, moist place.

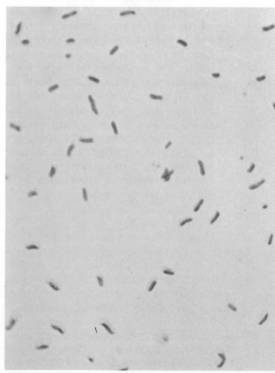

chest. Some of the germs at this early stage easily enter the blood and are carried to various other parts of the body. The germs of tuberculosis require an abundant supply of oxygen, and so the area where they thrive best, once they are distributed by the blood, is in the upper portions of the lungs. But the germs may also take up residence in such sites as the kidneys, the vertebrae, the ends of long bones, or the lymph nodes.

The presence of these germs, now that they reside in the body's tissues, sets in motion an immune reaction by which phagocytic cells of the body's defense system engulf many of the invading germs. In the course of this destruction of the germs, tiny areas of tissue are also destroyed. This deterioration calls for a healing process wherever the small areas of tissue destruction exist. And these tiny areas where healing occurs by scar formation and even by the deposit of calcium are called granulomas. At the center of each granuloma usually a few live germs of tuberculosis remain entrapped within the fibrous capsule of the granuloma. As we will see, it is these imprisoned germs which may cause serious difficulty at some later time.

This primary infection which we have just described occurs so frequently that it is estimated that 15,000,000 people in the United States have experienced it. The reason it is often not noticed is that the body's defense mechanism is usually equal to the situation and entraps the invading germs, as described above, before they have opportunity to cause systemic disease. In occasional cases, however, (approximately 10 percent of primary infections) the body's defenses prove inadequate because of poor general health, and therefore an active condition of tuberculosis develops in this early stage. This active form of the disease may involve either the lungs or some other organ of the body in which the unrestrained germs are located.

Physicians use a simple skin test (the tuberculin test) to determine whether a

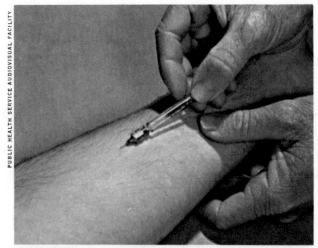

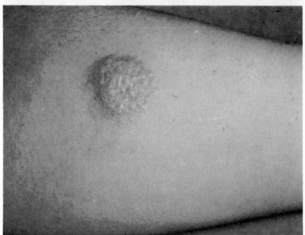

A positive tuberculin reaction indicates that tuberculosis germs have been present and that preventive treatment may be indicated.

person has had this primary infection with the germs of tuberculosis. When the test is positive it indicates that the germs of tuberculosis have already entered this person's body. Even if no evidences of the disease of tuberculosis remain, a positive test indicates that dormant germs are now encased in granulomas wherever they may be located.

Outcome of the Primary Infection. For most persons who have had this

285

primary infection, the dormant germs remain encapsulated in the granulomas for the remainder of life. However, such persons carry the risk that at some future time their body's defenses may lapse and allow the development of an active case of tuberculosis—so-called reactivation tuberculosis.

Reactivation Tuberculosis. Reactivation tuberculosis occurs in a minority of persons who have had the primary infection. The likelihood of such a person becoming ill with tuberculosis is greatest soon after his primary infection, and this likelihood decreases year by year thereafter.

Notice that we are now using the word *tuberculosis* instead of the word *infection*. The word *tuberculosis* implies an active disease in one or more of the body's organs. Reactivation tuberculosis may develop within weeks after the occurrence of a primary infection, or it may occur years later. It develops when the body's defense mechanisms become insufficient to the extent that certain of the dormant germs previously encapsulated in granulomas are now liberated and produce an active disease in that part of the body where they reside.

The usual manifestation of reactivation tuberculosis is an involvement of the lungs (pulmonary tuberculosis). The disease begins insidiously with loss of appetite, loss of body weight, night sweats, low-grade fever, cough, production of excess sputum, and the appearance of blood in the sputum. When untreated, the disease tends to become chronic and follows a downhill course, with the development of anemia, possible hemorrhages from the lungs, and other complications.

In the days before drug therapy became available for the treatment of tuberculosis, the mortality rate was high. The cases that survived were those in which the body's defenses were built up by such measures of healthful living as those promoted by Dr. Trudeau.

Now that effective medications are available, the prospects for successful treatment of reactivation tuberculosis are good. The program of treatment is described later in this section.

Extrapulmonary Tuberculosis. Tuberculosis is a systemic disease, but the symptoms and the sites of tissue destruction which occur in a given case depend upon which organ of the body is particularly affected. Inasmuch as the germs of tuberculosis require abundant oxygen, the lungs are the most common site of involvement. However, other organs of the body are involved in about 15 percent of cases of reactivation tuberculosis. Even when the lungs are primarily involved, other organs may share the involvement. The organ systems other than the lungs most commonly affected are the genitourinary organs, the musculoskeletal strutures (especially joints and bones), and the lymph nodes.

These involvements of other organs throughout the body may cause crippling defects, as when the vertebrae are affected, or may be life-threatening, as when the kidneys are involved. Inasmuch, however, as tuberculosis is a systemic disease, the same kinds of drug therapy which are effective in the treatment of tuberculosis lung involvement are also effective in the treatment of tuberculosis of other organs of the body.

Miliary Tuberculosis. Miliary tuberculosis is an occasional manifestation of this disease (about 1 percent of all cases) in which the individual's defense mechanisms prove so inadequate that the germs of tuberculosis seem to have free access to the entire body, being carried by the blood to all areas. When untreated, miliary tuberculosis uniformly causes death within a few weeks. The disease is not localized in any particular organ or organ system, for it affects the entire body. Even with the use of combined drug therapy, the mortality rate is still about 35 percent.

Prevention of Tuberculosis. In certain cases it is advisable to actively prevent tuberculosis rather than passively hope that the disease will not develop. Prevention is recommended for children and adolescents who have been in close contact (as within the family) with someone who has active tuberculosis. Prevention is also recommended for a person who has recovered from tuberculosis but who has never received the medications now used in treating this disease. Also, prevention is recommended for persons whose body defenses are now at low ebb and whose tuberculin skin test indicates that they have once had the primary infection with the germs of tuberculosis.

Prevention is accomplished by administration of one of the drugs otherwise used for the treatment of the disease, once established. Out of a total of about ten drugs now available for the treatment of tuberculosis, the one preferred for purposes of prevention is isoniazid. It is administered, of course, under the supervision of a physician.

Care and Treatment

The successful treatment of active tuberculosis by the use of drug therapy dates back to the late 1940s when streptomycin, an antibiotic drug, was first used for this purpose. Streptomycin is still useful in certain selected cases, but, as with most powerful drugs, the possibility exists of unfavorable side effects which limit its general usefulness. Now about ten drugs have been approved in the United States for the treatment of tuberculosis. Prominent among these are isoniazid, ethambutol, and rifampin. Experience during the several years that drug therapy has been used in the treatment of tuberculosis has developed certain general principles for the administration of these important drugs. It is now recognized that treatment is most effective when two or three drugs are used in combination rather than one singly. It is recognized now that a single daily dose of the drug or the combination of drugs is preferred to several doses in the same day. The use of these drugs is best continued over several months, even though the symptoms of the illness have disappeared. It is often necessary to persuade the patient in this matter, lest he become careless in the use of the medication because he no longer feels ill.

Formerly, patients with tuberculosis were treated in an institution for many months. Now, with the effective use of drug therapy, patients can live at home while being treated without serious danger of infecting other members of the family. Even so, it is recommended that the patient just beginning his course of treatment be cared for in a hospital for two or more weeks until his condition becomes stable enough that danger no longer remains of his transmitting the disease to other persons. The recommended period of treatment with the appropriate drugs is at least nine months.

TULAREMIA (RABBIT FEVER)

Tularemia is an infectious disease caused by the *Francisella tularensis*. This germ infects many kinds of animals and may be transmitted to humans by contact with infected animals, by the eating of inadequately cooked meat, or by the bite of insects. Wild cottontail rabbits are the usual source of the infection in the United States. Hunters, butchers, and housewives are at greatest risk of acquiring this disease.

The infection enters the human body through a break in the skin or through membranes, or by being swallowed or inhaled. The incubation period is three to seven days. The resulting illness may follow various patterns, depending on where the germs gained entrance to the body.

The usual manifestation consists of an ulcer of the skin or membrane, accompanied by painful enlargement and breakdown of the lymph nodes in the vicinity of the ulcer. Severe headache, high fever, and enlargement of the liver and spleen develop.

Less commonly, the disease may affect the lungs, the digestive organs, or the membranes surrounding the eyes.

Prevention. A vaccine is now available which is effective in preventing tularemia. Other than the use of the vaccine, prevention requires caution in the handling of wild rabbits, rodents, and even game birds.

Care and Treatment

Streptomycin is the antibiotic medication of choice for the treatment of tularemia. The usual program requires the intramuscular injection of streptomycin twice a day for about one week. The patient should be kept in bed, should receive a generous diet of easily digested food, and should drink adequate amounts of fluid. Application of an ice bag for about ten minutes out of each half hour to ulcerated areas or to swollen lymph nodes brings some comfort. When one or both eyes are affected, special treatment is required.

TYPHOID FEVER (INCLUDING PARATYPHOID FEVERS)

Typhoid fever is an acute, severe, systemic disease with principal involvement in the small intestine, which is caused by the typhoid bacillus *(Salmonella typhosa)*. The disease is unique to humans. Prior to 1900 it occurred frequently and caused many deaths in the United States. The incidence has steadily decreased in recent years until now only about 400 cases are reported each year in the United States and almost half of these are in persons who acquired their infection in some other part of the world. The decline in the incidence is the direct result of improved methods of sanitation to provide pure water, effective sewage disposal, and pasteurization of milk. Typhoid fever continues to be a frequent illness in parts of the world where unsanitary conditions exist.

The germs of typhoid fever enter the body through food or drink contaminated by bowel or kidney discharge from a typhoid fever patient or a car-

rier. One agent which transfers the germs to food is the common housefly.

The symptoms begin five days to five weeks after the germs enter the body. The onset is usually gradual, with a tired feeling and general weakness. There may be headache and nosebleed. The fever rises higher each day, until by the end of the first week it may reach 104° F. (40° C.)—higher in the evening than in the morning. The appetite is poor, the tongue is coated, and the teeth and lips are covered with a brownish deposit.

Diarrhea is common, especially at first; but there may be constipation instead. The stools have a very offensive odor. The abdomen is distended and tender to pressure. After seven to ten days, small, rose-colored spots may appear on the skin, most abundant over the abdomen but sometimes on the chest and back also. Near the beginning of the third week of illness, the fever usually begins to fall gradually.

During the early part of the disease the patient's face is flushed and the eyes are bright, but by the second week the expression becomes listless and dull. Cough is fairly common and, usually, the skin is dry. Sweating may occur late in the course of the disease.

The symptoms and severity of typhoid fever vary greatly. Serious complications may develop, the most serious being intestinal hemorrhage and intestinal perforation. When these occur, they usually come during the third week of the illness. The occurrence of intestinal hemorrhage is indicated by a sudden drop in temperature, a weak and rapid pulse, and a dark discharge from the bowel. Intestinal perforation is indicated by sudden pain in the abdomen (often on the right side), a rapid drop in temperature, a spread of the abdominal pain to include the entire abdomen, and a weak but rapid pulse.

In some cases of typhoid fever the symptoms are so mild that the patient feels it unnecessary to go to bed or to consult a physician. Even in these mild cases, however, danger of intestinal hemorrhage threatens. It is the mild

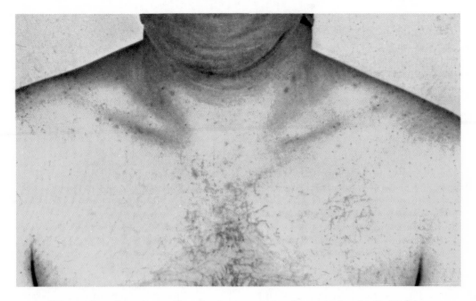

Rose-colored spots on the chest commonly characterize typhoid fever.

cases that create the greatest danger of transmitting the infection to susceptible persons, the reason being that the mildly ill person may be careless about the proper disposal of discharges from the bowel and the bladder.

Persons in reasonably good health but whose bodies still harbor the typhoid bacillus to the extent that it is present in their bowel or bladder discharges are called carriers. The person who has a very mild attack of typhoid fever is just as likely to become a carrier as one who has a severe attack. It is in the effort to eliminate carriers that health departments insist on laboratory tests being made after a person recovers from this disease. If the germs are still present in the body discharges, a course of treatment with the proper antibiotic drug will usually remedy the situation. One of the reasons that food handlers are required to have periodic examinations is to detect typhoid carriers, because many cases of the disease are traceable to food inadvertently contaminated by food handlers who are carriers.

In communities with poor sanitation, water is the more frequent means of transmitting typhoid fever. Food, especially milk, is the next most frequent offender. In urban areas, food that has been contaminated by typhoid carriers poses the greatest danger.

Prevention. The enforcement of proper methods of community sanitation is the best means of preventing typhoid fever. For individuals who care for typhoid fever patients or for those who may be traveling in areas where the disease is prevalent, immunization by the use of typhoid vaccine is urgently recommended. For those who rely on this protection, a yearly booster of the vaccine is necessary.

Paratyphoid Fever. There are two varieties of paratyphoid fever, caused by germs much like those that cause typhoid fever: paratyphoid A and paratyphoid B. Fever of either type tends to run a shorter course and tends to be less severe than typhoid fever, but the patient should receive similar care, and the same precautions should be taken against the spread of infection to other people.

Care and Treatment

Certain of the antibiotic drugs are effective in shortening the course of

289

typhoid fever or paratyphoid fever, in making the illness less severe, and in preventing serious complications. The antibiotic drug of choice is chloramphenicol. Ampicillin may be used as an alternative, but the response to this drug is not as prompt or as predictable as in the case of chloramphenicol. Even these drugs do not bring about the dramatic, sudden recovery usually expected from the use of antibiotic drugs in other types of infection.

Good nursing care is still the mainstay of treatment for typhoid fever. It is important, both for the comfort and recovery of the patient and also for carrying out those precautions that prevent the spread of the infection to other individuals. See chapter 24, volume 3, for instruction on nursing care for infectious diseases.

The patient should be kept in bed consistently from the time of onset of his symptoms until he recovers. He should use a bedpan instead of getting up to go to the bathroom. He should receive an adequate supply of fluid, even beyond what he may choose to drink. His diet should be adequate to maintain good nutrition and should consist chiefly of milk, cream, buttermilk, gruels, broths, pureed vegetables, thickened soups, poached and soft-boiled eggs, fruit juices, and simple desserts. The patient's mouth and teeth should be kept clean, liberal use being made of a dentifrice. High fever may be reduced by tepid sponge baths or alcohol rubs. Should it be necessary to administer an enema to bring about a bowel movement, great care should be taken to avoid undue pressure in administering the enema fluid. The physician's recommendation should be strictly followed in this matter. As a means of preventing bedsores, the patient's back should be rubbed with alcohol at least three times a day. The use of a very mild talcum powder after the alcohol rub is also helpful. The patient's position in bed should be changed frequently during the day, but he must be as-

sisted in making these changes so as to avoid undue exertion. If signs of intestinal hemorrhage or intestinal perforation appear, the physician should be notified at once.

Spirochetal Diseases

The spirochetes are spiral-shaped bacteria which move by rotating around a longitudinal axis. They are divided into many subclasses, but only three generally cause diseases in humans. These diseases are now described.

ENDEMIC TREPONEMATOSES

The endemic treponematoses occur in disadvantaged areas of the world and consist of three forms of illness caused by a spirochete practically identical with the *Treponema pallidum* which causes sexually transmitted syphilis. These diseases are pinta, bejel (endemic syphilis), and yaws.

Pinta (Carate; Azul). This form of treponematosis involves the skin only. It causes no disability except for its cosmetic defects (marked changes in the color of the skin). Pinta usually affects older children and teens between the ages of 10 to 20. It occurs in Central America and northern South America. The incubation period is seven to thirty days.

It is not exactly clear how the disease is transmitted from person to person. The first evidence is the development of a single, small papule, which gradually increases in size to make a plaque of elevated, reddened skin tissue. At this early stage the lymph nodes which drain the area of the initial lesion become enlarged and tender.

One month to one year later there develops a second stage of this illness characterized by a generalized enlargement of the lymph nodes. Numerous secondary lesions appear on the face, neck, and extremities. These are red in color at first, but on skin areas exposed to the sun they gradually become very dark (slate-blue). After another three

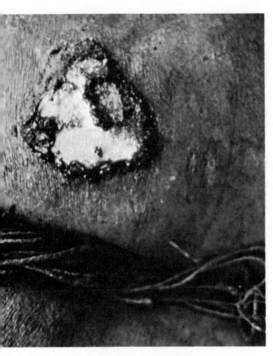

A typical case of yaws.

nent white blotches that cause disfigurement.

Bejel (Endemic Syphilis). Bejel is a disease of early childhood which affects skin, mucous membranes, and bones. It occurs in parts of Africa, Arabia, central Asia, and Australia. It is transmitted by mouth-to-mouth contact or by the sharing of eating and drinking utensils. The first evidence is the development of a lesion (mucous patch) of the membrane lining the mouth. The lymph nodes in the neck area become enlarged and tender. Later there often develops an inflammation of the periosteum (surface layer) of the leg bones. Later destructive lesions develop in the skin of the trunk and extremities. Another late manifestation is the destruction of the skin, membrane, and deeper structures of the nose and pharynx.

Yaws (Frambesia). Yaws affects the skin and bones of young children. This disease, occurring in warm, tropical parts of the world, has an incubation period of from three to four weeks. The spirochetes enter the tissues by way of insect bites, abrasions of the skin, or

months to a year, the secondary lesions lose their dark coloration, becoming brown or even white. It is these permanent

A yaws patient receiving an injection, an important early treatment.

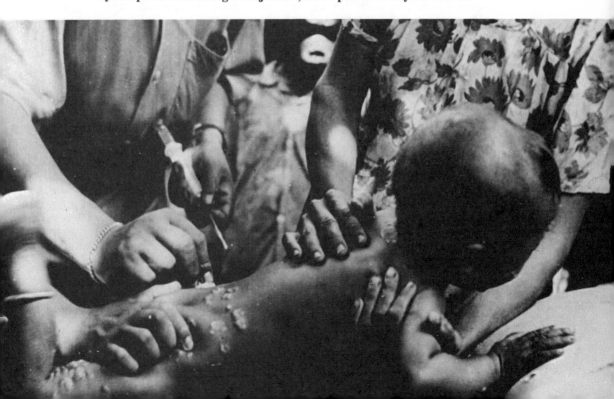

other injuries which break the skin. It is spread from person to person by direct contact with infected lesions or, possibly, by insects as intermediaries.

The first evidence of the disease is a skin lesion at the site of the innoculation of the germs. This initial lesion usually occurs on the leg and is called the "mother yaw." The lesion itches and the lymph nodes related to this area (usually in the groin) become enlarged and tender. The initial lesion heals slowly in about six months. In the second stage of the illness destructive lesions of the skin, bones, and joints develop. Those of the skin occur on the exposed parts of the body and, as they heal, leave scars and changes in the color of the skin. The secondary lesions may come and go for a period of five or more years. Inasmuch as this disease affects bones as well as skin, there may develop destruction of the nose, of the palate, or of the upper jaw. The illness is typically accompanied by fever.

Care and Treatment

The three illnesses mentioned above respond readily to the intramuscular injection of penicillin G benzathine, administered in a single dose of 2.4 million units for adults and half this dose for children. Even though this treatment eradicates the spirochetes causing the illness, the lesions, as they heal, leave scars.

LEPTOSPIROSIS

Leptospirosis is a systemic disease caused by any one of a group of *Leptospira* organisms. The severity of the disease varies from case to case, and the organ principally affected may be the liver, the kidneys, the heart, the meninges, or the lungs. The disease exists and is perpetuated in animals such as cattle, pigs, sheep, and dogs. The animals may or may not have symptoms. The disease is usually transmitted to humans by contact with the urine of an infected animal, the organisms entering through a break in the human's skin or through the membranes of his eyes or mouth. The organisms may survive in the soil for several weeks when deposited there by contaminated urine. They may enter the human body by contaminated drinking water.

The number of cases of leptospirosis in the United States average about 100 per year. The incubation period varies from seven to twenty-one days. The average fatality rate is 3 to 6 percent, but is much higher (15 to 40 percent) in elderly patients and in those with involvement of the liver (Weil's disease). Those who survive usually recover completely. The initial symptoms of the illness may consist of fever only in the less severe cases, or may involve chills and high fever, headache, muscle pain, vomiting, abdominal pain, chest pain, diarrhea, cough, and stiff neck. In some cases, a skin rash develops. In the more serious cases where the liver is primarily affected, there will be jaundice. With kidney involvement, the possibility of renal failure exists. Depending upon which organs are involved, there may be enlargement of the spleen, the liver, or the lymph nodes.

Inasmuch as the symptoms of this disease are general in nature, the illness may be easily confused with a viral infection. The diagnosis of leptospirosis may be confirmed by laboratory methods for determining the body's antibody response to *Leptospira* or by the identification of these organisms in a sample of blood, spinal fluid, or urine.

Care and Treatment

Penicillin or tetracycline appear to be helpful when administered in large doses during the first four days of the illness. Beyond this time, the antibiotic preparations are not helpful. During the course of the illness, which may last three or four weeks, good nursing care and specific attention to and treatment of the complications that may develop are important.

RAT-BITE FEVER

Rat-bite fever, as mentioned on page

278, may be caused either by a spirochete *(Spirillum minor)* or by a bacillus *(Streptobacillus moniliformis)*. When caused by the spirochete, the incubation period is usually more than ten days, while it is less than ten days when caused by the streptobacillus.

In the infection caused by the spirochete, the wound at the site of the animal bite usually heals quickly, only to become inflamed again at the end of the incubation period. The patient then develops swelling and tenderness of the lymph nodes related to the area of the animal bite and has a come-and-go type of fever for four to eight weeks.

The kind of rat-bite fever caused by a bacillus is mentioned on page 278.

Care and Treatment

Most cases respond well to intramuscular injections of procaine penicillin G, 600,000 units given twice each day for seven to ten days.

RELAPSING FEVER

This acute infectious disease is caused by spirochetes belonging to the species *Borrelia*. The disease occurs commonly in animals, especially rodents, and is conveyed from animal to human by ticks. It may be transmitted from person to person by infected lice. The disease is characterized by recurring periods of fever, each lasting a few days. The interval of time between the attacks is usually one to two weeks. There are from two to ten attacks in the series, with the attacks becoming less severe as the patient's immunity improves. A mild skin rash, followed by rose-colored spots, commonly occurs during the attacks. Jaundice may develop late in the course of an attack.

Care and Treatment

The spirochetes which cause relapsing fever are readily killed by antibiotic medications such as tetracycline and penicillin. Such treatment, when adequate, prevents future relapses. It happens, however, that when the medication acts too rapidly, the patient's condition is made worse temporarily. To avoid this type of reaction, the physician usually uses a slow-acting type of penicillin or else administers the antibiotic during the symptom-free period between relapses.

Rest in bed and good nursing care are important. The patient should receive adequate fluids each day with an easily digested, nourishing diet.

SYPHILIS (LUES VENEREA)

Syphilis is a serious and widespread disease caused by the spirochete *Treponema pallidum*. Because it is sexually transmitted (a venereal disease) it is described in chapter 31, volume 2.

Systemic Fungal Diseases

The systemic fungal diseases are sometimes called the mycoses. The causative organisms (fungi) are a little more complex than bacteria. There are many species of fungi. They lack chlorophyl but are able to synthesize proteins. They are largely parasitic or saprophytic, meaning that they derive most of their sustenance from plant or animal tissues or from decaying matter.

The systemic fungal diseases are not transmitted from person to person. Many of them are acquired by inhaling spores (the dormant phase) of the fungus.

The fungal diseases tend to run a chronic course. The typical symptoms include chills, fever, loss of appetite, weight loss, night sweats, indisposition, and mental depression. Most of these diseases do not respond to the commonly used antibiotic medications such as penicillin. Fortunately, however, most do respond to the antibiotic amphotericin B. Good nursing care and, in selected cases, specialized surgical procedures are important adjuncts.

Notice that this chapter deals with the systemic fungal diseases. The fungal infections of the skin are considered in chapter 25, volume 2.

BLASTOMYCOSIS

Blastomycosis is a systemic fungal disease which occurs primarily in the central and southeastern areas of the United States. There have been occasional scattered cases in various parts of Africa. A slightly different form of the disease occurs among coffee growers in Brazil. The disease is not contagious from person to person and is usually acquired by inhaling spores. The lungs are therefore primarily affected. In the more serious cases, the organism is spread by way of the blood to other parts of the body, including the skin.

In untreated cases, the disease progresses slowly toward a fatal outcome.

Care and Treatment

A carefully supervised course of treatment with amphotericin B is effective in controlling this infection. The results of treatment are best, of course, when treatment is begun early in the course of the illness.

COCCIDIOIDOMYCOSIS (VALLEY FEVER)

The natural habitat of the fungus that causes this disease is the desert soil of certain parts of California, Arizona, Utah, New Mexico, Nevada, southwestern Texas, adjacent areas of Mexico, and several sites in Central and South America. The disease enters the human body by inhalation of spores along with dust. The disease is most frequent between the ages of 25 and 55 and occurs more commonly in men than in women.

In the usual pulmonary type of the disease, influenzalike symptoms develop one to four weeks after the spores are carried into the lungs. This form of the disease ends spontaneously and requires no particular treatment.

In a small percentage of cases the organisms are carried by the blood from the lungs to various parts of the body. This is the so-called disseminated form of the disease. There often develop burrowing abscesses and draining cavities in the skin and even in the bones. Sometimes the meninges which cover the brain are involved. In this form of the disease, the mortality runs as high as 60 percent.

Care and Treatment

The usual case of the pulmonary form of the disease requires no particular treatment. But because of the seriousness of the disseminated form of coccidioidomycosis, intensive treatment with amphotericin B is recommended for the following situations: (1) a case of prolonged pulmonary coccidioidomycosis; (2) a case of the pulmonary infection occurring during pregnancy; (3) a case of pulmonary infection in which the patient is in a state of low resistance to infection; or (4) a case in which a surgical procedure is undertaken during an illness with coccidioidomycosis. The administration of the amphotericin B should be under the direct supervision of a physician.

CRYPTOCOCCOSIS (TORULOSIS)

This fungal disease is present in various parts of the world, including the southeastern part of the United States. It usually occurs in adults between 40 and 60 years of age, with males having the disease twice as frequently as fe-males. The most serious cases are those in which the central nervous system and its coverings are affected. The disease may also involve the lungs, skin, bones, and other organs. Evidence exists that the lungs are involved first, even in those cases in which the nervous system is affected. This type of fungus has been found in the excreta of pigeons. It is dust from such material

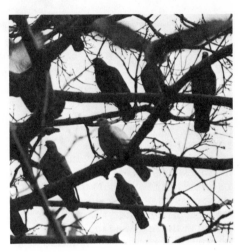

Dust from the excreta of pigeons may cause cryptococcosis.

that carries the organism into the delicate tissues of the lungs.

In untreated cases the disease makes slow progress and may continue with remissions and relapses for a matter of several years. Untreated cases in which the nervous system is affected usually end fatally within a few months.

Care and Treatment

Amphotericin B is the drug of choice in treating cryptococcosis. Infusions of this drug are given daily or on alternate days by injection into a vein, or into the cerebrospinal fluid channels in cases where the nervous system is involved.

HISTOPLASMOSIS

This disease is caused by a specific fungus, the ordinary habitat of which is

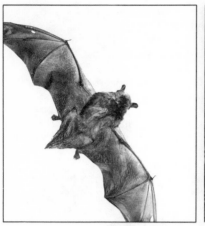 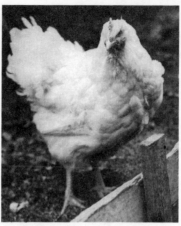 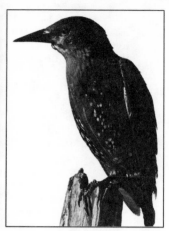

Soil contaminated by fecal droppings of bats, chickens, or starlings may harbor spores of histoplasmosis.

the soil, particularly soil which has contained fecal droppings of chickens, starlings, or bats. In the United States, histoplasmosis is prevalent in the Mississippi River valley and its tributaries. It occurs in river valleys of South America, Africa, and the Far East, but is rare in Europe. The infection is introduced into the body by inhalation of the spores of this fungus. Epidemics of the disease usually occur when the soil in contaminated areas is disturbed during such activities as construction, urban renewal, or cleanup campaigns involving parks or empty lots. The disease, therefore, is commonly observed in farmers, construction workers, and children. A striking feature is that the disease may be so mild as to pass unnoticed, or it may be so severe as to prove fatal.

The majority of persons who inhale the spores of this disease will not develop symptoms. When symptoms develop, they resemble those of the common cold or influenza. The relatively mild cases in which the infection is limited to the lungs are classed as primary histoplasmosis. In these recovery is spontaneous even without treatment.

In a small minority of cases the infection spreads to other parts of the body and is then described as disseminated histoplasmosis. This form of the disease occurs in those whose resistance

to infection is at low ebb. The liver is often affected in such cases, but other organs, such as the adrenal glands, may be involved. Several organs may be involved in the same case. These are the cases that urgently require intensive treatment, for the mortality rate in such untreated cases exceeds 90 percent. With adequate, intensive treatment, the mortality rate is less than 10 percent.

Care and Treatment

As with most other fungal infections, the drug of choice is amphotericin B adminstered daily by intravenous injection over a period of several weeks.

MADUROMYCOSIS (MADURA FOOT; MYCETOMA)

Maduromycosis is a chronic infection which affects the skin, underlying tissues, and even bone. It may be caused by any one or more of about twenty different types of fungi or by the *Nordcardia* bacteria. It is most common in tropical areas and does occur in southern United States.

The fungi which cause this disease live in the soil and enter the human tissues of the bare foot or leg after the skin has been broken by some injury. It may occur in other parts of the body when an area of broken skin comes into contact with contaminated objects, such as by carrying a dirty sack over the shoulder. At the site of the injury there occurs a firm, rounded, somewhat discolored, painless swelling. After a few weeks the swelling softens and ruptures, persistently discharging blood-streaked pus. As time goes on, more and more swellings form and break down, the entire foot enlarges to two to four times its normal size, the discharging openings persist, and the leg muscles shrink from disuse. All the tissues of the foot, including the bones, become involved; and bits of diseased bone are discharged in the pus at times. The affected area is usually not painful.

If the disease is not checked in its early stages, the crippled victim may suffer from it for ten to twenty years, finally dying from general debility or from some other infection that attacks him in his weakened condition.

Care and Treatment

The choice of treatment of maduromycosis becomes complicated by the fact that this illness may be caused by any one or more of several fungi or by a bacterium. The cases occurring in the United States are usually caused by a fungus which responds favorably to treatment by amphoteracin B. About half the cases, worldwide, are caused by the *Norcardia* bacteria, which respond to treatment by the sulfonamides. Other cases are caused by bacteria that cause actinomycosis and therefore are best treated by the use of penicillin or the tetracycline antibiotics. (For details see chapter 18, volume 3.) In cases in which the disease has persisted for many months, amputation of the affected foot or leg may become necessary.

SPOROTRICHOSIS

Sporotrichosis is a chronic fungal infection which occurs worldwide and is caused by a fungus which lives in decaying vegetation. The illness is common among those who work with plants. The organisms may gain entrance through a scratch in the skin or the penetration of a thorn. The organism thrives in such materials as sphagnum moss, often used as a mulch for plants.

The usual incubation period for the infection which gains entrance through the skin is a few days to two weeks. The skin lesion begins as a firm, elastic, movable nodule underneath the skin. As the nodule enlarges, it becomes inflamed and then breaks through the skin, forming an ulcer. Other nodules form along the lymph vessels related to the original infected area. The lymph vessels may become inflamed and thickened, feeling like cords beneath the skin. Nodules may form in scattered locations almost anywhere in the body, including bones, joint muscles, and various organs. The lungs may become involved as a result of inhaling the causative fungus.

In untreated cases in which the skin is primarily involved, the infection may persist several years without seriously affecting the individual's general health.

Care and Treatment

The use of the skin remedies is not effective in the treatment of sporotrichosis. The usual form of the illness responds well to the administration of potassium iodide taken by mouth. The treatment is started by the taking of ten drops of a saturated solution of potassium iodide three times a day after meals. The dosage is gradually increased to the point of the patient's tolerance. This should be continued for at least one month after the skin lesions disappear. Ulcers of the skin may require additional types of treatment.

When sporotrichosis affects the internal organs, the accepted treatment is the intravenous administration of amphotericin B given daily over a period of six to eight weeks.

Parasitic Infections

This chapter deals with diseases caused by the invasion into the human body of animal organisms of simple structure. They are larger than ordinary germs and obtain their nourishment from the human tissues.

The first division of the chapter considers the common diseases caused by protozoa. Protozoa constitute the lowest division of the animal kingdom. A protozoan consists of one cell or of a small group of undifferentiated cells held together loosely.

Malaria is the most important disease caused by the protozoa, but there are others. It is estimated that 500 million people live in parts of the world where malaria is common. Because of an upsurge of malaria prevalance in recent years on a worldwide basis, a reported 200 million are sick with the disease at any one time, and about one and one-half million die each year.

The chapter's second division deals with the diseases caused by multicelled worms. These disease-causing worms are not common in the United States, but are a great menace in certain other parts of the world. International travel and the importation of food make it important that these diseases be recognized and treated when they do occur.

A. Diseases Caused by Protozoa

AFRICAN TRYPANOSOMIASIS (AFRICAN SLEEPING SICKNESS)

Trypanosomiasis is a disease in which protozoa of the genus *Trypanosoma* have invaded the blood of the victim. Either one of two trypanosomes *(Trypanosoma gambiense* or *Trypanosoma rhodesiense)* are involved as causes of African trypanosomiasis. These protozoa are spindle-shaped, actively moving organisms of microscopic size, but larger than a red blood cell. In a case of trypanosomiasis, the protozoa may be found in the blood, the cerebrospinal fluid, and in certain tissues of the body, especially in lymph nodes. The trypanosomes are transmitted by the bites of tsetse flies *(Glossina),* which become infective within from eighteen to thirty-four days after biting a person or an animal who is sick with trypanosomiasis. Many species of wild or domestic animals can harbor the trypanosomes, some being made ill by them and some not. Animals form the usual reservoirs from which the organisms are transmitted to and by the tsetse fly.

The bite of the tsetse fly produces some irritation, and within two days the site is marked by a red nodule surrounded by a white zone. In a typical case, fever develops within two or three weeks; but its onset may be longer delayed. Fever may continue in an irregular way for months or years, or it may be relapsing in character with considerable periods of quiescence. Headache, neuralgic pains, sleeplessness, and loss of the ability to concentrate are common symptoms. Pink or reddish patches may appear from time to time on the trunk and thighs and persist for a few days. The lymph nodes in any or all parts of the body may become enlarged, but those most commonly and noticeably so are in the sides of the neck below and behind the ears. This last symptom is an important diagnostic sign.

In some cases the disease runs an acute course, with involvement of the brain and the development of convulsions, seizures, and coma. In other cases, the disease progresses slowly, with the patient becoming mentally and physically feeble. The peculiar lethargy that gives rise to the common name sleeping sickness occurs when the trypanosomes invade the central nervous system. When untreated, African trypanosomiasis ends fatally.

Prevention. The best methods of prevention consist of avoiding the possibility of being bitten by the tsetse fly. This precaution requires the use of insect repellents, the wearing of protective clothing which covers the wrists and ankles, careful screening of living quarters, and the use of mosquito netting while sleeping. A single intramuscular injection of the drug pentamidine is said to protect a person for a period of from two to six months from the Gambian form of the disease. It probably is not effective in protecting from the Rhodesian form. Some persons react unfavorably to this drug.

Care and Treatment

Trypanosomiasis is a life-threatening disease. Once the trypanosomes have entered the body, they are not readily eradicated. The effective medications are powerful drugs and carry considerable hazard of serious side effects.

The least hazardous of the several drugs that may be used for treatment is pentamidine. When used early, before the trypanosomes have invaded the central nervous system, a daily intramuscular injection of pentamidine continued for ten days will usually serve to eradicate the protozoa of the Gambian type of the illness.

For the Rhodesian type of trypanosomiasis, suramin (Antrypol) is the drug of choice, if treatment is begun before the nervous system is involved. Suramin is administered intravenously in a series of about five injections given on days 1, 3, 7, 14, and 21.

When the disease has already progressed to involve the brain, a more potent drug than the ones mentioned above is indicated. The drug of choice for both the Gambian and the Rhodesian types is then melarsoprol. This drug contains arsenic, and the schedule for its use provides sufficient drug to kill the trypanosomes in the various tissues of the body. The usual pattern of administration requires a daily intravenous injection for three days, same to be repeated after two weeks.

Relapses of the illness may occur even after treatment, and when these occur another course of treatment should be arranged. Even in the cases which seem to respond favorably, repeat tests of the blood and cerebrospinal fluid should be made at six months and at twelve months as a means of determining whether or not the trypanosomes have been eradicated.

AMEBIASIS (AMEBIC COLITIS; AMEBIC DYSENTERY)

Amebiasis is an infection of the large intestine caused by the one-celled parasite, *Entamoeba histolytica*. This parasite occurs in many parts of the world, and it is estimated that about 10 percent of the world's population are infected by it. The majority of persons who harbor this parasite do not have symp-

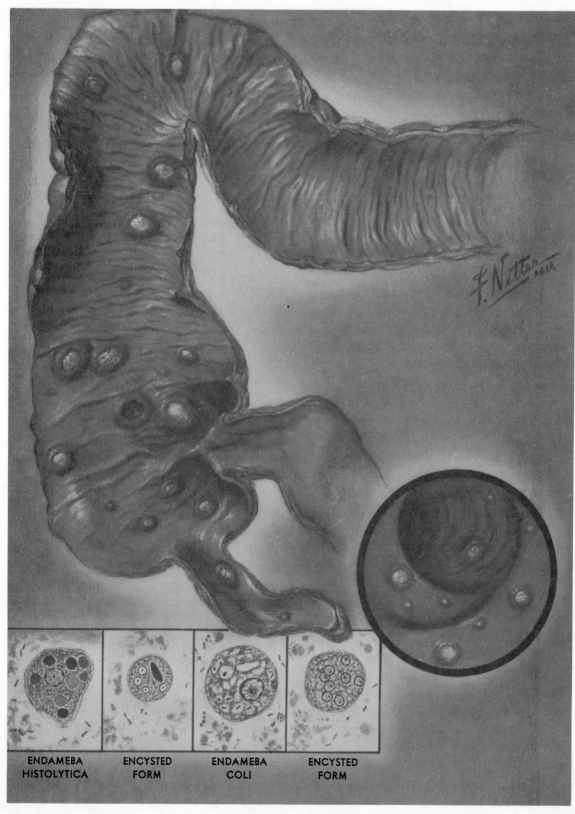

ENDAMEBA HISTOLYTICA   ENCYSTED FORM   ENDAMEBA COLI   ENCYSTED FORM

Amebic colitis (amebiasis).

toms, but they may excrete the cysts of this parasite by way of the feces and may therefore serve as carriers of the disease. The parasite gains entrance into the body through the mouth, being carried by contaminated foods or beverages.

In cases in which symptoms develop, the patient has cramping abdominal pain with intermittent diarrhea or constipation. The stools contain pus, mucus, and blood. The symptoms typically come on gradually.

Abscess of the liver is an occasional complication of amebiasis. An amebic liver abscess may develop without there having been any previous detectable intestinal symptoms. The parasites are carried from the intestine to the liver by blood flowing through the portal vein.

It is important, before beginning treatment for this condition, to make certain of the diagnosis, for the symptoms are very similar to those occurring in other infections of the large intestine which require a different form of treatment. The positive diagnosis for amebiasis depends on identifying the *Entamoeba histolytica* by microscopic examination of the stool. In making this examination, *Entamoeba histolytica* must be differentiated from the relatively harmless *Entamoeba coli,* which is similar in appearance.

Prevention. Prevention of amebiasis requires the protection of all food, water, and other beverages from contact with fecal or sewage materials. In areas in which sewage disposal and water supply are not handled according to modern sanitary standards, boiled water should be used for drinking. Vegetables and fruits should not be eaten raw unless they are the type that can be peeled.

Care and Treatment

Drugs effective in ridding the *Entamoeba histolytica* from a person's body are powerful and should be used only under the supervision of a physician. The drug presently most effective is metronidazole (Flagyl). The course of treatment requires taking the appropriate doses of the medication three times a day by mouth for a period of ten days. Following the completion of such a course of treatment, stool specimens should be examined to determine whether or not the parasite has been eradicated.

AMERICAN TRYPANOSOMIASIS (CHAGAS' DISEASE)

Chagas' disease is caused by the *Trypanosoma cruzi,* a protozoan which occurs chiefly in South America, Central America, Mexico and, occasionally, in the southern portions of the United States. The protozoa are transmitted by reduviid bugs (assassin bugs or kissing bugs), which usually attack the face at night. The protozoa are not directly transmitted by the bites, however, but are excreted in the bug's feces which are passed at the time of the bite, and then rubbed or scratched into the itching bite wound. Human beings, cats and dogs, and wild animals such as the opossum and armadillo are the usual reservoirs of the infection.

The disease is more severe in children than in adults. A continuously high fever is a common feature. Swelling of one side of the face and inflammation of the corresponding eye is a characteristic sign. Additional symptoms include swelling of the local lymph nodes, enlarged liver and spleen, nervous and mental disturbances, rapid pulse, and irregular heartbeat.

The acute phase of the disease is relatively brief, and in the majority of cases the patient appears to recover completely.

The chronic phase of the disease appears somewhat without warning one or more years after the acute phase of the disease. In this chronic phase there develops serious damage to the heart and, often, to the digestive organs. The complications affecting the heart and other organs become progressively worse and may lead to a fatal outcome.

Prevention. Prevention consists essentially of avoiding the bites of the

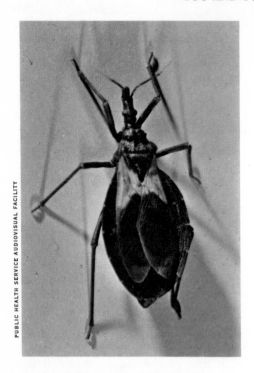

PUBLIC HEALTH SERVICE AUDIOVISUAL FACILITY

Kissing bug, vector of the parasite involved in Chagas' disease.

reduviid bugs by sleeping under a bed net, and by treating the walls of one's dwelling with residual insecticide sprays such as benzene hexachloride. The bugs often reside in cracks in plaster walls and in the thatched roofs of tropical dwellings.

Care and Treatment

No completely satisfactory treatment exists for American trypanosomiasis. Once damage to the body's organs has occurred, the changes are irreversible. The accompanying ailments of the heart and the digestive organs should be treated the same as such ailments caused by other diseases. The patient's general vitality should be preserved by his following a conservative way of life. The drug Lampit (Bayer 2502) has been used somewhat effectively in the acute phase of the disease. It is given in daily doses for a period of three or four months.

BALANTIDIASIS (BALANTIDIAL DYSENTERY)

Balantidiasis is similar in many respects to amebiasis but is less common and less severe, though more widespread geographically. The causative protozoan is *Balantidium coli,* the largest of the protozoa that cause human disease, it being about twelve times as long as the diameter of a red blood cell. A large proportion of infected individuals are healthy carriers of this parasite and suffer no symptoms. This is a common parasite of swine, and the infection is most common among people who have contact with these animals. Liver abscesses are not produced as a complication of this infection, as they are in amebiasis.

The symptoms consist essentially of abdominal pain and diarrhea. There may be a period of freedom from symptoms, followed by recurrence of the diarrhea after weeks or months. The diagnosis is confirmed by the microscopic identification of this protozoan in the stool specimens.

Care and Treatment

Balantidiasis is quite responsive to tetracycline taken as a medication four times a day for ten days.

GIARDIASIS

Giardiasis is an infection caused by the protozoan *Giardia lamblia,* which has been recognized in approximately 100 countries in various parts of the world. Giardiasis is one of the important causes of "traveler's diarrhea." Isolated cases and even epidemics of this illness occur also in the United States.

The principal source of infection by the *Giardia lamblia* is drinking water contaminated by fecal material that contains this protozoan. The cysts of the *Giardia lamblia* are not killed by the usual concentrations of chlorine used to purify domestic water. These cysts can be destroyed, however, by a temperature of 122° F. (50° C.) or by certain chemicals containing iodine.

A small percentage of people infected with *Giardia lamblia* have no symptoms. For others, the symptoms may be mild or severe, may last for a few days or may continue in chronic form for years. In many cases, the parasites and the symptoms disappear eventually, even without treatment. The usual symptoms consist of diarrhea with watery, foul-smelling stools, abdominal distension, and loss of weight.

The diagnosis is made by the microscopic identification of the *Giardia lamblia* in stool specimens.

Care and Treatment

The preferred medication is quinacrine hydrochloride (Atabrine), taken by mouth three times a day for a period of seven days in doses determined by the individual's size and age. Metronidazole and furazolidone are alternate drugs which may be used in cases in which quinacrine hydrochloride is not well tolerated.

LEISHMANIASIS

A group of diseases under the general heading of leishmaniasis are caused by various representatives of the genus of protozoa called *Leishmania*. These diseases are transmitted from animal to humans by the bites of various species of sandflies (*Phlebotomus*).

Espundia is the name given to one form of leishmaniasis (American Leishmaniasis) in which both the skin and the mucous membranes are attacked. In another form of the disease, the spleen and liver are chiefly involved, causing a disease called kala-azar. In still a third form, the parasites abound in and beneath the skin in one or more circumscribed areas, giving rise to slowly developing ulcers (oriental sores).

1. *Espundia (American Leishmaniasis)*. Espundia occurs chiefly in forest workers in various parts of Central and South America. Forest rodents harbor this disease, and the tiny parasites are transmitted to human beings by sand-

flies. Ten or more days after the bite of the sandfly a skin lesion develops at the site of the sandfly bite. This enlarges and permits the development of a secondary bacterial infection. The disease then spreads to cause ulcerative lesions of the nose, mouth, and throat. Often a destruction of tissue of these parts occurs, which brings about a disfigurement and impairment of normal function. Neglected cases progress slowly toward a fatal outcome.

Care and Treatment

For early cases of espundia, the injection of antimony sodium gluconate (stibogluconate sodium) into the margins of the lesions may bring about their gradual regression. In more advanced cases, intramuscular injections of antimony sodium gluconate may be beneficial. Antibiotic medications should be administered for the control of the secondary bacterial infections.

2. *Kala-azar (Visceral Leishmaniasis); Dumdum Fever*. In this form of leishmaniasis, the parasites occur in the blood and multiply extensively in the tissues of the spleen, liver, bone marrow, lymph nodes, skin, and small intestine. The symptoms include chronic irregular fever, emaciation, anemia, and enlargement of the liver and spleen. In women, a cessation of menstruation usually develops early in the course of the disease.

Peculiarly, the kala-azar victim, in spite of being feverish, weak, and emaciated, does not feel seriously ill. Probably not more than 5 percent of untreated kala-azar victims recover, but death is usually from some other infection rather than from the kala-azar itself. With suitable treatment, especialy if begun early, 95 or more percent of kala-azar victims can be saved.

Care and Treatment

Bed rest and nourishing food are important for preserving the patient's general vitality. Blood transfusions may be advisable in cases of severe

anemia. Secondary bacterial infections should be treated with the usual antibiotic medications. The preferred medication for the treatment of kala-azar is sodium stibogluconate adminstered daily by intravenous or intramuscular injection.

3. *Oriental Sore (Cutaneous Leishmaniasis); Tropical Sore; Delhi Sore.* A typical oriental sore begins

In one form of leishmaniasis the parasites causing it abound beneath the skin and give rise to sores.

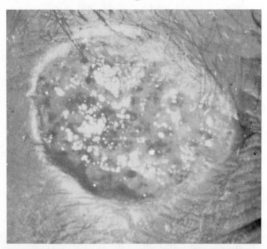

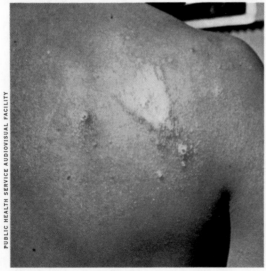

PUBLIC HEALTH SERVICE AUDIOVISUAL FACILITY

after a long incubation period as a small, itchy, slightly raised spot on the skin. It enlarges slowly and becomes scaly. When the scaly crust is removed, a moist, bleeding ulcer is revealed. The ulcer, having a scanty discharge, becomes crusted again from time to time and slowly increases in size, often reaching a diameter of more than 1 inch (2.5 cm.).

Within two months to a year or more, slow healing begins, usually in the center. When healing is complete, a somewhat depressed and contracted scar is left. When scarring is extensive, it may cause disfigurement or deformity. Oriental sores, however, are not fatal; and one attack usually protects the victim against future infection of the same sort.

As a rule the sores are neither painful nor dangerous, but secondary infection may make them so. Treatment is aimed as much toward prevention or control of the secondary infection as it is toward influencing the parasitic infection. While the description of the sore here speaks of it in the singular, a person may have several or many of them at the same time.

Care and Treatment

Injections of sodium stiboguconate into the margins of the sores performed three or four times on alternate days is usually helpful. Where numerous lesions are involved, it may be advisable to administer medication by intravenous or intramuscular injection. Secondary infections should be treated with appropriate antibiotic medications.

MALARIA (AGUE)

Malaria is an ever-present, tantalizing menace to those who live in the parts of the world where malaria-carrying mosquitoes (*Anopheles* mosquitoes) wait for their chance to pierce one's skin. Those who travel into such areas face even greater danger than longtime residents, for the residents have usually developed a certain degree of immunity.

The disease is actually caused by one or the other of four species of parasites of the genus *Plasmodium*. The *Anopheles* mosquito carries the parasite within its body and injects it in its sporozoite phase into the tissues of a human victim at the time of a mosquito bite. The sporozoites then migrate to the victim's liver, where they multiply and develop into the merozoite phase and from where they are released into the bloodstream. Within the red blood cells further development and multiplication occur, with the ultimate bursting of the red blood cells. This releases a new generation of the parasites, then free to enter other red blood cells or to be carried away by mosquitoes that now penetrate the skin's surface. The developmental cycle continues within the mosquito's body until it reaches the sporozoite phase and the parasite becomes available for injection into some other victim.

The various phases of the parasite's development within the red blood cells of a person's body proceed in precisely timed unison so that all the affected red blood cells release their cargoes of parasites at the same time. It is at this time of release that the patient experiences the typical symptoms of chills and high fever. The paroxysms of chills and fever recur in two- or three-day cycles, depending on which species of the parasite is involved in the particular case. The incubation period between the time of the mosquito bite and the first appearance of symptoms is ten days or longer. In occasional cases there may be a lapse of months before symptoms appear. If such a person has returned in the meantime to an area where malaria does not ordinarily occur, the possibility of malaria, when the symptoms first appear, may not enter the minds of the patient or his doctor.

Although the recurring paroxysms of chills and fever are the hallmark of vivax malaria, relapses also occur in ovale malaria, a rather rare infection. Falciparum malaria is the most serious form of malaria and is caused by the *falciparum* species of the *Plasmodium*.

The other usual symptoms of malaria include headache, muscle pains, enlargement of the spleen and of the liver, anemia, and increasing weakness. In untreated cases, the paroxysms of chills and fever tend to become less severe and less regular. But even after a person appears to have recovered from the disease, persisting parasites harbored in the liver (*P. vivax*) may cause a recurrent attack, months, or years later.

Blackwater fever is a serious complication of malaria, occurring usually in association with the falciparum form of the disease. It is characterized by the sudden development of high fever, jaundice, dark-colored urine (on account of a large content of decomposed hemoglobin), collapse, and the possibility of acute kidney failure. The fundamental problem is an extensive destruction of red blood cells, with the consequent liberation of hemoglobin into the blood plasma.

Prevention of Malaria. Persons living in a malarial zone or those visiting such areas should take the following precautions: (1) Cover all skin areas as far as possible with light-weight, loose-fitting clothing. (2) Live in a well-screened house. (3) Sleep under mosquito netting. (4) Apply mosquito repellents to exposed skin areas. (5) Take malaria-preventive medication by mouth.

The effectiveness of preventive medication has now become complicated by the development in some geographic areas of resistant strains of falciparum malarial parasites. Chloroquine is currently the drug of choice for preventing malaria in areas where the parasites have not developed resistance to this drug. Fansidar (a combination of sulfadoxine and pyrimethamine) is used successfully in areas where the parasites are resistant to chloroquine, but it is not yet available in the United States. For those planning to travel in a malarial area, the preventive medication should begin two weeks before entering the area and

305

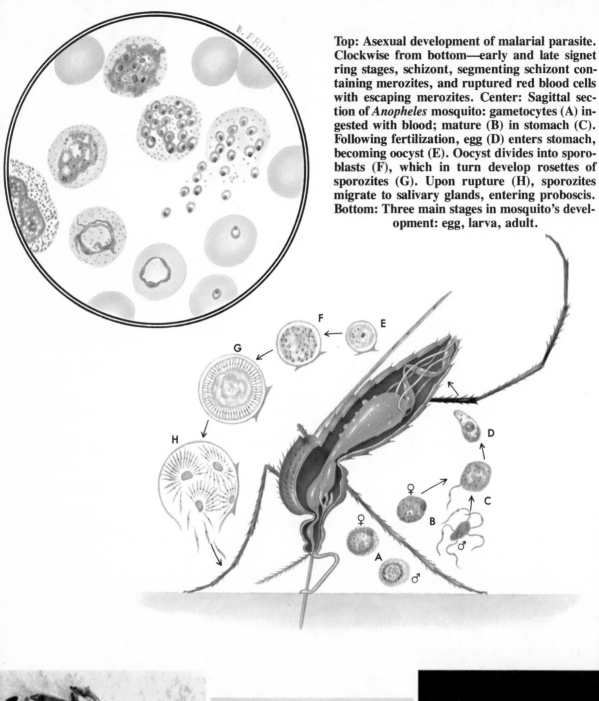

Top: Asexual development of malarial parasite. Clockwise from bottom—early and late signet ring stages, schizont, segmenting schizont containing merozites, and ruptured red blood cells with escaping merozites. Center: Sagittal section of *Anopheles* mosquito: gametocytes (A) ingested with blood; mature (B) in stomach (C). Following fertilization, egg (D) enters stomach, becoming oocyst (E). Oocyst divides into sporoblasts (F), which in turn develop rosettes of sporozites (G). Upon rupture (H), sporozites migrate to salivary glands, entering proboscis. Bottom: Three main stages in mosquito's development: egg, larva, adult.

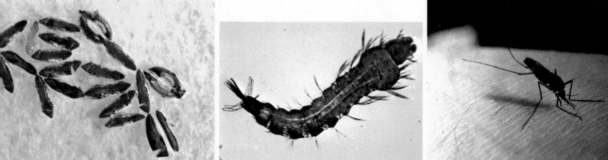

CHAS. PFIZER & CO., INC., PUBLIC HEALTH SERVICE AUDIOVISUAL FACILITY

should be continued for four weeks after leaving. Pregnant women should avoid traveling in malaria-infested areas if at all possible.

Care and Treatment

For the treatment of an acute attack of malaria, the same drugs, in heavier doses, are effective as are used for prevention (see above). For a patient suffering severe vomiting, the chloroquine may have to be given, temporarily, by intramuscular injection. The dosage and schedule of administration should be under a physician's supervision. Primaquine phosphate is used for prevention of relapses of *P. vivax* and *P. ovale* only.

Nursing care during the period of illness is important. The patient should be kept in bed. When the patient's temperature reaches or exceeds 104° F. (40. C.), cool sponges, alcohol rubs, or cool enemas will help to reduce it. The patient should avoid overexertion, even on the days when he has no chills and fever.

TOXOPLASMOSIS

Toxoplasmosis is a disease which occurs in a minority of the large number of people whose bodies harbor the protozoan *Toxoplasma gondii*. Its distribution is worldwide. The organism is also present, significantly, in cats and in many other forms of animal life, domestic and wild.

The *Toxoplasma gondii* enters the human body by either of two routes: (1) by the swallowing of undercooked pork, mutton, or beef containing the cysts of this protozoan, or the swallowing of contaminated material containing oocysts derived from cat feces, and (2) by the transmission from mother to unborn child of the protozoan in its trophozoite phase.

When cysts or oocysts of the *Toxoplasma gondii* are swallowed, they are soon transformed to the trophozoite phase and then circulated briefly in the blood, soon reaching the body's organs where they become encysted and remain viable but latent within the cells of the organ in which they reside.

Most people whose bodies harbor the *Toxoplasma gondii* can expect to live out their life-span without suffering any illness on this account. But there are four clinical manifestations of toxoplasmosis which can be caused by the trophozoite phase of this protozoan.

1. *Congenital Toxoplasmosis.* A mother can transmit the *Toxoplasma gondii* to her unborn child only when she has recently acquired this infection. It is only when the organisms are in their trophozoite phase and are circulating in the blood that they can pass through the placenta to infect the unborn child. When a woman has acquired this infection prior to her pregnancy, and there has been time for the organisms to become encysted in her body, she cannot transfer the parasite to the unborn child.

Fortunately, only a small percentage of unborn children thus infected will develop serious symptoms. But when the disease develops in this small percentage of infants it causes serious damage to the brain and threatens the life of the child. As a precaution, pregnant women should not eat undercooked meat and should avoid contacts, as far as possible, with domestic cats.

There is no effective treatment for congenital toxoplasmosis.

2. *Lymphadenopathic Toxoplasmosis.* This is the most frequent of the clinical manifestations of toxoplasmosis. It consists of an enlargement of the lymph nodes caused by the invasion of the *Toxoplasma gondii*. Lymph nodes in any part of the body may be involved, but the ones most commonly affected are those in the sides and back of the neck. Although the involvement of lymph nodes may be the only manifestation of the disease in many cases, there may be such associated symptoms as fever, pain in the muscles, sore throat, fatigue, and weakness. The en-

largement of lymph nodes may persist for many months, but usually it does not require specific treatment.

Care and Treatment

In severe cases, the use of such medications as pyrimethamine and one of the sulfonamides may be helpful. These drugs are usually most effective when used in combination.

3. *Ocular Toxoplasmosis.* Toxoplasmosis is probably the most common cause of the sight-threatening condition of chorioretinitis (posterior uveitis). This condition occurs typically in older children and young adults. It is believed that it usually occurs as a reactivation of congenital toxoplasmosis. The characteristics and symptoms of chorioretinitis are described in chapter 8, in this volume. Fortunately, ocular toxoplasmosis usually affects only one eye. In most cases the patient suffers loss of central vision in the affected eye.

4. *Toxoplasmosis in Immunosuppressed Patients.* In patients who have received a transplant of a tissue or or-

gan from some other individual, it is necessary to use medications to suppress the patient's immunity mechanisms so as to avoid the rejection of the transplanted tissue or organ. This leaves the patient, for the time being, without his usual defense against infectious diseases. If the patient under such circumstances is one who has previously acquired an infection with the *Toxoplasma gondii,* the latent organisms may now become activated, producing symptoms of toxoplasmosis. The manifestations in such a case are usually such serious conditions as encephalitis or other involvements of the brain and nervous system. This is a serious development and usually ends fatally if not treated aggressively. The parasite may be transmitted to the recipient of an organ transplant via an infected organ, such as a kidney.

Care and Treatment

The preferred medication is pyrimethamine used in combination with one of the sulfonamides.

TRICHOMONIASIS

The usual manifestation of trichomoniasis is an infection caused by the protozoan *Trichomonas vaginalis,* which affects the female sex organs and is therefore considered in chapter 30, volume 2.

B. Diseases Caused by Parasitic Worms (Helminthic Infections)

There are certain actual worms that can take up residence in the human body and cause various illnesses, some of which are life threatening.

Diseases Caused by Common Intestinal Worms (Nematodes)

HOOKWORM INFECTION (GROUND ITCH; ANCYLOSTOMIASIS)

Hookworms cause more cases of serious illness than do any other of the intestinal parasites. Hookworm disease is prevalent in many parts of the world

Hookworm (10 times actual size; ovum, 350 times).

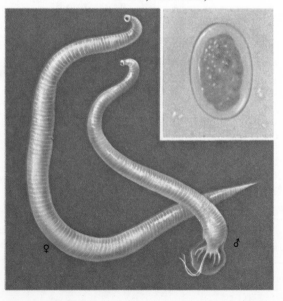

and is present in some sections of the United States.

Hookworms are small and slender, about half an inch (13 mm.) in length, the female being somewhat longer than the male. They live in the small intestine, where they attach to the intestinal lining and are nourished by drawing blood from the capillaries in the intestinal wall.

The female worms produce great numbers of eggs, which are expelled with the stools. Contact with warm, moist soil favors the hatching of the eggs and the rapid development of the young embryos. When a human's skin surface, such as bare feet or hands, comes in contact with the moist earth containing these almost microscopic young worms, they rapidly penetrate the skin and enter the blood vessels. They are then carried by the blood to the lungs. Here the young hookworms enter the air passages, make their way to the throat, are swallowed, and arrive in the intestine, where they develop into full-grown worms and attach themselves to the lining membranes. When fewer than a hundred worms are present in the intestine, there may be no symptoms. On occasion, more than 4000 worms have been found in the intestine of a single individual.

When the young worms first penetrate the skin of an individual, itching and burning develop, with the formation of small papules and blisters at the site of penetration. This symptom accounts for the common name of ground itch. During the time the immature parasites are passing through the lungs, there may be spells of coughing, with sore throat and bloody sputum.

While the parasites are attaching themselves to the intestinal wall and growing to maturity the characteristic symptoms are diarrhea, bloating, and abdominal discomfort. Later, as large numbers of hookworms begin to draw their sustenance from their human host's blood, the patient develops weakness, pallor, fatigue, weight loss, and anemia. The symptoms are especially severe when children are affected. In severe, untreated cases, a child's life is even threatened.

Care and Treatment

The essence of prevention is the proper disposal of all human bowel discharges so that the ground does not become contaminated. Keeping the hands out of the soil and the wearing of shoes by persons working with the soil helps to prevent the young worms from penetrating the skin.

For treatment mebendazole (Vermox) given twice a day for three days is the drug of choice. A physician should supervise this treatment, for attention must be given also to improving the patient's nutrition and to the anemia which he has probably developed. His diet should contain adequate protein.

PINWORM INFECTION (OXYURIASIS; ENTEROBIASIS)

Pinworm infection is more common in children than in adults. Pinworms live in the large intestine, especially in the rectum. They are usually present in large numbers, and females ready to lay eggs often crawl out through the

Pinworm (10 times actual size; ovum, 350 times).

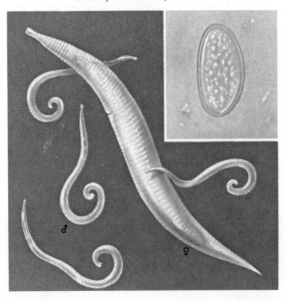

anus and lay their eggs upon the surrounding skin. This causes much itching in this region, especially at night.

These worms are small and white. The female, larger than the male, averages less than half an inch (13 mm.) long and lays large numbers of eggs. An infected child may reinfect himself by scratching the skin of the anal region and then handling food or objects that he puts into his mouth. Or he may infect other people who eat food handled by him. Underclothing and bedclothing become contaminated easily. It has proved difficult to clear up the infection in one member of a family unless the other members are treated at the same time.

If the skin around the anus is not kept clean, the eggs may hatch there and the immature worms migrate back through the anus into the rectum. Pinworm infection usually does not cause severe symptoms, aside from the itching, but there may be vague gastrointestinal discomfort, restlessness, and sleeplessness.

Care and Treatment

The drug of choice for this infection is pyrantel pamoate (Antiminth). It is administered by mouth in a single dose of 11 mg. per kg. of body weight, up to a maximum of 1 gram. An alternate single-dose drug is mebendazole (Vermox). It requires one tablet, regardless of weight, for children over two years of age and for adults.

For itching of the skin apply yellow oxide of mercury ointment or an ointment consisting of 1 percent phenol in petrolatum. The infected person should wear tight-fitting shorts day and night, or use any other effective method to prevent him from scratching the skin of the anal region. Bed linen and underclothing should be changed daily and passed through boiling water as a part of the laundering procedure. Toilet seats in the house should be scrubbed daily with soap and water.

All members of the family should cooperate by taking the regular single dose of the medication and by carefully washing their hands with soap and water after each bowel movement and before all meals. Their fingernails should be trimmed short and kept clean. All members should be warned to keep their fingers out of their mouths and advised to not scratch the skin of the anal region.

ROUNDWORM INFECTION (ASCARIASIS)

Roundworm infection is most prevalent in places with a warm, moist climate, but no part of the world is free from it. An estimated one fourth of the world's population, including one million Americans, harbor this parasite. The worm is from 6 to 14 inches (15 to 35 cm.) long, the female being larger than the male. It lives chiefly in the upper part of the small intestine, but may travel to other parts of the digestive tract. It may enter the stomach and be vomited up.

The females produce large numbers of eggs. Several weeks are required for the embryo worms to develop in the eggs. The eggs abound in places contaminated with fecal material, such as in leafy vegetables and drinking water. Children playing in contaminated dirt or handling contaminated pets may carry the eggs on their hands or under their fingernails. When they eat with unwashed hands or uncleaned finger-

Roundworm (actual size) and its ovum (enlarged 400 times).

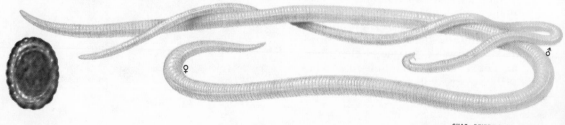

nails, or put their fingers into the mouth, the eggs are swallowed and arrive in the stomach or the intestine, where they hatch and liberate the tiny embryos. The embryos burrow into the intestinal wall and migrate to the lungs. Here they enter the air passages and make their way upward to the throat, and are then swallowed. In the intestine, the embryo worms develop into adults and reside there a long time.

During the migration of the immature worms through the lungs, symptoms of wheezing, cough, and fever may occur. Adult worms in the intestine may cause no symptoms if the worms are few in number. But large numbers of worms in the intestine may cause abdominal pain, fever, diarrhea, restlessness, and even convulsions, especially in children. The presence of worms may be discovered accidentally when an adult worm is vomited or passed in the stool. Otherwise the diagnosis is usually made by finding the eggs in the feces.

Care and Treatment

There is no effective treatment program for the phase of this infection in which the embryos are passing through the lungs. Only symptomatic treatment and good nursing care is indicated then.

For the removal of the adult worms from the intestine, the administration of the appropriate dose of mebendazole or pyrantel pamoate or piperazine citrate is effective. A single dose after breakfast on two successive days will cause the adult worms to release their attachment within the intestine so that they will be eliminated with the stool.

TAPEWORM INFECTION
See under Diseases Caused by Other Parasitic Worms, this chapter, pages 319-323.

THREADWORM INFECTION (STRONGYLOIDIASIS)
Threadworm infection is common in tropical and subtropical areas in all

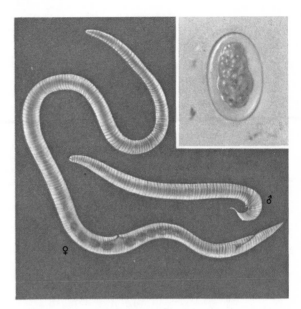

Threadworm (70 times actual size; ovum, 350 times).

parts of the world, including the southeastern United States. The larvae usually enter the body by penetrating the skin and migrate through it in much the same way as do hookworm larvae. Some of them, however, may complete much of their development in the lungs or the air passages, giving rise to symptoms resembling those of bronchitis or bronchial pneumonia. Infection of the intestines, which is the usual form, may produce no noticeable symptoms. There may be watery diarrhea. In occasional cases intestinal ulceration develops.

The adult worms resemble hookworms in general appearance, but are smaller. They are found in great numbers in the upper part of the small intestine. The anemia which they may cause is much less severe than that from hookworm infection. It is the larvae that are expelled from the intestine, and it is these that may contaminate the soil. In occasional cases, some of the larvae penetrate the walls of the intestine and cause an unusually severe illness. The diagnosis is confirmed by the finding of larvae by microscopic examination of stool specimens.

311

Care and Treatmenet

It is urgent that threadworm infection be treated promptly and adequately to avoid the danger of the potentially fatal complication occurring when the larvae penetrate the intestine. The medication of preference is thiabendazole, administered twice daily for two or three days in a dosage of 25 mg. per kg. (2.2 pounds) of body weight. It is important to continue stool examinations after the treatment has been completed to make sure that the parasites have been eliminated.

WHIPWORM INFECTION (TRICHURIASIS)

Whipworms are about one and a half to two inches (35 to 50 mm.) long. They get their common name from their shape, resembling a whip with a slender lash and a thicker handle. The small end of the lash is the head of the worm. Whipworms occur mostly in tropical areas where the level of sanitation is low. When they invade the human body, they live chiefly in the large intestine and rarely cause symptoms ex-

Whipworm (5 times actual size; ovum, 350 times).

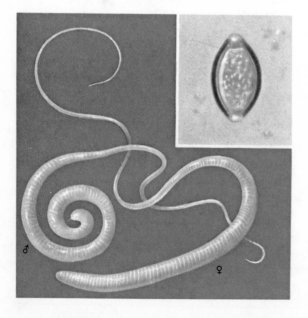

cept when present in large numbers. Then they may cause intestinal distress, diarrhea, and abdominal bloating.

Whipworm eggs pass out of the intestine and must develop over a period of several weeks as embryos within the eggs. The eggs must be swallowed in contaminated food or water, and thus enter the human body.

Care and Treatment

The treatment of whipworm infection is not as uniformly successful as with some other intestinal worms. The preferred medication is mebendazole (Vermox), which is taken by mouth in 100 mg. doses twice a day for three days. This medication is not recommended for children under the age of two or for pregnant women.

Diseases Caused by Other Parasitic Worms

DRACUNCULIASIS (GUINEA WORM INFECTION)

This parasitic infection is said to affect about 50 million people in various parts of Africa, in the Middle East, in northeastern South America, and in the Caribbean Islands. Humans acquire this parasite when they drink water contaminated by infected water fleas (copepods), which serve as the intermediate host. The embryo guinea worms occurring in contaminated water are barely large enough to be visible to the unaided eye. The water becomes contaminated when infected persons are wading or immersed in the water. An embryo must first enter the body of a copepod for a period of preliminary development. Once the embryo enters the human body by way of contaminated drinking water, it grows to a length of 1 to 2 feet (30 to 60 cm.). It is a smooth, slender, white worm and lies in an irregularly coiled position in the connective tissues beneath the skin. Its development requires several months to a year.

312

As maturity approaches, the worm migrates to those parts of the body most frequently in contact with water, usually the legs and feet. At maturity the head end of the worm approaches the skin's surface and excretes an irritating and toxic substance which causes a blister to form. When this blister ruptures, a slightly raw area with a small opening in its center becomes apparent. Whenever cool or cold water comes in contact with this area, the worm discharges a milky cloud of coiled embryos through the opening in the skin. The worm's head may protrude through this opening slightly, especially when most of the embryos have been discharged.

Prior to the time when the Guinea worm approaches the skin's surface and prepares to discharge embryos, it causes few or no symptoms in the infected person. The most marked symptoms occur at the time of the blister formation and consist of itching, vomiting, diarrhea, dizziness, and difficulty in breathing. Secondary infection of the ulcerated area is common and may even cause abscess formation.

If a worm dies within the human tissues or is broken during attempts at removing it, serious infection often occurs.

Care and Treatment

The worm may be removed by three methods: (1) It is still common practice to place a silk thread around the worm's head at the time it protrudes from the skin opening. By gently drawing on this thread, with care to avoid breaking the worm, it may be gradually withdrawn over a period of a week or two. (2) A physician may be able to enlarge the skin opening through which the worm's head protrudes and loosen the tissues enveloping the worm sufficiently to extract it. (3) Recently the drug niridazole (Ambilhar) has been used to kill the adult worm. After a course of treatment with this drug, the worm can be withdrawn quite readily. The dosage is 25 mg. per kg. of body weight each day for seven days. Preferably, the daily quota of the drug should be divided into three parts and administered at four- or five-hour intervals.

FLUKE INFECTION (TREMATODIASIS)

Several kinds of flukes (trematodes) are parasitic in man and animals. The infections result from the ingestion of uncooked or insufficiently cooked fish, crustaceans, and vegetation—the intermediate hosts of the trematodes. Four of the common health problems caused by flukes are now considered:

1. *Blood Fluke (Schistosomiasis; Bilharziasis).* Blood fluke infections occur in many tropical or subtropical regions. They may be caused by any one of four somewhat similar parasites, the adult forms of which look like small, slender worms: *Schistosoma mansoni, Schistosoma japonicum, Schistosoma haematobium,* and *Schistosoma mekongi.* Schistosomiasis is not endemic in the U.S.A.

If body discharges containing the eggs of these parasites find their way into water, the eggs hatch and the tiny young parasites swim about until they find a suitable snail to harbor them. In the snail's body they undergo further development. Once more they escape into the water, where they await an opportunity to come into contact with and penetrate the skin of some human or other warm-blooded animal. Their penetration in considerable numbers causes an irritation sometimes called swimmer's itch. They may also enter into their victim's body should he happen to drink water containing them.

Having entered the body, the parasites travel by way of the blood or lymph channels. They seem to prefer the small veins of the bladder, the liver, or the mesentery of the intestines as a place in which to congregate. Eggs are laid in these small veins. The eggs produce a lytic enzyme which enables many of them to work through the walls of the veins into the lumen of the bladder or the intestine, from which

313

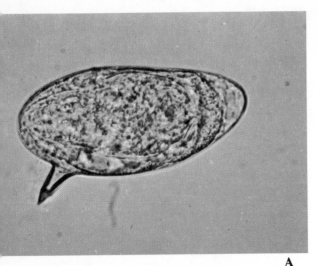

A

One of the parasites responsible for
bilharziasis: A. egg; B. young; and
C. adult form.

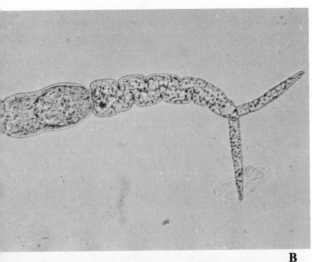

B

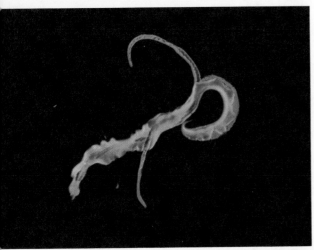

C

they are expelled in the urine or the feces.

Those cases in which the bladder is affected are characterized by blood in the urine. The illness tends to become chronic and to lead to general debility and the formation of bladder stones.

When the intestine is involved there may be diarrhea, with mucus and blood in the stools. The illness is more severe than that affecting the bladder, the symptoms in this type including spells of fever, abdominal pain, loss of appetite, chills, cough, and enlargement of the liver and spleen. Frequently the patient suffers from hemorrhoidlike growths at the anus, and these may require surgical treatment. The dysenteric stools abound with the eggs of the parasites. In the later stages of the disease the liver may become damaged with fibrosed eggs, and collections of eggs in various parts of the body may cause firm swellings or large abdominal tumors.

Prevention. Make sure of the sanitary disposal of human excreta. Boil all questionable drinking water. Avoid bathing or wading in or otherwise coming in contact with the water of rivers, canals, ponds, or rice fields in geographic areas in which blood flukes occur.

Care and Treatment

The treatment of blood fluke infection should be under the direction of a physician, for the drugs effective in eradicating these flukes are potent drugs and frequently cause toxic side effects. The drug niridazole is preferred for illnesses caused by the *Schistosoma mansoni* and the *Schistosoma japonicum;* metrifonate is the preferred drug for illnesses caused by the *Schistosoma haematobium.* These drugs are available from the government Center for Disease Control, Atlanta, Georgia 30333. Recently oxamniquine has been licensed in the United States for the treatment of *Schistosoma mansoni.* In advanced cases it is often advisable for certain of the affected tissues to be removed by surgery. Nursing care is important, and the patient's general health needs to be promoted by a well-balanced diet and by freedom from overexertion.

2. *Liver Fluke (Clonorchiasis).* In some parts of the Orient, particularly where raw fish forms a part of the diet, as many as half the population may be infected with liver flukes; but only a few of the victims may be made noticeably ill thereby. In light infections, mild indigestion may be the only symptom. In severe cases, an enlarged liver, swelling of the tissues, and recurring attacks of jaundice are typical. The discovery of the flukes' eggs by microscopic examination of the patient's stools confirms the diagnosis.

Adult liver flukes live in the small bile ducts of the liver. The eggs pass with the bile into the intestine and thence to the outside. They do not hatch unless they find their way into water, and usually not until they are swallowed by some freshwater snail, in whose body the first stage of development occurs. The next stage takes place in or on the body of some freshwater fish, in which the embryo becomes encysted. Carp seem to be especially susceptible. Humans become infected by eating raw or insufficiently cooked fish. The infection may persist for several years, even though no new parasites enter the victim's body.

Prevention of Liver Fluke Infection. Make sure of the sanitary disposal of bowel discharges. Avoid eating raw or insufficiently cooked fish.

Care and Treatment

The treatment of liver fluke infection is generally not satisfactory. Patients with symptoms may be treated with chloroquine phosphate, administered in 250 mg. doses three times a day for six weeks. This drug frequently causes side effects affecting the eyes and the intestines. Even this drug does not kill the adult worms, but it does reduce the production of

eggs. Praziquantel is the drug of choice, but is available only on an investigational basis in the United States.

3. *Fascioliasis (Liver Rot).* This is most commonly a disease of sheep and cattle, but it may also affect humans. It is caused by the *Fasciola hepatica,* a comparatively large liver fluke. The eggs pass out of the body in the feces, spend their first stage of development in the bodies of snails, and then attach themselves in the form of cysts to certain water plants, usually watercress or other green vegetation. If the cysts happen to be swallowed by sheep or by humans, they become active, penetrate the wall of the intestine, grow to maturity in the bile ducts, and produce more or less liver damage.

Fascioliasis may cause vomiting, joint pains, abdominal pain, jaundice, itching, diarrhea, and an irregular fever; but it is seldom fatal. Diagnosis is made by finding the eggs in the stools.

Care and Treatment

Praziquantel gives prospect of becoming the drug of choice for fascioliasis, but at the time of writing it is still being evaluated. At present the best available drug is bithionol, administered in doses of 30 to 50 mg. per kg. (2.2 pounds) of body weight on alternate days for a total of 10 to 15 doses. Bithionol can be obtained from the Center for Disease Control, Atlanta, Georgia 30333.

4. *Lung Fluke Infection (Paragonimiasis; Endemic Hemoptysis).* Lung flukes are found in many parts of the Far East, in West Africa, and in Central and South America. The disease which they cause in humans is transmitted by the eating of raw, salted, or wine-soaked freshwater crabs or crayfishes which happen to be infested with the cyst of this particular parasite. When a living cyst is swallowed, it begins its development in the intestine. Later it penetrates the intestinal wall

and the diaphragm and migrates to the lung.

In a typical case, the symptoms develop gradually. They include a chronic cough and vague distress in the chest and an abundant, sticky, reddish-brown sputum which, on microscopic examination, is found to contain many red blood cells and eggs of the parasite. The victim occasionally spits blood and may become very anemic. The disease may be diagnosed by the finding of eggs in a sample of the patient's sputum, but most frequently in the feces because the eggs are swallowed.

Care and Treatment

Other than good nursing care, the treatment of paragonimiasis requires the use of a powerful drug. Bithionol is the preferred medication, which is administered in doses of 30 to 50 mg. per kg. (2.2 pounds) of body weight on alternate days for 10 to 15 doses. This drug may be obtained from the Center for Disease Control, Atlanta, Georgia 30333. Praziquantel may replace bithionol as the preferred drug as more drug-evaluation data are obtained.

GNATHOSTOMIASIS

This infection occurs principally in Thailand and Japan. It is caused by a worm which normally lives in the tissues of the stomach of dogs and cats. The eggs are expelled in the feces of these animals. After hatching in water they pass through two intermediate hosts. The larvae occur in freshwater fish, frogs, and eels, which, in turn, may be eaten by ducks and chickens. Humans become infected by eating uncooked fish, duck, or chicken.

Once these parasites have entered the human body, they migrate through various tissues, including the internal organs. The usual result is only a painless swelling surrounding the parasite.

Care and Treatment

Other than the surgical removal of the parasites, there is no treatment for this ailment.

LARVA MIGRANS

In occasional cases the larvae of one or the other of certain forms of worm parasites that normally live in the tissues of such animals as dogs and cats invade the human body and die there. These are not capable of perpetuating their life cycles in human tissues. They are called larva migrans because they *migrate* from their site of entry once they have entered human tissues.

1. *Visceral Larva Migrans (Toxocariasis).* The eggs of the *Toxocara* roundworms of either dogs or cats are shed from the bodies of the animals in their feces and remain viable in the soil for as much as several weeks. When these eggs are swallowed by young children who put dirt in their mouths, they move to the intestine, where the eggs produce larvae. The larvae penetrate the intestine and are carried by the blood to the various organs: the liver, lungs, heart, eye, skeletal muscles, and even the brain. The resulting symptoms include loss of weight, fever, irritability, wheezing, cough, enlargement of the liver, and itching of the skin. Seizures may occur when the brain is involved.

Deaths from this illness are rare. The condition is self-limited, and no specific treatment is effective.

2. *Cutaneous Larva Migrans (Creeping Eruption).* In this case it is the larvae of the dog and cat hookworm *(Ancylostoma)* that cause the difficulty. The larvae invade the human skin and migrate by producing tunnels in the skin until they die there. This produces severe itching and scratching, which often permits secondary infections. Without treatment the larvae may persist in the skin for weeks or months.

Care and Treatment

Wet dressings of aluminum acetate (1:20) solution are helpful when applied to the involved skin area. Local applications of anesthetic ointment will help to relieve the itching. Antibiotic medication is advised when the

skin area becomes severely infected. Spraying of the advancing end of the larva's burrow with ethyl chloride until the superficial layer of skin becomes frozen will cause a blister to form and result in the death of the larva. Thiabendazole taken by mouth in doses of 25 mg. per kg. (2.2 pounds) of body weight, taken morning and evening for five days, is the systemic medication of choice.

LOIASIS (CALABAR SWELLINGS)

This disease is prevalent in West and Central Africa. It is caused by a worm belonging to the filarie called *Loa loa,* which is transmitted by deer flies of the genus *Chrysops*.

The mature form of the *Loa loa* migrates in the body, chiefly in the connective tissues. The migration may cause itching, prickling, or creeping sensations, and temporary swellings or puffiness—the Calabar swellings—in various parts of the body. An especially vulnerable area is beneath the conjunctiva of the eyeball.

Ordinarily this disease is not of serious consequence, except for the itching of the skin and the anxiety it causes.

Care and Treatment

Diethylcarbamazine (Hetrazan), administered in gradually increasing

Wuchereria bancrofti, a parasite responsible for elephantiasis.

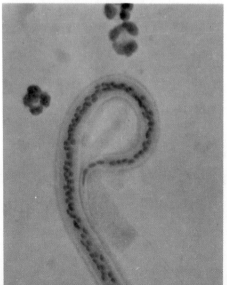

doses, is the drug of choice. This may cause an allergic reaction to the tissues of the parasites that are being destroyed, hence the use of small doses at the beginning of the period of therapy. The initial dose for an adult is 50 mg. taken by mouth. On the second day, three 50-mg. doses may be administered. On the third day, three 100-mg. doses are given and, finally, for the remaining seven days, 200 mg. doses are given three times a day. For the allergic reaction, the use of antihistamine medications is helpful.

Cold, wet dressings applied over the areas of skin irritation may give some comfort.

LYMPHATIC FILARIASIS (ELEPHANTIASIS)

Filariasis is a disease which occurs in tropical countries of southern Asia and the Far East. It is caused by either one or two kinds of worms *(Filarioidea):* (1) *Wuchereria bancrofti* or (2) *Brugia malayi*. These organisms are small, extremely slender worms, most of the adults varying between 1 and 3 inches (2.5 and 7.5 cm.) in length, though adult females of one species sometimes reach a length of 20 inches (50 cm.). In some tropical countries, more than half of the population harbor these worms.

In the adult form the *Filarioidea* live in the human lymphatic system and discharge their offspring (microfilariae) usually at night.

The night-swarming microfilariae are taken into the bodies of mosquitoes which bite infected persons. In the mosquito's body the embryos undergo partial development. When the infected mosquito bites another person, some of the parasites escape into the victim's skin. Within this person's body they find their way into the lymphatic tissues and gradually grow to maturity and then begin the production of new multitudes of microfilariae.

Oddly, the presence of millions of microfilariae in the blood causes no distress. It is the adult worm that causes symptoms, many of them brought on by irritation or obstruction of the

317

lymphatic tissues and vessels.

In those cases in which symptoms occur, the parasite goes through an incubation period of several months before the victim develops fever and pain originating in the lymph nodes and lymph vessels. The symptoms last from seven to ten days and then spontaneously disappear, only to recur from time to time. The involvement of the lymph nodes may actually develop into abscesses.

The late development which may occur many years after the initial infection involves a plugging of the lymph vessels by the bodies, even though they may be dead, of the adult worms. It is this development that carries the name of elephantiasis, a stage of the disease characterized by an abnormal swelling of the tissues that would normally be drained by the obstructed lymph vessels. The legs are most often affected. Other parts of the body that may be affected are the feet, the arms, the scro-

tum, the breasts, and the vulva. The chief drawbacks in connection with the development of elephantiasis are the awkwardness and repulsive appearance caused by the swelling. These are, in some cases, so extensive as to make it impossible for the victim to work or even to move about without help. No cure for elephantiasis is known, once this complication develops.

Prevention. There are three obvious parts to the program of preventing infections with the *Filarioidea:* (1) guarding healthy people against the bites of infected mosquitoes, (2) keeping infected people from being bitten by mosquitoes, and (3) extermination of the insects. Success in this program has proved difficult in most localities.

Care and Treatment

The control of filariasis has been aided in recent years by the use of diethylcarbamazine (Hetrazan), which causes a marked reduction of the microfilariae in the blood and probably also kills or injures some of the adult worms. The course of treatment lasts three or four weeks, during which time doses of 2 mg. per kg. (2.2 pounds) of body weight are given three times a day. During such a course of treatment the patient may experience a rather severe allergic reaction to the dying parasites. The use of antihistamine medications at such a time may help to relieve the allergic reaction.

ONCHOCERCIASIS (RIVER BLINDNESS)

This disease occurs in central Africa and in Central America—in the latter mainly in southern Chiapas, Mexico, and in Guatemala. It is caused by one of the filarial parasites called *Onchocerca volvulus,* the mature parasite being transmitted by the bite of the blackfly (buffalo gnat) of the genus *Simulium.* The presence of the mature parasites in the tissues causes itching and local inflammation, with the formation of slowly growing nodules surrounding the parasites beneath the skin. These nodules are firm to the

Enormous swelling of the legs commonly characterizes elephantiasis.

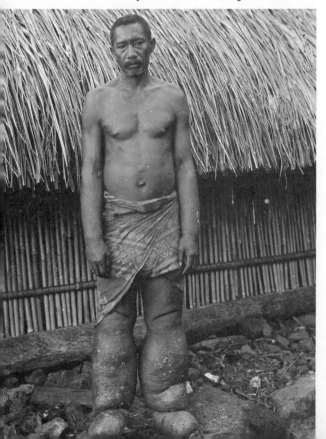

touch and swarm with microfilariae, which do not circulate in the blood. The nodules may cause pain but usually only itching. In the course of time, various structures in the eyes may be attacked, with the danger of resulting blindness. This complication usually occurs only after the disease has persisted for several years.

Care and Treatment

Nodules occurring in accessible areas should be removed by minor surgery. The most effective drug for the control of this disease is suramin, which must be administered with caution because of the possibility of kidney damage. The usual program of administration consists of a test dose of 100 mg. given by vein. If this is tolerated, it is followed by five weekly intravenous injections of 1 gm. of the drug.

TAPEWORM (CESTODE) INFECTION

The tapeworms, or cestodes, are long, flat, thin worms with segmented bodies. Unlike other worms that may inhabit the human body, the tapeworms lack digestive organs. They absorb their food through their entire surface as they attach themselves to the lining membrane of the intestine of the human or the animal in which they reside. The attachment organ has sucking discs, and some also have hooklets for holding onto the intestinal lining. The old segments gradually drop from the back end as new segments are formed near the head. The segments that drop off and escape with the feces often contain great numbers of eggs. These may be eaten by some lower animal along with its food. In the stomach and intestine of this animal, the eggs hatch into larvae, which migrate into the muscles or other parts of the animal's body and become encysted or dormant there, not developing further until the infected flesh of the animal is eaten by a human or some other suitable host.

1. *Beef Tapeworm (Taenia saginata) Infection*. Infection with the beef tapeworm occurs in all parts of the world in which it is the custom to eat raw or undercooked beef. In the majority of cases symptoms are unnoticed. In others, they include abdominal discomfort, diarrhea, weight loss, nausea, and a greater-than-usual appetite. The diagnosis is usually made by finding the worm segments in the feces. Several of these are shed daily, and this makes their recovery fairly easy. Often, the segments rupture and discharge their eggs at the time they are expelled from the body. The eggs may then occur in the stool or on the skin area surrounding the anal opening. Surprisingly, adult beef tapeworms may grow within the intestine to a length of up to 30 feet (nearly 10 meters).

Care and Treatment

The preferred medication for ridding the intestine of the beef tapeworm is the drug niclosamide (Yomesan), which is given in a single dose of 2 grams (for adults) on an empty stomach. This single treatment will

Beef tapeworm. Note how segments break off the tail end.

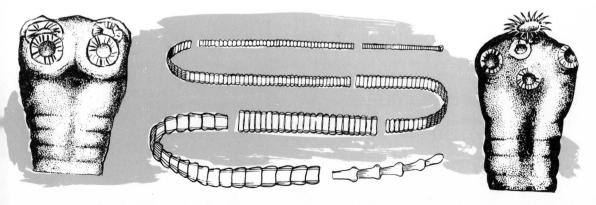

cause the eventual elimination of the worms in about 90 percent of cases.

2. *Dwarf Tapeworm (Hymenolepis nana) Infection.* This is the most common tapeworm infection in the southeastern United States and is seen more frequently in children than in adults. This tapeworm has both a direct and indirect life cycle, involving insect intermediate hosts. Infection is usually by transfer of eggs from anal skin to the mouth by the fingers. The parasite is common in mice. Eggs in mouse droppings contaminate cereals and grains and thus may spread infection. The infection is diagnosed by the finding of tapeworm eggs in feces. The drug niclosamide, repeated in two weeks, is effective treatment.

3. *Fish Tapeworm (Diphyllobothrium latum) Infection.* This is the largest of the tapeworms infecting man. It may grow to a length of nearly 40 feet (12 meters). The segments may be half an inch (13 mm.) in breadth, and one worm may have 3000 or more segments. The eggs of this worm are laid and must hatch in water; and the larva is eaten by a water flea (cyclops), which in turn is eaten by a fish. Humans are infected by eating raw or undercooked fish.

In many cases there are no noticeable symptoms, but there may be abdominal pain, loss of appetite, nausea, and loss of body weight. Within the human intestine, the worm requires a large quota of vitamin B_{12}, thus depriving the host of this important vitamin. This loss may cause anemia and nervous symptoms to develop in some persons. The diagnosis is made by finding the worm eggs in stool specimens.

Fish tapeworm disease occurs in many parts of the world, and in the United States is transmitted particularly by freshwater fish, including pike and yellow perch.

Care and Treatment

Niclosamide (Yomesan) is the drug of choice. It is administered in a single dose of 2 grams (adult dose) on an empty stomach.

4. *Pork Tapeworm (Taenia solium) Infection.* The pork tapeworm lives in the intestinal tract of humans, where it may remain alive for even several decades. It may become as long as 22 feet (7 meters). It may have as many as 1000 segments. The eggs which it produces are infective both to humans and to hogs, the hog serving as the intermediate host in the life cycle of this worm.

Pork tapeworm infections occur worldwide, but are most common in Russia, Eastern Europe, Asia, Africa, Mexico, and South America. Relatively few cases occur in the United States now because of the strict program for inspection of meat.

The pork tapeworm produces two distinct types of disease, depending upon whether it is the larvae of the tapeworm or the eggs that are swallowed by the human subject.

Type I, Adult Pork Tapeworm Infection. This type is similar in many ways to other forms of tapeworm disease. It is acquired by the eating of inadequately cooked pork which happens to contain the larvae of the pork tapeworm. The resulting young tapeworm then attaches itself to the lining of the intestine where, if untreated, it remains for years. This adult worm produces eggs. These eggs, contained in old worm segments, pass through the intestine to the outside and then are potentially infective to both humans and hogs.

The symptoms are relatively mild and may consist of abdominal pains and general weakness. The tapeworm segments, as they break away from the adult worm, pass through the remainder of the intestinal tract. In the meantime, many of the segments discharge the eggs which they contain, and these will be contained in the feces or they may adhere to the skin surrounding the anal opening. The diagnosis of this condition depends on finding the typical segments that are passed, or less fre-

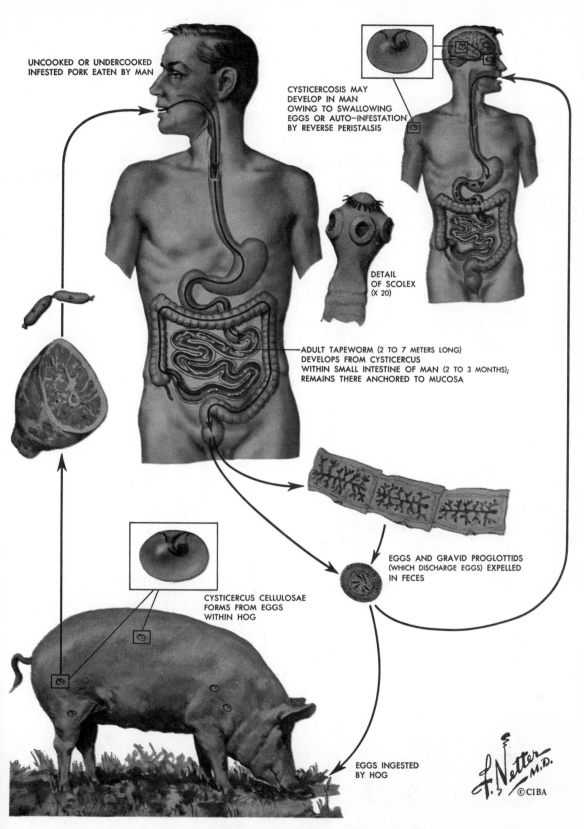

UNCOOKED OR UNDERCOOKED
INFESTED PORK EATEN BY MAN

CYSTICERCOSIS MAY
DEVELOP IN MAN
OWING TO SWALLOWING
EGGS OR AUTO—INFESTATION
BY REVERSE PERISTALSIS

DETAIL
OF SCOLEX
(X 20)

ADULT TAPEWORM (2 TO 7 METERS LONG)
DEVELOPS FROM CYSTICERCUS
WITHIN SMALL INTESTINE OF MAN (2 TO 3 MONTHS);
REMAINS THERE ANCHORED TO MUCOSA

EGGS AND GRAVID PROGLOTTIDS
(WHICH DISCHARGE EGGS) EXPELLED
IN FECES

CYSTICERCUS CELLULOSAE
FORMS FROM EGGS
WITHIN HOG

EGGS INGESTED
BY HOG

©CIBA

LIFE CYCLE OF THE PORK TAPEWORM

quently eggs in the feces or from skin scrapings of the area around the anus.

Care and Treatment

The preferred drug for killing the adult pork tapeworm is niclosamide (Yomesan) given in a single, 2-gram dose. This should be followed in four hours by the administration of a purgative as an aid to flushing the dying worm through the remainder of the intestine.

Type II, Cysticercosis. This form of pork tapeworm disease is acquired when the eggs of the pork tapeworm are swallowed. The usual source of the eggs is food contaminated by egg-containing human feces from an infected person. So-called autoinfection is also a possible source when a person who harbors the adult pork tapeworm is careless to the extent that he carries the eggs by finger contact from the anal region to his mouth.

A. Echinococcus granulosis (magnified 23 times). B. Sectional view of a hydatid cyst.

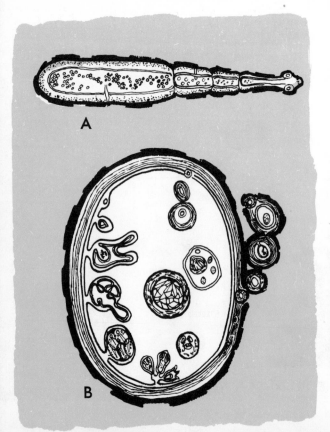

A

B

Once the eggs are swallowed, they hatch in the stomach or in the upper intestine, releasing the larvae form of the pork tapeworm. The larvae then penetrate the wall of the intestine and are carried by the blood to various tissues throughout the body. They may lodge in the tissues beneath the skin, in the skeletal muscles, or in the heart, liver, eye, brain, or lungs. The most common site of lodgment is in the muscles of the tongue, the neck, or the trunk. Wherever these larvae happen to lodge, within a period of two or three months they become encysted within a fibrotic capsule which grows to a diameter of $1/4$ to $3/4$ inch (6 to 18 mm.). This encysted larva is called a cysticercus, and the larvae may remain alive within it for as much as five years. Eventually, however, the larvae die and the body tissues then react toward the cysticercus as to any foreign body.

The usual symptoms of cysticercosis are muscle pains, weakness, and fever. But when cysticerci develop within the brain, there may be symptoms which simulate brain tumor or encephalitis, and there may be convulsive seizures.

The diagnosis of the cysticercosis type of pork tapeworm infection (type II) is made either by the X-ray evidence of the calcified remains of the encysted larvae or by a positive complement fixation test made in the laboratory.

Care and Treatment

There is no medication which will remove the encysted larvae once they become scattered throughout the body's tissues. Troublesome lesions are sometimes removed by surgery.

5. *Hydatid Disease (Echinococcosis).* Hydatid disease occurs in certain sheep-raising regions. The adult tapeworm lives in the intestines of dogs, foxes, and wolves, which animals become infected by eating the carcasses of sheep containing the larval forms. Infection of humans is with the larval form, and usually results from swallowing food accidentally contaminated with dog feces or from putting

contaminated fingers into the mouth.

When a person thus swallows the eggs, they hatch in the intestine. The young worms spend but a short time there, and then burrow into the tissues. Most of those that survive lodge in the liver, where they cause the formation of cysts filled with fluid and lined with a membrane that may produce large numbers of immature worm heads. A cyst may develop in the lung, in bone, in the heart, or in the central nervous system. Some cysts act like malignant tumors and produce a serious illness.

Prevention. Prevention of hydatid disease requires care in handling sheep dogs and in disposing of sheep carcasses.

Care and Treatment

The only medication which has given promise, thus far, of killing the larvae of this tapeworm is mebendazole. At the time of writing, however, the use of this drug is still in the experimental stage. When the cysts become large enough or when they are located in such a site as to produce symptoms, they may be removed surgically.

TRICHINOSIS (TRICHINIASIS)

Trichinosis is a disease caused by the invasion into the human body of the larvae of the *Trichinella spiralis,* a worm which occurs in the bodies of carnivorous animals in almost the entire world. Trichinosis is contracted by eating raw or insufficiently cooked flesh of animals (usually hogs but occasionally bear) in which the *Trichinella* is encysted in dormant form. In a few cases the infection has been transmitted by meat other than pork, which was chopped on the same chopping block that had been used to chop pork.

When infected meat is eaten, the embryo worms are liberated in the stomach and the intestine, where, in about three days, they grow to full size, most of them becoming imbedded in the intestinal membrane. They do not lay eggs that pass out of the intestine, but produce great numbers of young

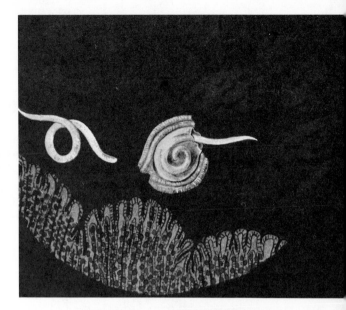

Trichinae in stomach (the worms shown much enlarged).

Trichinae encysted in muscle.

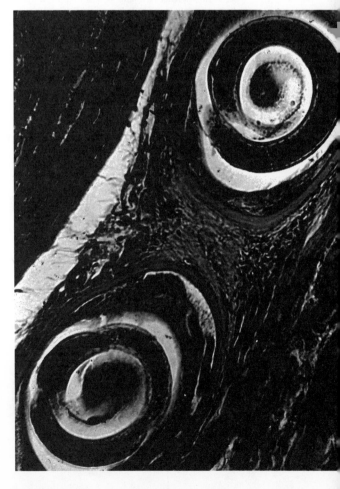

worms, most of which are deposited into the tissues and are carried throughout the body by the blood and lymph circulations. They finally become encysted and lie dormant in the muscle tissue as tiny coiled worms. They are not equally abundant in all muscles; the diaphragm gets more than its proportionate share of them.

After infected meat is eaten, six or seven days are required for the full development of the first brood of young embryos, which are then ready to migrate in the body. The production of embryos continues for some time. Bowel symptoms, such as discomfort and diarrhea, may occur at the time the worms are multiplying in the intestine.

Different symptoms develop while the young worms are migrating. These may be so severe that death results in some cases. Fever, chills, and abdominal and muscle pains are common. The patient suffers muscle tenderness while the embryos are becoming encysted, with swelling of the muscles and the overlying skin.

The worms may lie dormant in the muscles as long as 20 years, but the symptoms of their presence largely disappear after the first few weeks or months. The most serious cases are those in which the nervous system is involved.

During recent years, the number of cases of trichinosis in the United States has declined significantly. This decrease is partly due to laws that forbid the feeding of uncooked garbage to pigs. The overall mortality rate from this disease is now probably less than 2 percent in the United States.

Prevention. Once the organisms have entered a person's body, there is no way to stop the progress of this disease, so prevention of infection is of vital importance. For those who eat pork, the only safe procedure is to make sure the meat has been thoroughly cooked or else frozen to low temperature prior to cooking. No practical method exists by which meat handlers can detect the presence of trichinella in pork.

Care and Treatment

No completely satisfactory remedy has been found for trichinosis. In most cases, the disease is self-limited. Thus the care of the patient during the period when symptoms are present consists largely of good nursing care, including hot baths to relieve the pain in the muscles as far as possible. The drug thiabendazole has been used to kill the encysted larvae in the tissues of laboratory animals. When used in humans, it has afforded prompt relief of symptoms, but there may be such side effects as vomiting and fever. In the more serious cases where the nervous system is involved, a short course of the corticosteroid drug prednisone may be beneficial.

SECTION VI

First Aid;
Poisoning;
Emergencies

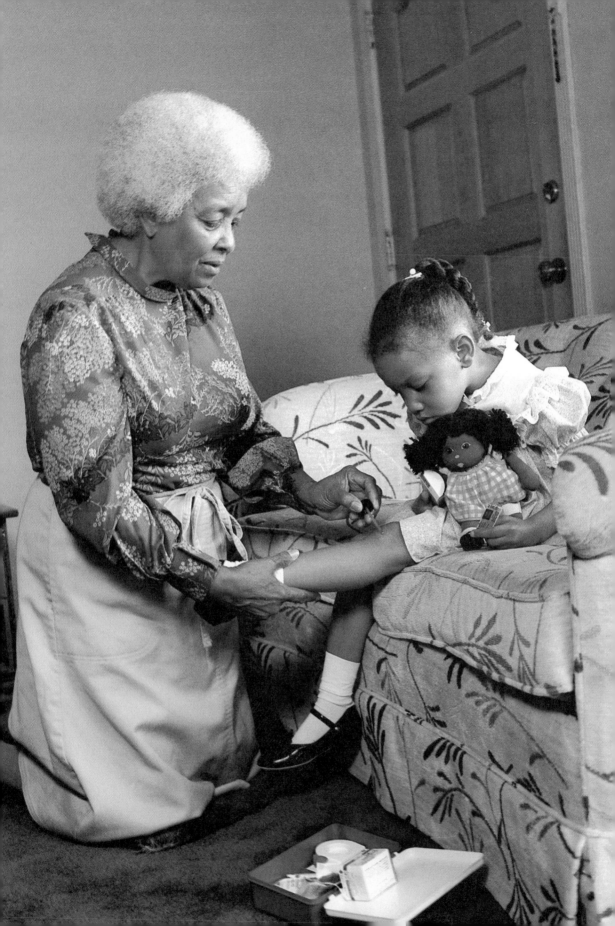

First-aid Kits and Home Medicine Chests

The prevalence of accidents in and around the home and on highways makes first-aid kits a necessity in every household and in every car. Extensive experience indicates that a small transportable emergency kit for the home should contain at least the following articles, most of which can be purchased at the drugstore:

Box of adhesive bandages about 1 x 3 inches (2.5 x 7.5 cm.) in size.

Box of adhesive bandages half as wide as the above.

Sterile gauze squares, about 3 x 3 inches (7.5 x 7.5 cm.), preferably in individual packages—at least a dozen.

Pieces of sterile gauze about one yard (meter) square, in individual packages—at least three.

Triangular bandages—at least three.

Roller bandages, 1-inch (2.5 cm.) and 2-inch (5 cm.) widths.

Some approved variety of burn ointment.

Small bottle of aromatic spirits of ammonia.

Small bottle of antiseptic solution.

Scissors, medium size.

Wire or thin board splints—at least two long and two short.

The kit to be carried in the car need not include so many articles. The following are recommended:

One roll of 1-inch (2.5 cm.) width adhesive tape.

Six small adhesive bandages.

Six 3 x 3 inch (7.5 x 7.5 cm.) sterile gauze squares, packaged separately.

One yard square (meter) of bandaging material (muslin).

One tube of approved variety of burn ointment.

One small bottle of antiseptic.

Kits to be carried in the car should be kept in canvas rolls or metal containers. Those for the home may also be kept in metal cases or boxes. Avoid the tendency to keep articles for home first-aid use lying around in different drawers or piled on shelves. Places specified for these articles should not be used for anything else. The materials should be kept in good order in the case or box, arranged so that any desired article can be found without unpacking everything in the kit, and the separate packages should be wrapped in such a way that unused material will not be soiled by handling.

The bottle of aromatic spirits of ammonia should be replaced with a new one every year to ensure full strength always. Certain antiseptics also contain a volatile substance which makes periodic replacement of them likewise necessary, perhaps even every six months.

Various manufacturers put up special individual packages or kits, often of sizes and shapes convenient for packing into cases for first-aid use. Also these kits are packed so as to prevent contamination or spoilage, generally with printed directions for use on the outside of each package. If you are willing to spend a little more to obtain your first-aid supplies in such forms, you will probably feel repaid in the long run. Your druggist will doubtless be able to show you samples.

Home Medicine Chests

In some homes, the first-aid kit and the home medicine cabinet are combined, but it is better to have a separate medicine cabinet, preferably in the bathroom. The ordinary small cabinet usually installed above the lavatory and kept more or less full of toilet articles will not serve the purpose adequately. Separate shelves out of reach of children, or preferably a separate cabinet equipped with a lock, should be built and kept solely for medicines and treatment supplies. The following is a suggested list of contents—sizes and measurement being given in both standard and metric units, which, however, in most cases are not precisely equivalent:

Home Medicine Chest: Suggested Contents

Absorbent cotton, sterile—4 oz. or 100 gm.
Activated charcoal—4 oz. or 100 gm.
Adhesive tape, 1-inch (2.5 cm.) width—1 roll.
Antiseptic, one bottle.
Antiseptic soap.
Aromatic spirits of ammonia—2 oz. or 50 ml.
Aspirin tablets.
Baby oil.
Bedpan.
Boric acid ointment, 5 percent—2 oz. or 50 mg.
Calamine lotion—4 oz. or 100 ml.
Clinical thermometer, mouth style.
Earache drops—1 oz. or 25 ml.
Enema kit.
Epsom salts—1 pound or 500 mg.
Eucalyptus oil—2 oz. or 50 ml.
Gauze roller bandage, 1-inch (2.5 cm.)—1 roll.
Gauze roller bandage, 2-inch (5 cm.)—1 roll.
Glycerin—8 oz. or 200 ml.

Hot-water bottle.
Hydrogen peroxide, 8 oz. or 200 ml.
Ice bag.
Lysol, 4 oz. or 100 ml. (label as poison).
Medicine droppers—two.
Milk of magnesia—8 oz. or 200 ml.
Mineral oil—1 pint or 500 ml.
Mustard powder—4 oz. or 100 gm.
Nose drops.
Oil of cloves—1/2 oz. or 10 ml.
Petrolatum (vaseline)—4 oz. or 100 gm.
Potassium permanganate crystals—2 oz. or 50 gm.
Razor blades (stiff-backed).
Rubbing alcohol—1 pint or 500 ml.
Safety matches.
Safety pins, medium size—one dozen.
Scissors, medium size.
Syringe, soft rubber—2 oz. or 50 ml. size.
Syrup of ipecac—2 oz. or 50 ml.
Tylenol tablets.
Zinc oxide ointment—1 oz. or 25 gm.
Zinc stearate powder—2 oz. or 50 gm.

The list of items and the amounts given above are only general suggestions. There may be other articles or substances which your experience will prove necessary for your family. On the other hand, some in this list you may not require. You would be unwise to keep your medicine cabinet cluttered up with items or substances which you seldom use. The nearer you are to a drugstore and the more convenient it is for you to buy what you need, the fewer the articles you will need to keep readily on hand at home.

Special Classes of Medicines

Certain home remedies which householders usually include in a medicine chest deserve special mention:

Analgesics. These are pain relievers, often more harmful than beneficial. Aspirin is probably the least harmful, but it is one especially to be kept out of the reach of children, as it constitutes the most common cause of child poisoning. Oil of cloves for tooth ache is another common analgesic.

Antacids. These are used to counter excess acid in the stomach. Magnesium carbonate, aluminum hydroxide, and magnesium trisilicate are the commonly used antacids and constitute the active ingredients of commercial preparations obtainable at drugstores. Baking soda (sodium bicarbonate), though often used as an antacid, is not recommended for this purpose.

Antiseptics. For superficial wounds which may become infected, present usage favors thorough cleansing with soap and water in preference to chemical antiseptics. However, many persons still feel more secure against infection if they apply an antiseptic preparation such as can be obtained from the drugstore. The reader may check with his pharmacist for a recommended brand. Also available commercially are disinfectants useful for decontaminating articles used in caring for wounds. Lysol solution is a well-known example. The householder or first-aid worker will of course recognize that these preparations are not to be administered internally.

Cathartics. A continuous use of cathartics entails the risk of developing the carthartic habit. But an occasional dose of Epsom salts or milk of magnesia for constipation will do little or no harm. However, *even the simplest cathartic may be hazardous if taken when a person has abdominal pain.* In case such pain is due to an inflamed appendix the use of a cathartic may dangerously aggravate the condition.

Emetics. These are substances that produce vomiting. To induce vomiting have the victim drink lukewarm water (plain or containing a little salt, baking soda, or soap) after which the first-aider places his finger in the victim's throat, causing him to gag and thus to vomit. If syrup of ipecac is available, it may be used as directed on page 334, PROCEDURE E, *To Induce Vomiting.*

Hypnotics. These are sleep producers. Their common or habitual use is recognized as harmful. They should be used only as prescribed by a physician.

Stimulants. In conditions such as poisoning, shock, or heat exhaustion the patient, if conscious, may be given a teaspoonful of aromatic spirits of ammonia in a glass of cool water. Also a drink of warm coffee may be given; however, for reasons stated elsewhere (see chapter 54, volume 1, pages 491-493), this beverage, like other stimulants, is not recommended for nonmedicinal use. A warm, strong coffee enema may be given to even an unconscious patient suffering from the above-mentioned conditions.

Caution With Poisons

The home medicine cabinet may contain a few substances that are poisonous, including even "safe" preparations if taken in excess. Treatment for poisoning is outlined in the following chapter.

It is dangerous to take any substance the nature or identity of which is not absolutely clear. If bottles or packages lose their labels, the contents should be flushed down the toilet. Keep your medicine chest in good order; it could mean the saving of a life.

Poisonings

General Considerations

It is estimated that more than a million cases of poisoning occur each year in the United States, with about 6000 deaths. A large percentage of poisoning cases occur in children, and of these children, 80 percent are between the ages of 1 and 4. The most common cause of poisoning in children is the taking of many tablets of flavored, chewable baby aspirin.

Among adults, barbiturate medicines come first, with methyl alcohol (wood alcohol) and the various kinds of denatured alcohols coming second.

Even newborn babies are not immune. Boric acid solutions have been used accidentally as diluent in babies' formulas, causing a number of deaths.

Widespread knowledge of first-aid procedures, prompt and efficient action by physicians in general, and recent development in all major cities of poison-control centers have greatly reduced deaths from accidental poisoning. In view, however, of still high percentages of children involved in accidental poisonings, parents also must join hands in helping to prevent these accidents. Therefore the inclusion of vital information on this subject as a separate chapter in *You and Your Health*.

Prevention Rather Than Cure. One's conduct, particularly at home, is determined largely by habit. Habits of taking precautions and avoiding risks are life-saving in the long run, whereas habits of carelessness and attitudes of "It can't happen to me" form the prelude to misfortune. To prevent poisoning accidents, first, recognize the hazards and, second, adopt and enforce policies for the home and members of the family which remove the conditions under which such accidents can occur.

How to Poison-proof Your Home

The American Medical Association provides the following list of seven precautions, which, when put into effect, will eliminate practically all danger of accidental poisoning:

1. Make sure to keep all drugs, poisonous substances, and household chemicals out of the reach of children. (Remember children can climb.)

2. Do not store nonedible products on shelves used for storing food.

3. Keep all poisonous substances in their original containers; don't transfer them to unlabeled containers.

4. When medicines are discarded, destroy them. Don't throw them where they may be reached by chil-

NOTE: The following section on first aid for poisoning conforms to the recommendations made at the Joint Symposium of the American Academy of Clinical Toxicology, the American Association of Poison Control Centers, and the Canadian Academy of Clinical Toxicology, held in 1976.

331

POISONS

dren or pets. Flush them down the toilet.

5. When giving flavored or brightly colored medicine to children, always refer to it as medicine—never as candy.

6. Do not give or take medicine in the dark.

7. *Read labels* before using chemical products.

Poison-proof Instructions for Specific Rooms

The Kitchen. More poisonings occur here than in any other room in the house—an estimated 34 percent. Poi-

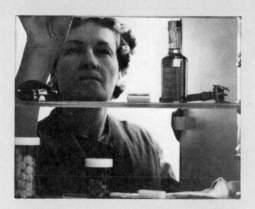

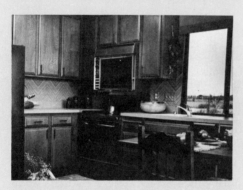

son-proof your kitchen, therefore, by keeping all dangerous household agents by themselves, separate from food, in their original containers and properly labeled, and out of reach of children.

The Bedroom. Here about 27 percent of all poisoning accidents take place. From what? Mothballs, cosmetics, cleaning agents stored in the closet, and from sleeping pills and other medicines placed on the night stand.

How to poison-proof the bedroom? Two simple directives to follow: (1) Keep all poisonous agents and medicines in their proper containers and stored in places inaccessible to children; and (2) keep medicines where they cannot be reached "conveniently" by a person too sleepy to be aware of what he is doing.

The Bathroom. This is the location for about 15 percent of all poisoning ac-

cidents. Poison-proof by keeping all medicines in a locked cupboard and placing the key well out of reach of children.

The Living Room. This is the locale of some 9 percent of all poisoning accidents. How can one poison-proof this room? Do not allow cosmetics, cleaning agents, and medicines to accumulate here, where they don't belong anyway.

The Garage, Yard, and Basement. Cans of petroleum products, solvents, pesticides, and those magic chemicals used around the car, house, and yard are kept here—substances which cause about 16 percent of all poisoning accidents.

Poison-proof by keeping all chemicals in plainly labeled containers and stored out of the reach of children. Many a child's life has been in danger because he mistook some household solvent in an unlabeled pop bottle as good to drink.

General Symptoms of Poisoning

These are often confusingly similar to the symptoms of some of the infectious diseases and include loss of appetite, pain in the abdomen, a feeling of being sick at the stomach with a tendency to vomit, and diarrhea.

Also, a poison victim's skin may be cold, clammy, and blue-colored. There may be loss of consciousness and even convulsions.

First Aid for Poisoning

The outcome of a case of poisoning depends a great deal on the way it is handled by the first person who renders help—very often the mother of a child. Speed being the essence of success, the judgment of the first-aider is of prime importance.

THE EMERGENCY CALL

Once poisoning is suspected, place an emergency call at once for a physician, the emergency squad of the fire department, or **the poison control center of your nearest city.** Preferably this call should be placed by a second responsible person so that the first-aider can devote all his time to the care of the patient. In placing the call, give as much information as possible: the patient's name, any clue as to the nature of the poison (such as the wording of the label on the container), the patient's symptoms, and the patient's exact present whereabouts. The person placing the call should ask for instructions on how to care for the patient until help arrives or while the patient is being taken to an emergency room.

First Aid for Poisons Injected Through the Skin

This includes poisoning by snakebite or by the sting of an insect. For first-aid procedures see under *Bites* in this volume, pages 362-366, and under *Stings* in this volume, pages 413, 414.

First Aid for Poisoning by Skin Contact

Contact with substances spilled on the skin may cause not only burns but systemic poisoning by absorption of the chemical through the skin. For first-aid procedures, see under *Burns— Burns Caused by Chemicals* on page 372 of this volume.

First Aid for Poisoning by Inhalation

When the victim has breathed a poison gas (such as carbon monoxide), remove him from the room or area in which he has inhaled the gas and administer artificial respiration as necessary to keep him breathing. (See under *Respiratory Failure* in this volume,

**In any case of poisoning
CALL POISON CONTROL CENTER
in your area without delay.**

pages 407-409.) Call for trained help. If a tank of oxygen is available, waft a stream of the oxygen gas under the victim's nose so that he breathes it.

First Aid for Poisoning by Mouth

Try to learn the nature of the poison or the medicine that has been swallowed. Give all such information to the doctor, the emergency squad, or the poison control center when making the emergency call previously mentioned. Save the container, if available, and any remaining portion of the poison or medicine. Save the stomach contents if and when the patient vomits. All of these items are to be examined by the doctor or the poison specialist who takes over the case.

The particular kind of first aid for a person who has swallowed a poison or taken an overdose of medicine depends on his present condition and on the kind of poison or medicine swallowed.

So there comes next a listing of the five general procedures, designated as A, B, C, D, and E, each adapted to a particular situation. The first-aider should check through these and choose the one that fits the case he is handling. If in doubt on which procedure to use, he can refer to the *Alphabetical Listing of Specific Poisons* which begins on page 335.

General Procedures for Poisonings by Mouth

PROCEDURE A. *When the victim is unconscious.* Call for trained help. Administer artificial respiration as necessary to keep the patient breathing. (See under *Respiratory Failure* in this volume, pages 407-409.) Do not give fluids while the patient is unconscious. Do not force the unconscious patient to vomit; but if he does so spontaneously, turn his head so that the vomitus drains out of his mouth. Save the vomitus for later examination.

PROCEDURE B. *When the victim has swallowed a petroleum product* such as kerosene, gasoline, benzine, paint thinner, fuel oil, and naphtha. Call for trained help. Arrange to take the victim to a hospital as soon as possible because of the great danger of a serious type of pneumonia.

Remove any contaminated clothing and wash the underlying skin. Keep the victim quiet and warm. Use artificial respiration as necessary to keep the victim breathing. (See under *Respiratory Failure* in this volume, pages 407-409.) If a tank of oxygen is available, waft a stream of the oxygen gas under the victim's nose so that he breathes it. **Do not force the victim** to vomit except under a doctor's order and supervision. Give a glass of milk to drink so as to dilute the stomach contents. Give egg white or crushed banana by mouth to soothe the inflamed membranes.

PROCEDURE C. *When the victim has swallowed a corrosive poison* such as strong acid or alkali. Common examples are lye, caustic soda, drain and toilet-bowl cleaners, and electric dishwasher detergents in either solid or liquid form. There may or may not be burns on the lips and around the mouth. The severe damage occurs inside the mouth and in the lining of the esophagus.

Call at once for trained help. Plan for hospitalization. Dilute the caustic agent at once by giving the victim a drink of milk (or water if milk is not at hand). Remove any contaminated clothing and wash the underlying skin. Do not try to make the victim vomit. Irritations of the lining membranes may be soothed by having the patient swallow cream or

egg white. Keep the victim quiet and warm. Use cracked ice to relieve thirst.

PROCEDURE D. *When the victim is having convulsions.* Do not try to prevent the patient's movements but do what is necessary to keep him from injuring himself. (See *Convulsions* in this volume, page 380.) Do not give fluids by mouth. Do not force the patient to vomit; but if he vomits spontaneously, turn his head so that the material drains from his mouth.

PROCEDURE E. *When the victim is conscious, is NOT having convulsions, and has NOT swallowed a petroleum product or a corrosive poison.* Three principles are followed here: (1) Dilute the poison in the victim's stomach by having him drink milk or water. (2) Induce vomiting to empty the stomach. (3) Give activated charcoal to absorb the poison that remains in the stomach.

To induce vomiting. Have the patient swallow the proper dose of syrup of ipecac: 1 tablespoonful (15 ml.) for a child or 2 tablespoonfuls (30 ml.) for an adult. Follow this by 2 glasses or more of water or milk. If vomiting does not occur within 15 minutes, the first-aider inserts his finger and gently tickles the back of the patient's throat. If syrup of ipecac is not available, have the patient drink fluid and then tickle his throat.

Vomiting should be induced even though it has been several hours since the poison was swallowed. The vomitus should be saved for later examination. If the patient is reclining, turn his head as he vomits so as to prevent choking.

Activated charcoal should be administered after the vomiting to absorb what remains of the poison. One or two tablespoonfuls of activated charcoal (powder) are stirred into a glass of water and given to the patient to drink. If the patient vomits again, have him drink another dose of the activated charcoal. Activated charcoal is a harmless potion available at drugstores and is effective in absorbing most poisons and medicines.

Alphabetical Listing of Specific Poisons

POISONS

BY ACIDS—STRONG ACIDS

Immediately after swallowing a strong acid the victim experiences pain in the mouth, throat, and abdomen. The membranes of the lips and mouth appear white, and the patient experiences intense thirst. If the victim vomits, the vomitus appears as "coffee grounds."

What to Do

Follow PROCEDURE C on page 334.

BY ALCOHOL—ETHYL ALCOHOL

(See also *Intoxication, Alcoholic,* page 403, this volume.)

It is this type of alcohol that is contained in alcoholic beverages as well as in many medicines prepared as "tinctures."

Symptoms of poisoning by ethyl alcohol: drunkenness which includes an initial state of excitement, followed by depression, nausea, vomiting, and unconsciousness. When the amount of alcohol in the body fluids becomes dangerously high, the body's vital functions are impaired. When death occurs, it is from paralysis of the breathing mechanism.

What to Do

1. Cause the patient to vomit as explained under PROCEDURE E on page 334.
2. Keep the patient warm.
3. Make sure that he continues to breathe. Use artificial respiration if necessary. (See *Respiratory Failure,* pages 407-409, this volume.)
4. Give a simple stimulant. If the victim is unconscious, administer strong lukewarm or cold coffee by rectum, in which case the caffeine contained in the coffee will serve as a stimulant.

If the patient is conscious, allow him to drink strong coffee or a glass of water containing one teaspoonful of aromatic spirits of ammonia.

BY ALCOHOL—METHYL ALCOHOL (Wood Alcohol)

Methyl alcohol is commonly present in paints, paint thinners, paint removers, and "canned heat." One tragic complication of methyl alcohol poisoning is the common occurrence of blindness resulting from damage to the optic nerves.

In addition to the symptoms of intoxication (drunkenness), the victim may have headache, pain in the abdomen, nausea, vomiting, and blindness.

What to Do

1. Rinse out the victim's stomach by causing him to vomit. See *To Induce Vomiting* under PROCEDURE E, page 334.
2. Protect the patient's eyes from light.
3. Make sure that breathing continues even though this may require artificial respiration. (See *Respiratory Failure*, page 407, this volume.) Administer pure oxygen if available.
4. Arrange for care by a physician or for hospitalization.

BY ALDRIN *(See By CHLORDANE.)*

BY AMMONIA

Ammonia is kept commonly about the house to be used as a cleaning agent. When ammonia is swallowed, it causes burning of the mouth, of the esophagus, and of the stomach, followed by thirst and nausea. The fumes of strong ammonia, when blown in the face or when inhaled, cause severe irritation of the membranes of the eyes, throat, and air passages.

What to Do

Ammonia is a powerful irritant and corrosive. Follow PROCEDURE C on page 334. When the fumes have irritated the eyes, wash the eyes freely

335

POISONS

while holding the lids open and using several quarts of water. Afterward the pain may be soothed by placing a few drops of dilute boric acid solution beneath the eyelids.

BY AMPHETAMINES

The group of amphetamines includes Benzedrine, Dexedrine, and Methedrine. They are used to reduce appetite and weight and to combat fatigue and depression. They are commonly involved in drug abuse under such names as ''pep pills,'' ''bennies,'' and ''speed.'' Overdosage causes serious symptoms and possible death.

What to Do

Follow PROCEDURE E on page 334.

BY ANILINE

When aniline has been swallowed, nausea and vomiting occur. Systemic symptoms include shallow breathing, low blood pressure, weak and irregular pulse, convulsions, and unconsciousness.

What to Do

When aniline has been absorbed through the skin, this skin area should be cleaned with soap and water. If the poison was swallowed, the stomach should be emptied by vomiting. (See *To Induce Vomiting* under PROCEDURE E on page 334.) A dose of Epsom salts (one to two tablespoonfuls in a glass of water) should be given to hasten the removal of the poison from the digestive organs. The victim's most urgent need is an adequate supply of oxygen.

If pure oxygen is available, arrange for the patient to breathe this. If his breathing becomes difficult, use artificial respiration. (See *Respiratory Failure*, page 407, this volume.)

BY ANTIFREEZE (See By *Ethylene Glycol*, page 339.)

BY ARSENIC

Arsenic is contained in many insecti-cides, rodent poisons, and crop sprays, as well as in some paints, dyes, and cosmetics.

In the usual case of acute arsenic poisoning the symptoms resemble those of food poisoning. Vomiting may occur within fifteen minutes and intense diarrhea, with watery stools, within one or more hours. There develops a sense of tightness in the throat and of intense pain in the abdomen. There may be muscle cramps, inability to pass urine, unconsciousness, convulsions, and eventual collapse.

What to Do

Until a trained professional person takes over the case, follow PROCEDURE E on page 334.

The most effective subsequent treatment, to be administered by a physician, is the injection of dimercaprol (''BAL,'' British antilewisite). This is given by injection in gradually decreasing doses over a period of several days.

BY ASPIRIN AND OTHER SALICYLATES

Aspirin is the most common cause of poisoning among young children. Symptoms may develop slowly. They include rapid breathing, vomiting, extreme thirst, sweating, fever, and mental confusion. In severe cases there may be unconsciousness or convulsions. Because the symptoms are not distinctive, the diagnosis of aspirin poisoning usually centers around a clue that the child or other victim has taken this drug. When aspirin poisoning is suspected, a physician should be consulted at once.

What to Do

For the emergency treatment, follow PROCEDURE E on page 334. Call for professional assistance.

BY ATROPINE, BELLADONNA, AND STRAMONIUM

Atropine eye drops and belladonna preparations occasionlly cause poisoning in children. Stramonium is found in

POISONS

Jimsonweed (thorn apple, stinkweed) and certain other plants. The seeds are especially toxic, as they contain atropine, scapolamine, and hyoscyamine.

First symptoms are burning and dryness of the mouth, flushing, fever, intense thirst, and visual disturbance (the pupils are widely dilated). Weakness, dizziness, staggering gait, mental confusion, excitement, and delirium follow.

What to do

Arrange for trained help as quickly as possible. For first aid, follow PROCEDURE E on page 334. Use artificial respiration as necessary to keep the patient breathing. (See under *Respiratory Failure* in this volume, pages 407-409.)

BY BARBITURATES

The barbiturates include many drugs used as sedatives. These are commonly kept in the family medicine cupboard or in dresser drawers. The usual victim

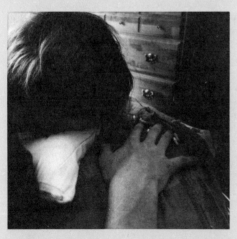

is one who takes the medicine out of curiosity. Barbiturates are often taken by depressed persons and with suicidal intent.

An overdose of one of the barbiturates depresses the nervous system (causing stupor or unconsciousness) and causes a slowing of breathing, a fall in blood pressure, and a final state of shock. Before these symptoms of mental and physical depression set in, however, there is often a short period of excitement during which the patient may act intoxicated.

What to Do

If the victim is still conscious, follow PROCEDURE E on page 334. If the victim is already in a stupor, forced vomiting is not recommended. Call the doctor. First-aid measures while waiting for the doctor or for transportation to the hospital include artificial respiration and the administration of oxygen, if possible. (See under *Respiratory Failure* in this volume, pages 407-409.)

BY BENZEDRINE (See *By Amphetamines.*)

BY BENZENE (See *By Kerosene, Gasoline, Benzene, and Naphtha.*)

BY BENZENE HEXACHLORIDE (BHC) (See *By DDT.*)

BY CARBON MONOXIDE

Carbon monoxide is a poison gas contained in automobile exhaust and given off by improperly vented heating devices. Poisoning may occur when people least suspect the possibility of danger.

The symptoms include headache, faintness, dizziness, weakness, difficult breathing, and possible vomiting, followed by collapse and unconsciousness. The skin, either entirely or in patches, often appears cherry-red.

What to Do

Remove the victim at once from the source of the poison gas. Carry him so that he does not exert himself, for his system is already handicapped for lack of oxygen. Then keep him warm and give artificial respiration as necessary. (See *Respiratory Failure* in this volume, pages 407-409.)

Inhalation of pure oxygen is often helpful. Request help promptly from a physician, the fire department, or the police emergency squad. In making the request, specify the need for oxygen. The victim should be kept at

337

POISONS

complete rest for many hours even after he begins to recover.

BY CARBON TETRACHLORIDE

Carbon tetrachloride is commonly available around the house in cleaning fluids, fire extinguisher fluid, paint remover, or as a general solvent. Poisoning may occur from drinking the fluid (usual victims, children) or by inhaling the fumes as when used for dry cleaning, or as a result of some prank.

Early symptoms include headache, pain in the abdomen, vomiting, and diarrhea. There may be the appearance of intoxication; later, convulsions and loss of consciousness may develop.

What to Do

When the fumes have been inhaled, the patient should be removed to an area where fresh air is available. He should be given artificial respiration as necessary. (See *Respiratory Failure* in this volume, pages 407-409.) When the carbon tetrachloride has been swallowed, repeated drinking of large amounts of water and repeated vomiting are advised. Do not give milk to drink or other liquids containing fat.

The victim should be placed under a physician's care because of the probable damage to kidneys and liver.

BY CHLORDANE (See *By DDT*.)

BY CHLORINATED COMPOUNDS (See *By DDT*.)

BY COCKROACH POISON (See *By Phosphorus*.)

BY CYANIDE

Chemical combinations of cyanide are present in silver polish, rodent poisons, and other preparations used about the garden. Cyanide is one of the most rapid-acting of the various poisons. Very few cases of genuine cyanide poisoning survive. Poisoning results quickly from swallowing a substance containing cyanide, from inhaling cyanide as a vapor, or by ab-

sorbing it through the skin or a small wound.

With large doses, death occurs quickly on account of paralysis of the organs of breathing. With smaller doses, there is difficulty in breathing, mental confusion, vomiting, and diarrhea. Violent convulsions may occur.

What to Do

Work quickly. Induce vomiting immediately with a finger down the victim's throat. If amyl nitrite ampules are available (such as some persons carry for relief of pain from the heart), break one of these ampules into a handkerchief and allow the victim to breathe the fumes for fifteen to thirty seconds. Repeat this procedure after two minutes.

The effective treatment for cyanide poisoning is the administration of a solution of sodium thiosulfate by vein. It is seldom that this can be administered in time to save the victim's life. If the dose of poison is small, the patient can be treated for shock and can be given pure oxygen to breathe if facilities are available.

BY DDT AND OTHER CHLORINATED ORGANIC INSECTICIDES

This class of insecticides includes many that are used in the garden and on the farm such as aldrin, benzene hexachloride, chlordane, DDE, DDT, DFDT, dieldrin, heptachlor, lindane, methoxychlor, and toxaphene. These can cause poisoning by being taken into the mouth, by being inhaled, or by direct contact with the skin. Although these poisons seldom prove fatal, they do cause damage to the brain and to the liver.

Poisoning by these insecticides causes aching limbs, nervous irritability, slowing of the thought processes, twitching of the muscles, convulsions, and unconsciousness.

What to Do

If the poison has been taken by mouth, have the victim drink three or four glasses of warm water and then induce vomiting by placing your finger far back in the victim's throat. Repeat this several times to rinse the stomach. Avoid using cathartics, oily preparations of any kind, or epinephrine (adrenaline). When paralysis of respiration occurs, give artificial respiration. (See *Respiratory Failure* in this volume, pages 407-409.)

It is advisable to hospitalize the victim so that a physician can give proper medication to control convulsions and to prevent liver damage.

BY DEPILATORIES

Commercial preparations for removing superfluous hair commonly contain thallium acetate, which is highly poisonous, or barium sulfide and sodium sulfide, which are moderately poisonous. Children are the usual victims in this type of poisoning. Symptoms appear several hours after the poison has been taken. Those involving the digestive organs include abdominal pain, vomiting, and diarrhea which may be bloody. Damage to the nervous system causes unusual sensations, drooping of the eyelids (one or both), crossing of the eyes, facial paralysis, and possibly delirium and convulsions. These poisons also cause damage to the liver and kidneys.

What to Do

It is important to empty the stomach quickly. If available, give the victim 1 percent solution of sodium iodide to drink (three or four glasses). Then promptly induce vomiting by tickling the victim's throat. If sodium iodide is not available, have the victim drink three or four glasses of milk. Combat shock by keeping the victim warm and elevating his legs above the level of his body. Give much water to drink to reduce damage to the kidneys. Strong coffee (lukewarm or cool) by enema may help by its stimulating action.

BY DETERGENTS

Reports from poison control centers indicate an increasing number of incidents in which children have swallowed detergents. Although the symptoms in such cases of poisoning may be serious, actual cases of death are rare.

Symptoms include vomiting, restlessness, difficult breathing, mental confusion, muscle weakness, convulsions, possible collapse, unconsciousness, and death due to paralysis of the breathing muscles.

What to Do

For poisoning by a simple detergent, cause the patient to vomit by the use of syrup of ipecac as instructed in the paragraph *To Induce Vomiting* under PROCEDURE E on page 334. Follow this by having him drink milk or egg white to soothe the inflamed membranes. Assist breathing, if necessary, by artificial respiration. (See *Respiratory Failure* in this volume, pages 407-409.)

For stronger detergents such as those prepared for automatic dishwashers, these being caustic in their effect on the tissues, follow PROCEDURE C on page 334.

BY DFDT (See *By DDT.*)

BY DIELDRIN (See *By DDT.*)

BY DYES (See *By Aniline.*)

BY EPN, TEPP, OMPA (See *By Parathion.*)

BY ETHYL ALCOHOL (See *By Alcohol—Ethyl Alcohol.*)

BY ETHYLENE GLYCOL (Antifreeze).

Ethylene glycol is used extensively in industry as a solvent. In pure form it is used as a coolant and antifreeze for cars. It is a sweet, colorless, slightly syrupy liquid. When taken by mouth it causes a form of drunkenness but with no odor of alcohol on the breath. Symptoms include vomiting, pain in the abdomen, rapid breathing, rapid pulse, elevated blood pressure, and evidence of damage to the kidneys. When as much as a third of a glass (80 ml.) has been ingested, death may occur within 12 to 36 hours.

What to Do

Arrange for professional care and hospitalization at the earliest possible moment.

Rinse out the victim's stomach by causing him to vomit. (See *To Induce Vomiting* under PROCEDURE E, page 334.) Give abundant water to drink. Keep the victim warm; use artificial respiration if necessary to keep him breathing (see *Respiratory Failure* in this volume, pages 407-409); and waft a stream of pure oxygen gas in front of his nose if oxygen is available.

BY FLUORIDE (See *By Sodium Fluoride.*)

BY FOOD

Inasmuch as food is taken into the digestive organs, the mucous membranes of which are highly absorptive, it is understandable that poisoning can easily result when food contains any poisonous substance. By nature, some plant leaves, roots, and fruits contain poisonous ingredients; these in turn may be eaten by birds, animals, or fish, making their flesh poisonous as food.

Food contaminated by germs and improperly refrigerated, or canned food improperly cooked and containing spores of bacteria, may be a cause of poisoning. Thus there are many kinds of food poisoning and food infection. The common ones, along with methods of emergency treatment, are here described.

A. *By Botulism*. This is the most serious type of food poisoning. It results from a germ (*Clostridium botulinum*) common in gardens and on farms and probably present on all vegetable products. Poisoning does not result from eating freshly prepared garden products, for it takes a period of time for the germ to develop its poisoning capabilities. Conditions become right when garden products are improperly canned, stored for a while, and then served without first being cooked at

boiling temperatures for at least twenty minutes. Canning procedures are quite critical.

Gas-containing, off-color, off-smelling foods or foods from bulging cans should not be eaten, nor even tasted.

Symptoms of botulism usually occur within eighteen hours after the contaminated food has been eaten, possibly longer, depending on the amount of toxin ingested. Serious symptoms consist of dim vision, double vision, and difficulty in talking and swallowing because of paralysis of the muscles of the larynx and throat. The toxin produced by this germ is very damaging to the body's organs and produces death in about 70 percent of untreated cases.

What to Do

Medical care should be arranged at once. It is not possible to reverse the damage already done, but if the victim can receive the antitoxin prepared especially for this disease early in its course, his chances of survival are better than after the disease is established.

B. *By Mushrooms*. Several varieties of mushroomlike plants are poisonous. Many persons claim they can tell the difference between the poisonous and the edible. Danger of making a mistake, however, indicates the only safe course lies in obtaining mushrooms from commercial sources. The poisonous mushroom itself contains the toxin that damages the body's cells and causes death in more than half the cases of ingestion.

Symptoms occur several hours after the poisonous mushrooms have been eaten. They include abdominal pain, vomiting, and diarrhea, progressing in many cases to shock, convulsions, unconsciousness, and death after several days.

What to Do

Arrange medical aid as soon as the condition is suspected. First-aid treatment consists of absolute bed rest and, if the victim is not already vomiting, of emptying the stomach by in-

ducing vomiting. (See *To Induce Vomiting* under **PROCEDURE E** on page 334.) **Keep the victim warm and quiet to reduce the danger of shock.**

C. *By Salmonella Infection (Salmonellosis)*. This is caused by a group of bacteria known as the salmonellas, introduced into the body by contaminated food, especially meat and meat products, but also eggs, especially duck eggs. Contamination may be caused by disease in the animal itself or by careless handling of food. This type of infection often involves several persons who have eaten food from the same source.

Symptoms develop eight to twenty-four hours after the contaminated food has been eaten. These consist of abdominal cramps, nausea, watery diarrhea, and possibly mild fever associated with chilling.

The acute phase of the illness lasts about two days. Some mild and some severe illnesses may occur among persons infected at the same time and place.

What to Do

It is questionable if an effort should be made to terminate the diarrhea, for this is a natural means of ridding the body of the toxins which the contaminating germ produces. However, pectins absorb toxins, hence the common employment of apple juice, scraped raw apple, blackberry juice, et cetera, as home remedies for diarrhea may help. For severe cases medical advice should be arranged.

D. *By Shellfish*. This is caused by eating shellfish which have absorbed poisonous substances from their food. The same kind of shellfish may produce this poisoning at one time of year but not at another, though the danger is not limited to a specific season. Shellfish from Pacific coastal areas should not be eaten between May 1 and October 31, if at all, since shellfish, including crabs, are scavengers and are frequently infected with coliform organisms, including typhoid.

The symptoms include paralysis of certain muscles, including those of the neck, chest, and diaphragm, thus causing impairment of breathing. The digestive organs may also be affected, and there is often a reddish-blue skin rash with severe itching.

What to Do

Medical attention is urgent in these cases, for sometimes the swelling of the tissues of the larynx interferes suddenly with breathing. Epsom salts may be given as a cathartic to hasten the removal of the poison from the intestines. Because the victim is already emptying his stomach spontaneously, it is usually not necessary to induce vomiting.

E. *By Staphylococcus*. This type of food poisoning results from the rapid multiplication of the Staphylococcus bacterium in food allowed to remain for a while at room temperature before serving. It can be prevented by rigid surveillance of food handlers to prevent gross contamination as from infected fingers, and by adequate refrigeration of food once it has been prepared. These germs, when allowed to multiply, produce a highly poisonous toxin which is not destructible by subsequent cooking of the food.

Symptoms consist of nausea, vomiting, abdominal pain, and diarrhea, of abrupt onset soon after eating the offending food, such as cream pastries. Many a banquet has been broken up in this way. The illness is often confused with "intestinal flu." Death seldom occurs, although in severe cases the victim's condition approaches the stage of shock.

What to Do

There is no specific treatment. The victim usually recovers spontaneously.

BY GASOLINE (See *By Kerosene, Gasoline, Benzene, Naphtha.*)

BY HAIR REMOVERS (See *By Depilatories.*)

POISONS

BY HEPTACHLOR (See *By DDT.*)

BY INSECTICIDES (See *By Arsenic; By DDT; By Moth Repellents; By Nicotine; By Parathion; By Phosphorus; By Sodium Fluoride.*)

BY IODINE

Iodine is contained in a popular antiseptic preparation, Betadine, used for cuts and breaks in the skin. When such an iodine-containing preparation is taken internally, the victim becomes thirsty, pale, nauseated, and may have blood in the stool. There may be painful urination and/or convulsions.

Evidences of iodine poisoning are a brownish stain on the lips and on the lining of the mouth and a yellow or blue color in the vomitus.

What to Do

First, get the victim to drink a lot of fluid—milk, barley water, starch solution, or a thin mixture of flour stirred into water—three or four glasses of it. Then make him vomit by placing your finger far back in the victim's throat. He should then drink more of one of the fluids mentioned above or take a liberal drink of egg white.

BY IRON (FERROUS AND FERRIC COMPOUNDS)

As little as three grams of ferrous sulfate has proved fatal in children. Serious shock may ensue (as late as twenty to forty-eight hours afterward) because of the corrosive effect of the poison on the gastrointestinal tract. Vomiting, abdominal pain, diarrhea due to the local caustic action, weakness, rapid pulse, pallor, and cyanosis may develop rapidly.

What to Do

While waiting for professional help, have the victim drink a demulcent such as milk or milk of magnesia. Induce vomiting by syrup of ipecac (see *To Induce Vomiting* under PROCEDURE E on page 334 of this volume). Shock should be treated in the hospital emergency room.

BY KEROSENE, GASOLINE, BENZENE, NAPHTHA

The usual accident resulting in this type of poisoning occurs when a child discovers a container partly filled with clear fluid and, on impulse, drinks it. The symptoms depend on the effect of the poison on the brain and lungs. At first there may be a stage of excitement, followed by mental depression and unconsciousness. The greatest danger comes from irritation of the lungs as the poisonous substance is carried there after being absorbed into the blood. Death, when it occurs, is due to this damage to the lungs.

What to Do

Follow PROCEDURE B on page 334 of this volume.

BY LEAD

Lead may be taken into the body by eating substances which contain lead, by inhaling lead-containing fumes, or by absorption of lead through the skin. For children, the usual cause is the swallowing of dried paint, as when a teething child bites the paint on his crib or on his toys. Fortunately, lead is not used as commonly in paints now as in former years.

For adults, lead poisoning is usually related to occupation—as with painters, storage-battery workers, and those who handle tetraethyl lead in the gasoline industry. Consumption of alcohol makes the nerves more prone to the adverse effects of lead poisoning.

Symptoms may be acute or chronic, depending on the amount of lead and the rate at which it has been taken into the body. Most symptoms relate to the digestive organs or the nervous system: metallic taste, dry throat, thirst, pain in the abdomen, vomiting, constipation, headache, drowsiness, convulsions, and paralysis of certain muscles, particularly the extensors of the wrist. Anemia is typical of chronic lead poisoning.

What to Do

For the acute case. Even though the

victim may have already vomited, have him drink two to four glasses (less for a small child) of water containing one tablespoonful of magnesium sulfate (Epsom salts) per glass.

Then induce vomiting as under PROCEDURE E, page 334. After the victim vomits, have him drink a little more of the magnesium sulfate solution and retain it.

Early care consists in keeping the victim warm in bed. Continued care should be carefully supervised by a physician, who will arrange a chemical treatment designed to remove lead from the body's other tissues and to prevent permanent damage to the patient's kidneys.

Treatment for chronic lead poisoning should be supervised by a physician.

BY LINDANE (See *By DDT*.)

BY LYE

Poisoning by lye is tragically common among small children. Lye is contained in drain-pipe cleaner, some washing powders, and some paint removers.

The first symptom is burning pain extending from the mouth, through the esophagus, to the stomach. Swallowing becomes difficult. Membranes of the mouth and throat first appear white, then brown, then ulcerated with bleeding surfaces. The victim's pulse and breathing are rapid. If he survives, scar formation later produces stricture (narrowing) of the esophagus.

What to Do

Follow PROCEDURE C on page 334 of this volume.

BY MALATHION (See *By Parathion*.)

BY METHOXYCHLOR (See *By DDT*.)

BY METHYL ALCOHOL (See *By Alcohol—Methyl Alcohol*.)

BY MOTH REPELLENTS CONTAINING NAPHTHALENE

Mothballs and moth repellents are a frequent cause of poisoning in children because of their easy accessibility. Products which contain naphthalene may cause severe damage to liver and kidneys.

Symptoms of naphthalene poisoning are cramps in the abdomen, nausea, vomiting, burning pain on passing urine, discoloration of the urine (brown or black), mental depression, convulsions, and unconsciousness.

What to Do

Early treatment requires emptying the stomach (see *To Induce Vomiting* under PROCEDURE E on page 334) and then giving large amounts of fluid to decrease the concentration of the poison in the kidneys.

Avoid giving the victim any oily or fatty substances by mouth. Avoid the use of castor oil and of foods high in fats. Epsom salts as a cathartic may help to rid the body of the poison. The physician in charge may find it necessary to arrange a blood transfusion to combat anemia.

BY MUSHROOMS (See *By Food—By Mushrooms*.)

BY NAPHTHA (See *By Kerosene, Gasoline, Benzene, Naphtha*.)

BY NAPHTHALENE (See *By Moth Repellents*.)

BY NARCOTICS OVERDOSE

The narcotic drugs are those which dull the senses, relieve pain, soothe the feelings, and induce sleep. These drugs

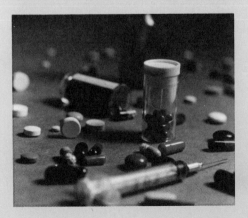

POISONS

commonly lead to addiction. They include heroin, morphine, meperidine, methadone, propoxyphene, cocaine, codeine, and opium. Although the addict develops a certain tolerance for his drug, the serious danger of overdose threatens addicts as well as nonaddicts.

The effect of an overdose, depending on the amount taken and on individual susceptibility, varies between mild stupor and deep coma.

Typically there will be a combination of three symptoms: (1) stupor, (2) "pinpoint" constriction of the pupils of the eyes, and (3) reduced breathing.

What to Do

Call a physician or the fire department's emergency squad. For first aid, stir one or two tablespoonfuls of activated charcoal (powder) into a glass of water and have the patient drink this. (See *Activated Charcoal,* page 334.) Repeat until the patient has drunk two or three glasses of the activated charcoal slurry (less for a small child). If the patient vomits, give more of the activated charcoal for him to retain in his stomach. Keep the patient warm. Give artificial respiration (see *Respiratory Failure* on pages 407-409 of this volume) and pure oxygen to breathe as necessary to maintain respiration. The doctor can administer a specific antagonist drug (naloxone) to offset the effect of the narcotic.

BY NICOTINE

Many of the insecticides commonly used about the garden contain nicotine, as in "Black Leaf 40." This is a very potent poison, interfering, as it does, with the transmission of nerve impulses.

Absorption of nicotine is very rapid and causes symptoms of a hot, burning sensation in the upper digestive organs due to its local caustic action. The fatal dose is relatively small, usually causing death quickly from stoppage of the heart or, a little later, from failure of the respiratory functions. Convulsions may occur in the meantime.

What to Do

Follow **PROCEDURE E on page 334 of this volume. If activated charcoal, as specified in PROCEDURE E, is not available, strong tea may serve as a substitute. Even when activated charcoal has been used, the victim should be given strong tea to drink after the vomiting has ceased. The physician in charge may find it advisable to use certain drugs to maintain the victim's heart action. As for nursing care, the victim should be kept warm in bed. He may also require artificial respiration and resuscitation of the heart. (See *Cardiac Arrest* in this volume, pages 373, 374; also *Respiratory Failure* in this volume, pages 407-409.**

BY PARATHION AND OTHER ORGANIC PHOSPHATE INSECTICIDES

This group of poisons not only includes parathion but also malathion, EPN, TEPP, and OMPA. These have come into wide use for destroying insect pests in crops. Cases of poisoning usually occur among farmers who use these insecticides or among persons or children who live close to where they are used. Persons in these categories should be educated concerning the dangers of these agents and the proper means of protection against poisoning. Poisoning can be caused by inhalation, by absorption through the skin, or by swallowing. The use of protective clothing and the custom of immediate washing of the skin after contact with the poison will serve to prevent many accidents.

Early symptoms of poisoning are dizziness and a feeling of tightness in the chest. At this same early stage, the eye pupils become small. Two or more hours later the symptoms include nausea, abdominal cramps, vomiting, diarrhea, and muscular twitching. In unfavorable cases unconsciousness, convulsions, and death follow.

What to Do

Call for help by having someone

POISONS

phone the emergency squad of your fire department or the poison control center of your nearest city. Using rubber gloves, the first-aider should remove the victim's clothing and wash contaminated skin areas with soap and water. If the poison has been swallowed, then follow PROCEDURE E on page 334 of this volume.

The drug atropine, or atropine plus one of the drugs now available as an antidote for the organic phosphates (such as "2-PAM"), are usually life-saving. These drugs must be administered by a physician. Beyond this, keeping the patient breathing is the important item. Artificial respiration may be required for several hours. (See *Respiratory Failure* in this volume, pages 407-409.)

BY PESTICIDES (See *By Arsenic; By Cyanide; By DDT; By Moth Repellents; By Nicotine; By Parathion; By Phosphorus; By Sodium Fluoride.*)

BY PHOSPHATE (See *By Parathion.*)

BY PHOSPHORUS

Phosphorus was formerly commonly contained in rat poisons and roach poisons. It may also be contained in some fireworks, but those containing phosphorus are now largely outlawed.

Phosphorus poisoning causes burning pain in the mouth, esophagus, and stomach. Diarrhea, nausea, and vomiting with the taste and breath odor of garlic occur. The vomitus and later the stools and urine may appear luminous because of their content of phosphorus. Damage to the liver and kidneys is extensive.

What to Do

Call for professional help. If there has been skin contact with the phosphorus compound, wash the skin thoroughly. If the poison was swallowed, keep the victim warm; use artificial respiration as necessary to keep him breathing (see *Respiratory Failure* on pages 407-409 of this vol-

ume). Do not allow the victim to take fats or oils by mouth. Emergency-room care usually involves rinsing the stomach with a dilute solution of copper sulfate or a dilute solution (1:1000) of potassium permanganate.

BY RAT POISON (See *By Phosphorus.*)

BY ROACH POISON (See *By Phosphorus.*)

BY RODENT POISON (See *By Arsenic; By Cyanide.*)

BY SALICYLATES (See *By Aspirin.*)

BY SALMONELLA (See *By Food—By Salmonella Infection.*)

BY SHELLFISH (See *By Food—By Shellfish.*)

BY SILVER POLISH (See *By Cyanide.*)

BY SODIUM FLUORIDE

Ant powders and roach powders often contain sodium fluoride. This white powder resembles in appearance baking soda, baking powder, or flour. Cases of poisoning therefore often result when the cook or housewife fails to read the label or carelessly stores the product with foodstuffs. If untreated, the victim may die within eight hours.

Symptoms include excessive production of saliva, abdominal cramps, vomiting of blood, failure of respiration, and heart failure (convulsions may occur). The kidneys are subject to severe damage.

What to Do

Get the victim to drink lime water, milk, or powdered chalk stirred into water. Then induce vomiting with syrup of ipecac as instructed in *To Induce Vomiting* under PROCEDURE E on page 334 of this volume. After vomiting, the victim should drink more lime water, milk, or chalk slurry. Keep the victim quiet and warm. From here on the victim should be under a physician's care.

POISONS

BY STAPHYLOCOCCUS (See *By Food—By Staphylococcus.*)

BY STRYCHNINE

Death by strychnine poisoning is terrible, and the symptoms, even in cases which survive, are most alarming.

Strychnine poisoning causes involuntary spasms of the muscles and generalized convulsions. Typically, the muscles contract in a way that pulls the victim's body into a grotesque arched position with head pulled backward between the shoulders. There is usually difficulty in breathing.

What to Do

Call at once for professional help. The first effort must be to control the convulsions. Keeping the victim quiet in a darkened room with absence of all distracting stimuli will help. It may be necessary for the physician to give an anesthetic intravenously or by rectum to control the convulsions before the stomach can be emptied. Using a stomach tube, rinse the stomach with several glassfuls of activated charcoal slurry (one to two tablespoonfuls of the activated charcoal powder to the glass). Artificial respiration (see *Respiratory Failure* on pages 407-409 of this volume) with the administration of oxygen may be necessary.

BY THALLIUM (See *By Depilatories.*)

BY TOADSTOOLS (See *By Food—By Mushrooms.*)

BY TOXAPHENE (See *By DDT.*)

BY TRANQUILIZERS

The consequences of overdoses of tranquilizers or the ingestion of these by mistake are not as serious as in the case of barbiturates. The usual symptoms of overdose of a tranquilizer are deep sleep or unconsciousness. In occasional cases, convulsions may develop after the initial period of sleep. There may also be depression of breathing and a dangerous drop in blood pressure.

What to Do

The case should be cared for by a physician or in a hospital emergency room. Emptying the stomach by stomach tube and administering counteractive drugs are the usual procedures.

BY WOOD ALCOHOL (See *By Alcohol —Methyl Alcohol.*)

First Aid for Emergencies

What This Chapter Contains

This chapter contains instructions on how to deal with common emergencies until a doctor takes charge of the patient. The material is arranged as indicated in the following skeleton table of contents for the chapter.

In searching for information on any emergency not listed below, please use the General Index at the back of any volume of *You and Your Health*.

The Purpose of This Chapter

An emergency is anything that immediately threatens the physical welfare or the life of a person. It is the purpose of this chapter to give concise instruction to persons, not medically trained, on how to render proper emergency care to someone suddenly taken ill or injured.

It is not expected that the reading of this chapter will make anyone proficient enough to take a job in a hospital. Nor will it enable anyone to give all the care that an emergency case may need. In most of the emergency situations considered, however, the suggested care will tide the patient over until a paramedic or a physician can take charge. And this concept typifies the intent of the chapter—to enable any person, medically trained or not, to become a friend in need and thus, perhaps, to save a life.

In many cases of emergency what is not done is just as important to the victim's welfare as what is done. Many times throughout this chapter the reader is warned about what he should *not* do.

The word *emergency* implies to most people that time is of the essence, that what is done must be done at once, that speed at all costs is required. Not necessarily true. A rapid appraisal of the seriousness of a situation is, of course, important. Certain conditions, such as copious bleeding, must be handled quickly and properly before life ebbs away. But in other conditions blind haste may entail greater danger than judicious delay. Many a life has been snuffed out because a person with a broken neck was handled carelessly while being removed from a wrecked car. Often an injured person's prospects of survival are reduced by crowding him into a cramped position in the back seat of a passenger car rather than waiting for an ambulance.

So this chapter is designed to help the person who must handle an emergency to be reasonable in what he does and to act in harmony with the best interests of the victim. Of course you can't carry this big book with you wherever you go. You should, however, prepare yourself for possible emergencies by becoming familiar with the instruction in this chapter, especially if you are interested in first-aid work, if you are active in outdoor recreation, if you or your associates are engaged in hazardous pursuits, or if you are responsible for the welfare of children.

By studying a few items each day and by reviewing a few of the old ones, you will soon become familiar with what to do. This knowledge may enable you to save life—possibly at some unexpected time, possibly soon.

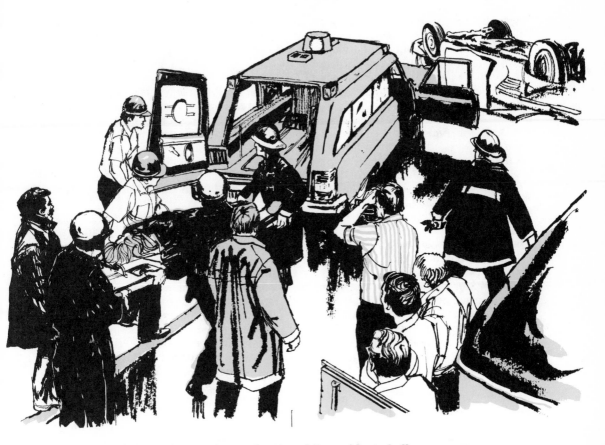

Possibility of an unexpected automobile accident challenges every citizen to preparedness as a first-aider.

First Things to Do in a Grave Emergency

Persons suddenly injured or stricken with illness do not have labels on them telling what the trouble is and what help should be given. So the person who renders aid must evaluate the circumstances and the condition of the victim and decide what to do. The better trained this person is and the more careful and accurate his observations, the better care he will be able to give. Suppose that *you* are the person who must give emergency care to someone suddenly taken sick or injured. Don't waste time in bemoaning your lack of training. Get on with the job and do the best you can; that is all that can be expected of anyone.

If other people are around, you may ask yourself, Am I the best qualified to give aid? If not, then let the better qualified person take charge while you follow his instructions. But unless you know that someone else can render better emergency care than you can, take over and tell others what to do without thought of hurt feelings. If someone else tries to replace you, question his qualifications. You be the judge of who is best able to give emergency care. While in charge, do not let others disregard your instructions. Use a firm voice, and ask for the help you need.

The following suggestions are intended to help you think logically when handling an emergency.

A. *Keep calm.* Even though you feel

nervous, put on the act of being calm and deliberate. This will help you to think clearly and will help the victim, if conscious, to avoid psychological panic that might throw him into shock. Keeping calm also inspires the confidence of those helping you.

B. *If the emergency consists of a sudden illness,* try to get in touch with a doctor. Send someone else to phone while you continue caring for the victim. Have this person tell the doctor about the circumstances and the victim's present condition and ask for advice on what to do. If a doctor cannot be reached, direct the call to the emergency room of a hospital.

C. *When poison has been swallowed,* place an emergency call at once for a physician, the emergency squad of the fire department, or a poison control center. Preferably this call should be placed by a second responsible person so that the first-aider can devote all his time to the care of the patient. In placing the call, give as much information as possible: the patient's name, any clue as to the nature of the poison (such as the wording on the label on the container), the patient's symptoms, and the patient's exact location. The person placing the call should ask for instructions on how to care for the patient until help arrives or while the patient is being taken to an emergency room. For further information on first aid for poisoning, see the previous chapter, beginning on page 333.

D. *When the victim has been burned,* follow the instructions beginning on page 369 of this chapter, on how to care for the particular kind of burn with which you are concerned.

E. *In case of an accident,* it may be more important to have someone call an ambulance than to phone for a doctor. Ambulance crews are trained in first aid and therefore can do the best for the victim while taking him to the nearest hospital. If you are in an iso-lated area where an ambulance cannot reach you soon, call for a policeman or a sheriff.

F. *Don't be in a hurry to move an injured person* unless it is essential for his safety. First, try to determine the nature of the problem. In some serious illnesses and injuries, moving the victim without proper equipment or before first aid is rendered may cause death. Do not allow the injured person to sit up, much less to stand or try to walk.

G. *When a person is not breathing,* begin giving artificial respiration at once. This is of first priority, for one may die within a matter of three or four minutes without air. Mouth-to-mouth breathing, in which you force your own breath into the patient's mouth and thus into his lungs (while holding his nostrils closed), is the simplest and most effective method of artificial respiration. For further instruction on giving artificial respiration, see the item RESPIRATORY FAILURE beginning on page 407 of this chapter.

H. *Next in importance is to check for bleeding.* The simplest way to control continued loss of large amounts of blood from an injured part is to place a clean cloth right into the wound and exert firm, continuous pressure. For additional instruction on the control of bleeding, see the item BLEEDING beginning on page 366 of this chapter.

I. *When the victim is unconscious,* care for him as best you can right where you are until conditions are favorable for moving him. Make sure that he continues to breathe, either naturally or by artificial respiration. Don't try to rouse an unconscious person. Don't try to give him fluids by mouth. Remove loose objects such as false teeth so that these will not interfere with his breathing. Keep him covered to conserve his body heat. For further information see the item UNCONSCIOUSNESS in this chapter beginning on page 417.

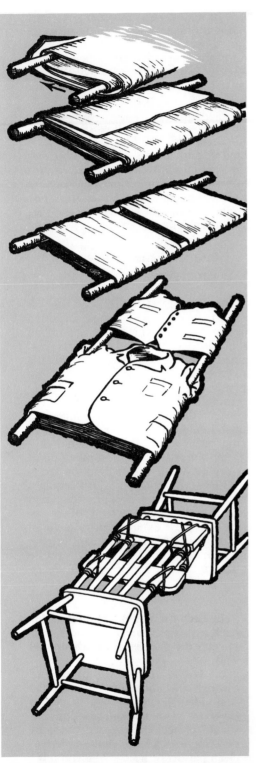

J. *Look for evidences of fractured bones*. The most serious possibility here is that of a broken neck or a broken back. See the item FRACTURES beginning on page 392 of this chapter.

K. *General care of the waiting victim*. While waiting for instructions from a doctor or while waiting for the ambulance to arrive, follow certain principles of general care such as these:

1. Loosen tight clothing which may constrict the victim's neck or waist.

2. Do not administer any form of alcoholic drink.

3. Conserve body heat by covering the victim with a blanket or with coats. Be mindful of the danger of burning the skin of an unconscious person by the use of heating devices. (See the item SHOCK beginning on page 410 of this chapter, and the item CIRCULATORY SHOCK in chapter 9, volume 2.)

4. When the victim vomits, turn his head gently to one side to avoid the danger of his choking on the vomitus. If he is lying on the ground, dig a little trench into which the vomitus may flow or lay a sheet of newspaper beside his head. Using a handkerchief or paper tissue, gently wipe away the remaining vomitus from the victim's face and lips.

L. *When the time comes to move the victim,* take care so as not to change the relative position of the parts of his body. His body should be kept straight and horizontal, not allowed to sag, jackknife, or twist. If the victim must be moved from where his body rests on the highway, he can be slid lengthwise on a blanket. The blanket for this sledding purpose can be placed under the victim by rolling him gently to one side while half of the blanket is tucked under him. Then, by rolling him to the opposite side, the tucked portion of the blanket may be straightened.

Another way of transporting an injured or very sick person is by the use of an improvised stretcher made from two poles placed through the arms of two jackets, the jacket arms having

Examples of how improvised stretchers for moving an accident victim can be made.

351

EMERGENCIES

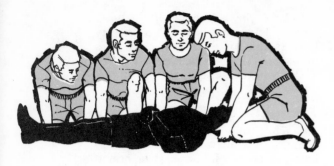

Cooperative effort, carefully synchronized, is essential in moving the victim of an accident.

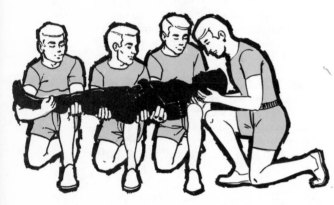

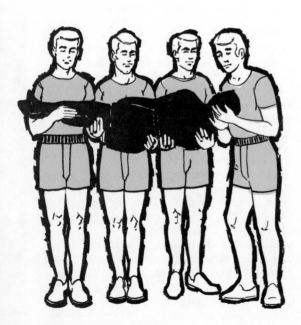

been turned wrong side out.

Still another proper way to move an injured person is by the cooperative effort of four persons who work carefully together as they lift and move the victim. Three take their position on one side of the victim, one at his shoulder, one at his hip, and one at his knees. If one side is injured, they work from the uninjured side. The fourth person is located at the victim's head, and his one responsibility is to lift the head in unison with the other three persons in such a way that the head does not change position in relation to the victim's shoulders.

Common Emergencies and Emergency Procedures

ABDOMINAL INJURIES

We consider here injuries sustained by violence in which the abdominal wall has been torn open or has sustained a stab wound. Gunshot wounds are considered on page 396 of this same chapter.

Abdominal injuries are serious because of the possibility of damage to the abdominal organs, the possibility of hemorrhage within the abdominal cavity, and the grave danger of infection of the organs and tissues within the abdomen. Every abdominal injury requires careful examination by a physician and definitive treatment which often involves surgical exploration. The function of the first-aider is to care for the victim until an ambulance arrives or the patient is received at a hospital emergency room.

What to Do

1. Keep the victim lying flat on his back with a pad under his knees so as to relax the muscles of the abdominal wall.

2. If the intestines protrude through the abdominal wound, the first-aider should not try to return these to their normal position but should protect the exposed tissue by covering with a clean cloth, a piece of clean plastic, or a sheet of metal foil.

3. The protective covering should be held in place by a bandage firmly applied but not tight enough to interfere with the circulation of blood in the tissues.

4. When the abdominal injury consists of a stab wound but no protrusion of abdominal organs, the wound should be covered by a clean pad of cloth or a bandage.

5. Do not give fluids or solid foods lest such interfere with the surgical procedure that may have to be performed.

6. Keep the patient warm by covering him with a blanket or coats.

ABRASIONS

An abrasion is an injury to the skin caused by scuffing or forceful scraping. Usually the outer part of the skin is lost at the time of the injury so that the area oozes straw-colored fluid or blood. A skinned knee is a common example.

Small particles of dirt, sand, or other foreign substances are often ground into the injured area. An abrasion has usually been grossly contaminated, and the wound must have proper cleansing as quickly as possible.

What to Do

1. Cleanliness comes first. To begin, the operator should wash his own hands with abundant soap and water.

2. Remove clothing from the injured area and wash the skin area around the site of injury. Use a clean cloth or gauze and abundant soap and water. In washing, make strokes away from the injured area, not toward it.

3. Starting with a new piece of clean cloth or gauze, wash the injured area itself with soap and water or swab it with an antiseptic solution such as pHisoHex. Be gentle but thorough. Remove the dirt that has been ground into the wound. Use forceps (sterilized by passing quickly through a flame) to remove the particles of dirt, and scissors (sterilized) to snip off tags of skin or torn tissue.

4. Apply some mild antiseptic solution (as hydrogen peroxide) either by pouring the liquid into the wound or by gently dabbing some on with sterile gauze soaked in the antiseptic solution.

5. Cover the injured area, preferably with a nonadherent dressing or sterile gauze held in place by a bandage.

6. It is advisable to have a booster dose of tetanus toxoid administered at a hospital.

7. Replace the dressing with a fresh one after twenty-four hours or at any time when it becomes unduly soiled. If the bandage tends to stick to the injured area, soak it loose by the use of hydrogen peroxide solution.

8. If the injured area becomes unusually painful or swollen or if radiating red streaks appear, consult a physician for treatment of the infection.

9. Alternating hot and cold applications will increase the circulation of blood through the affected area, thus aiding in the control of infection and hastening the process of healing. For details, see the item BRUISES in this chapter, number 3 of What to Do, page 369.

ACCIDENT, AUTOMOBILE

The main characteristic of injuries from motor vehicle accidents is that they are multiple—several parts or organs of the body are injured at the same time. The part of the body most commonly injured is the head.

The gravest mistake a first-aider might make at the site of a motor vehicle accident is to act too hastily. Unless the injured person is in danger from fire or from oncoming traffic, it is best not to move him until such time as adequate help is available.

What to Do

Keep in mind the first-aider's order of priorities. *First*, attention to the victim's breathing; *second*, attention to the possibility of bleeding; *third*, attention to the danger that the victim may choke on his vomit; and *fourth*, preparation of the patient for

EMERGENCIES

transportation to a hospital.

1. To facilitate breathing, an unconscious victim should be turned to lie on his side *(unless it appears that he has a severe injury of the back or of the neck)* and his mouth cleared of dirt, stones, and false teeth (if present) so that he can breathe easily through his mouth. Using a handkerchief, grasp his tongue and pull it forward, thus preventing it from falling back into his throat and interfering with breathing. If the chest has been seriously injured, check for any opening in the chest wall through which air might be passing as the victim breathes. If so, this "sucking wound" should be covered at once with anything available to prevent the passage of air through the wound. Use a folded cloth or a folded newspaper and bind this firmly to the chest wall so the patient will breathe through his mouth without losing air through the wound. If the victim does not breathe, artificial respiration should be administered, preferably by the mouth-to-mouth method.

2. Next, look for severe hemorrhage. Do not bother yet with mild bleeding and superficial wounds. Concern yourself, rather, with blood that may be spurting from a severed artery or welling up into a deep wound. Usually this can be controlled by direct pressure over the area or by a firmly applied bandage, preferably white.

3. Keep the injured person's mouth and nose free from obstruction by vomitus. Otherwise, fatal choking may ensue. Turn the victim on his side, or, if he is lying face down, turn his head to one side so that the vomitus will flow away from his face.

4. If the accident victim has been severely burned, the burned area should be covered lightly with whatever soft cloth may be available such as a handkerchief, a shirt, or a sheet. Never should a blanket be placed in direct contact with a burned area of the body.

5. While awaiting the arrival of the ambulance, keep the injured person's body warm by covering it with one or two blankets or extra coats.

6. In preparing an injured person for transportation to the hospital, keep in mind that his back or neck may have been broken and handle the victim accordingly. Moving him carelessly may permanently damage the spinal cord.

7. If possible, arrange for someone to accompany the victim to the hospital—someone informed as to the nature of the accident and the first-aid measures already used. Otherwise, this information should be jotted down and sent along with the victim.

ASTHMA ATTACK

In asthma an abnormal condition of the membrane-lined tubes which serve the lungs interferes with breathing. These tubes (the bronchi) become swollen and congested and contain an unusual mount of mucus. The patient experiences more difficulty in expelling air from the lungs than in drawing it in.

The typical picture is that of a child, sitting upright in bed with his arms extended at his sides, pressing downward against the bed. His skin appears blue because he cannot bring the normal amount of air into and out of his lungs. His efforts at breathing are accompanied by characteristic wheezing, particularly distressing when air is being forced out of the lungs. The large veins of the neck are conspicuous, and the heart is pounding rapidly.

In approximately half the cases, asthma is caused by the patient's sensitivity to certain pollens or dust in the air, or to certain foods or drugs. In the remaining half, asthma seems to result from infections of the organs of breathing, the patient having become sensitive to the products of the germs causing the infection.

What to Do

The successful treatment of asthma varies from case to case, depending upon the cause. Here we are concerned more with relieving the symptoms of asthma at the time of an attack than with the long-range cure of the disease. For additional information, consult the General Index for the item, *Asthma*.

If the patient has had previous asthmatic attacks, he probably has learned to use a medication for the control of his symptoms. If so, this medication should now be administered to relieve the acute attack.

For the immediate treatment of asthma, other than by medication, try giving the patient a drink of hot milk, Postum, or just plain hot water. This may relax the tissues in the air passages.

A steam inhalation accompanied by a hot foot bath may bring relief. If no mechanical vaporizer is available, moist air may be provided by conducting steam from a pan of boiling water through a paper cone to the area of the patient's face. Care must be taken not to burn the face or the sensitive membranes of the nose.

If these simple remedies do not relieve the attack, a physician should be consulted by phone, or the patient should be taken to a hospital emergency room where he can receive such medication as epinephrine which will relieve the obstruction in the air passages.

BANDAGING METHODS

Why a Bandage? A bandage is an external cover designed to protect an injury from contamination during the healing process. Examples are the small, ready-prepared adhesive bandage available at the drugstore; or its larger counterpart, a sterile gauze bandage designed to be held in place by a cloth wrapping. A bandage may also be used in cases of fracture or deep injury to hold splints in place or to prevent movement of the injured part. Another use is to exert firm pressure on the underlying tissues, helpful, for example, in the control of bleeding.

Principles of Bandaging. A bandage should be snug but not so tight as to impede the circulation of blood. Even for one experienced in bandaging, the question of how tight is so difficult to answer that he may have to remove and replace a bandage a time or two in order to find the happy medium. Even then, the swelling of tissues may decline and the bandage become too loose, or the injured tissues may swell and the bandage become too tight. A bandage applied to the leg, the arm, or the finger should be double-checked occasionally to make sure the tissues beyond the bandage are warm and of normal color.

When a bandage is used to hold a wet dressing in place, the cloth of which the bandage is made may become moist and shrink and thus make the bandage tighter. This possibility emphasizes again the need for occasional checking.

It may be advisable to place strips of adhesive tape over a bandage to keep it from shifting. These can extend beyond the bandage so as to anchor it to the skin. The loose end of the bandage can be fastened either by the use of adhesive tape or, in the case of a roller bandage, by tearing or cutting the bandage down the center for a few inches, tying the loose ends together with a simple knot, and then using them as straps, one passing in one direction and one the other, to serve as a final tie.

Kinds of Bandages:

A. *The Roller Bandage.* This is made of muslin cloth or of gauze prepared especially for bandages and designed to stretch slightly so that it conforms to the shape of the part being bandaged. Roller bandage material, because usually sterile when packaged, can be applied safely to a wound which has been cleansed. Roller bandage material comes in various widths from about one-half inch to four inches, the narrower widths being used for fingers and toes. The accompanying drawings indicate how roller bandages can be applied to various parts of the body.

Roller bandages may need to be reinforced by the use of adhesive strips, either to hold the roller bandage in place or to add support to the injured part as,

355

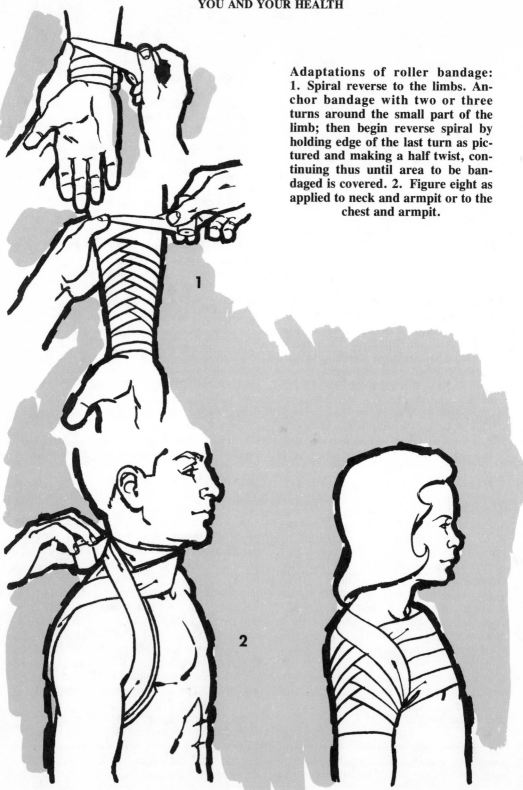

Adaptations of roller bandage: 1. Spiral reverse to the limbs. Anchor bandage with two or three turns around the small part of the limb; then begin reverse spiral by holding edge of the last turn as pictured and making a half twist, continuing thus until area to be bandaged is covered. 2. Figure eight as applied to neck and armpit or to the chest and armpit.

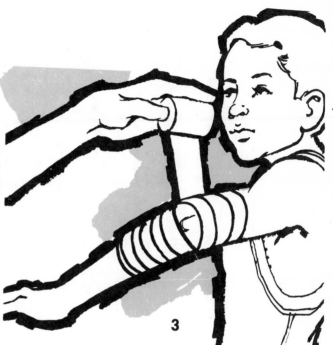

Roller bandages continued: 3. Figure eight to the elbow. This is especially suitable whenever a single bandage needs to be applied above, across, and below the elbow or knee. 4. Multiple cranial.

3

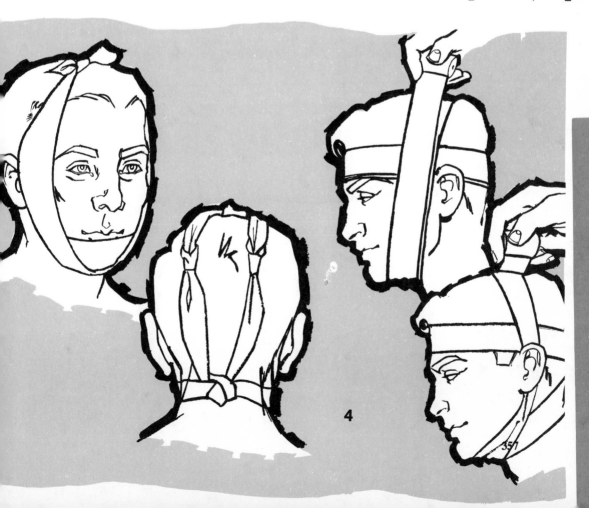

4

E
M
E
R
G
E
N
C
I
E
S

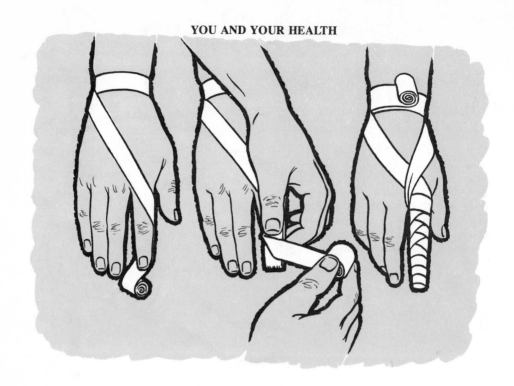

Narrow widths of roller bandages can be used effectively for bandaging a finger, the spiral and recurrent loop technique being used.

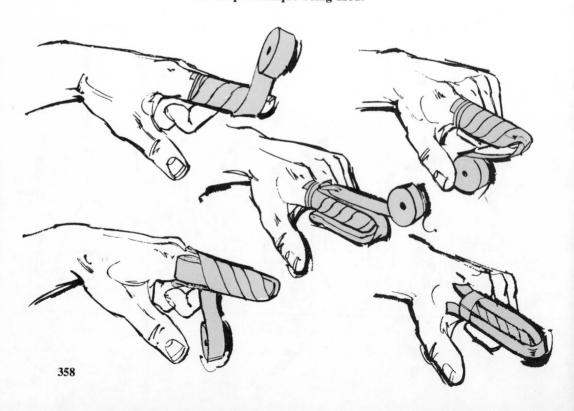

358

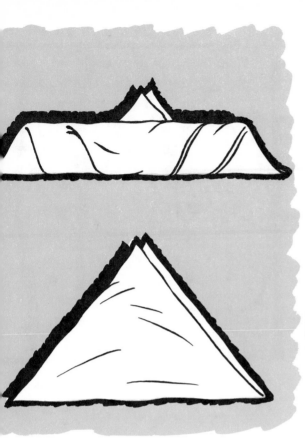

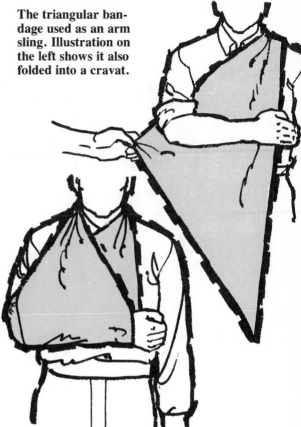

The triangular bandage used as an arm sling. Illustration on the left shows it also folded into a cravat.

for instance, in the case of a sprained ankle.

B. *The Triangular Bandage*. The triangular bandage has several uses, as indicated in the accompanying drawings. This bandage is usually made from a piece of muslin, the size varying with the particular use in each case.

C. *The Cravat Bandage*. The cravat bandage is made from a triangular piece of cloth such as is used for the triangular bandage. The width of the cravat is determined by the number of times the cravat is folded (see illustration). The cravat may be used to bandage the head, the neck, the eye, or the ear. It may also be used for injuries to the hand or forearm, the ankle and leg, or for fractured ribs, as well as for application of a tourniquet. See accompanying drawings here and on next two pages.

Note: A tourniquet should be used only in extreme cases of severe bleeding which cannot be controlled by other means. It is dangerous inasmuch as it shuts off the entire blood supply to the part of the body beyond the tourniquet (see TOURNIQUET on pages 416, 417 of this same chapter).

D. *Gauze Pads or Rolls*. Sterile gauze pads can be obtained from the drugstore in packages which can be easily kept in the first-aid kit. Usually when a gauze pad or roll is applied to a wound, it is held in place either by adhesive tape or by a roller bandage. Convenient ready-made bandages of gauze and adhesive tape are available in various small sizes at the drugstore or in most markets. This type of bandage is commonly and conveniently used for abrasions, lacerations, and open wounds. In the case of a wound involving the palm of the hand, it is convenient to place a roll of sterile gauze in the victim's palm with the fingers grasping the roll loosely. The hand is then bandaged in this position by the use of a roller bandage.

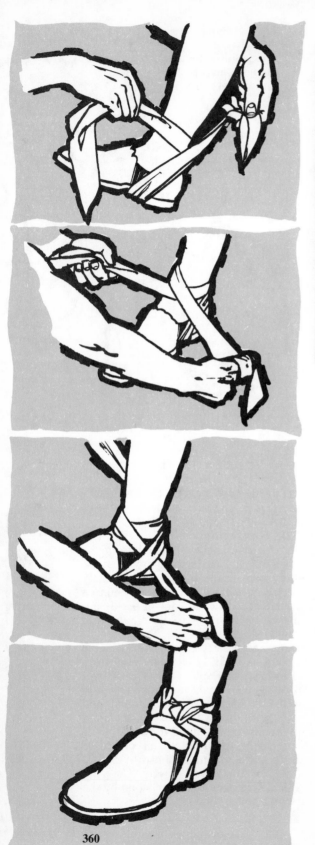

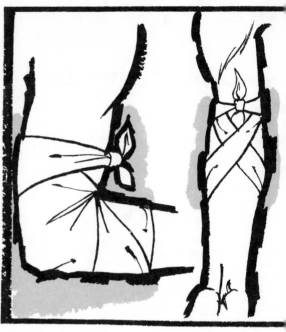

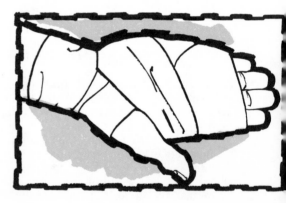

The cravat, made by folding the triangular bandage at least twice, makes an ideal bandage for immobilizing the joint in case of a sprained ankle. It may also be used for injuries to the arm, hand, and other areas.

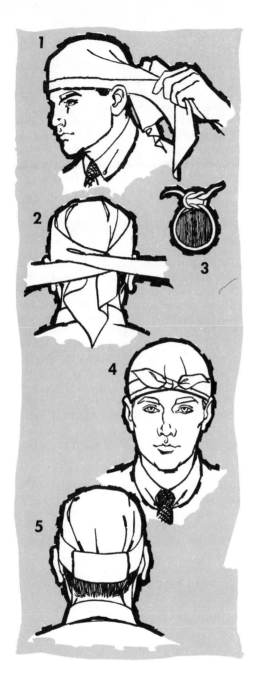

How to apply an open triangular bandage to the chest: 1. Pass apex of triangle over shoulder to the back on injured side and drop base downward in front so that its midpoint is directly below shoulder. 2. Carry ends around to back and tie below the same shoulder. 3. Bring longer end of the knot up and tie to apex hanging over the shoulder and down the back, thus completing the bandaging operation.

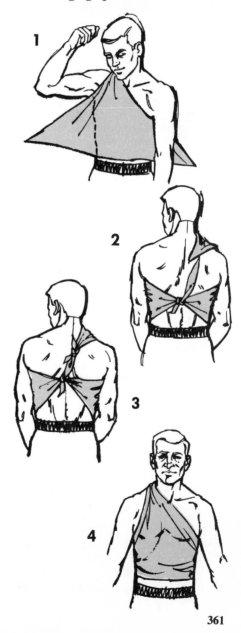

Bandage to the head: 1. Fold two-inch hem along base of triangle. With hem to the outside, pull two ends backward (above ears) making bandage snug across forehead. 2, 3, 4. Cross ends at the back (do not tie) and bring them round again to the front and tie in the center of the forehead. 5. Pull apex of triangle downward at back, making bandage fit snugly over the head; then fold upward and tuck in.

361

BITES

(See also the item STINGS, pages 413, 414.)

A. ANIMAL BITES (including DOG BITE)

B. SNAKE BITE

C. SPIDER BITE

D. TARANTULA BITE

E. TICK BITES

A. *Animal Bites.* Here we include bites by dogs, cats, and wild animals such as squirrels and bats which, when they bite, abrade the skin, puncture it, or tear the flesh. These bites are especially serious because of the strong probability that infection has been introduced. Also, the dread disease of rabies may be transmitted to the human by the bite of an animal. Dogs are by no means the only animals that can transmit rabies, it now being recognized that wild animals such as bats, foxes, and others can be infected with this disease and can transmit it to humans through their saliva at the time of a bite.

What to Do

The extent of an animal bite cannot be judged by the appearance of the wound, for the animal's teeth may have done more damage than is apparent.

1. Wash the wound thoroughly with running water to remove as much of the animal's saliva as possible. Continue the washing for at least five minutes, using a clean cloth or gauze sponge with soap or detergent solution. After washing, rinse the wound thoroughly with running water.

2. Cover the wound with a clean dressing and keep the injured part at rest while the victim is being transported.

3. Take the victim to a doctor's office or to the emergency room of a hospital as quickly as possible and give complete information on the circumstances of the animal bite.

4. The rapidity of the development of rabies symptoms depends on the location of the wound. No treatment can cure the disease after symptoms occur. It is presumptuous to delay treatment after possible exposure.

5. The protective treatment consists of a series of intramuscular injections of a special vaccine (diploid cell vaccine) given over a period of twenty-eight days. For further details, see chapter 16, volume 3.

B. *Snakebite.* Snakebites are becoming more common in the United States because of increased interest in outdoor activity. There are four kinds of poisonous snakes in the United States, the bites of which endanger life: (1) rattlesnakes, (2) water moccasins (cottonmouths), (3) copperheads, and (4) coral snakes. The first three are called pit vipers, and these cause 98 percent of the poisonous snakebites in the United States. Pit vipers strike quickly, whereas coral snakes hang on after they bite, moving their jaws in a chewing motion as they sink their fangs into the victim's flesh. The following precautions will help you when hiking to avoid being bitten by a snake:

1. Do not hike alone.

2. Wear protective clothing: boots, trousers, gloves.

3. Do not try to surprise or corner a snake.

4. Do not play with poisonous snakes.

5. When you can't see where you are about to step, prod the ground with a stick.

6. Do not reach into blind holes or rocky ledges.

7. Beware of old piles of wood or rocks and old buildings.

What to Do

First aid for the bites of poisonous snakes is summarized in the accompanying copy of a poster from the American Red Cross. A bite by a nonpoisonous snake may be treated like any simple puncture wound. See the item WOUNDS, PUNCTURE in this same chapter, pages 419, 420.

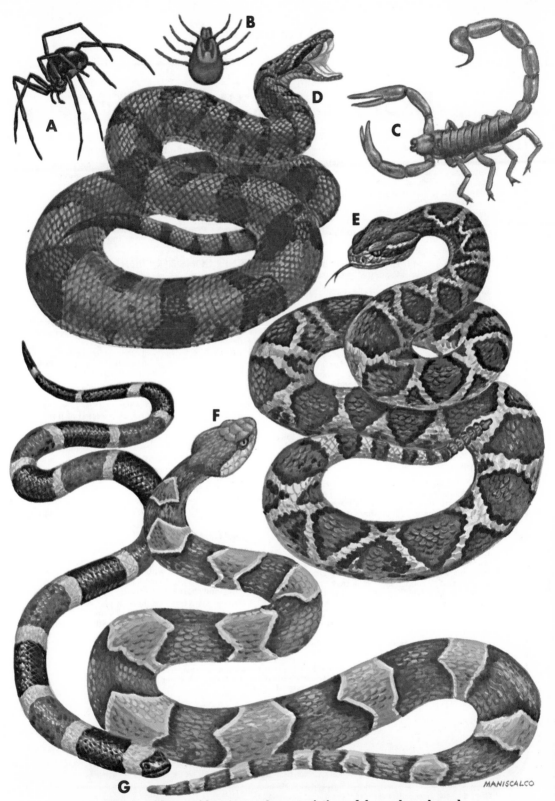

A. Black widow spider (note characteristic red hourglass-shaped mark on underside of the abdomen); B. tick; C. scorpion; D. cottonmouth; E. rattlesnake; F. copperhead; and G. coral snake.

FIRST AID FOR SNAKEBITE

POISONOUS OR NONPOISONOUS

Poisonous or nonpoisonous, a snakebite should have medical attention. A snakebite victim should be taken to a hospital *as quickly as possible,* even in cases when snakebite is only suspected.

FIRST AID

1. As stated above, *get the victim to a hospital fast.* Meanwhile, take the following general first aid measures:
   - Keep the victim from moving around.
   - Keep the victim as calm as possible, preferably lying down.
   - Immobilize the bitten extremity and keep it at or below heart level.

   If a hospital can be reached within 4 to 5 hours and no symptoms develop, this is all that is necessary.

2. *If mild to moderate symptoms develop, apply a constricting band* from 2 to 4 inches above the bite but NOT around a joint (i.e., elbow, knee, wrist, or ankle) and NOT around the head, neck, or trunk. The band should be from ¾ to 1½ inches wide, NOT thin like a rubber band. The band should be snug, but loose enough to slip one finger underneath. Be alert to swelling; loosen the band if it becomes too tight, but do not remove it. To ensure that blood flow has not been stopped, periodically check the pulse in the extremity beyond the bite.

3. *If severe symptoms develop, incisions and suction should be performed immediately.* Apply a constricting band, if not already done, and make a cut in the skin with a sharp sterilized blade through the fang mark(s). Cuts should be no deeper than just through the skin and should be ½ inch long, extending over the suspected venom deposit point (because a snake strikes downward, the deposit point is usually lower than the fang mark). Cuts should be made along the long axis of the limb. DO NOT make cross-cut incisions; DO NOT make cuts on the head, neck, or trunk. Suction should be applied with a suction cup for 30 minutes. If a suction cup is not available, use the mouth. There is little risk to the rescuer who uses his mouth, but it is recommended that the venom not be swallowed and that the mouth be rinsed.

IF THE HOSPITAL IS NOT CLOSE (cannot be reached within from 4 to 5 hours)

1. Continue to try to obtain professional care by transportation of the victim or by communication with a rescue service.

2. *If no symptoms develop,* continue trying to reach the hospital and give the general first aid described above.

3. *If ANY symptoms develop,* apply a constricting band and perform incisions and suction immediately, as described above.

OTHER CONSIDERATIONS

1. *Shock:* Keep the victim lying down and comfortable and maintain body temperature.

2. *Breathing and heartbeat:* If breathing stops, give mouth-to-mouth resuscitation. If breathing stops and there is no pulse, cardiopulmonary resuscitation (CPR) should be performed by those trained to do so.

3. *Identifying the snake:* If the snake can be killed without risk or delay, it should be brought, *with care,* to the hospital for identification.

4. *Cleansing the bitten area:* The bitten area may be washed with soap and water and blotted dry with sterile gauze. Dressings and bandages can be applied, but only for a short period of time.

5. *Cold therapy:* Cold compresses, ice, dry ice, chemical ice packs, spray refrigerants, and other methods of cold therapy are NOT recommended in the first aid treatment of snakebite.

6. *Medicine to relieve pain:* A medicine *not containing aspirin* can be given to the victim for relief of pain. DO NOT give alcohol, sedatives, aspirin, or other medications.

7. *Snakebite kits:* Keep a kit accessible for all outings in snake-infested or primitive areas.

SYMPTOMS

1. *Mild to moderate* symptoms include mild swelling or discoloration and mild to moderate pain at the wound site with tingling sensations, rapid pulse, weakness, dimness of vision, nausea, vomiting, and shortness of breath.

2. *Severe* symptoms include rapid swelling and numbness, followed by severe pain at the wound site. Other effects include pinpoint pupils, twitching, slurred speech, shock, convulsions, paralysis, unconsciousness, and no breathing or pulse.

The information on this poster is based on a report prepared for the American Red Cross by the National Academy of Sciences-National Research Council.

American Red Cross

Snakebite prevention practices that can eliminate needless illness and worry may be learned in a Red Cross first aid course. Call your chapter to enroll.

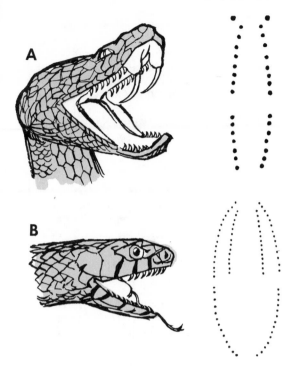

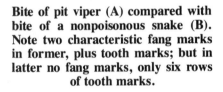

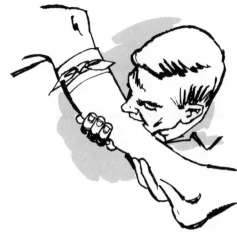

Emergency treatment for snakebite includes suction of wound. This can be done by mouth after making an X-shaped incision across the fang marks left by the bite.

Bite of pit viper (A) compared with bite of a nonpoisonous snake (B). Note two characteristic fang marks in former, plus tooth marks; but in latter no fang marks, only six rows of tooth marks.

C. *Spider Bite*. The spider which causes the greatest discomfort and harm is the female black widow spider, found throughout the Americas. The bite produces a sharp pain locally, followed in about thirty minutes by rigidity of the muscles of the abdomen and abdominal cramps. Weakness, severe pain in the limbs, and even convulsions (especially in children) may come later. The outcome depends on the amount of venom injected, the general vitality of the victim, and the promptness with which treatment is administered. The mortality rate is about 5 percent, with most deaths occurring in children.

What to Do

1. Take the victim to a hospital as quickly as possible. Local treatment at the site of the spider bite is not effective.

2. Warm baths may help to relieve the muscle pain.

3. Antivenin prepared especially for black widow spider bites should be injected intramuscularly as promptly as possible.

D. *Tarantula Bite*. Tarantula bites may be painful but are usually less serious than bites by the black widow spider.

What to Do

1. For a minor involvement, apply cold compresses to the area of the bite.

2. For a more serious involvement in which systemic symptoms develop, apply a constricting band to the affected arm or leg as described in item 2 of First Aid for Snakebite on page 364. Be prepared to give artificial respiration by the mouth-to-mouth method if necessary to keep the victim breathing (see pages 407-409).

E. *Tick Bites*. The bite of a tick not only produces discomfort in the local

365

area where the tick's head is buried in the skin, but it may also transmit infections, some of which are serious.

What to Do

In attempting to remove a tick, one risks the danger that the body will break away, leaving the head still embedded in the skin. To avoid this, turpentine may be applied to the exposed portion of the tick. Or, touching the tick with an extinguished matchhead (still hot) may cause the insect to release its grasp. Another method is to cover the tick and the skin immediately surrounding it with petrolatum (vaseline) or heavy oil. This closes the insect's breathing pores, usually forcing it to dislodge within half an hour. As a last resort, the insect may be removed from the skin by careful manipulation with tweezers, rotating the head counterclockwise.

Following removal, the skin area should be scrubbed with soap and water for about five minutes. If the victim develops a fever within the next few hours, a physician should be consulted, because this symptom may indicate that the tick has transmitted disease-producing germs.

BLEEDING (HEMORRHAGE)

The control of severe bleeding is important as a life-saving measure.

There are two main kinds of bleeding: external and internal. In external bleeding, blood escapes to the outside as when tissues are torn by a cut or by crushing injury. In internal bleeding, blood escapes from a blood vessel into the tissues or into one of the body cavities. A person may die from internal bleeding even though not a drop of blood escapes to the outside.

A person may lose as much as two or three pints of blood and still survive. If a large artery has been severed and bleeding is rapid, it does not take long for this much blood to be lost. The treatment of such bleeding, therefore, must be prompt.

The loss of significant amounts of blood, whether it be by external bleed-ing or internal bleeding, causes certain changes in the body functions. These occur even in a case of internal bleeding and may serve as an aid in determining that bleeding is taking place. For these general symptoms of bleeding, see chapter 6, volume 2. For the meaning of bleeding as it occurs in various parts of the body, see the General Index and the subheadings under the entry *Bleeding*.

A. *External Bleeding.* An injured person should be examined completely as soon as possible to determine whether he is losing blood. Clothing must be removed from parts of the body where blood is seen seeping through.

What to Do

1. Apply direct pressure at the point of bleeding. A sterile gauze dressing, a clean sanitary napkin, or a freshly laundered piece of cloth should be placed over or into the wound and held there firmly. Only the amount of pressure necessary to stop the bleeding should be used, for excessive pressure may interfere with the blood supply to other parts. If such pressure controls the bleeding, a bandage may be necessary to hold the temporary dressing in place until the patient reaches the hospital. When pressure over the wound does not control the bleeding, see the next item.

2. Use pressure points to control persistent bleeding, particularly when blood comes in spurts as when an artery has been severed. The accompanying diagram shows the locations in the body where the arteries run near enough to the surface to be closed off by pressure from the outside. Bleeding from a large artery will seldom stop of its own accord, for the flow of blood is too brisk to permit the formation of a blood clot. In such a case, pressure over the proper pressure point may need to be maintained until a physician ties off the bleeding artery. Obviously, the control of bleeding at a pressure point applies only to

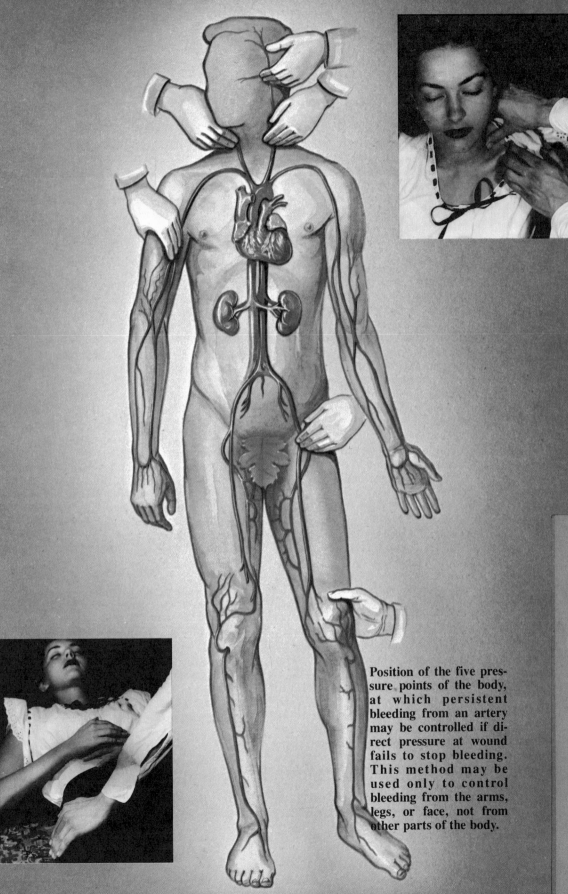

Position of the five pressure points of the body, at which persistent bleeding from an artery may be controlled if direct pressure at wound fails to stop bleeding. This method may be used only to control bleeding from the arms, legs, or face, not from other parts of the body.

bleeding from an arm, a leg, or the face. Do not try to control the bleeding of the head, neck, or body by applying pressure at pressure points.

3. Apply a tourniquet as a LAST RESORT when severe bleeding from an arm or a leg cannot be controlled by the methods mentioned above. Use of a tourniquet can result in permanent injury to the arm or leg, with the probability of amputation. If blood is being lost so rapidly, however, as to endanger life, it is better to run the risk of amputation than to permit the victim to bleed to death. A wide band of cloth such as is used for a bandage or such as may be torn from a sheet or a shirt is folded to make a strip three or four inches wide and consisting of about four layers of cloth. This is wrapped snugly twice around the bleeding arm or leg. It should be placed as close as possible to the bleeding wound, between it and the victim's heart. The free ends of the band of cloth should be tied with an overhand knot. A short, strong stick or similar article that will not break is placed on the knot and two additional overhand knots are tied on top of the stick so as to hold it in place. The stick is then twisted, tightening the tourniquet, until bleeding stops. One or both ends of the stick are then tied to the limb in such a way that the twisting cannot unwind.

See the item TOURNIQUET in this same chapter, pages 416, 417.

When a tourniquet is applied to an injured person, written notation should accompany the patient to the hospital indicating that a tourniquet has been applied and the time of application. The information can be written on the victim's forehead with an indelible pencil or lipstick if no paper is available. The tourniquet should remain exposed where it may be seen by hospital attendants and not forgotten.

4. Prevent or treat shock. Excessive loss of blood increases the probability of shock. As a precaution, the patient should be placed in a reclining position and kept comfortably warm. If bleeding is from an arm or a leg, this part should be elevated so as to reduce the blood pressure in it and thus favor control of the bleeding. If the victim is conscious, encourage him to take liquids by mouth. Avoid coffee, however, or any other stimulant, because stimulants raise the blood pressure and thus increase the tendency to bleed.

B. *Internal Hemorrhage.* Internal hemorrhage results from damage to or rupture of one of the internal organs such as the liver or spleen; from the rupture of an oviduct (as in tubal pregnancy); from the severing of a blood vessel (as in gunshot); from disease within a lung; from rupture of varicose veins in the esophagus; or from erosion into a blood vessel as by an ulcer in the stomach or intestine.

Bleeding from the lungs is usually indicated by coughing up of bright-red, frothy blood. Bleeding from the stomach may be indicated by vomited blood—red if the blood is recent, and dark and clotted if the blood has been acted on by the digestive juices. Bleeding into the intestine may be evidenced by the passing of jet-black stools. Bleeding near the anal opening causes the stools to be streaked with bright-red blood.

What to Do

Often the only adequate treatment for severe internal bleeding is appropriate surgery. While waiting for the doctor, the victim should be kept warm, with his feet and legs elevated above the level of his body to prevent or control the condition of shock.

BRUISES (CONTUSIONS)

A bruise, or contusion, is an injury to the deeper tissues in which the skin is usually not broken. It could be caused by a blow from a fist or a club, by a pinch, or by impact against a solid object as in falling or in being struck by some moving object. In a typical case the small blood vessels are broken in the bruised tissues and blood escapes into these tissues, causing them to swell and become dark in color. It is this blood in the tissue spaces that causes a bruised area, as it heals, to appear "black and blue" (ecchymosis). In addition to the first-aid treatment for ordinary bruises, separate consideration for two special cases—black eye and bruised fingertip—follows:

What to Do

1. As soon as possible after the injury, bathe the bruised part with cold compresses wrung from ice water, or else immerse the bruised part (such as hand or foot) repeatedly in an ice water bath for a few minutes at a time. This limits the amount of blood that escapes into the tissues and thus reduces the amount of swelling that will occur.

2. If it is one of the extremities that has been bruised, keep the part elevated so that it is approximately level with the body. Also, keep the injured part at rest for several hours. These measures have the effect of reducing the flow of blood in the part and thus of limiting the amount of swelling.

3. By the next day after the injury it is time to use measures that increase the flow of blood through the area of injury so as to promote healing and to remove the dark coloration as quickly as possible. This is accomplished by the use of contrasting heat and cold. If the injury involves a part of the body that can be immersed in water, use a hot foot bath or hot arm bath, as the case may be, gradually adding hot water to increase the temperature as much as the patient can stand. After about three minutes, place the part quickly and briefly (about half a minute) in ice water. This sequence should be repeated several times at each treatment, with about four treatments a day. If the main part of the body or the head is involved, use applications of hot compresses (being careful to avoid burns), followed briefly by a compress wrung from ice water.

A. *Black Eye.* The tissues around the eye are soft and thus bruise easily when pinched against the margins of bone which surround the eye socket. The treatment of black eye is the same as that for bruises in other parts of the body—cold compresses during the first twenty-four hours and contrasting hot and cold thereafter.

During the process of healing, a black eye can be made less conspicuous by using cosmetics designed to obscure discolorations of the skin. In a severe contusion, blowout of the floor of the orbit may occur, leading to double vision. Such an injury requires surgical correction. A black eye developing after a severe head injury may be a sign of skull fracture.

B. *Bruised Fingertip.* A common and painful form of bruise results from a fingertip being caught in a door or injured by the blow of a hammer. The greatest tissue damage in this case occurs beneath the fingernail. The injury is more painful than bruises in other areas because the fingernail limits the amount of swelling as blood escapes into the tissues.

The same kind of treatment by cold hand baths and then hot and cold, as outlined in "What to Do" 1 and 3 above, is helpful here. In addition, a great deal of suffering can be prevented by drilling a small hole through the fingernail so as to permit the escape of the accumulated blood beneath the nail. A simple way to make this hole is to unbend a paperclip and then, while grasping it with pliers, heat the end of the clip in a flame. While hot, the end of the paperclip is carefully forced through the nail, burning a small opening in the nail as it goes and, presently, permitting the bloody fluid beneath the nail to escape.

BURNS
A. BURNS CAUSED BY HEAT
B. BURNS INVOLVING THE LUNGS OR AIR PASSAGES
C. BURNS CAUSED BY CHEMICALS

369

D. BURNS CAUSED BY ELECTRIC CURRENT

E. BURNS CAUSED BY RADIATION

Burns vary in severity from minor ones to serious, life-threatening injuries. Burns severe enough to attract attention affect more than 2 million Americans each year. Of these, about 75,000 are serious enough to require hospital care and 10,000 end fatally. Burns constitute America's third leading cause of accidental death.

A surprisingly high number of burns are sustained by young children, and many of these are caused by contact with hot fluids (scalds). Hot tap water drawn from a household faucet is a frequent offender.

In severe burns the patient's life is in danger because of shock, loss of fluid, disturbance of chemical balances, and systemic infection.

A. *Ordinary Burns Caused by Heat.* The severity of a burn (and, thus, the method of its treatment) depends upon the depth to which the tissues have been injured. The victim's eventual welfare depends also on how much of the body's surface has been involved. For purposes of treatment, burns are conveniently classified as first-degree, second-degree, and third-degree.

First-degree Burns. In a first-degree burn only the outer layer of the skin is damaged. The victim suffers pain, redness of the skin, and possible swelling of the tissues, but no blisters. Mild sunburn or mild exposure to steam, hot water, or direct heat are examples. No scar is formed when healing occurs.

What to Do

Treatment for a first-degree burn is simple, centering merely around the relief of pain. It is best accomplished by applying a nongreasy ointment which contains a mild anesthetic to deaden the pain. If such ointment is not available, the burned area may be patted lightly with a paste prepared by stirring baking soda into

water. Immersing the burned part in cold water also helps to relieve pain.

Second-degree Burns. In a second-degree burn the deeper layers of the skin are involved as well as the surface

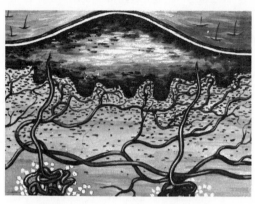

Diagrammatic views of the skin following local burns: A. The surface layer of the skin (epidermis) has separated and tissue fluid has accumulated to form a blister. B. A slightly more severe burn in which part of the epidermis has been destroyed. C. A still more severe burn in which all the epidermis is missing and portions only of a sweat gland and a hair follicle are seen.

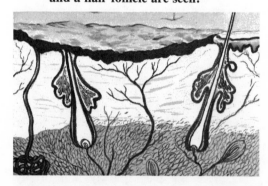

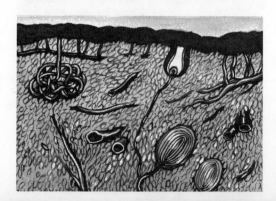

layer. Tissue fluid escapes into the damaged tissues, causing blisters which are easily broken. Because of a breakdown of the skin's surface layer, the development of infection becomes a serious possibility. An extensive second-degree burn can cause serious systemic effects, shock and infection being the worst complications. Inasmuch as the skin is not totally destroyed in a second-degree burn, it is still capable of satisfactory healing without extensive scar formation.

What to Do

If large parts of the body are involved in a second-degree burn, the victim should be transferred to a hospital. Extensive burns can cause complications such as shock and infection. Competent medical care is imperative.

First-aid instructions given here for second-degree burns are intended only for burns that cover a relatively small part of the skin's surface and, also, for the immediate care of a more extensive burn until the victim can be transferred to a hospital. The treatment should be aimed toward (a) the prevention of shock, (b) the relief of pain, (c) the control of infection, and (d) the proper care of the wound.

To reduce the danger of shock, the victim should be placed in a reclining position with his feet slightly elevated. He should be kept comfortably warm but not overheated. In view of the possibility of the tissues swelling, all finger rings and bracelets and other items that might cause constriction should be removed, even from parts not directly involved in the burn. The victim should be given reasonable amounts of fluid by mouth every 15 or 20 minutes—this to replenish the amount of fluid lost from the burned area and also to make it easier for the kidneys to handle their extra load of toxins. Half-normal saline solution (one level teaspoon of salt to a quart of water) may be given orally, especially if hospital care is delayed and the victim is vomiting.

Pain is most safely relieved by immersing the affected part in cold water, if this is feasible, adding chips of ice to the water to keep it cold. Or, clean compresses wrung from ice water and changed frequently can be laid over the burned area. Oil or greasy ointments should not be used.

Clothing should be removed from the burned part or cut away from the burned area. In a severe burn when fragments of clothing still adhere to the burned tissue, a clean dressing can be placed over the area without removing all fragments until such time as the victim arrives at the hospital. When the burn area is relatively small and it seems feasible for the first-aider to clean the wound, he may do this gently, using warm water and sterile soap. Effort should always be made to avoid contaminating the wound. Dressings should be either sterile surgical dressings, or portions of light cloth which have been recently ironed. Aside from keeping the wound clean, infection is best controlled by using antibiotic drugs under a physician's direction.

Third-degree Burns. A third-degree burn, by definition, involves destruction of the entire skin thickness of the involved area. In severe cases the deeper tissues, such as muscle, may also be damaged or partially destroyed. Inasmuch as the skin is destroyed in this type of burn, it cannot be expected to regenerate at the center of the wound. It is in such injuries that skingrafting is advised as soon as the danger of infection is under control. Otherwise, the tissues at the margins of the injury contract as they heal, causing heavy scars which become misshapen by strictures.

What to Do

The general plan for handling the victim of a third-degree burn is the same as that for a second-degree burn. Shock should be combated by keeping the patient in the reclining position with his feet slightly elevated,

EMERGENCIES

even while he is being transported to the hospital. Very little should be done to the burned area except to remove foreign material from the wound and keep it covered with clean cloths or sterile dressings. Also, even during the period of first aid, the patient should receive frequent drinks of water. If he is given any medicine, such as one or two aspirin tablets for the relief of pain, the time and amount of the medicine should be noted on a piece of paper and this pinned to the patient's clothing or covering sheet for the doctor's information.

B. *Burns Involving the Lungs or the Air Passages.* Many severe burns caused by explosions or blasts of hot air include damage to the air passages and lungs. These tissues are usually not burned in the sense that they have been overheated. Rather, they have usually suffered damage from smoke inhalation and the irritating chemical substances in the smoke. Such damage is indicated by singed hairs inside the nostrils, persistent coughing, hoarseness of the voice, and spitting of blood or particles of carbon. There may be such swelling of the lung tissues as to endanger the victim's life. Persons whose lungs have thus been damaged should be observed closely in the hospital for several days, even though they may feel reasonably well in the meantime.

C. *Burns Caused by Chemicals.* In these cases it is some chemical substance rather than high temperature that causes the tissue damage. It used to be assumed, unfortunately, that the first thing to do in a case of chemical burn is to apply a chemical antidote for the substance causing the burn. Experience has taught, however, that in all chemical burns the first effort should be to flood the involved area with plain water. Otherwise, valuable time is lost while finding a proper neutralizing agent. Chemical manufacturing plants have installed emergency shower facilities in strategic locations.

What to Do

1. Flood with running water the portion of the victim's body which includes the burned area. Do not wait to remove clothing.

2. After thorough flooding with water, remove the clothing from the involved area and treat the burned tissue with mild neutralizing solutions if the nature of the original chemical is known. In burns by acid, treat the area with a dilute solution of ordinary soda (2 tablespoonfuls to the quart of water). If the burn has been caused by an alkali, treat the area with a solution of vinegar which has been diluted half and half with water. Burns by carbolic acid (phenol) should be flooded with ordinary alcohol (rubbing alcohol is good). Then rinse the area with plain water.

3. When an eye is involved in a chemical burn, the eyelid should be held open while a gentle stream of water is used to irrigate the eye. After such rinsing with water, a mild ophthalmic ointment may be placed under the eyelid if such is available.

4. The subsequent treatment of chemical burns, after the initial washing and neutralizing of the chemical agent, is the same as for burns caused by heat.

D. *Burns Caused by Electric Current.* Damage to tissues caused by passage of an electric current occurs at the sites of entrance and exit of the current. The tissue damage is often much greater than can be seen by examining the skin at the site of the injury. It may take several days for the full extent of the tissue damage to become apparent. The greatest danger to life is interference with the action of the heart and the breathing apparatus. Damage to the heart is caused by the passage of the electric current through the chest, while that to the organs of breathing is caused by injury to the respiratory center in the brainstem.

What to Do

If the victim is still in contact with

the electric curcuit, the obvious first thing to do is to break the contact. This must be done carefully lest the rescuer also receive the current and become a victim. For instructions, see page 410 of this same chapter which considers SHOCK BY ELECTRIC CURRENT.

Once the electric current is no longer passing through the victim's body, attention must be given to the action of his heart and lungs. If he is not breathing or if his heart is not beating, artificial methods of resuscitation must be begun at once. See the item CARDIOPULMONARY RESUSCITATION on pages 374, 375 of this chapter.

Minor electrical burns of the skin and underlying flesh are treated as are ordinary burns caused by excessive heat. Extensive electrical burns may require skin grafting.

E. *Burns Caused by Radiation.* Radiation burns may be caused by excessive exposure to X rays or from careless contact with radioactive substances as used in nuclear reactors, cyclotrons, linear accelerators, and atomic bombs. (For a general discussion of the hazards of exposure to radiation, see item NUCLEAR EXPLOSION on pages 405, 406 of this chapter.) The damage caused by exposure to radiation may be delayed so that the symptoms occur days or weeks after the exposure. The degree of injury depends upon the amount of radiation absorbed, upon the rate of absorption, and upon the particular part or parts of the body exposed to the radiation.

What to Do

First-aid treatment of a radiation burn involving the superficial tissues of the body is similar to that for burns caused by heat. In addition, attention should be given to the systemic effects of the radiation. On general principles, transfusion of blood is advisable to help in combating the associated anemia. Exposure to radiation also reduces a person's resistance to infection. Thus, antibiotics or other means of combating infections should be used.

CARDIAC ARREST (HEART STOPPAGE)

There are many conditions in which the heart stops beating (cardiac arrest), some so serious that the heart will not beat spontaneously again regardless of what is done. In others, the heart will resume its beating, either spontaneously or in response to stimulation.

When the heart stops beating, the circulation of blood ceases. Various cells of the body, particularly certain ones in the brain, are so dependent upon a continuous circulation of blood that they become permanently damaged if deprived of blood for more than about six minutes. The role of the first-aider, then, is to institute artificial circulation of blood, as described below, so as to keep blood circulating through a victim's body until such time as it can be determined whether the heart will resume its normal function of propelling blood.

It used to be thought necessary in case of sudden cardiac arrest to make an incision in the chest and actually reach in and squeeze the heart in order to keep the blood circulating. It is now recognized, however, that the circulation of blood can be maintained in a case of cardiac arrest by exerting intermittent, external pressure on the chest sufficient to force the blood out of the heart and into the blood vessels that distribute it throughout the body. The valves within the heart prevent the blood from flowing backward and so, when the pressure on the chest is released, other blood will enter to replace what has been moved on its way.

What to Do

HEART RESUSCITATION; ARTIFICIAL CIRCULATION

1. Lay the victim on his back on a firm foundation, such as on the floor.
2. The operator works at the victim's side.
3. The operator applies pressure

EMERGENCIES

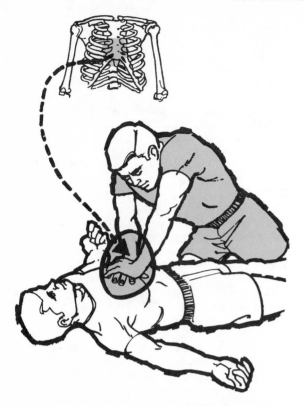

4. After each downward pressure, the operator's hands should relax to permit the victim's chest to expand again. Make sure that you do not exert an unreasonably great amount of pressure, for it is possible to break the victim's ribs if too much pressure is used.

5. Continue this procedure until the victim's heart begins beating spontaneously, or, at least, for as long as one hour. If the patient is transported to a hospital in the meantime, the procedure should be continued even while the patient is being moved.

CARDIOPULMONARY ARREST

Usually, when a person's heart stops beating, his breathing also ceases. The reverse is not necessarily true, however. Many a person ceases to breathe even though his heart is still beating (such as in drowning). In a case in which the heart is not beating, then, it is usually necessary to give artificial respiration at the same time the procedure for heart resuscitation is being used.

What to Do

CARDIOPULMONARY RESUSCITATION (CPR); BASIC LIFE SUPPORT

It is not easy to administer artificial respiration at the same time that the procedure for heart resuscitation is being used. If two rescuers are available, one can take care of the artificial respiration (mouth-to-mouth method) while the other performs heart resuscitation by making intermittent pressure on the victim's breastbone. The lungs should be filled with air at intervals of about five seconds.

If only one rescuer is available, it is advised that he discontinue his intermittent pressure on the breastbone after each twelve cycles, long enough to take time out to blow air into the victim's lungs twice. He then resumes the intermittent pressure on the breastbone for another twelve cycles. For the method of mouth-to-mouth

over the lower third of the victim's breastbone, releasing it and exerting it again in a rhythm of about one cycle per second. The amount of pressure to be applied varies with the age of the victim. For babies, the pressure should be gentle, exerted through the tips of the operator's fingers as they press against the center of the baby's breastbone. There is danger of pressing so hard that the heart is bruised. For children of about 10 years of age, pressure should be exerted by the heel of one hand against the child's breastbone. For adults, one of the operator's hands is placed over the other so that pressure is exerted by both hands sufficient to move the breastbone approximately two inches toward the victim's spine (pressure of about 70 pounds). The operator can time his pressure strokes by counting slowly, "One little second, two little seconds," et cetera, so that the pressure is exerted at about one-second intervals.

artificial respiration, see the item **RESPIRATORY FAILURE** in this same chapter, pages 407-409. Also notice there the accompanying diagrams which illustrate artificial respiration.

CHEST INJURIES
   A. FRACTURED RIBS
   B. FLAIL CHEST
   C. PENETRATING WOUNDS

When the chest is compressed as in a fall or by impact in an automobile accident, the ribs or the bones to which the ribs attach are often fractured. The serious consequences of chest injury relate to the possibility that the broken end of a rib may pierce a lung or the heart, that the blood vessels within the chest may be severed, or that the chest wall may be pierced so that air entering through the wound may allow a lung to collapse.

A. *Fractured Ribs*. With a fractured rib, the patient suffers severe pain at the site of injury each time he inhales. This causes the patient to take shallow breaths and to avoid coughing. In severe injuries a sharp end of a rib may pierce a lung. When this happens, the victim often coughs up bright-red, frothy blood.

What to Do

1. **Evaluate the probable seriousness of the injury. If it seems that several ribs are broken, see the next item, B. *Flail Chest*. If the victim appears to be in shock and if it seems that there may be injury to the vital organs within the chest, try to obtain professional help at once. If the skin of the chest is broken and there appears to be an opening into the chest cavity, see item C. below, *Penetrating Wounds*.**

2. **If pain on taking a breath is the patient's principal symptom, and there appear to be no other complications, try to give the patient comfort as he breathes by placing a firm-fitting binder (a broad bandage) entirely around his chest below the**

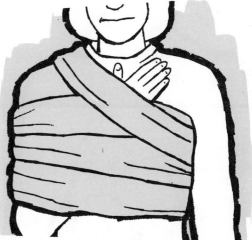

A person with a broken rib may receive some comfort from the application of a broad bandage to the chest which may even include the arm on the injured side.

armpits. In some cases greater comfort can be obtained by including the arm of the injured side within the binder as indicated in the accompanying illustration.

3. **Breathing is easier in such cases when the victim lies down with his head and shoulder slightly higher than his hips.**

B. *Flail Chest*. In this situation, so many ribs are fractured that part of the chest wall no longer has rigid support. When the victim attempts to inhale, the injured area sinks and thus interferes with the filling of the lungs. When the victim exhales, the injured area bulges outward.

What to Do

This is a serious injury and the victim must have skilled medical help as promptly as possible. In the meantime, the weak area of the chest should be stabilized by applying a binder or pressure dressing with cravat binder so that the weakened area does not bulge with each exhalation. The victim should be kept in a reclining position, even during transporta-

E
M
E
R
G
E
N
C
I
E
S

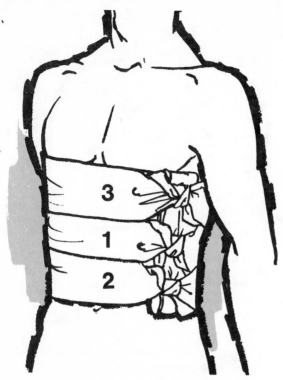

How to apply cravats as rib binders or pressure dressings: First place padding vertically across ribs where knots are to be tied. Bind wide cravat (1) around body over fracture, making sure all air is expelled from lungs. Repeat with second cravat (2) below and a third (3) above, overlapping a little in each case.

tion, with the head and shoulders elevated slightly.

C. *Penetrating Wounds, Sucking Wounds.* Penetrating wounds of the chest made by a knife or a bullet or any other object that passes from the outside through the chest wall, carry the danger of admitting air into the space around the lung each time the patient inhales. As air enters through the wound it accumulates between the chest wall and the lung, causing one lung to collapse and thus interfering with the usual process of breathing. There is usually a characteristic suck-ing sound as air enters the chest through such a wound.

What to Do

A pressure dressing should be applied immediately to this type of wound so that air can no longer enter the chest cavity. Use a layer of vaseline-impregnated gauze or plastic sheeting next to the skin and cover it with a firm bandage. Ask the patient to "breathe out" while the bandage is made secure.

CHOKING (STRANGLING)

Choking or strangling occurs when a person accidentally draws a foreign body or a bolus of food into his air passages. It may occur when a child at play draws a small object into his larynx.

The person who chokes makes a great effort to breathe. He is unable to speak. His head is thrown back, his eyes protrude, and his face becomes bluish red. If his air passages have become completely closed, he soon collapses and will die within a few minutes if he does not receive help.

Food-choking is said to be the sixth most common cause of accidental death, causing more deaths than are caused by accidents with firearms or by airplane accidents. In middle-aged and elderly people, death from choking on food is easily mistaken for death by heart attack.

The classic victim of choking on food is an elderly person who wears dentures, who is eating steak or beef at the time, and who has possibly had an alcoholic drink before the meal. The dentures and the drink of alcohol contribute because they hinder the person in his judgment of the size of the bolus of food he can properly swallow. Choking then occurs when the lump of meat lodges in the throat behind the tongue and closes the combined passage for food and air.

What to Do

First aid may be rendered to a choking victim by three approved

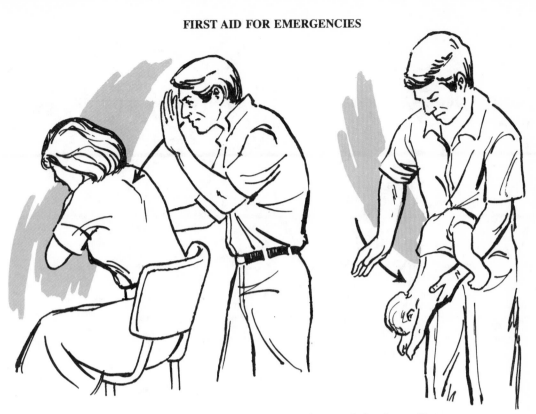

Delivering back blows to a choking victim can bring immediate relief if the obstruction is not lodged too firmly. Notice the method for handling an infant.

maneuvers: (1) *Back Blows*, (2) *Epigastric Thrust* (the Heimlich maneuver), and (3) *Finger Probe*. Any one of these may work successfully in a given case.

1. *Back Blows.* This maneuver requires the operator to use the heel of his hand to deliver a series of rapid whacks to the victim's spine between his shoulder blades. The maneuver may be used with the victim standing, sitting, or lying on his side. The blow should be forceful enough to jar the victim's body and thus dislodge the object obstructing his air passages. A gentle modification of the maneuver may be used in the case of an infant by supporting the infant, face down, on one's forearm (see accompanying illustration). Only when he is unable to breathe at all should his head be held low.

2. *Epigastric Thrust (the Heimlich maneuver).* Some air remains within the lungs even when a person's air passages are closed as in choking. The epigastric thrust maneuver is designed to force this residual air out of the lungs so quickly that it pushes the material trapped in the throat upward into the mouth, thus removing the hindrance to the flow of air. This maneuver is accomplished by exerting swift pressure upward through the soft tissue of the epigastrium. The epigastrium is that part of the front portion of the body wall located just below the breastbone and between the lower ribs as they curve downward and outward. Such pressure forces the diaphragm upward, thus compressing the lungs and forcing the air upward through the air passages.

The maneuver can be performed with the victim standing, sitting, or

377

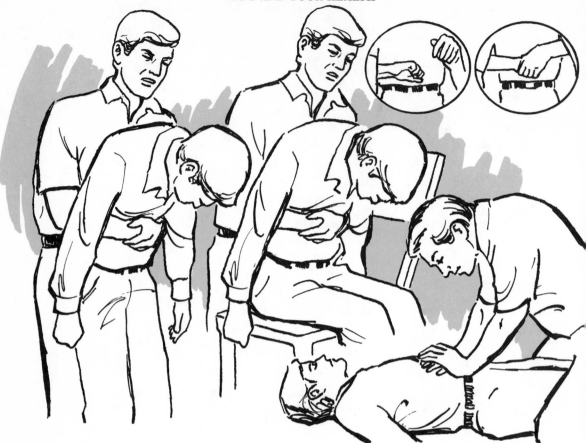

lying on his back. When the choking person is standing or sitting, the operator works from behind. He wraps his arm around the victim's waist, placing the thumb side of one fist against the victim's abdomen just above the navel and just below the ribs. He then grabs his fist with his other hand and makes a quick upward thrust (see accompanying illustrations).

When the victim is lying on his back, the epigastric thrust is performed as the operator kneels beside the victim or straddles the victim's hips. He places one of his hands on top of the other with the heel of the lower hand located slightly above the victim's navel and just below the ribs. The operator then rocks forward as he makes a quick upward thrust in the midline of the victim's body.

3. *Finger Probe*. This maneuver is especially useful when it is certain that a bolus of food or other firm object has become lodged in the victim's throat. Open the victim's mouth widely, grasp the tip of his tongue through the fold of a handkerchief, and pull the tongue well forward. Pass the forefinger of the other hand over the tongue and along the side (not the middle) of the victim's throat far enough to reach the edge of the obstructing object. (If the finger were pushed into the midline of the victim's throat, it migh push the obstructing object farther into the air passages.) Then with a sweeping motion, bring the object forward into the victim's mouth.

After the choking victim has received first aid, even though he appears to be breathing normally again,

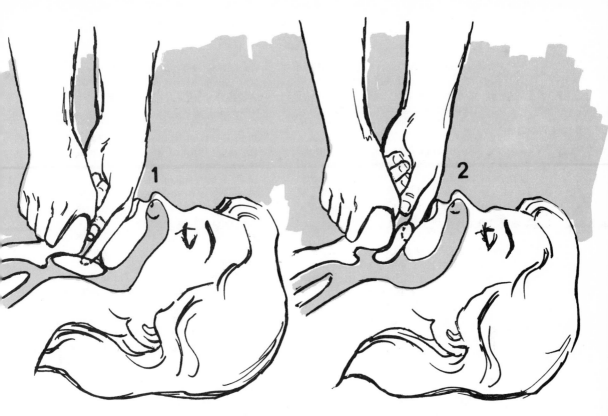

The epigastric thrust (opposite page) or the finger probe (above) may be required to dislodge obstructions which cannot be removed by blows to the back. In using the finger probe, care must be taken to prevent pushing the obstruction farther into the air passages.

it is important that he be seen by a physician. The reason for this imperative is to determine whether the obstruction to the airways has been completely removed and whether the maneuvers used to restore his breathing have caused any damage to his tissues.

COLD INJURY (FROSTBITE)

Cold injury so severe as to cause freezing of the tissues is called frostbite. It may occur in such exposed parts of the body as the ears, nose, hands, or feet. Just before the tissues become frozen, they may appear violet-red in color. Once freezing has occurred, color changes to gray-yellow.

What to Do

1. Avoid rubbing the frozen parts, and do not resort to the outmoded treatment of massaging with snow to bring about thawing.

2. After placing the victim in a warm room, remove all items of clothing that constrict the frozen part of the body, such as boots, gloves, or socks.

3. Immerse the frozen part in warm water (not hot) and attempt to raise the temperature of the frozen tissues gradually to normal body temperature. When the nose or the ear is frozen, use compresses wrung from warm water to thaw the frozen part.

4. Try to improve the victim's general condition by keeping him warm and giving him hot drinks (not liquor).

5. After the frozen part has thawed, keep it dry and avoid the use of wet dressings.

6. Take special precautions to

avoid pressure of heavy bedclothing or other objects against the part that was frozen. The part may need to be protected by a "cradle" placed over it, keeping the bedclothes from touching it.

7. Encourage the victim to move the part that was frozen, for this will increase blood circulation through these tissues. If it was his foot, he should avoid standing on it until the tissues are completely healed.

CONVULSIONS (EPILEPSY)

A consideration of the convulsive disorders, their significance and causes, appears in chapter 4, volume 3. In the present chapter we are concerned with the first-aid handling of a person who has a convulsion.

What to Do

1. Place the victim on something wide and soft such as a bed or a thick rug so that he will not be injured on account of his involuntary motions— if on a bed, stand guard so that he will not fall off.

2. Loosen his clothing so as to reduce the danger of choking or harm caused by the twisting of garments.

3. Put something blunt and soft (such as a small roll of cloth) between the victim's teeth so as to hold the jaws apart and thus reduce the danger of his biting his tongue.

4. Place the victim on his side rather than on his back, for, particularly in the case of a child, danger of vomiting exists and the possibility that he may choke on the vomitus. Do not leave the patient face down because of the danger of smothering. Always keep his face turned to one side.

5. Breathing is usually interrupted for brief periods during a convulsion. If breathing stops completely for more than a minute or two, administer artificial respiration. See the item RESPIRATORY FAILURE on pages 407-409 of this same chapter.

NOTE: Do *not* put anyone with convulsions in the bathtub. The thrashing movements of the convulsion can cause injuries here. Furthermore, it is difficult to care for a person in a bathtub.

6. In convulsions associated with high fever, as in cases of heatstroke or the beginning of an illness marked by fever, take measures to reduce the body temperature as quickly as possible. This is best done by wrapping the patient in a sheet wrung out of cold water. Then allow an electric fan to play on the wet sheet. This will cause rapid evaporation of the moisture in the sheet and will have a cooling effect. Cool sponging of the victim's skin with a damp cloth produces a similar effect.

7. Convulsions not associated with fever typically last for only a short time. The first-aider's effort in such a case is to protect the victim so that he will not injure himself during the convulsion. After the convulsion the individual should be permitted to rest quietly until he feels reasonably normal again.

8. When repeated convulsions occur, one after the other, arrange for medical help or transport the patient to the emergency room of a hospital.

CROUP

See chapter 17, volume 1, for a discussion on croup.

CUTS

A cut, in contrast to a puncture wound, usually lies open, bleeds easily, and is less likely to become infected. Such a wound is caused by a knife, a razor, broken glass, or any sharp edge.

What to Do

Treatment depends on the size and location of the cut. Simple cuts can be safely treated at home. Deeper or more extensive cuts, particularly those in which nerves and blood vessels may be involved, require the services of a physician. For simple cuts, care may be given as follows:

1. Bleeding should be controlled first. In simple cases, firm pressure

over the wound through a sterile surgical dressing or a freshly laundered handkerchief may control the bleeding. In severe cases it may be necessary to insert a clean dressing into the wound and exert pressure on this.

2. Wash the surrounding skin area thoroughly with soap and water, sponging the soapy water away from the wound rather than into it.

3. Gently inspect the wound for dirt or foreign material. If any is found, remove it by irrigating with sterile salt solution or by gently sponging with sterile gauze.

4. If the wound requires suturing (stitching) or additional care by the physician, cover it with a clean dressing and keep the injured part quiet until the physician is available. If the cut is relatively small, the edges may be held together without suturing by holding them next to each other while applying a butterfly-shaped strip of adhesive tape (one cut down to a narrow width at the point where it crosses the cut).

5. Protect the wound during healing by a sterile dressing of appropriate size and type.

6. When excessive swelling occurs during healing or when the area becomes unusually tender and red or, particularly, should there be red streaks extending away from the wound, consult a physician at once for treatment of the infection.

DELIRIUM

The definition, causes, and symptoms of delirium, together with the general principles of treatment, are considered in chapter 4, volume 3. In the present chapter we consider the emergency treatment of a person who becomes delirious.

What to Do

The primary responsibility of the first-aider in caring for a patient with delirium is to make sure that no harm comes to the patient during the period of delay before medical supervision takes over. The patient should be kept in a quiet, relaxed environment. If there is long delay, make sure that the patient receives adequate fluid. Beyond this, effort should be directed to obtaining professional care so that the actual cause of the delirium may be determined and specific treatment administered.

DELIVERY OF A BABY (EMERGENCY DELIVERY)

Occasionally circumstances prevent the attendance of a physician at the delivery of a baby. In such an emergency, it becomes necessary for someone to help the mother through the childbirth and to take care of her and the newborn baby.

When time and circumstances permit, the following items should be made ready before the baby is actually born:

1. A basket or bassinet lined with soft blankets in which to place the baby.

2. A piece of plasticized sheeting about four feet (1.25 meters) square to protect the bed on which the mother lies.

3. One or two clean sheets.

4. One or two medium-sized towels, freshly ironed with a very hot iron and folded so their inner surfaces have not been touched by hands.

5. A small supply of sanitary napkins, kept clean in their original package.

6. Three or four strips of cloth tape about one-half inch (about 1 cm.) wide and at least 10 inches (25 cm.) long. The ordinary cotton binding tape which a seamstress uses is satisfactory. Otherwise, strips of cloth torn from a sheet or a handkerchief will do.

7. A medium-sized pair of scissors for cutting the umbilical cord.

8. A basin measuring at least 10 inches (25 cm.) in diameter.

Getting the Patient Ready. The expectant mother should lie on her back near the edge of the bed in such a position that the person who cares for her at this time can lean over her as the baby is being born. Her knees should

E
M
E
R
G
E
N
C
I
E
S

be raised, and some provision should be made for her to brace her feet in a manner to enable her to "bear down" effectively at the time of each labor pain.

If time permits, the rubber sheet should be placed beneath the cloth sheet under the patient's hips. The patient's genital area (the area surrounding her vulva) should be gently but thoroughly washed with soap and hot water. To avoid contaminating the birth canal, the washing strokes should be away from the vulva and downward toward the rectum.

CAUTION

Do not try to keep the baby from being born even though the doctor has not arrived or even though the mother is still on her way to the hospital. Unfortunately, some have tried to delay the birth by holding a towel against the baby's head or by having the mother cross her legs. Such efforts may result in injury to the baby or mother.

The Baby's Birth. Usually, it is the crown of the baby's head that can be seen first as the baby is pushed through the birth canal. With the mother lying on her back, the baby faces downward, obliquely toward the right or toward the left. As the baby's head comes through the mother's vulva, it stretches to their limit the tissues that form the outlet of the birth canal, sometimes causing them to tear. When this occurs, the tear is toward the mother's anus. Sometimes the attendant can prevent this tearing by covering his hand with a freshly laundered towel and gently working the tissues of the vulva past the baby's head.

Once the baby's head has been born, the most difficult part of the birth procedure is over. The baby's head can be supported slightly by the attendant's hand while the shoulders and body complete their passage through the birth canal. Mucus should be wiped away from the baby's nose and mouth.

Baby's First Cry. At this point in the delivery, the baby is still attached to its mother by way of the umbilical cord, which is fastened to the placenta (afterbirth) which has not yet been delivered. The umbilical cord is normally long enough so that the baby can be moved easily in the immediate vicinity.

It now becomes important for the baby to take its first breath. To bring this about, the baby should be held upside down, suspended from its ankles which are held securely between the attendant's fingers. The baby's skin is very slippery and great caution should be taken lest the attendant lose his hold. With the baby thus suspended, the attendant's other hand should be used to wipe away remaining mucus from the baby's nose and mouth (using a clean towel or freshly laundered handkerchief). The baby should then be rubbed briskly up and down his back. This normally causes the baby to cry and thus to take its first breath.

Tying the Umbilical Cord. Once the baby has cried, a clean towel should be placed across the mother's abdomen and the baby laid on the towel, crosswise to its mother's body. Now is the time to tie the umbilical cord. It is for this procedure that the pieces of cotton tape or narrow strips of cotton cloth mentioned above are used. Never use string or yarn for this purpose, because it tends to cut the tissues of the umbilical cord. Place one of the tapes around the umbilical cord at a point about three inches (7.5 cm.) from the attachment of the umbilical cord to the baby's body. As the first tie is drawn tightly, the soft tissues of the umbilical cord will move aside slightly so that the tape will actually compress the blood vessels within the umbilical cord. Be deliberate in making this tie. As a precautionary measure, place another tape next to and below (closer to the baby) the first one.

Place a third tape around the cord still farther away from the baby (about two inches [5 cm.] beyond the first tape) and tie this one also.

Using the medium-sized scissors, cut

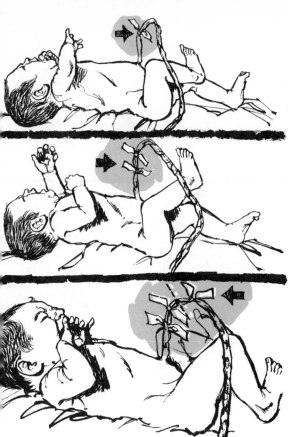

Three ties preparatory to cutting umbilical cord: (1) three inches from navel; (2) close to and below 1; (3) two inches above 1, cut to be made between 1 and 3.

the cord between the outer two tapes. A small amount of blood will ooze from the cut ends of the umbilical cord. If more than a small amount of blood escapes from the baby's end of the umbilical cord, another tape should be tied around the stump of the cord. The baby is now completely separated from its mother and can be wrapped comfortably in a soft blanket and placed alongside the mother's body or in the basket or crib that has been prepared.

The Afterbirth. The attendant's attention is now directed to the delivery of the afterbirth (placenta), which usually passes through the birth canal about 15 minutes after the baby has been born. The afterbirth can be guided by taking hold of the end of the umbilical cord; but the umbilical cord should

not be used as a means of pulling on the afterbirth to extract it. As it passes through the vulva, a small gush of blood usually accompanies it. The afterbirth should now be placed in a basin and set aside for the doctor to examine as a means of making sure that the delivery has occurred normally.

Preventing Bleeding. The power for the delivery of a baby is derived from the forceful contraction of the muscle in the wall of the mother's uterus (womb). Now that delivery is completed, the muscle of the uterus will possibly relax as a consequence of fatigue. Normally, it should remain firm in order to prevent the further loss of blood.

Immediately after the passing of the afterbirth, the attendant should place his hand on the mother's abdomen just below her umbilicus (navel). Here he can feel a large mass. This is the uterus, much larger now than it will be a few days later. By massage right through the abdominal wall, the uterus can be caused to contract firmly. Frequent examination through the abdominal wall to determine the condition of the uterus should continue for about an hour after the delivery of the placenta. If at any time it begins to relax and permit further bleeding (becoming larger and softer), the massaging should be resumed. As a precautionary measure, have the mother hold her hand over the uterus and report if it is relaxing.

Continuing Care. After the afterbirth has been expelled, two or three sanitary napkins, fresh from their container, should be used to cover the mother's genital area. These should be covered by a folded towel. These do not need to be fastened in place other than by the pressure of the patient's thighs. She should be allowed to rest now, but it should be made certain that she remains warm. If she tends to chill, a hot-water bag can be placed beside her with a blanket placed between the bag and her gown.

The early care of the baby should be

383

under a doctor's directions. Drops of a mild antiseptic solution, usually an antibiotic, are placed in the baby's eyes. The baby should be permitted to nurse relatively soon.

DISLOCATIONS OF THE ANKLE, ELBOW, FINGER, HIP, JAW, KNEE, SHOULDER, THUMB, TOE, AND WRIST

In a dislocation of a joint, one of the bones which forms part of the joint becomes misplaced. For example, in a ball-and-socket joint, the ball portion of the joint slips out of the socket portion. The bones that form a joint are normally held in place by the fibrous capsule of the joint and by ligaments that span the joint. In a dislocation, the capsule and one or more of the ligaments are either stretched or torn.

It is often difficult to tell the difference between a dislocation and a fracture. In such a case, it is wise to treat the injury as though it were a fracture, awaiting the time when a physician can make an examination and treat the injury appropriately.

A. *Dislocation of the Ankle*. This is usually associated with one or more fractures in the area.

What to Do

A severe injury of the ankle in which parts of the joint have obviously slipped out of place should be treated as a fracture, and this procedure requires the services of a physician. See the general instructions under the item FRACTURES OF BONES in this same chapter, pages 392, 393.

B. *Dislocation of the Elbow*. Dislocation here is usually caused by a twisting of the forearm or by a fall on the hand. It causes great pain, inability to bend the elbow, and an obvious deformity as compared with the shape of the other elbow.

What to Do

Obtain the services of a physician

as soon as possible. If the patient must be transported, the entire forearm should be secured to a splint with the elbow in as straight a position as feasible.

C. *Dislocation of the Finger*. This impairment occurs in various injuries in which one of the joints of the fingers is forced beyond its usual range of motion.

What to Do

This dislocation is one of the easiest to set. Using his two hands, the first-aider can grasp the dislocated finger both above and below the disabled joint. He then pulls steadily and firmly as though he were trying to make the finger longer. Thereupon the bones usually snap back into normal position.

D. *Dislocation of the Hip*. The ligaments which normally hold the hip joint in place are strong, but because of the rather wide range of motion of this joint, dislocations do occur under great stress, as when the victim, in a fall, suddenly thrusts his weight on a foot or

In preparing to transport a case of hip dislocation, strap the patient to a firm board with a pillow placed beneath his knees.

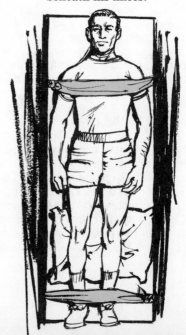

knee. The hip is a ball-and-socket joint, and the head of the hipbone (femur) may move out of its socket in any of several directions. Because of the danger of injury to structures of the joint or those in the vicinity, any attempt by a first-aider to set a dislocated hip is not recommended.

What to Do

1. Transport the victim as quickly as possible to a hospital or to a physician's office.

2. If an ambulance is not available and a car must be used, strap the victim to a firm board, with a pillow beneath his knees, as indicated in the accompanying illustration.

E. *Dislocation of the Jaw.* A person may suffer dislocation of the jaw from opening his mouth widely, as in yawning, or from being struck on the chin while his mouth is open. Usually both sides of the jaw are dislocated at the same time. This is a painful injury and the victim is unable to close his mouth.

What to Do

If the attempt to set a dislocated jaw proves successful, the jaw snaps back into normal position so quickly and with so strong a pull of the muscles that the victim may unintentionally bite the person helping him. In preparation, therefore, the attendant should wrap both his thumbs with several thicknesses of cloth and then proceed as follows:

1. With both thumbs on the victim's lower molar teeth, one thumb on each side, exert steady pressure and, at the same time, lift the tip of the jaw with the third and fourth fingers.

2. Continue to exert this firm pressure as the victim attempts to relax his chewing muscles. Keep telling the victim, "Let me move your jaw."

3. As the operator feels the jaw moving into place, he should slip his thumbs sideways into the space between the patient's teeth and cheeks to avoid being bitten.

4. Once the jaw returns to normal, a wide bandage should be applied around the jaw and over the top of the head to give the jaw support while the stretched ligaments are healing.

F. *Dislocation of the Knee.* A complete dislocation of the knee joint is unusual, caused only by major violence.

What to Do

In such severe injuries to the knee, the injured parts should be splinted in as comfortable a position as possible and the victim transported to the hospital.

G. *Dislocation of the Shoulder.* This serious type of dislocation is probably the most common. It is caused by a fall on the shoulder or by the body's weight being thrust on the elbow or hand. Such dislocation may be associated with a fracture of one or more bones. Also the nerves or blood vessels in the vicinity may possibly be damaged.

Because the attempt to set a dislocated shoulder may damage nerves and blood vessels in the area, it is preferable for a physician rather than a first-aider to do this. Furthermore, because of the ever-present danger of fracture-dislocation, X rays are usually taken before correction is attempted.

What to Do

1. Arrange a sling for the arm of the injured side.

2. Transport the victim to a hospital or a physician's office.

H. *Dislocation of the Thumb.* This injury is more serious than a dislocated finger.

What to Do

Dislocation of the thumb usually requires a surgical procedure for correction. In any case, a physician's services are usually necessary.

I. *Dislocation of a Toe.* Dislocation of a toe is usually the result of a blow on the end of the toe.

E
M
E
R
G
E
N
C
I
E
S

What to Do

The correction of the dislocation of a toe involves the same procedures as for setting a dislocated finger. See above.

J. *Dislocation of the Wrist*. The wrist joint is a complex one in which the bones of the forearm and the hand, as well as the several bones of the wrist proper, combine to permit great flexibility. Dislocation of some of these bones is usually combined with tearing of the ligaments and with one or more fractures of bone. A dislocation of the wrist is recognized by comparing the shape and position of the injured wrist with that of the victim's other wrist.

What to Do

1. Because a dislocation of the wrist usually involves one or more fractures of bone, the first-aid treatment is the same as that for fracture of the forearm. See the item *Fracture of the Forearm* on page 393 of this same chapter.

2. A physician will order an examination of the area by X ray. He will then decide what is the best way to treat the fractures and at the same time will restore the bones to their normal positions.

DIVING, RELATED EMERGENCIES

Diving into the water from the shore or from a springboard is a usual accompaniment of swimming. Its danger lies in the possibility of striking the head against something solid, like a rock or the floor of the swimming pool.

What to Do

The first-aider should restrain his impulse to get the diver out of the water quickly, for danger lurks that the diver's neck may have been injured—even broken. Should the victim be hurriedly pulled out of the water, his spinal cord could be injured or even severed, thus condemning him to lifelong paralysis.

Instead of removing the victim quickly, let a good swimmer keep him afloat (lying on his back in the water) until help comes to support him properly and bring him out of the water without tension on his neck. If the victim has stopped breathing, it is even possible to administer mouth-to-mouth respiration while he is still floating in the water. To remove him from the water, place a rigid stretcher, a surfboard, a door, or a wooden plank under him and then lift him gently, keeping his body motionless while he is placed on the shore or in a waiting ambulance so that his neck or spinal cord will suffer no additional damage.

For further directions on handling this type of accident, see the item HEAD INJURY on page 397 of this same chapter.

Deep Diving. Equipment now available makes it possible for amateurs to dive to depths of more than 100 feet (30 m.). It is estimated that scuba divers number at least a million in the United States alone. Possible failure of equipment which provides air or oxygen for divers, danger of becoming entangled in weeds or caught in rocks, and the possibility that inexperienced divers will take risks greater than justified make drowning the principal cause of death in underwater accidents. See the item DROWNING, pages 387-389.

Decompression Sickness (The Bends). Those who dive to depths of greater than 30 feet (10 m.) face the danger of decompression sickness (caisson disease) and its possible serious consequences. This problem occurs when a diver remains too long at great depths and then ascends to the surface without allowing sufficient time for the gases dissolved in the fluid of his body to reach a new equilibrium. Thus bubbles of gas develop in his tissues and may cause serious aftereffects.

Symptoms of decompression sickness include pain in the joints, pain in the chest with cough and difficult breathing, paralysis of certain muscles, disturbances of vision, and dizziness—these beginning to appear soon after the diver emerges from the water.

What to Do

Treatment of decompression sickness involves use of pressure equipment, which may not be easily available. Official lifeguards and other authorities in areas where diving is common are usually informed on the location of such equipment and can help in transporting the victim to such a center.

In treating decompression sickness, the victim is placed in a tank constructed for this purpose and the air pressure within the tank is increased to simulate the pressure to which he was subjected while diving. The pressure is then gradually reduced, over a period of a few hours, allowing the patient's tissues to make a gradual adjustment.

DROWNING

Drowning is listed as America's fourth leading cause of accidental death, accounting for about 7000 casualties per year.

A swimmer in danger of drowning often panics. He thus makes it dangerous for another swimmer, even though skilled, to rescue him lest he cling to his rescuer so tenaciously as to pull him under too. It is better therefore to throw an imperiled swimmer a rope or a life preserver than to attempt a person-to-person rescue, or perhaps reach for him with an oar or pole.

If the person in danger has been injured while in the water, great caution should be used in removing him. It is relatively easy to keep the average person afloat with his mouth and nose above water; however, once attempt is made to remove him, the buoyancy which the water imparts is lost and the struggle to lift him may even aggravate his injury. It is best to keep an injured person afloat until suitable equipment arrives, even though this may mean administering mouth-to-mouth respiration while the victim is still in the water. The acceptable way to remove an injured person from the water is to place a firm stretcher or wooden door or wide plank underneath him to keep his body straight while he is being lifted out of the water.

Many factors may contribute to the hazard of drowning, even with experienced swimmers. One, formerly mysterious but now understood, is hyperventilation. This danger threatens a swimmer when he takes several deep breaths just before swimming underwater, thereby releasing from his body a large portion of carbon dioxide which, under normal circumstances, would stimulate his continued breathing. Thus the swimmer loses his desire to breathe and falls in danger of losing consciousness while still holding his breath. Another circumstance in which this same tragic series of events may occur is that of diving repeatedly with very short intervals between dives. Here again the diver may breathe so vigorously between dives as to nearly rid his body of carbon dioxide and thus lose his urge to breathe to the extent that he loses consciousness while under water and fails to surface for another breath.

What to Do

If there is anyone else at the scene, send him at once to summon help, preferably a rescue squad. Do not leave the victim yourself, but stay with him and keep him breathing.

1. Keep the victim breathing. This is the rescuer's primary occupation, and he must work to this end even while the victim is still in the water and even later while he is being taken to the hospital. If the victim is still breathing on his own, well and good. If not, artificial respiration must be administered as outlined below.

2. Begin artificial respiration at once if the victim is not breathing. Allow not more than 10 seconds for clearing debris or mucus or water out of the victim's mouth and then begin mouth-to-mouth resuscitation.

3. Place the victim's head in exten-

EMERGENCIES

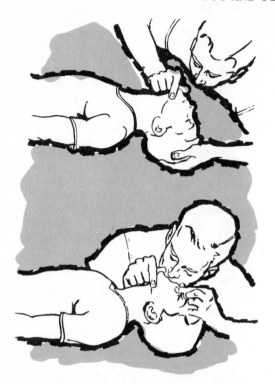

In mouth-to-mouth artificial respiration the victim's chin is kept tilted upward. (For other illustrations of this method see *Respiratory Failure* in this chapter.)

sion (chin up) as illustrated in the accompanying drawing. This tends to keep the air passages open so that air can enter his lungs.

4. Fill your own lungs with air and then breathe this into the victim's mouth while holding his nostrils closed either by your cheek against the openings or by your thumb and finger. This forced air should cause the victim's chest to expand. If the victim is a child, remember that the capacity of his lungs is small. Be careful, therefore, not to overinflate them, but give small, short puffs. Do not waste time trying to get water out of the victim's lungs before you begin to breathe into his mouth.

5. If the victim's mouth is clenched shut, as sometimes occurs in the case of a drowning person, separate his lips and breathe into his mouth anyway, allowing your breath to pass between his teeth. After filling the victim's lungs with your own breath, take your mouth away while he expels this air. This he will do on his own without your having to compress his chest and even though he is unconscious.

6. Be alert to the possibility that the victim may vomit. If he does, simply turn his head to one side, clean out his mouth as quickly as possible, and continue breathing air into his lungs. Vomiting simply indicates that the victim is short on oxygen. Furthermore, he may have swallowed considerable water, which is now being regurgitated.

7. It is common for a drowning person to have a convulsion. Do not let this alarm you, and do not let it interrupt the mouth-to-mouth resuscitation any longer than absolutely necessary.

8. When the rescue squad arrives, allow those with experience to take over giving artificial respiration, a task sometimes accomplished by a mechanical device administering pure oxygen to the victim.

9. While continuing mouth-to-mouth respiration, feel high on the side of the victim's neck for the pulsation of his carotid arteries. If you feel none, presumably the victim's heart has stopped. It then becomes necessary for you or someone helping you to stimulate heart action. This is done by applying pressure over the lower third of the victim's breastbone, releasing it, and exerting it again in a rhythm of about one cycle per second. The amount of pressure to be applied varies with the age of the victim. For babies, the pressure should be gentle, exerted through the tips of the operator's fingers as they press against the center of the baby's breastbone. For children of about 10 years of age, pressure should be exerted by the heel of one hand. For adults, one of the operator's hands is placed over the other so that pressure is exerted by

both hands sufficient to move the breastbone approximately two inches (5 cm.) toward the victim's spine (pressure of about 70 pounds). The operator can time his pressure strokes by counting slowly, "One little second, two little seconds," et cetera, so that the pressure is exerted at about one-second intervals. If you have an assistant, make sure that the mouth-to-mouth breathing is not interrupted during this procedure. If you are working alone, compress the breastbone twelve times and then take time out to blow air into the victim's lungs two times. Then repeat this procedure.

10. The attempt to revive a victim of drowning should be continued for *at least* an hour before giving him up as dead.

11. A person who has been rescued from drowning in salt water has suffered the loss of body fluid because of the osmotic action of salt water. He therefore needs to have water administered to him by mouth. In a freshwater accident the rescued person is not in need of additional water.

12. Even when a person is saved from drowning and begins to breathe on his own, nursing care, preferably in a hospital, will be necessary for many hours after the incident. Many persons who have been saved from drowning remain seriously ill for hours or even days after the incident. During this time they need supervision by a physician.

FAINTING

Fainting is characterized by a temporary loss of consciousness. In its common form it results from a reduction in the blood supply to the brain. For a discussion of its various causes see chapter 9, volume 2.

What to Do

For the common type of fainting, place the victim in a horizontal position with the feet elevated slightly above the level of his body. Apply cold water or a cold compress to his face and head. Clothes fitting tightly at the neck or the waist should be loosened. If a bottle of aromatic spirits of ammonia is available, open it and hold it near the patient's nose. If unconsciousness lasts more than a minute or two, call a doctor. Meanwhile, keep the patient covered warmly.

In the usual case the patient will re-

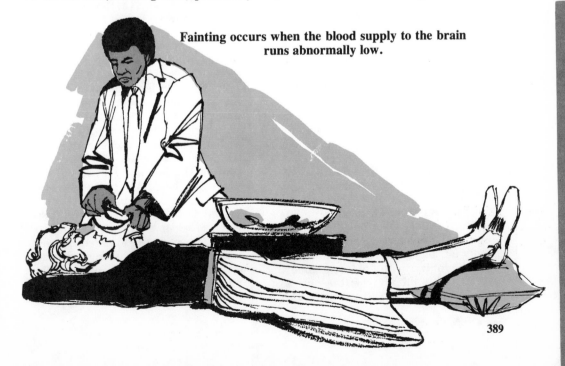

Fainting occurs when the blood supply to the brain runs abnormally low.

E
M
E
R
G
E
N
C
I
E
S

389

gain consciousness quickly. He may have a headache for a while after the episode. It is best to keep him warm and in a reclining position for an hour or so or until the doctor releases him.

FECAL IMPACTION
See chapter 17, volume 2.

FOREIGN BODY IN THE EAR CANAL, EYE, NOSE, SKIN, STOMACH, OR THROAT

A. *Insect in the Ear Canal.*

What to Do

1. Hold a lighted flashlight near the ear in a darkened room. The light may encourage the insect to leave the ear canal.

2. Tilt the victim's head slightly so that the affected ear is uppermost. Then pour slightly warmed glycerine, olive oil, cooking oil, or mineral oil into the ear canal and allow it to remain a few minutes. This should suffocate the insect so that it will not resist being removed. Then irrigate the ear gently with warm water, using a small rubber syringe to introduce the water into the ear canal and holding a basin under the ear to catch the water as it flows out.

3. If this does not remove the insect, consult a physician.

B. *Hard Object in the Ear Canal.*

What to Do

1. Tilt the head so that the affected ear points downward. Then pull the external lobe of the ear in various directions. Ideally this may cause the foreign body to fall out. If not, then proceed as follows:

2. Dip a small artist's brush or the clean blunt end of a matchstick into white glue or any other quick-drying adhesive mixture. Then, while pulling upward and backward on the ear lobe so as to straighten the ear canal, carefully introduce the sticky end until it makes contact with the foreign body. Wait a few minutes for the glue to dry, allowing the brush or matchstick

to fasten to the foreign body. Then gently remove, pulling the foreign body out.

3. If the foreign body cannot be removed by this gentle means, consult a physician. Never introduce a sharp object into the ear canal because of the danger of seriously damaging the eardrum.

C. *Foreign Body in the Eye.* If there is any possibility that a splinter of steel or any other small foreign object has penetrated the eyeball, a physician should be consulted at once. See chapter 8, volume 3.

If it is a cinder or dust particle that has found its way between the eye and the eyelids, proceed as follows:

What to Do

1. Have the victim close both eyes for a few minutes. The discomfort of the irritation will cause tears to flow from both eyes. In fortunate cases, this extra flow of tears will wash out the offending particle. The eye should not be rubbed.

2. If the foreign particle is still present, then grasp the lashes of the upper eyelid and draw the upper lid out and down over the lashes of the lower lid. Release the upper lid and allow the lower lashes to serve as a brush to wipe out the foreign particles. It helps, sometimes, for the victim to blow his nose during the procedure.

3. If the foreign body still remains, fill a medicine dropper with plain water or with sterile salt solution and gently rinse the space between the eyeball and the eyelids by grasping the eyelashes, one lid at a time, and holding the lids away from the eye slightly as the fluid flows underneath.

4. The last resort before taking the patient to the doctor is for the first-aider to wash his hands thoroughly with soap and water and then turn the patient's eyelids wrong side out, one at a time, as he searches for the particle of foreign material. This turning of the lids is accomplished

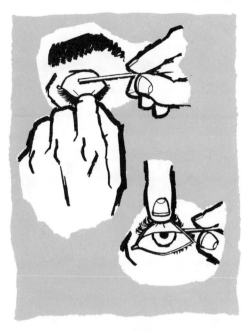

In turning upper eyelid wrong side out, first pull eyelid down over eye and place matchstick across it; then fold eyelid upward and backward over the matchstick.

easily in the lower lids by simply grasping the eyelashes. For the upper lid, it is best to use a slender pencil or a matchstick, as shown in the accompanying illustration, to help turn the upper lid wrong side out. Once the foreign object is discovered, it may be removed by gently touching it with the corner of a clean handkerchief and brushing it out of the eye.

5. If it is discovered that the foreign body is lodged in the substance of the cornea (transparent tissue at the front of the eye), a physician should be consulted at once.

D. *Foreign Body in the Nose.* Children sometimes force a bean, a kernel of corn, or an object of similar size into one of the nostrils.

What to Do

A foreign body in the nose can usually be seen by having the child tip his head backward. Inasmuch as the na-

sal cavity is narrow from side to side and tall in the vertical direction, it is usually possible to slip a loop of fine wire either above or beneath the object and gently withdraw it by pulling it forward through the nostril. If this is not successful, solicit the help of a physician.

E. *Foreign Body in the Skin.* A foreign body in the skin usually consists of wood (a splinter), metal, or glass. If the object is small and close to the surface, it can usually be removed at home. If it penetrates the deeper tissues or is underneath a fingernail or toenail, a physician should be consulted. In such cases the physician usually considers protection against tetanus (lockjaw) to be necessary. When a wound becomes infected after a foreign body has been removed, a physician should be consulted.

What to Do

1. The first-aider should wash his hands thoroughly with soap and water and also the patient's skin in the area of the splinter.

2. A needle and a small forceps should be sterilized by passing the operational ends through a small flame.

3. Use the needle to enlarge the opening in the skin through which the splinter passed. When the end of the splinter is exposed, it can be grasped by the forceps and the splinter gently removed.

4. Wash the area a second time with soap and water and cover it with a sterile dressing or an adhesive-gauze bandage.

F. *Foreign Body in the Stomach (Swallowed Object).* It is common for small children to swallow coins, marbles, keys, bobbie pins, and even safety pins. An object without sharp points will usually pass on through the gastrointestinal tract within a few hours or at least a few days. Open safety pins and bobbie pins sometimes become lodged in the intestine and may even

EMERGENCIES

perforate the wall of the intestine, with serious consequences. In such cases a physician must be consulted. He will use X ray to locate the object and may find it necessary to perform surgery for its removal.

G. *Foreign Body in the Throat.* When a child puts a small object in his mouth and it slips beyond his control, it either lodges in the pharynx (throat), passes into his air passages leading to the lungs, or is swallowed. Here we are concerned with the first possibility.

What to Do

If the child is able to get his breath by allowing the air to pass around the foreign body, keep him as quiet as possible in a reclining position while he is taken to the doctor. If the foreign body completely obstructs the child's breathing, you may try the expediency of holding him upside down while slapping him between the shoulder blades—this in the hope of causing him to use what air remains in his lungs for a cough which may dislodge the foreign body. Other than this, follow the instructions in the item CHOKING on pages 376-379 of this same chapter.

FRACTURES OF BONES

The exact means of caring for a fracture will depend upon the whereabouts of the injured person. Fractures should always be set by a physician, particularly open fractures, and preferably in a hospital. The first-aider's duty, then, consists of caring for the victim while waiting for the ambulance or for instructions from a doctor.

What to Do

The treatment for shock, the application of cold cloths or an ice bag to the injured area to relieve pain, the bandaging of an open fracture, and the proper splinting of the injured part in preparation for transportation of the victim are the principal responsibilities of the first-aider.

In case of an open fracture, the

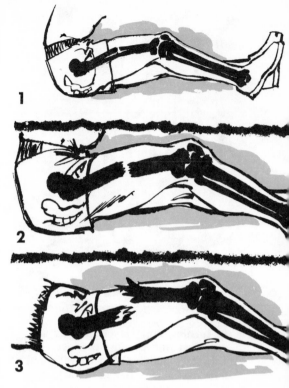

Three types of fractures: 1. "greenstick," 2. closed, 3. open.

first-aider should attempt first to control bleeding. (See the item BLEEDING in this same chapter, pages 366-368.) If bleeding is profuse, he should cover the wound with sterile surgical dressings or with clean cloths and bandage these snuggly in place.

Great caution should be taken to avoid moving the victim any more than necessary. Splints and proper supports should be applied to the injured person where he lies, so that when he is moved he will face no danger of greater damage to his tissues by any action of the sharp ends of the broken bones or by the stretching of tissues that would ordinarily be supported by the bones now broken.

Splints can be made from whatever is available—boards, sticks, magazines, newspapers, or pieces of corrugated carton. A splint should reach above and below the site of the injury far enough to prevent movements of the fragments of the broken bone. If an arm or a leg has been broken, the part should be gently straightened and placed in as natural a position as possible before the splint is applied. Strips of cloth, neckties, leather belts, or bandages may be used to fasten the splint in place. See the accompanying diagrams on the next two pages for the methods of applying splints to the various parts of the body.

CAUTION

If it is the back, the neck, the pelvis, or the skull that is injured, great precautions must be taken before moving the patient at all.

What to Do

A. *Fracture of the Arm*. In a fracture of the arm (between the shoulder and elbow) the injured member should be splinted to the body as indicated in the accompanying drawing (1).

B. *Fracture of the Back*. The grave danger in handling a person with a broken back arises from possible damage to the spinal cord in fracture dislocations, an injury which could produce lifelong paralysis. Plan your handling of such a victim before you move him at all. Commandeer the help of at least three other persons in placing the victim on a stretcher. For the proper method of lifting an injured person under these circumstances, see the diagrams on page 352 of this same chapter. The spine must not be bent, twisted, or overextended. In a fracture of the spinal column at any level, the victim must be transported on his back with small bolsters to support the small of the back and the neck. In placing him on the stretcher, which should be made rigid if not already so, make sure that the four people who handle him move in complete unison so as to reduce the danger of damage to the spinal cord. Patient should be firmly attached to the stretcher to obviate accidental fall and further injury. See drawing (3).

C. *Fracture of the Forearm*. In this case, after taking care of other complications such as shock and bleeding, the injured forearm is splinted and then placed across the victim's chest as indicated in the accompanying drawing (2).

D. *Fracture of the Hip*. This fracture is very serious, particularly in elderly people. Treatment requires a physician's services and hospital care. For transporting a person with a broken hip, a firm splint must be used for the entire length of the victim's body and injured leg, fastened as indicated in the accompanying diagram (4). Tying both limbs together is also a method of splinting.

E. *Fracture of the Leg*. After taking care of the possibility of shock and controlling bleeding, if present, prepare the victim for transportation by splinting his leg as indicated in the accompanying drawing (5).

F. *Fracture of the Neck*. A broken neck is a most serious injury and often results in the death of the victim. The possibility of a broken neck must always be borne in mind when handling an accident case where the victim has been thrown against some solid object. It is preferable not to move such a person until an ambulance crew arrives. If such help is not available, then the victim should be handled as recommended for broken back: The victim is placed on a stretcher, lying on his back, with a small bolster under his neck. One of the four people who assist in moving the victim must be commissioned to hold the head at all times so that it remains in line with the rest of the body—this to prevent further injury to the spinal cord at the site of the break.

G. *Fracture of the Pelvis*. Most

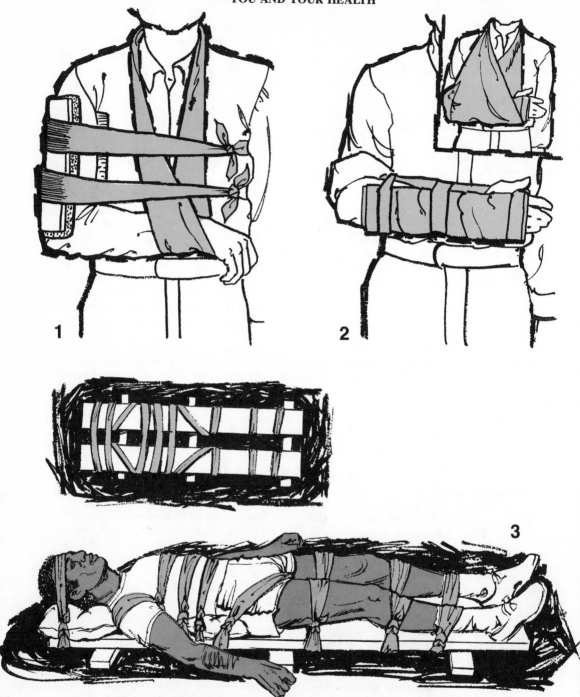

Methods of splinting and transporting fracture cases: 1. Arm splint. Injured member is splinted, placed in sling, and strapped to body. 2. Forearm splint. Injured member is splinted and placed in sling. 3. Back splint (also neck). Victim is secured full-length to stretcher with bolsters at neck and small of back.

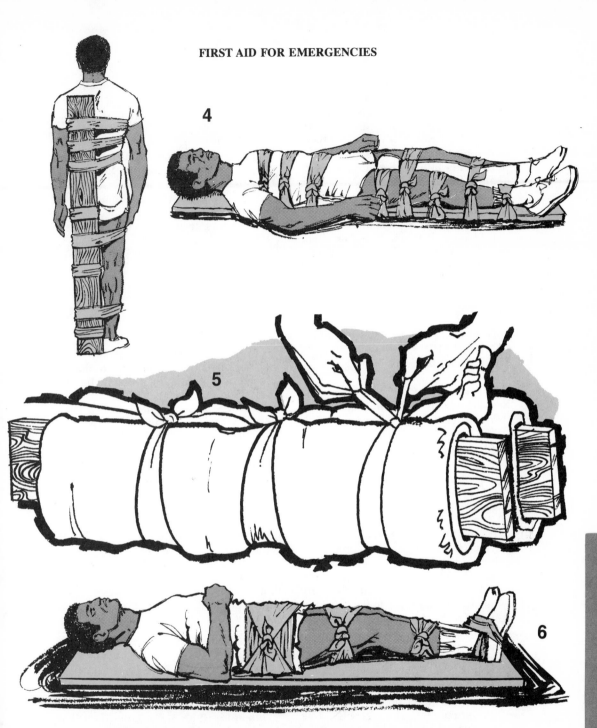

Methods of splinting and transporting fracture cases (continued): 4. Hip splint. A firm splint must extend the entire length of victim's body. Both legs bound together helps also as a splint. 5. Leg splint. Make entire length of leg rigid with padded splints on both sides. 6. Pelvis splint. Bandage knees together, also ankles, and place broad bandage firmly around hips. If transported, victim must be secured firmly to a board.

EMERGENCIES

fractured pelvises are caused by automobile accidents. They are usually associated with other serious injuries, often of the internal organs. Combating shock is usually a major problem in handling such a case. Before transporting the injured person it is preferable to place a large bandage around his pelvis to support it in corset fashion. As a preparation for transportation, the victim should be placed on a firm stretcher or large board and his legs fastened securely together and to the stretcher or board so as to avoid movement of the broken bones, as indicated in the accompanying drawing (6).

H. *Fractures of the Ribs*. See under CHEST INJURIES on pages 375, 376 of this same chapter.

I. *Fractures of the Skull*. See the item HEAD INJURY on page 397 of this same chapter.

GUNSHOT INJURY

The severity of a gunshot wound depends upon many factors, the most important being which part of the body was injured. Other factors include the size, the shape, and the speed of the penetrating missile. When a single bullet passes through the body or part of the body, the wound of entrance is smaller than that of exit. Injury by shotgun at close range causes more damage to the tissues than that by a single bullet from a rifle. The wound caused by a shotgun blast may contain fragments of clothing, perhaps some of the wadding of the shell, and individual pieces of shot.

The extent of damage caused by gunshot cannot be determined by examining the surface wound itself. The wound is usually contaminated, and the victim should receive protection against tetanus. All such injuries should be tended by a physician. The responsibility of the first-aider is to control serious bleeding, if present, and to take the usual steps necessary to avoid shock. (See the item WOUNDS,

PUNCTURE on pages 419, 420 of this same chapter.)

What to Do

1. Keep the patient in a reclining position and take the usual precautions to control shock by keeping the patient quiet and warm.

2. Do not attempt to probe the wound or remove the bullet or other foreign material that may have penetrated the tissues.

3. Cover the wound with a sterile dressing or clean cloth and then bandage.

4. Arrange at once for a physician to take over the care of the patient.

HAND INJURY

Injury to the hand may be caused by being crushed, as when a car door is closed on the hand or a finger; by contact with machinery, as by a moving saw blade; by encounter with a sharp instrument, as a straight-edge razor; or by a penetrating foreign body, as by gunshot.

The human hand is a very complicated "organ." It contains nerves, blood vessels, tendons, bones, and small muscles. The future usefulness of an injured hand depends on the care and thoroughness with which the injured parts are preserved and repaired. In a serious hand injury, the first-aider's function is not to attempt to repair the damage, but to care for the victim while he is being transported as quickly as possible to the emergency room of a hospital or to a doctor's office.

What to Do

1. Elevate the injured hand above the level of the victim's heart and maintain it in such a position. This aids the control of bleeding and reduces the swelling of the injured tissues.

2. Control serious bleeding by local pressure through a pad of sterile gauze or a clean cloth.

3. Do not probe the wound or try to remove debris, for this may dam-

age delicate structures that are still intact or that can be repaired by the doctor. Do not remove fragments of tissue or portions of fingers still attached.

4. Place a suitable-sized roll of bandage or a pad of cloth or gauze in the palm of the injured hand and gently bend the fingers around it. Separate the fingers slightly by placing gauze or bandage material between them and then cover the entire hand with a sterile towel, cloth, or unused plastic bag.

5. Support the hand and arm by a pillow or other object and keep it elevated as much as possible while the victim is being transported.

HEAD INJURY

The seriousness of a head injury centers around the possibility of damage to the brain or bleeding within the cranial cavity, leading to compression of the vital centers. Head injuries, common in traffic accidents, in falls, and in any incident of violence, are generally more serious in childhood because of a child's more fragile skull.

The types of head injury and the possible complications are discussed in chapter 4, volume 3. The instructions which follow are intended for the first-aider as he cares for the victim at the site of injury and during transportation:

What to Do

1. Keep the victim of head injury lying down and covered with blankets or coats so as to conserve his body heat and thus reduce the danger of shock.

2. As far as possible, treat the victim at the site of the injury until the arrival of an ambulance crew or until advice is received from a physician.

3. If there is strangling, gently turn the victim's head to one side so that the mucus or blood or vomitus may escape from the corner of his mouth and thus reduce interference with his breathing.

4. If bleeding from the scalp occurs, cover the wound with a clean cloth held gently in place by a bandage. Avoid undue pressure over the scalp wound because of the possibility of skull fracture.

5. If an ice bag is available, pad it and place it near the victim's head.

6. When it is necessary to move the victim, do it with the least possible movement of his body and with the victim always lying flat.

7. Observe the victim closely for a period of at least 24 hours. Make note of any deepening of his stupor or return to unconsciousness after he has once been conscious. Advise the doctor of any such change, for this may indicate bleeding inside the skull.

PRECAUTIONS

1. Do not permit the victim of a head injury to sit up or walk around. In his confused mental condition he may insist on walking, but this should be prevented.

2. Do not try to rouse the victim of head injury from his unconsciousness.

3. Do not administer any alcoholic drink.

4. Do not give stimulants.

5. Do not give any sedative or pain-relieving medicine (even aspirin) to a head injury victim not fully conscious.

6. Do not leave the victim of a head injury unattended.

7. Do not restrain the victim too much. If he wishes to lie on his side, permit him to do so. Excessive restraint may cause the injured person to become violent.

HEART ATTACK

For a complete discussion of coronary heart disease and the heart attack with which it may be associated, see chapter 8, volume 2.

A heart attack may come as a complete surprise, or the victim may have known for some time that he had heart disease or high blood pressure. The exact symptoms vary from case to case, and some of the usual symptoms may be absent in a particular instance.

E
M
E
R
G
E
N
C
I
E
S

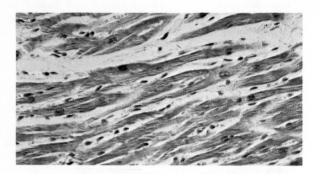

A microscopic view of the muscle contained in the wall of a normal heart.

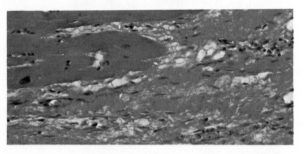

A microscopic view of a portion of the heart wall in which healing has occurred following a typical "heart attack" caused by the occlusion of a branch of a coronary artery. The lighter areas consist of scar tissue; the darker structures are remaining heart muscle fibers.

In the usual case of heart attack the patient is incapacitated with intense discomfort which originates in the chest, or even in the region of the upper part of the abdomen, and radiates to the left shoulder and left arm. He may feel that his chest is being squeezed. Often the discomfort is so intense that the patient can hardly breathe. He becomes weak. He may be nauseated and may vomit. He often perspires freely. His skin may be moist and cold. The skin may appear pale and dusky. He often expresses fear of impending death. The discomfort usually persists for half an hour or more.

With good care, many victims of heart attack survive. In some cases death occurs soon after the attack strikes. The function of a first-aider in caring for a victim of heart attack is to place him under the most favorable conditions until he can receive specialized, professional care.

What to Do

1. If the victim's heart has actually stopped beating (if you feel no pulse at the wrist or no heart sounds when you place your ear on the skin of the left side of his chest) follow the instructions for cardiac arrest as given on pages 373, 374 of this same chapter.

2. In any event, send someone for help while you yourself remain with the victim. Place an urgent call for the fire department rescue squad, an ambulance, or a doctor. Make the message urgent, stating that a person is having a heart attack. Provide name, address, and telephone number.

3. Place the victim in a half-reclining position with his head and shoulders elevated slightly. Keep him in this position until trained help arrives.

4. Insist that the victim remain absolutely at rest, not even moving a finger.

5. Loosen the victim's clothing where it might constrict his neck or waist.

6. Allow the victim to breathe fresh air. If a tank of oxygen is available, play a gentle stream of oxygen over the victim's face so he can breathe it.

7. If the victim has had previous similar attacks, he may be carrying nitroglycerine tablets as recommended by his doctor. If so, one of these should be placed under his tongue (not swallowed).

8. When trained help arrives, follow instructions.

9. Allow the patient to be transferred to the emergency room of a hospital or, if available, to a hospital coronary care unit.

HEAT CRAMPS

Heat cramps result from a depletion of salt in the body when a physically active person is exposed to high surrounding temperature. He loses the salt from his body by excessive perspiration. The symptoms consist essentially of painful contractions of the muscles, especially in the calves of the legs and in the abdomen.

What to Do

Prevention and treatment of heat cramps consists of adequately replacing by mouth the salt (sodium chloride) and water lost by perspiration. In the more severe cases, recovery can be hastened by the administration in the hospital of sodium chloride solution by vein. In many industrial plants where high temperatures prevail, employees are encouraged to take salt tablets routinely, so that their bodies do not become depleted of salt, and to drink water freely. Salt tablets, either five-grain or ten-grain, are available at the drugstore. Some prefer to take coated salt tablets to avoid the nausea which sometimes occurs from taking plain salt tablets.

HEAT EXHAUSTION (HEAT PROSTRATION)

Heat exhaustion is the second most severe of the three heat diseases, being more severe than heat cramps but less severe than heatstroke. A careful differentiation must be made between heat exhaustion and heatstroke, inasmuch as treatment for the two conditions differs markedly. Heat exhaustion occurs in persons exposed to hot weather or conditions of excessively high temperature who have not previously been accustomed to such high temperature. In this condition, large quantities of blood accumulate in the skin in the body's automatic effort to combat the external high temperature. This accumulation of blood reduces the amount available for the heart's pumping action so that not enough remains to provide the needs of the brain.

The chief symptom of heat exhaustion is a tendency to faint. It is associated with sweating, dizziness, extreme weakness, paleness (in contrast to the redness of the skin occurring in heatstroke), brief loss of consciousness (which may give the impression of ordinary fainting), clammy skin (which feels cool), weak pulse, and shallow breathing. The patient's body temperature as measured by a thermometer under the tongue is usually about normal.

What to Do

1. Lay the victim down in a cool place and in as comfortable a position as possible. Remove his external clothing and loosen any clothing that fits tightly. Place moist cloths on his forehead and wrists and, if available, play the airstream of an electric fan over his body.

2. Elevate the victim's feet and legs and massage the tissues of the legs with strokes toward the body so as to move stagnant blood into the body's active circulation.

3. If the victim does not rouse promptly, hold an open bottle of aromatic spirits of ammonia near his nose to act as a stimulant.

4. If the victim is now conscious, he may be given salt tablets by mouth or a glass of salt solution (salt dissolved in water, 4 tsp. per quart). If he is unconscious, he may be given a weaker solution by enema (2 tsp. per quart) with the salt solution retained in his bowel.

5. As the victim recovers, he should be kept quiet in a cool place, still in a reclining position. He should be instructed to avoid high temperatures for several days to come.

HEATSTROKE

Heatstroke (sometimes called sunstroke) is the most serious of the three forms of heat disease and carries a mortality rate of almost 50 percent. The basic cause is failure of the body's heat-regulating mechanism. It seems that conditions of extreme heat and high humidity overwhelm the brain's heat controls. Sweating ceases and internal

E
M
E
R
G
E
N
C
I
E
S

399

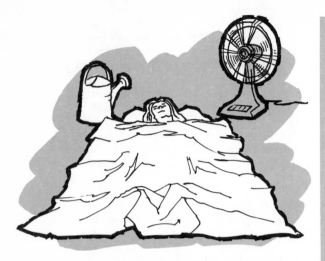

First-aid treatment for heatstroke calls for reducing the victim's body temperature as quickly as possible.

body temperature rises to dangerous levels—as high as 106° F. (41° C.) or higher. Other symptoms are collapse and a flushed dry skin which feels hot to the touch. Early in the course of the condition, the flushed, red skin is the most important indication of heatstroke. Later, however, if the circulation of blood is reduced, the color of the face may become deathly gray.

Heatstroke constitutes a serious emergency, and medical aid should be called at once. Even while waiting for the ambulance, effort should be made to reduce the victim's body temperature before permanent damage is done to the tissues of his body.

What to Do

1. Remove the victim's clothing and place him in a tub of very cold water (containing ice if possible). If a tub is not available, sprinkle his body with water and then fan his skin. An ice water enema carefully administered may be helpful.

2. Massage the arms and legs to assist in the circulation of the blood. The strokes of the massage should be toward the victim's trunk.

3. Check the internal body tem-

perature at frequent intervals (by a thermometer under the tongue), and judge the progress being made in reducing the temperature. By the time the body temperature becomes as low as 100° F. (38° C.) the extreme measures for reducing temperature (immersion in a tub of ice water or the use of ice water enema may be discontinued. Continue, however, to check the victim's temperature; and if it rises again, resume the more drastic measures.

4. If hospital facilities are available, salt solution should be administered by vein.

5. Allow for a prolonged period of slow recovery with medical supervision.

HERNIA, STRANGULATION OF

A hernia consists of the protrusion, usually of the intestine and related structures, through a weak place in the abdominal wall, most commonly in the vicinity of the groin. The protruded structures pass through the muscle layers but not through the skin. Thus a bulging mass is obvious on examination.

When the weakened area in the abdominal wall fits so tightly around the protruding tissues that the blood supply to this portion of the intestine is impaired, the hernia is said to be incarcerated. This condition is accompanied by pain, extreme tenderness, nausea, and vomiting. If the condition persists until the tissues begin to deteriorate from lack of blood supply, the hernia is then said to be strangulated.

What to Do

In the early stages of obstruction, a reasonable attempt should be made to return the herniated bowel to its normal location. The victim should lie on his back with hips slightly elevated. The attendant should then flex the victim's knee on the affected side, bringing the knee toward the chin. This should relax the abdominal muscles sufficiently to allow the herniated tissues to slip back into their normal position. Or the victim can assume a kneeling-lying position in bed (face down with face and shoulders on the pillow with hips elevated by way of kneeling).

If this treatment does not restore the herniated tissues to their normal position, the case then becomes an emergency. Arrangements should be made promptly for hospitalization and appropriate surgery.

HICCUP

See chapter 6, volume 2, for a discussion of hiccups.

What to Do

Many remedies are listed for hiccup, but none is universally satisfactory. The relief of persisting hiccup may even tax the ingenuity of a physician. In most cases, however, the ailment will respond to one of the following simple remedies:

1. Apply ice to the back of the victim's neck.
2. Have the victim swallow small pieces of ice.
3. Grasp the victim's tongue with a napkin in hand and pull it firmly forward.
4. Place the puckered opening of a medium-sized paper bag over the victim's mouth and nose, holding it tightly in place while the patient breathes for a minute or two into the bag. This exercise will increase the amount of carbon dioxide in the patient's lungs, a buildup which, of itself, may terminate the series of hiccups.
5. Have the person drink a glass of warm water slowly.

IMPACTION, FECAL

See chapter 17, volume 2, for a discussion on this problem.

INFECTION

For a general discussion of infection and infectious diseases, see chapter 15, volume 3.

In the present chapter we are concerned with the treatment of infections in wounds caused by injury. Infection is the greatest enemy of the healing of a wound. Infected wounds not only heal more slowly but heal with greater scar formation than uninfected ones.

For several reasons wounds caused by injury are more susceptible to infection than those produced by surgical procedures: (1) Injuries commonly occur in a germ-laden environment. (2) A wound caused by injury is usually jagged, containing many areas of devitalized tissue which foster the survival and multiplication of germs. (3) An injury usually destroys or harms the local blood vessels, thus reducing the supply of blood to the injured tissues and limiting their ability to combat the invading germs by the usual means of tissue resistance.

What to Do

1. To combat infection in cuts and minor wounds, the first-aider is directed to instructions outlined under CUTS, pages 380, 381, and under WOUNDS, page 419, in this same chapter.
2. The prevention of infection following serious injury requires that drugs which hinder multiplication of bacteria (antibiotics) be administered to the victim under the direction of a physician. He will continue the administration of such drugs, perhaps for several days.
3. It is important, in a case of serious injury, that the physician do a thorough job of cleaning the wound, removing all foreign material, cutting away the fragments of tissue which have been seriously damaged, and suturing as necessary.
4. It is important that proper steps be taken early for the prevention of tetanus. It must be assumed that all deep wounds are potentially contaminated with the spores of tetanus. See chapter 2, volume 2.
5. Even while drugs to combat infection are being administered, it is helpful to build up the patient's tissue resistance to infection by a simple procedure of hydrotherapy such as a

series of contrast baths. This procedure stimulates the circulation of blood through the injured tissues. First, the injured part is immersed in hot water, with the temperature gradually increased by adding more hot water as the patient's tolerance increases, for a period of three minutes. Then the part is plunged into another container, this one filled with ice water, and held there for about fifteen seconds. It is then returned to the hot water for another three-minute period, and so on, alternating thus between hot and cold water for about fifteen minutes per treatment. About four such treatments should be given each day.

INJURY, SEVERE (TRAUMA)

Injuries such as occur from a fall, an explosion, or from being crushed may be just as serious as those sustained in an automobile accident. Both external parts and internal organs of the body can be injured at the same time.

What to Do

Severe injuries, regardless of their cause, require the same kind of first-aid treatment. For this, see the item entitled ACCIDENT, AUTO-MOBILE on pages 353, 354 of this same chapter.

INSANITY

In various kinds of mental derangement the patient reacts unnaturally and may become dangerous to himself and to others. If already hospitalized such a patient will of course be cared for appropriately. But if the problem occurs in the home, the disturbed person's family will need to know how to handle it. First and foremost, those caring for the patient should be deliberately calm and positive in dealing with him while a physician's counsel is being sought. Realizing that a mentally disturbed person is not responsible for his present conduct, they will not resort to ridicule or harshness. Usually a disturbed person will respond cooperatively to a positive approach, even though his

words may indicate resentment. Although physical restraint and coercion are to be avoided as far as possible, extreme cases may demand such emergency measures, even with the help of a police officer.

The common forms of mental derangement, with suggestions on how to handle them, are now listed:

A. *Acute Psychosis*. Patients having this affliction lose contact with reality. They may become violently aggressive and even attempt assault or homicide.

What to Do

The patient with acute psychosis should be placed in a psychiatric hospital. When the condition develops without warning, perhaps at home, it may be necessary to arrange for the help of a police officer in order to control or subdue the patient. He should be under constant supervision, not being left alone for even a few seconds. All weapons and objects that might be used for harm should be removed from his room. Those caring for him should not allow him to come between them and the exits of the room. His threats of harm should be taken seriously, and he should be treated accordingly. As far as feasible, physical restraint should be avoided in favor of firm supervision. Under appropriate treatment by a physician, this acute phase is of short duration.

B. *Alcoholic Hallucinosis*. This is a complication of chronic alcoholism and is characterized by the patient's hearing and seeing things that are not real. The patient is in danger here because his hallucinations usually take the form of accusations by people around him and threats to his own safety. These may lead him to suicide or homicide.

What to Do

The care of a patient with alcoholic hallucinosis is the same as that for the patient with acute psychosis. See the preceding item.

C. *Delirium*. This is a form of excitement in which the patient may act out of context to reality and may even experience hallucinations. The many causes of delirium include influence of drugs, development of organic brain disorders, head injury, severe infections with fever, and the early stages of recovery from surgery.

What to Do

First, give attention to the underlying causes of the delirium and remedy them if possible. Beyond this, simply give constant supervision to prevent the patient from doing harm to himself.

D. *Depression*. In this form of mental ailment, the patient slows down both mentally and physically. He has poor appetite and loses interest in surrounding activities. He is apprehensive and troubled with sleeplessness. The greatest danger here is possible suicidal attempts, any mention of which by the patient should be taken seriously. For further information on depression, see chapter 5, volume 3.

What to Do

Such a case requires close nursing supervision, preferably in a hospital.

E. *Hysteria*. Hysteria is a conversion reaction. See chapter 5, volume 3. The manifestations of hysteria may imitate almost any disease, including mental disorder.

What to Do

Careful study of the case by a physician is necessary to differentiate hysteria from the disease it may imitate. The immediate care of the patient requires a combination of firmness and kindness.

INTOXICATION, ALCOHOLIC

For a consideration of alcoholic intoxication, see chapter 6, volume 2. In the present chapter, we are concerned with what to do in helping the intoxicated person to "sober up."

What to Do

1. Empty the person's stomach by helping him to vomit. This may be accomplished by having him drink two or three glasses of warm salt water (1 tsp. of salt to the glass).

2. Administer a large dose (1 Tbsp. of crystals in a half glass of water) of Epsom salts.

3. Keep the patient's body warm. Because alcohol produces a surface sensation of warmth, it is easy for an intoxicated person to become chilly without realizing it and to develop pneumonia.

4. When possible have the patient drink a mixture of 1 teaspoonful of aromatic spirits of ammonia in a glass of water. This stimulant helps to offset the depressant effect of the alcohol.

5. Under no circumstances should sedatives be given to a person under the influence of alcohol.

LACERATIONS

A laceration differs from a cut in that a cut is produced by a sharp instrument, whereas a laceration is made by something blunt such as a shell fragment, which tears the tissues and produces a wound with uneven edges. Usually bleeding from a laceration is not as profuse as from a cut of similar size. Often the terms are used synonymously.

What to Do

Treatment for a laceration is much the same as that for a cut (see CUTS in this same chapter, pages 380, 381). Usually with a laceration the control of bleeding is not difficult. If bleeding is profuse and, particularly if blood is spurting from a torn artery, follow the usual method of control. (See BLEEDING, page 366, of this same chapter.) For the routine care of laceration, proceed as follows:

1. Wash the surrounding skin area with soap and water, sponging the skin away from the wound rather than toward it.

2. Gently inspect the wound, re-

moving the dirt and foreign material by flushing the wound with sterile salt solution or, if this is not available, with soap solution.

3. If there are pieces of ragged tissue in the wound, snip them away, using medium-sized scissors and forceps.

4. If the wound is extensive, needing perhaps to be sutured (the skin edges stitched together), arrange for care by a physician. In the meantime, cover the wound with a clean dressing and keep the injured part inactive. If the wound is small, the edges may be held together, after the wound has been thoroughly cleansed, by narrow strips of adhesive tape or by an adhesive gauze bandage. (Steristrips are ideal.)

5. Should excessive swelling develop during the healing process or should the area of the wound become unusually tender and red, consult a physician at once for treatment of the infection.

6. In case of an extensive laceration, particularly one contaminated by street dirt or fragments of clothing or other foreign material, report the incident to a physician and arrange for protection against tetanus.

LIGHTNING, INJURY BY

Being struck by lightning can produce serious damage similar to electric shock from any other cause. To avoid this danger, be alert to an impending thunderstorm and take necessary precautions. When a storm strikes, seek indoor shelter or the inside of a closed car. Do not take shelter under a tree. Avoid contact with metal objects. If caught in an open area, curl up on the ground or squat with your feet close together.

What to Do

For emergency treatment in case an individual is struck by lightning, see the item SHOCK BY ELECTRIC CURRENT, pages 410, 411, in this same chapter.

MOTION SICKNESS

This term includes seasickness, airsickness, car sickness, and similar instances of temporary illness caused by the rhythmic motion of travel. Some people are more susceptible to motion sickness than others, presumably because their organs of equilibrium are more sensitive. Usually it is possible for a person to become accustomed to a kind of travel which formerly made him ill.

Symptoms of motion sickness usually include dizziness and nausea. They may also include pallor, clammy perspiration, headache, and vomiting.

Some people are more susceptible than others to motion sickness.

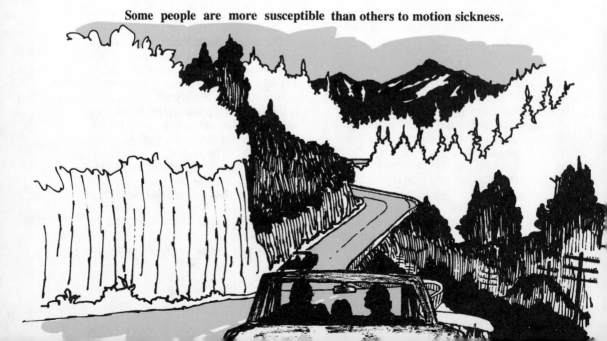

What to Do

1. Breathe fresh air, if possible, while you ride. When traveling by plane, a draft of air from the overhead vent, directed against one's face, will usually help.

2. Avoid moving your eyes from side to side as you ride in a car. Keep your eyes fixed on the road ahead. In a plane, fix the eyes on some given spot in the plane.

3. Avoid any kind of overindulgence before traveling. A hearty meal just before departure makes a person more susceptible to motion sickness.

4. If you are particularly susceptible to travel sickness, see your doctor before departure and have him prescribe one of the modern motion sickness remedies. Start taking the remedy as prescribed several hours before the time of departure, thus allowing time for your organs of equilibrium to be stabilized.

NOSEBLEED
See chapter 9, volume 3.

NUCLEAR EXPLOSION (NUCLEAR ATTACK)

There are three phases of injury by nuclear explosion: (1) blast injury, (2) heat injury, and (3) nuclear radiation.

1. *Blast Injury.* This is produced by the push-pull effect of the shock wave that emanates from the site of the explosion. It is this shock wave that uproots trees, collapses houses, and produces destruction by mechanical force. As far as a human injury is concerned, the blast produces all conceivable types of traumatic injury by throwing people against solid objects or by causing them to be crushed under falling materials.

2. *Heat Injury.* The amount of heat produced by a nuclear explosion is almost inconceivable, having been estimated as high as 1,800,000° F. (1,000,000° C.) at the center of the blast. It is this heat that causes extensive fires and the severe burns so typical among victims of nuclear explosion. The amount of light produced at the same time is so great as to cause blindness if the eyes are unprotected and the explosion, with its accompanying "ball of fire," is viewed.

3. *Nuclear Radiation.* Damage to human tissues by radioactivity is subtle. Rays can penetrate deeply into the tissues and cause severe damage to various organs and organ systems.

Degrees of Radiation Injury. The effects on the human body of nuclear radiation vary with the degree of radiation to which the individual is exposed. These may be summarized as follows:

1. With the highest doses, the principal effects of radiation are on the nervous system. Convulsions and coma occur within a few minutes, and death occurs, regardless of efforts at treatment, within a few hours.

2. In somewhat lower doses of total body radiation, it is the organs of digestion that suffer first. Nausea and vomiting begin soon after the exposure and are later accompanied by persistent diarrhea, which results from damage to the lining of the intestines. Even with good hospital care, the victim's condition is soon complicated by damage to the blood-producing tissues of the body. With such extensive damage to both the digestive organs and the blood-producing tissues, survival is impossible. Death usually occurs in about two weeks.

3. With still lower doses of total body radiation, it is the blood-producing tissues which suffer major damage. Some of these cases recover; others die within a few weeks. It is in this third group that we have the only genuine hope of successful treatment.

What to Do

1. Keep the victim at rest as much as possible.

2. With a radiation-detecting instrument, measure the amount of contamination by radioactive sub-

stances that may be present on the victim's clothing, skin, and hair. Discard contaminated clothing at the earliest possible moment. Radiation contamination of the skin may be largely removed by thorough washing with soap and water. (Carefully discard all the water used for this purpose.) It may not be possible to remove contamination from the victim's hair merely by washing. In some cases it is advisable to shave all the hair. Failure to decontaminate the victim of radiation injury has the effect of prolonging and intensifying the damage to his tissues.

3. As far as possible, the victim should be cared for in a hospital where frequent laboratory tests can be made to determine the degree of his radiation injury and the progress, if any, being made. This is especially important in cases where the radiation received has been relatively mild and the damage centers largely around injury to the blood-forming tissues.

4. Initial care in the hospital includes keeping the patient comfortable with sedatives, restoring his body fluid, and maintaining the proper balance of chemical substances within his blood.

5. Later hospital care includes the use of blood transfusions and the control of infection. The damage to the blood-forming tissues makes it impossible for the victim to produce his own antibodies and to combat infection. It is of prime importance, therefore, that he be kept in an environment as nearly germ-free as possible.

PARALYSIS

Paralysis consists of a failure on the part of a muscle or a muscle group to respond to nervous activation. In other words, the muscle or the muscle group becomes useless to the individual. Different types of paralysis and their various causes are detailed in chapters 6, volume 2, and 4, volume 3. See the General Index to find descriptions of the various manifestations of paralysis.

In the present connection we are concerned with the type of paralysis typically associated with a stroke. In this, the loss of activity of the muscles involved comes suddenly and often involves either one whole side of the body or, at least, sizeable muscle groups. It is in this type of suddenly occurring paralysis that the first-aider has an important function to perform until the patient can be cared for in a hospital or until he comes under the direct supervision of a doctor.

What to Do

Paralysis cannot be suddenly relieved as if by magic. Because of its sudden occurrence and because the patient is incapacitated, good reason exists for anxiety—on the part of the patient, if he is conscious, and also on the part of the family members.

1. Keep calm and avoid unnecessary handling of the paralyzed part of the patient's body. Any attitude or activity that increases the patient's blood pressure may aggravate the condition causing the paralysis.

2. When lifting or transporting the patient, always protect the paralyzed part of his body.

3. Nothing should be given to the patient by mouth until it is determined whether his throat may be paralyzed.

4. If the patient is unconscious, he may choke on his own saliva. He should therefore be placed on his side, preferably with the paralyzed side downward.

5. If the patient has difficulty in breathing, make sure that his airway is not obstructed by misplaced false teeth or by relaxation of his tongue. See the method of opening the patient's airway as described under RESPIRATORY FAILURE, beginning on the next page.

6. The most important factor in caring for a patient just paralyzed is gentle nursing care.

POISONINGS

See chapter 22, volume 3.

POISON IVY, POISON OAK

See chapter 25, volume 2.

RECTUM, PROLAPSE OF

Prolapse of the rectum consists of a protrusion of some or all of the tissues of the rectum beyond and through the anal opening so that they are easily seen and felt.

What to Do

The protruding tissue can usually be replaced by covering it with toilet paper and pressing upward. If this does not suffice, have the patient kneel and bend forward so that his head touches the floor. Resulting relaxation of the abdominal muscles, along with simultaneous pressure against the protruding tissue, usually causes the tissue to slip back into place. To hold it in place, the patient may wear a sanitary napkin for a while.

For children, the tendency to prolapse of the rectum is usually outgrown once they discontinue the practice of bearing down heavily when defecating. Toilet seats of appropriate size should be provided for children, since the use of an adult seat favors prolapse. For adults, a change in toilet habits may be necessary, such as going to the toilet when a strong urge first develops rather than waiting for a more convenient time. Also, if the fecal material tends to be hard and firm, drinking more fluid each day and including in the diet articles which have greater bulk will be helpful.

In extreme conditions of rectal prolapse, it is usually advisable to have a surgical repair of the tissues that have become weakened.

RESPIRATORY FAILURE (BREATHING FAILURE; RESPIRATORY ARREST; PULMONARY ARREST)

When for any reason a person stops breathing or becomes a victim of asphixiation, the cells of his body begin at once to suffer for lack of oxygen. Some of the cells of the brain, if deprived completely of their continuing supply of oxygen, will be permanently damaged after about six minutes.

Two of the body's organs normally work together in providing a continuous supply of oxygen to the body's cells: the lungs, which derive oxygen from the air, and the heart, which propels the oxygen-laden blood to all parts of the body.

Some of the conditions which cause interruption of breathing or of heart action are temporary. In such cases, life can be saved if the first-aider can keep the victim's lungs active by artificial respiration or can keep his blood moving by resuscitation of the heart until such time as these vital processes resume on their own. For the method of keeping the blood circulating, see CARDIAC ARREST on pages 373, 374 of this same chapter. For the method of resuscitating the heart and the lungs at the same time, see the item CARDIOPULMONARY ARREST on page 374 of this same chapter. The present item deals with the method of keeping the lungs active.

In any case of severe accident or of unconsciousness, see if the victim's chest is moving as he breathes. If not, begin artificial respiration at once as described below. Act fast.

What to Do
ARTIFICIAL RESPIRATION;
MOUTH-TO-MOUTH BREATHING

1. If the victim is in a room filled with smoke or gas, move him to a place where there is fresh air.

2. Lay the victim on his back on the ground, on the floor, or on a table.

3. Wipe any foreign material out of his mouth, using your fingers or a handherchief. Allow not more than ten seconds for this.

4. Place one hand under his neck and lift, at the same time tilting his head as far back as reasonable so that the front of his neck is stretched and his chin points upward.

5. Place your mouth firmly over the victim's mouth and blow hard

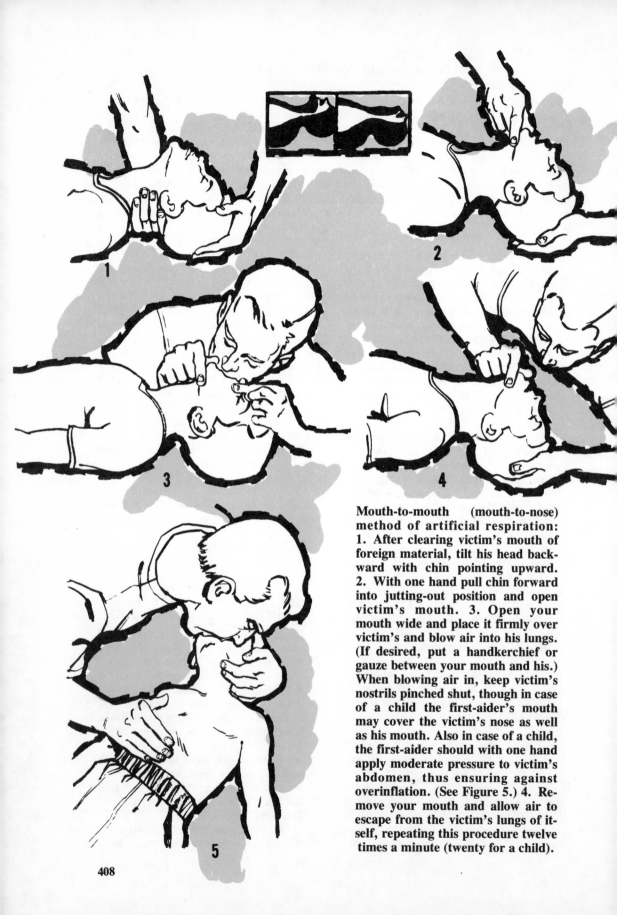

Mouth-to-mouth (mouth-to-nose) method of artificial respiration: 1. After clearing victim's mouth of foreign material, tilt his head backward with chin pointing upward. 2. With one hand pull chin forward into jutting-out position and open victim's mouth. 3. Open your mouth wide and place it firmly over victim's and blow air into his lungs. (If desired, put a handkerchief or gauze between your mouth and his.) When blowing air in, keep victim's nostrils pinched shut, though in case of a child the first-aider's mouth may cover the victim's nose as well as his mouth. Also in case of a child, the first-aider should with one hand apply moderate pressure to victim's abdomen, thus ensuring against overinflation. (See Figure 5.) 4. Remove your mouth and allow air to escape from the victim's lungs of itself, repeating this procedure twelve times a minute (twenty for a child).

enough to blow air into his lungs and make his chest rise. In doing this, you must close his nostrils either by pinching them closed or by placing your cheek against his nostrils as you blow into his mouth. If the victim is a small child, you may place your mouth over both his mouth and nose, thus making it unnecessary to close his nostrils separately. *Remember that a child's lungs do not hold as much air as those of an adult. Therefore, be careful not to overinflate a child's lungs.*

6. Remove your mouth from the victim's face and listen for the sound of escaping air. The patient should exhale on his own even though unconscious. If no air escapes, it must be that you did not succeed in forcing air into his lungs in your first attempt. In this case pull his chin forward (so that his lower teeth are ahead of his upper teeth) and try again. Make sure that the chin is pointing upward.

7. If you still cannot blow air into the victim's lungs, turn him on his side and slap him several times between the shoulder blades in hope of jarring loose whatever foreign material may be obstructing his air passages. In the case of a child, hold him by the feet, head down, and slap him sharply between the shoulders; then wipe his mouth clear of any obstructing material.

8. Once you succeed in blowing air into the victim's lungs, repeat this every five seconds (twelve times per minute), taking your face away betweentimes so that he may exhale.

9. Now you have time between breaths to summon help. Send someone to call an ambulance or a rescue team.

10. Have someone else find coats or blankets to cover the victim to keep him warm while you keep on breathing into his lungs.

11. Keep up the mouth-to-mouth breathing until the victim is able to breathe on his own or for at least an hour or until a physician pronounces the victim dead.

SHOCK, ANAPHYLACTIC (ALLERGIC SHOCK)

Anaphylactic shock is a state of collapse that occurs in certain persons who, by some previous contact, have become sensitive to certain medications (as penicillin) or to certain substances as may be contained in food, venoms, pollens, or dusts. The means of contact with a substance to which a person is sensitive may be by the administration of a medication, by the eating of a food (fish, shellfish, or berries are common offenders), by the sting of an insect (such as a bee, wasp, hornet, or yellow jacket), or by the breathing of pollens or dusts.

The severity of the symptoms of anaphylactic shock vary from person to person and depend on the amount of the offending substance absorbed. In mild cases the patient experiences itching and burning of the skin and membranes of the eyes and throat. Wheals of urticaria (hives) may appear on the skin. In more severe cases he suffers generalized swelling of the skin and membranes, with consequent difficulty in breathing. In very severe cases, the victim lapses into coma.

What to Do

Anaphylactic shock requires emergency treatment. The definitive treatment is the injection, preferably by vein, of a solution of epinephrine. But this is usually not available at the location where the victim is stricken. Hence the first-aider's primary concern is either to summon a medical emergency unit or to transport the victim promptly to the emergency room of a hospital or to a doctor's office. In the meantime the first-aider should carry out the general procedures used for a person in shock as a means of sustaining him. Make it as easy as possible for the patient to breathe. Keep the patient quiet and calm. Have him remain in a supine (lying, face up) position. Elevate his feet about twelve inches above his body. Keep him warm but not excessively so.

SHOCK, CIRCULATORY

This, the common type of shock, is a serious condition and requires appropriate treatment. The causes, usual manifestations, and emergency treatment of circulatory shock are given in chapter 9, volume 2.

SHOCK BY ELECTRIC CURRENT

Serious damage can result from the passage of an electric current through the human body. Such accidents occur when a person is struck by lightning, when he makes contact with defective electrical equipment, or when he comes in contact with "live" electric wires or devices. The amount of damage depends on the current (its voltage and amperage), on whether the victim is well grounded (as when he stands on a metal surface or when he is in water or in damp surroundings), or on the particular tissues of the victim's body through which the current passes. The current usually follows the most direct route from the point of entrance to the point of exit from the body. Ordinary domestic current in homes is exceedingly dangerous if the individual is well grounded, as in the bathtub or in contact with a plumbing fixture. Actual damage may vary all the way from a mild unpleasant tingling sensation to severe burns, paralysis of breathing, and stoppage of the heart.

Prevention of Electric Shock

Because of the possible serious consequences of electric shock, extreme care should be exercised, particularly at home, to remove the possibility of shock.

1. Ground all electrical appliances, particularly those in which water is used (such as washers). Modern home wiring provides for a third contact where the extension cord is plugged into the service outlet. This is the "ground" contact. If the service outlet has no such provision, a ground connection can be improvised by running a wire from the frame of the appliance to the nearest water pipe.

2. Keep all electrical equipment in good repair. If a shock is obtained on touching such equipment, make sure to repair it before using it again.

3. Avoid laying extension cords on the floor where walking on them may break the insulation.

4. Do not touch any electrical equipment (not even the light switch) while taking a bath or while otherwise in contact with plumbing fixtures.

5. Avoid using electric tools (such as electric garden equipment, electric shop equipment or electric machine tools) while standing on a wet surface or on the damp ground. If dampness is unavoidable, wear rubber shoes and dry gloves.

6. Never touch a swinging wire or try to pick up a wire or electric cable that may be lying on the ground. Such a wire or cable may be connected to the power line, and your contact with it may complete the circuit, making you a victim of electrocution.

What to Do

If the victim of electric shock is still in contact with the source of electricity, remove him from this contact (see opposite) or, preferably, shut off the current. If he has grasped a live wire, it may be that muscle contraction due to the passage of the current makes it impossible for him to release his hold.

CAUTION!

1. Extreme danger attends any attempt to free the victim from his contact with the electric current; the rescuer may make a similar contact and become a second victim. If possible, pull the switch to cut off the current. Otherwise, insulate yourself thoroughly by standing on a dry board or some other dry, nonconducting material and then with hands thickly insulated by dry newspaper, several layers of dry woolen cloth, or a sheet of rubber, separate the victim from the electrical contact.

2. Send someone to call a rescue squad or an ambulance.

3. If the victim is not breathing,

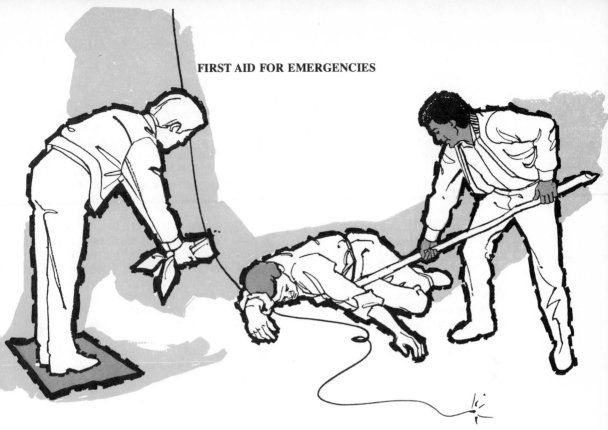

Precaution to be observed in removing a victim of electric shock from contact with the current: Rescuer should insulate himself by use of a dry wooden pole, rubber sheet, or dry cloth and prevent grounding by standing on a dry board.

start mouth-to-mouth type of artificial respiration at once and continue as long as he does not breathe spontaneously (even while en route to the hospital) or until a physician pronounces him dead. (See the item RESPIRATORY FAILURE on pages 407-409 of this same chapter.)

4. If the victim's heart is not beating, see the items CARDIAC ARREST and CARDIOPULMONARY RESUSCITATION on pages 373 and 374 of this same chapter.

5. Even after the victim has resumed breathing, keep him quiet, warm, and lying down for at least an hour or until the physician gives orders otherwise. Strangely, some persons become excited after they regain consciousness from an electric shock and do themselves permanent or even fatal damage by trying to walk around.

See also the item BURNS BY ELECTRIC CURRENT on pages 372, 373 of this same chapter.

SMOKE INHALATION

A major hazard of firefighting is the damage caused by the breathing of smoke. News items relating to fires frequently mention the number of people who suffer from smoke inhalation without giving details on the seriousness of the condition.

Smoke from burning buildings has become progressively more noxious in recent years due to the use of plastics and synthetics, both in building structures and in furnishings. Smoke from burning buildings now contains many irritating gases which do actual damage to the tissue of the lungs and the air passages. The symptoms of smoke inhalation consist largely of difficulty in breathing. The problem may develop immediately or may be delayed for as long as two days. Carbon monoxide

411

poisoning is also common in such cases. In severe cases pulmonary edema and/or bacterial pneumonia may develop. Persons who have inhaled smoke should be observed for at least two days even though they exhibit no immediate symptoms.

What to Do

The essential consideration in treating a person who has inhaled smoke is to maintain an adequate source of air or oxygen. As his breathing becomes handicapped, he may not receive as much oxygen as his body demands. Wafting a stream of oxygen beneath his nostrils is helpful. The attending doctor may order medication to reduce the swelling of tissues lining the patient's air passages. In extreme cases, a mechanical respirator may be necessary.

SPINAL CORD INJURIES

The spinal cord is the downward continuation of the brain. Many of the nerves that supply the various parts of the body both for sensation and for motor control are attached directly to the spinal cord and emerge between the vertebrae. Violent accidents pose the danger that vertebrae of the back or of the neck may have been broken and the spinal cord injured.

The structure of the spinal cord resembles that of the brain rather than that of the nerves. When the spinal cord is pinched or severed, all of the nerves below the level of injury are forever after useless, and the muscles that these nerves supplied can no longer be controlled by the brain. Paraplegia, in which the victim's legs are paralyzed, is the result of a severing of the spinal cord in the upper part of the back.

What to Do

For the first-aid handling of injuries in which the spinal cord may have been damaged, see the item FRACTURES OF BONES on pages 392, 393 of this same chapter, and the item SPINAL INJURIES in chapter 4, volume 3.

SPORTS INJURIES

Understandably these injuries continue to increase as the population's participation in sports increases. The greatest increase in sports participation in recent years has been in the unsupervised sports, such as skiing.

What to Do

For instruction on the first-aid handling of injuries that may result from participation in sports, see the General Index under such headings as Bandaging Methods; Dislocation; Diving, Related Emergencies; Drowning; Fractures; Injury, Severe; Sprain; and Strains.

SPRAINS

For a definition and description of sprains, see chapter 21, volume 2. The joints most commonly sprained are the ankle, the knee, and the wrist.

What to Do

It is advisable that a physician examine a sprained joint for any possible associated fractures. The physician will also advise on how long the patient should avoid using the sprained joint.

1. Immediately following the injury in which a joint is sprained, the application of a cravat bandage to support the joint helps to relieve the patient's discomfort. For the method of applying such a bandage, see pages 359-361 in this same chapter. A cravat bandage should not be left in place for long, however, because of a tendency for swelling in the vicinity of the injured joint that would make the cravat bandage too tight.

2. While a sprained joint continues to be swollen (which may be a few hours or even several days), it should be supported by an elastic bandage which allows for a reasonable amount of swelling. This bandage should be applied firmly but not so tightly as to interfere with the circulation of blood.

3. Once the tendency to swelling has ceased, a firmer support may be

applied, such as a strapping of adhesive tape. This should be applied by someone who has been trained in the use of adhesive bandages. Otherwise, the patient's blood circulation might be endangered.

4. During the first one to three days after the injury, or while a tendency for the joint to swell still persists, an ice bag can be applied to the injured joint. This tends to relieve pain and reduce swelling. The ice bag should be covered with a cloth so as not to come in direct contact with the skin.

5. Once the tendency to swelling has ceased, heat should be applied rather than cold. This increases the circulation of blood through the injured tissues and thus hastens healing.

6. For a sprained wrist, the forearm and hand should be carried in a sling. For a sprained knee or ankle, the patient should be kept in bed for the first day or two or until he can walk with crutches. Even then, the injured part should be supported in a horizontal position for at least fifteen minutes out of each hour.

STINGS
A. STINGS BY BEES, HORNETS, WASPS, AND YELLOW JACKETS
B. STINGS BY MARINE ANIMALS
C. STINGS BY SCORPIONS

A. *Stings by Bees, Hornets, Wasps, and Yellow Jackets.* Usually these stings are relatively harmless even though they produce painful swelling, redness, and itching at the site of the sting. Several stings at the same time, however, may inject sufficient venom into the victim's tissues to make him quite ill.

The serious fact in connection with stings by bees, hornets, wasps, and yellow jackets is that a few persons are sensitive to the toxins injected by these insects to the extent that anaphylactic shock develops. In such cases we deal with a life-threatening situation.

1. For those occasional cases in which anaphylactic shock develops, see page 409 of this same chapter for the method of emergency treatment.

2. In the usual case of a bee sting, the first procedure is to remove the stinger which includes the venom sac that the bee has deposited in the skin of the victim. Don't pull it out by grasping it with fingernails or tweezers, for thus you may squeeze more venom into the tissues. Try instead to scrape the stinger off gently with an object such as a knife blade, or loosen it with a needle so that you can remove it by sideways motion. Hornets and wasps do not leave a stinger in the skin. They are able to sting repeatedly.

The sting of a honeybee produces an allergic reaction characterized by swelling, redness, and itching. (Note stinger of honeybee left in center of affected area.)

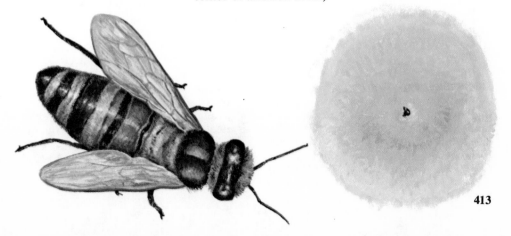

413

EMERGENCIES

3. Place an adhesive bandage over the site of the sting and soak this with a strong solution of Epsom salts.

B. *Stings by Marine Animals.*

1. *Catfish.* The saltwater catfish has a barbed stinger at the base of its large dorsal fin, the barb being strong enough to penetrate shoe leather. Accidents usually occur when a fisherman attempts to remove the catfish from a hook, the sting, of course, being inflicted on the hand. The principal dangers are possible allergic reaction or infection.

What to Do

Treat the sting of a catfish the same as a snakebite. There is no antivenin available. See the item *Snakebite* on pages 362-365 of this same chapter.

2. *Jellyfish.* The sting of the jellyfish is inflicted by long tentacles, usually on the victim's leg. The sting causes a feeling of illness which may last for several hours. An allergic reaction occurs in an occasional case.

What to Do

Treatment consists of soaking the affected foot and leg in diluted ammonia water (about 4 oz. [120 ml.] to a gallon [4 liters] of water). After soaking it from ten to fifteen minutes in the diluted ammonia water, soak it in hot water to which Epsom salts has been added (6 ounces [180 gm.] to a gallon [4 liters] of water). This tends to relieve the pain. After the soaks, the part should be kept slightly elevated above the level of the body. If the glands in the groin become painful, an ice bag should be applied here for about 20 minutes out of each hour.

3. *Stingrays.* When a stingray is accidentally stepped on, its whiplike tail can inflict a painful lash, the stinger being located near the base of the animal's tail. The sting produces a painful swelling of the leg. The area may become black and blue, and serious infection may develop. Damage is caused both by the injection of venom and by the injury to the tissues, with possibility of infection.

What to Do

1. Spread the wound open and wash it thoroughly with cold water.

2. Apply a firm bandage around the leg, as for snakebite, about two inches above the injury. Do this as soon as possible and make it firm enough to retard the spread of the poison through the superficial tissues but not so firm as to obstruct the flow of blood in the deep vessels. It should be possible to place one's finger beneath the bandage after it has been fastened in place.

3. Remove any remains of the stinger that may be still within the wound.

4. Arrange a hot bath for the injured leg, continuing it for as long as one hour or more and adding hot water as necessary to keep the temperature as high as the victim can reasonably tolerate. This helps to destroy the venom.

5. It is advisable to have a physician examine the wound in case it needs to be sutured and in case the victim may benefit by antibiotics to combat the infection.

C. *Stings by Scorpions.* Two species of scorpions frequent the southwestern states, the stings of which are serious but not usually fatal. The stings of scorpions in Africa and Asia are more serious and often fatal. The situation is most serious in the case of a child; the younger the child, the greater the danger of death.

What to Do

Antivenin prepared especially for scorpion stings is the only satisfactory treatment. A doctor should be contacted at once to see if antivenin is available. Otherwise, keeping the patient quiet and warm are the important things. The patient may experience dizziness, vomiting, increased production of saliva, and even shock.

STRAINS

A strain of the back or of a leg occurs when a person makes a vigorous, unexpected movement or when he uses his muscles improperly in heavy lifting. It involves an actual tearing of some of the muscle structures or their ligaments and tendons. The person may or may not be aware of the damage at the time it occurs. In some cases the symptoms of pain, muscle stiffness, and spasm develop later.

A. *Strain of the Back.* This usually involves the lower part of the back. But painful situations in the lower back may develop also from causes other than the tearing of the muscle structures; so it is desirable to have a physician evaluate the exact cause. For a back strain, the immediate treatment is as follows:

What to Do

1. Keep the victim in bed in the most comfortable position possible, in order to rest the involved muscles.
2. Apply heat and gentle massage to the painful area.
3. Once the muscle spasm relaxes, arrange for a supportive strapping of the lower back by the use of a two-inch (5 cm.) adhesive tape. The proper placing of the supportive strapping requires the skill of a medically trained person.

B. *Strain of the Leg.* This injury commonly happens to athletes or to someone not in good physical shape who might suddenly lift his weight by rising on the toes of one foot. The damage involves either the large muscles in the calf ("Charley horse") or a tearing of the large tendon at the back of the heel. Such accidents can also occur as a result of missing a step while descending a stairway.

What to Do

First relax the muscle spasm by gentle massage. Then apply a long strip of two-inch (5 cm.) adhesive tape along the back of the calf of the leg, running it under the heel and reinforcing it by shorter cross-strips running part way (not all the way) around the leg. This gives support to the damaged structures during healing. In severe cases it may be necessary for the injured person to use crutches for a few days, during which time he should avoid raising his weight on the toes of his foot. If a muscle or tendon is torn, the leg will become black and blue. Surgical treatment may be necessary for the most severe cases.

STROKE, APOPLECTIC

The causes, symptoms, and prevention of the usual kind of stroke are detailed in chapter 4, volume 3. In the present chapter we are concerned with the first-aid treatment of a person who suffers a stroke. Only the emergency care is given here. The person who has a stroke is entitled to long-range care and rehabilitation.

What to Do

1. Consult a physician or arrange for a person with a stroke to be taken to a hospital.
2. In the meantime lay the victim down in a comfortable position with his head and shoulders slightly elevated.
3. Loosen tight clothing.
4. Apply cold compresses (cloth wrung out of ice water) or an ice bag to the forehead and face.
5. Keep the victim quiet and do not encourage conversation even though he may be conscious.
6. If he vomits, turn his head to one side and take special care that the vomitus does not enter his air passages. This is particularly important inasmuch as the muscles of his throat may be partially paralyzed.
7. Give no stimulants and no other medicines except on a physician's special order.
8. If the victim has convulsions, place a rolled piece of cloth between his teeth so that he will not injure his tongue.

EMERGENCIES

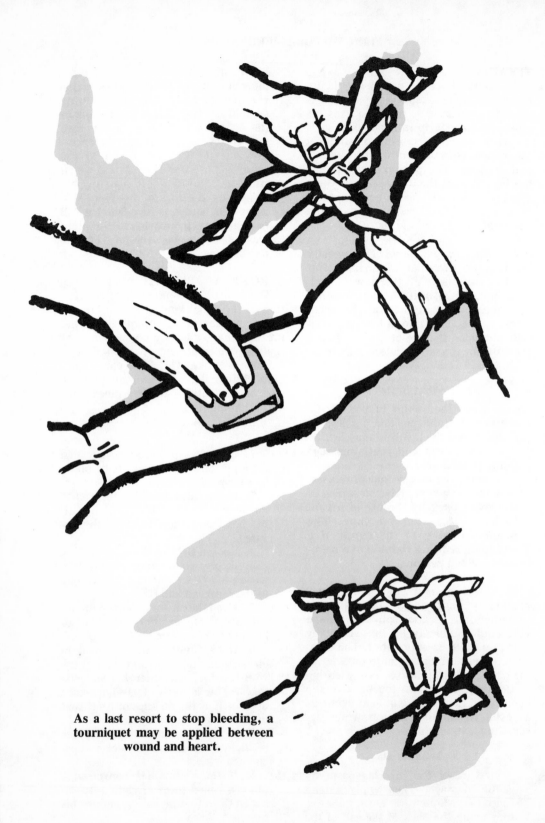

As a last resort to stop bleeding, a tourniquet may be applied between wound and heart.

SUICIDAL THREAT

The greatest mistake in dealing with a suicidal threat is to assume that the person does not mean what he says. You may save his life by taking reasonable precautions. Thoughts, threats, and attempts at suicide occur in some forms of insanity, particularly in cases characterized by depression, and also if the individual becomes seriously discouraged or thwarted.

What to Do

Arrange for continuous, 24-hour supervision of the individual for as long as necessary. Remove all objects or instruments from the surroundings which might be used in carrying out the threat. Arrange for professional help in seeking to find the basic cause of the depression and to devise ways for correcting it.

TOURNIQUET

The reason for mentioning a tourniquet here is to point out its dangers.

A tourniquet is a strong band of cloth or leather placed around an arm or a leg and usually twisted tight with a stick to control hemorrhage or to retard the spread of poison as in snakebite.

A tourniquet is dangerous because if made tight enough to prevent the flow of blood and thus to prevent hemorrhage in an injured area beyond the tourniquet, it will also cut off all the blood supply to the part beyond. These tissues then suffer for lack of blood and in many cases suffer permanent damage.

It used to be taught that a tourniquet to control hemorrhage should be loosened every twenty minutes to allow the blood to flow to the tissues beyond the tourniquet. It has been found, however, that this loosening usually starts the hemorrhage again and that in the long run the victim does not fare as well as when the tourniquet is left in place until he arrives at the hospital.

Concerning the use of a tourniquet for hemorrhage the first-aider faces this decision: If a hemorrhage in an arm or leg is so severe as to endanger the victim's life without the use of a tourniquet, then the tourniquet should be applied and made tight enough to stop the bleeding. The price that the victim will probably have to pay, however, is that his arm or leg will have to be amputated because of the damage done to the tissues by the placing of a tight tourniquet. In other words, it is a decision between the patient's life and the loss of a limb. See pages 366-368 under BLEEDING in this same chapter for other means by which severe bleeding may be controlled.

To control the spread of a toxin, as in snakebite, it is better to speak of the use of a "tight bandage" than to speak of the use of a "tourniquet." The tight bandage should not be made so tight as to prevent the flow of blood in the deep vessels. It should be just tight enough so that the first-aider can put one finger under the bandage after it has been applied.

UNCONSCIOUSNESS

Unconsciousness is one of the most baffling conditions that a first-aider faces. If the first-aider arrives after a person has become unconscious, he may not have the advantage of knowing the circumstances that caused the condition. See chapter 6, volume 2, for a consideration of the causes and types of unconsciousness.

What to Do

A. *Unconsciousness, Cause Unknown.*

1. If the unconscious person is not breathing, use the mouth-to-mouth type of artificial respiration. See the item RESPIRATORY FAILURE on pages 407-409 of this same chapter.

2. In the presence of witnesses, examine the contents of the victim's pockets (wallet) for a clue as to his unconsciousness. He may be carrying a card or wearing a bracelet saying that he is a diabetic or, for some other reason, subject to blacking out.

3. If the victim's face is red and flushed and his pulse strong, assume that he may have had a stroke and

417

treat him accordingly. See the item on STROKE, APOPLECTIC, on page 415 of this same chapter.

4. If the victim's face is pale and his pulse weak, check for bleeding and for head injury. Assume that he is in shock and keep him lying down, his head lower than his body.

5. If the victim's lips are blue, check both his heartbeat and his respiration. If the heart is not beating, see the item CARDIAC ARREST on pages 373, 374 of this same chapter.

6. Keep the unconscious person warm by covering with a blanket.

7. If the victim vomits, take special precaution by turning his head to one side, and make sure that he does not choke on the vomitus.

B. *Unconsciousness in Diabetic Coma.* In diabetes two kinds of unconsciousness can occur—the one when a person does not have a sufficient amount of insulin in his tissues (diabetic coma) and the other when he has too much insulin (hypoglycemic coma or insulin shock). (See below.) In diabetic coma the person lapses into unconsciousness gradually, his face is flushed, his lips appear red, and his skin is dry. The telltale symptom is the odor of acetone (which smells similar to nail-polish remover) on the victim's breath.

CAUTION. Do not confuse this form of unconsciousness with that caused by alcoholic intoxication. See under INTOXICATION, ALCOHOLIC in this chapter (page 403) and in the General Index.

What to Do

The only satisfactory remedy for diabetic coma is to give the victim an injection of insulin. Unless the victim carries this with him, the first-aider must await the arrival of an emergency unit, or the patient must be taken to the emergency room of a hospital. In the meantime, treat the victim as though he were in shock: Keep him covered and warm, keep his legs slightly elevated, and give fluid by

rectum if enema equipment is available. Do *not* give sugar or any form of carbohydrate.

C. *Unconsciousness From Too Much Insulin (Hypoglycemic Coma or Insulin Shock).* This situation is very much the opposite of the preceding one. In this condition, hypoglycemia, a diabetic patient has probably taken his usual dose of insulin but has failed to eat the amount of food which would use up the insulin he has taken. He appears pale, his skin is moist. He appears to be in shock, and there is *no* odor of acetone on his breath.

What to Do

1. If you are sure of the cause of the unconsciousness, place sugar on the patient's tongue, allowing it to dissolve slowly. Or give orange juice in small amounts by teaspoon even though the patient is unconscious.

2. In any event, summon professional help or call an ambulance.

D. *Unconsciousness From Stroke.* In this case the victim may have collapsed rather suddenly. He may be unconscious, or he may be simply stuporous and confused. The face is usually red and congested. The pupils of the eyes may be unequal in size, and there may be difficulty in speech if the unconsciousness is not complete. There may be a weakness of muscles on one side of the face or on one side of the body.

What to Do

See STROKE, APOPLECTIC on page 415 of this same chapter.

E. *Unconsciousness From Uremia.* This disorder is caused by an inability of the kidneys to function normally. Unconsciousness usually develops gradually after the person has been ill for some time with kidney disease or heart disease.

The patient usually suffers headache and mental confusion. The skin appears pale yellow and is cold and dry.

There is an odor about the patient similar to that of stale urine. The pulse is rapid and full.

What to Do

A first-aider can do very little in this case except to summon medical help and arrange for hospital care.

VOMITING

The causes and significance of vomiting are discussed in chapter 6, volume 2. We are here concerned with the immediate treatment of this symptom.

What to Do

1. Put the patient to bed with a hot water bottle at his feet. (The hot water bottle should be no hotter than can be applied to the first-aider's face.)

2. Restore fluid. Clear broth, thin gruel, 7-Up, or ice-cold milk may be acceptable. Otherwise, frequent small sips of water are helpful in restoring the fluid lost by vomiting.

3. Provide light food as tolerated. As the patient improves, he may be able to take a soft-boiled egg on hot milk toast.

4. Consult a physician if the vomiting continues in spite of bed rest.

WOUNDS

A wound consists of a break in the skin in which the deeper tissues such as muscle and bone may or may not be damaged.

What to Do

In the care of wounds the primary objectives are to prevent or minimize infection and to promote healing. Most important in preventing infection is a thorough cleansing of the wound, both in its interior and on the surrounding skin surface. First, of course, the clothing in the vicinity of the wound must be removed. Then thoroughly wash the skin of the surrounding area, directing the cleansing strokes away from the wound rather than toward it. Next, give careful attention to cleaning the interior of the wound, flushing it gently with sterile salt solution or soap and water. Remove all foreign matter and fragments of devitalized tissue (by the use of forceps and scissors, an operation preferably done under local anesthesia by a doctor). The doctor will use his judgment as to whether to pull the edges of the wound together by the use of sutures (stitches). Place a sterile dressing (preferably sterile surgical gauze) over the wound and cover it with a bandage to hold it in place.

Another important consideration in the care of wounds is to arrange for the prevention of tetanus. See chapter 18, volume 3.

WOUNDS, PUNCTURE

Puncture wounds are those in which the injury has been inflicted by a small object which has penetrated the deeper tissues without tearing the skin more than enough to admit the object that caused the damage. In these, the skin may close tightly around the opening.

The particular hazard of puncture wounds centers around the exclusion of air from the damaged tissues. This situation favors the development of one of the most deadly infections—tetanus. The tragedy of tetanus infection is that once the symptoms develop (a few days following injury) treatment (by prevention) is no longer effective and death is very probable. The time to treat tetanus (by prevention) is immediately after a penetrating injury is sustained. Better still is to maintain one's immunity to tetanus by the immunization shots which a physician is prepared to give.

The typical puncture wound is one sustained by stepping on a rusty nail. The danger of tetanus infection is particularly great when the injury occurs in the environment of a farmyard or where there may be contamination by street dirt.

What to Do

Every puncture wound should be considered serious and should receive the attention of a physician. He may find it necessary to enlarge the skin opening so as to cleanse the interior of the wound more thoroughly. Simple cleansing of the wound, however, is not sufficient to remove the danger of tetanus. The only satisfactory way to prevent this dread disease consists of receiving a tetanus immunization, which only the physician can administer. For more information see chapter 18, volume 3.

SECTION **VII**

Home
Treatments

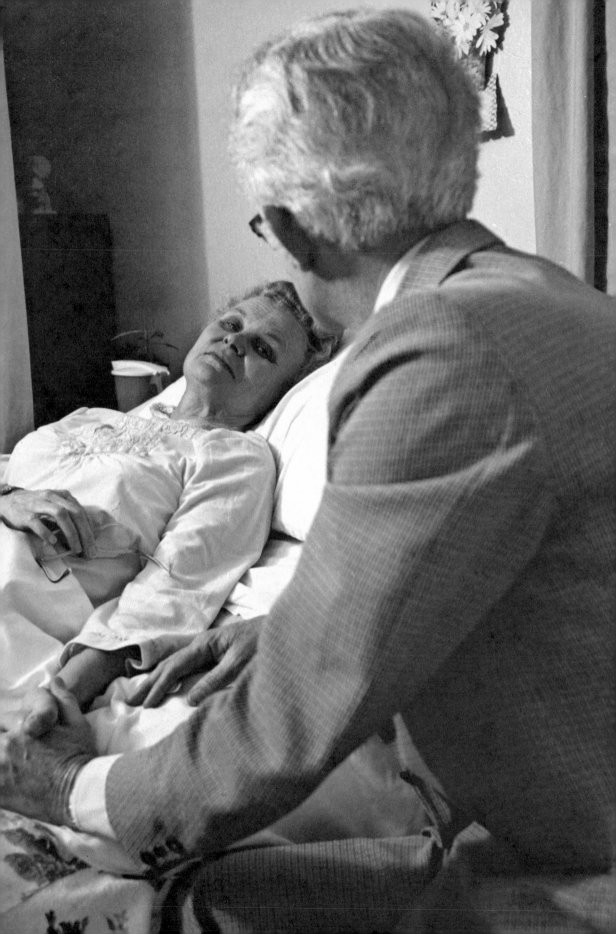

Section VII

CHAPTER *24*

When Someone in Your Home Is Ill

In many cases it is best for a seriously ill person to be cared for in a hospital. There facilities for precise diagnosis are provided. On the other hand, there are times when it is desirable instead to care for an ill person at home, such as following a stay in the hospital. Home care can even have its advantages. The patient benefits by being spared the bustle of a hospital and profits by the loving care and close attention that relatives can give.

This chapter deals with the patient partially or completely confined to bed at home. It is generally assumed that the patient is not to be up and out of bed because of the seriousness of his condition. It should be emphasized, however, that for most patients confined to bed, getting up and around is most important in the period of convalescence. To what extent such activity should be encouraged depends upon the medical condition of the patient, and of course in most cases upon consultation with the patient's physician. At first, and particularly with partially paralyzed patients, care should be given to prevent falling. Sometimes it is necessary to insist that the patient not get up unless someone stands by. Many of the principles and instructions given in this chapter apply during the period of convalescence.

The essence of care for a sick person is to place him in circumstances most favorable for his rehabilitation. By rehabilitation we generally mean one of three things: (1) return to the patient's usual way of life; (2) adoption of a way of life which eliminates the conditions that have caused his present illness— an improved pattern of living; or (3) development of a satisfying life program which makes allowance for the persisting limitations that his illness has caused and yet enables him to live productively.

Rehabilitation occurs gradually. It involves the process of healing: the restoration of torn tissues, the mending of a broken bone, or the development of immunity to an infection. And because of delay in the process, the patient faces the hazard of discouragement or even depression. It is here that the family environment is particularly helpful. Being part of the family group, engaging by proxy in the activities of family members, receiving the love and encouragement of dear ones—these often contribute more to rehabilitation than do medicines or counsel sessions.

Home care for a sick person does not

423

replace professional supervision; it complements it. Depending on the nature of the patient's illness, there may be need for supervision, not only by the physician, but also by other qualified health professionals. The visiting nurse, the physical therapist, the occupational therapist, the speech therapist, the psychologist, the social service worker, the vocational counselor, the chaplain—any one or more of these may be needed in a given case. The family members most involved in the care of the patient must work in close cooperation with these professionals.

The patient being cared for at home must be taught and encouraged to share in the responsibility for his rehabilitation. He should not be allowed to become content to let others wait on him. He must do as much for himself as his condition permits. Only as he learns to be independent and to function in his own right, can his recovery be complete.

The Home Environment

The room in which a sick person lives and receives care has much to do with his comfort and speed of recovery. Some homes are arranged more favorably than others for the care of a sick person. Thus the exact arrangement will have to be adapted to the individual case.

Ideally, the room chosen should be pleasantly decorated, should admit sunlight when desired, should have provision for heating and cooling as needed, should provide ventilation without causing a draft, and should be near a bathroom or toilet. The room should be clean and in order, each needed article kept in its designated place. Food should not be kept in the room, and all used dishes and soiled linen should be removed promptly after use. A potted plant or a few flowers may be permissible, but none with a strong odor.

The room should be aired once or twice a day, even in cold weather, by opening wide the doors and windows. At such times the patient should be well covered, if in bed, or should wear adequate clothing if sitting up or walk-

Choice of a home sickroom must take into account factors such as ventilation, sunlight, and bathroom facilities.

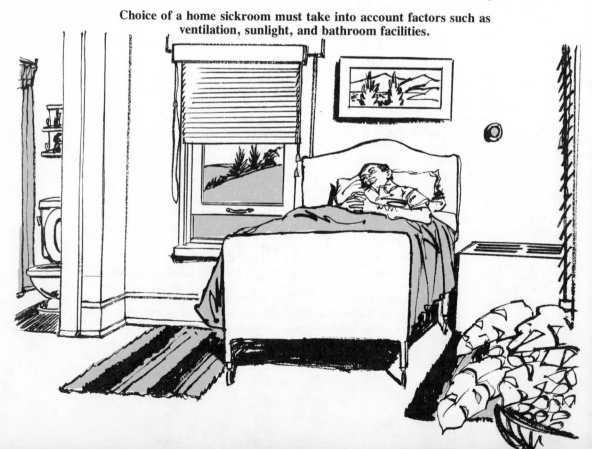

ing about the room. The bed should be so placed as to keep strong light from shining directly into the patient's eyes, but in a position to permit a pleasing view, if possible.

The Helper

If it is not possible to hire an experienced nurse, it is essential to select as the patient's helper a member of his family or some other person who has genuine concern for the patient's needs. The helper must follow the doctor's orders, which may be quite numerous and detailed. It may be best to write them down to avoid forgetting something or making a mistake. The helper should be a pleasant person, kind and considerate, but should go about his duties in a matter-of-fact way so as not to give the impression that the patient is seriously ill. If the patient cannot be left alone, a substitute should occasionally relieve the helper. This is true even when the sick person is a child under the care of his mother.

Beds and Bed Making

A comfortable bed is of extreme importance. It may be desirable to rent or purchase a hospital-type bed which can be mechanically raised and lowered. In the case of children and helpless older patients, it may be necessary to have side rails attached to the bed or by some other means to prevent the patient from falling out of bed.

A bed can be made firm by placing a sheet of plywood under the mattress. The mattress should be comfortable, having no humps or hollows. It is desirable to turn the mattress occasionally to help prevent its becoming misshapen. The mattress should be protected by a full-size pad or by a blanket that can be easily washed.

Sheets should be sufficiently wider and longer than the bed to allow for tucking them in securely. The lower sheet should be placed over the mat-

To raise home patient's bed to desired height remove casters and set legs on wooden blocks hollowed out to hold legs securely. (See inset.) Note also placement of waterproof covering and manner of tucking in corners of sheet.

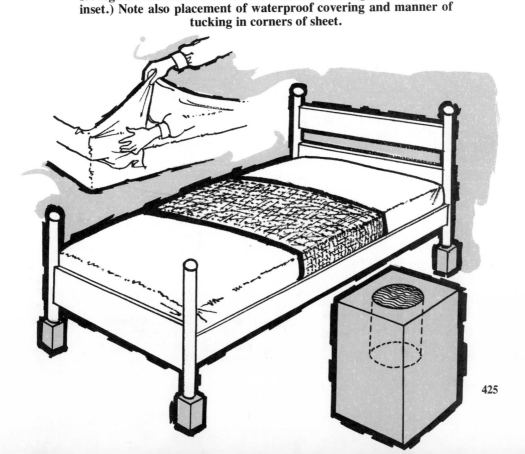

tress pad and snuggly tucked in at the top, bottom, and sides with smooth, square corners. Be sure to make this sheet tight; otherwise it will tend to wrinkle.

Should the mattress need to be protected from discharges, a smaller, plastic sheet may be placed over the lower sheet. When this is done, care should be taken that the plastic sheet is free from wrinkles and that it has no cracks which would allow leakage. The plastic sheet should cover only the midportion of the bed. (See the illustration.)

A drawsheet, just an ordinary sheet folded once lengthwise, should be placed with its folded edge toward the head, crosswise of the bed, and over the plastic sheet (if a plastic sheet is used), overlapping it a few inches both above and below, with the end at one side of the bed being left longer than at the other.

Where no plastic sheet is needed, a drawsheet is still a great convenience. It is then placed immediately over the lower sheet. It can be drawn to one side or the other, giving the patient a cool, smooth spot on which to lie; or, in case of accidental soiling of the bed, can be changed with little inconvenience to the patient and without having to remake the bed.

The upper sheet is then placed on the bed, with the upper end six to eight inches above the head of the mattress. It should be smoothed carefully and tucked in at the bottom with smooth, square corners. Then the blankets are placed with the upper ends about eight inches below the top of the mattress. The bedspread is then arranged with its upper end about three inches above the upper end of the blankets, this margin being turned in to protect the blankets. The lower end is tucked under the mattress, with square corners, and the sides left hanging. The upper sheet is then turned back over the spread about one foot. Then, with well-shaken pillows in place, the bed is ready for the patient. The overlying bedding usually needs to be loosened to give room for the feet when the patient lies face up

and when he turns. A device to keep the bedding lifted off the feet may be desirable.

Changing the Bed Linen

The linen on the patient's bed should ordinarily be replaced with fresh linen daily. In the case of serious soiling, at least part of the linen will need to be changed between times.

If the patient can be about the room part of the time, he should be seated comfortably in a chair while the bed linen is being changed. But for the bedridden patient, unable to leave the bed, the following procedure for changing the linen is recommended (see accompanying illustrations):

Have the clean sheets close at hand. Loosen the bedding on all sides, remove the spread, also the top blanket if there are two. Then gently draw out the soiled top sheet from the remaining blanket beneath (1). The patient, if not helpless, can help by holding this blanket. Then move the patient to one side of the bed and turn him with his face toward the edge of the bed on that side.

Remove the pillow and bring the blanket up close around the patient. Grasping the drawsheet on the vacant side of the bed, roll it tightly to the middle of the bed and a little beyond, bringing the roll next to the patient's back. The plastic sheet, if there is one, should be similarly rolled and brought next to the patient. Finally the lower sheet on the vacant side of the bed is rolled throughout its entire length, and the roll is brought up snugly next to the previous roll or rolls (2).

Now, working from the vacant side of the bed, take the clean bottom sheet, folded or rolled lengthwise, and spread it out to the middle of the bed. Tuck in the edges as in an unoccupied bed and bring the fold or roll up close to the rolls of soiled linen. Draw the plastic sheet, if one is used, back over the clean bottom sheet. Then fold and place the clean drawsheet, tucking it in at your side and spreading it up to the patient's back, with the free end still rolled or folded (3, 4).

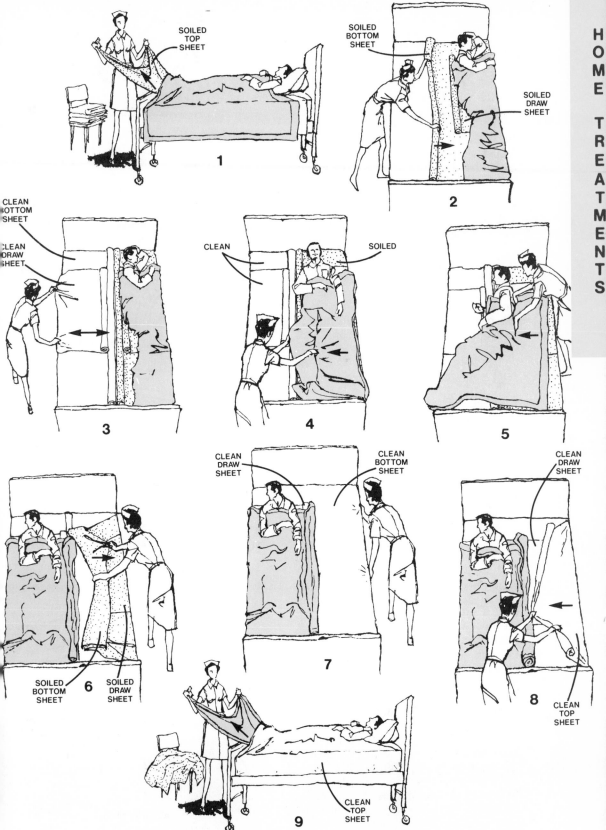

1 — SOILED TOP SHEET

2 — SOILED BOTTOM SHEET · SOILED DRAW SHEET

3 — CLEAN BOTTOM SHEET · CLEAN DRAW SHEET

4 — CLEAN · SOILED

5

6 — SOILED BOTTOM SHEET · SOILED DRAW SHEET

7 — CLEAN DRAW SHEET · CLEAN BOTTOM SHEET

8 — CLEAN DRAW SHEET · CLEAN TOP SHEET

9 — CLEAN TOP SHEET

427

Procedure for changing sheets when patient cannot be moved from the bed. See description in this chapter for details to be followed in the progressive steps here illustrated.

Lift the patient's feet, with knees flexed, over the closely rolled bedding, and, going to the other side of the bed, gently turn the patient back over the rolled sheets onto the fresh, smoothed portion, keeping the covering blanket in place (5). Then quickly remove the soiled bedding and draw the fresh bedding into place on this second half of the bed and tuck it in snuggly all around (6, 7). Place the clean top sheet over the blanket, and then, holding the sheet in place, slide the blanket out from under the sheet and lay it on top of this upper sheet (8, 9). If a second blanket is to be used, it can now be placed on the first one. Arrange the bedspread as before directed and tuck all in at the foot, being careful not to cause discomfort by drawing the bedding too tight over the patient's feet.

The patient can make use of several pillows of various sizes to add wonderfully to his comfort. They make comfortable positions possible by lessening the muscular tension. For example, when the patient is lying on his back with his knees flexed, a pillow under the knees and another for the feet to rest against are helpful. A weak or helpless patient turned on one side appreciates a pillow tucked against his back to support it, and a tiny pillow slipped under the abdomen helps. When the patient is lying on his side, flexing the upper knee a little more than the under one and placing a pillow between his knees is restful and relaxing. When the patient is able to sit up in bed, a kitchen chair nicely serves the purpose of a back support. Turn it upside down with the legs against the head of the bed so that the back forms an inclining plane (see accompanying illustration). Pad it well with pillows. (When a regular hospital bed can be obtained, this improvisation is unnecessary.)

If the patient is weak, a pillow under each arm while he is sitting up in bed makes him more comfortable; and, again, pillows as knee supports and foot rests are useful. One must be careful, however, in making a patient com-

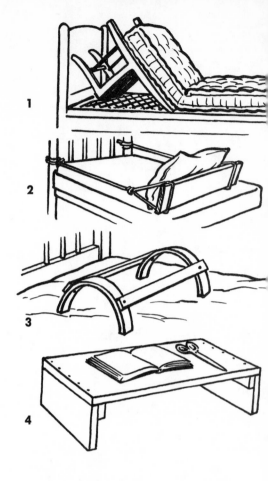

Types of bed-comfort aids: 1. Improvised back support. 2. Cushioned footrest. 3. Cradle to hold bedclothing off sensitive surfaces. 4. Portable worktable. Below: closeup of footrest.

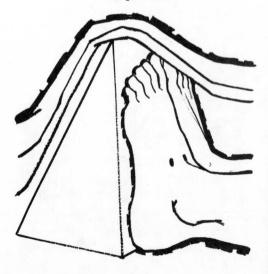

fortable, not to allow him habitually to assume a position which may cause shortening of the muscles, such as may occur from keeping the knees bent for long periods. It may be that a little discomfort is good, for then the patient will call for frequent changes of position which help to prevent deformities and possible damage to the skin.

Personal Care

The daily care of the patient begins in the morning when the face and hands are washed, the teeth are cleaned, and the hair is brushed. The patient may also use the toilet. Then the bed is smoothed, the pillows are shaken, and the patient is made ready for breakfast.

If a record is being kept of the patient's temperature, take a reading before the patient brushes his teeth or drinks water. To get an accurate temperature reading at any time of the day, the thermometer should not be placed in the patient's mouth sooner than 15 minutes after his taking a drink or for at least half an hour after a meal. Mouth breathing or breathing cold air will also affect the temperature reading. If a mercury thermometer is used it should be shaken down at least two degrees below the normal temperature level; then the bulb of the thermometer is placed well under the patient's tongue. The patient must hold his lips firmly closed for two minutes while the thermometer is in place. After being used, the thermometer should be rinsed in cool water and disinfected by dipping it in alcohol. The normal temperature of a person in health is approximately 98.6° F. (37° C.) though it usually varies some during the 24 hours.

With an unconscious patient, the temperature cannot be taken by mouth. The thermometer is then placed either in the rectum or in the axilla (armpit).

For taking an adult's temperature by rectum, have the patient lie on his side. Then lubricate the thermometer with petrolatum or oil and insert it into the rectum about two inches, holding it there for two minutes. As the thermometer is removed, it is wiped dry with cleansing tissue and the thermometer reading recorded. The thermometer is then washed with detergent and disinfected with alcohol. Temperature taken by rectum will normally be about a degree higher than that taken by mouth.

To take the temperature by axilla, first wipe the armpit dry and place the thermometer in it, holding it there for five minutes by pressing the arm tightly against the side of the chest. Temperature taken by axilla is about one degree lower than that taken by mouth.

It is easy to count the patient's pulse while taking his temperature by mouth. The pulse is most conveniently felt on the thumb side of the front of the wrist. Place two fingers over this area so that the beats can be felt plainly; then notice the time by watching the second hand on a watch. Count for half a minute and multiply by two. The pulse rate varies greatly with different individuals, but 72 to 80 per minute is usual. Any irregularity in the pulse may be significant and should be noted and reported to the physician.

Sometimes it is important to know

Patient's pulse can be conveniently counted at same time temperature is being taken.

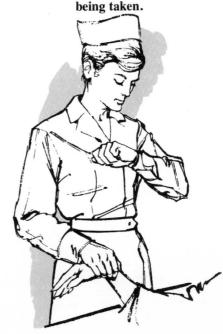

the rate of a patient's respiration. Normally an adult breathes between 12 and 20 times a minute. In pneumonia the number may run up to 40 to 50. Respirations are best counted for a full minute.

Bacteria are always present in the mouth, and, mingled with mouth secretions and mouth particles, will form a coating on the teeth unless frequently removed. The teeth should be cleaned, preferably after eating. Unless too helpless, the patient will probably prefer to clean his own teeth. The helper should spread a towel under the patient's chin, put the toothpaste on the brush, and hold a glass of tepid water for the patient. A patient unable to sit up can help himself by turning his head to one side and using a shallow basin for disposal of the used water. He should also brush his tongue, which is often coated, and rinse his mouth afterward with a mild mouthwash. For a patient unable to wait on himself, the helper should carefully cleanse the patient's mouth by using small swabs, which can be made by winding a bit of absorbent cotton on a wooden applicator or a toothpick. Cleanse the tongue, the gums, the teeth, and the crevices between the teeth, first dipping the swab in a good mouthwash, then discarding each swab after using it.

In illness characterized by high fever, and in cases where the patient breathes through his mouth, the lips often become parched and the mouth dry. This may be prevented or greatly alleviated by frequently moistening the lips with water or by applying glycerine or petrolatum jelly to them. Drops of water may be frequently placed on the tongue.

Every patient, even though bedridden, should be encouraged to do as much as possible for himself, performing such duties as shaving and combing the hair. Of course the helper will, when necessary, provide assistance. There is a fine line between allowing the patient to be discouraged because of his helplessness and forcing him beyond what he is actually able to do.

The helper needs to be tactful in such matters by offering encouragement as well as assistance.

The woman patient with long hair may require help in keeping her hair from becoming tangled. The hair should be thoroughly brushed and combed in the morning and again in the evening. A towel should be laid over the pillow and the patient's head turned to one side. Divide the hair into two portions, parting from the forehead to the nape of the neck. Begin brushing rather slowly at the ends of the hair, holding firmly with the hand above until all tangles are removed. Then comb gently, and braid near the ear, as firmly as is consistent with the patient's comfort. Tie the end of the braided strand of hair. The other side should be dressed in the same way from the opposite side of the bed. Never work across the patient. If the hair is heavy, the patient may be too fatigued to have the hairdressing completed at one time; but it should never be neglected for a whole day.

Normal Bowel Habits

For patients partially or completely confined to bed exercise is limited or not even possible. Constipation or lack of bowel movement is not uncommon. To maintain normal bowel habits is of great importance both for the comfort and health of the patient. Here are some suggestions which have proved helpful:

Have a regular time for going to stool. If at all possible have the patient go to the bathroom or use a commode. The patient should be encouraged to drink plenty of water, a glass on awakening, one between breakfast and lunch, and one between lunch and the evening meal. A last glass may be taken sometime before bedtime.

The diet, where possible, should provide a generous intake of bulk or dietary fiber. Whole grain cereals, whole grain bread, fruit with skins when possible, and vegetables, especially green, leafy vegetables, will be most helpful. Should a special diet be necessary, fiber may be given as a medicine and thus provide a physiologic laxative.

How to Give an Enema

Occasionally it may be necessary to give an enema to avoid severe constipation. Whenever possible, the patient should be encouraged to use the bathroom or a commode as the enema is given. Chemical enemas are convenient and require a minimum of time and effort. These are conveniently packaged and available at any drugstore. The substance contained in a tube is injected into the rectum, and this has the effect of stimulating bowel action.

For those who wish to use a water enema to meet the needs of a bed patient, a certain amount of equipment must be available. The bed should be protected by means of a plastic sheet covered with a large towel. Have the patient lying on his back with the knees flexed. The patient's gown should be raised above the hips as one rim of a bedpan is placed under the patient's hips in a way that allows the open portion to protrude toward the patient's heels. After placing the bedpan, the patient's back should be supported with a pillow. A newspaper spread over the patient's knees and legs forms a protection to the upper sheet should the water be expelled with force.

Bring to the bedside a roll of toilet tissue, vaseline, a plastic bucket, and an enema can or enema bag holding the solution to be injected. The solution should be warm—about 100° F. (38° C.) unless otherwise ordered by the doctor. A saline enema (about two teaspoons of table salt per quart of water) is preferable in most cases. Any other type of enema should be ordered by a doctor. To avoid too great force in the injection, the enema can or bag should be no more than two or three feet above the level of the patient's hips.

The solution is allowed to flow into the patient's rectum at a moderate rate. If the patient has a desire to expel the solution as soon as the enema is begun, stop the flow for a minute, lower the can or bag, and begin again slowly. Better results are obtained if the solution can be retained for a few minutes and then expelled gradually. An adult patient should be able to retain one or two quarts of the enema solution. The injection may need to be repeated if good results are not secured with the first injection. Always lift the patient's hips with one hand before removing the bedpan, as the skin easily adheres to it. The bedpan should be covered immediately when removed and emptied without delay.

Special attention should be given to the cleansing of the skin about the rectum after a bowel movement. The use of toilet paper alone may not be sufficient. It is important to keep the area clean and dry to prevent skin damage or irritation.

The bedpan may be used for ordinary bowel movements and for emptying the bladder in women patients. It should be remembered, however, that lying over a bedpan for a bowel movement or even for emptying the bladder is an abnormal position for these functions. Often more straining and work is required than in the normal sitting position over the toilet seat or over a bedside commode.

Showering or Bathing

Unless a patient is unable to leave his bed, he should be encouraged to shower daily. This routine gets him out of bed, provides exercise and relief from lying, and is simple and easy. A stool may be placed in the shower so the patient can sit while showering, if necessary. If the patient can be helped in and out of a bathtub, bathing may even be preferred to showering. The patient's bed may be made while he is in the tub.

A bed patient should have a bath of some sort every day, and a soap bath at least every other day. A plain sponge bath of warm or cool water may be given on alternate days. A description detailing the procedure for bathing a bed patient follows:

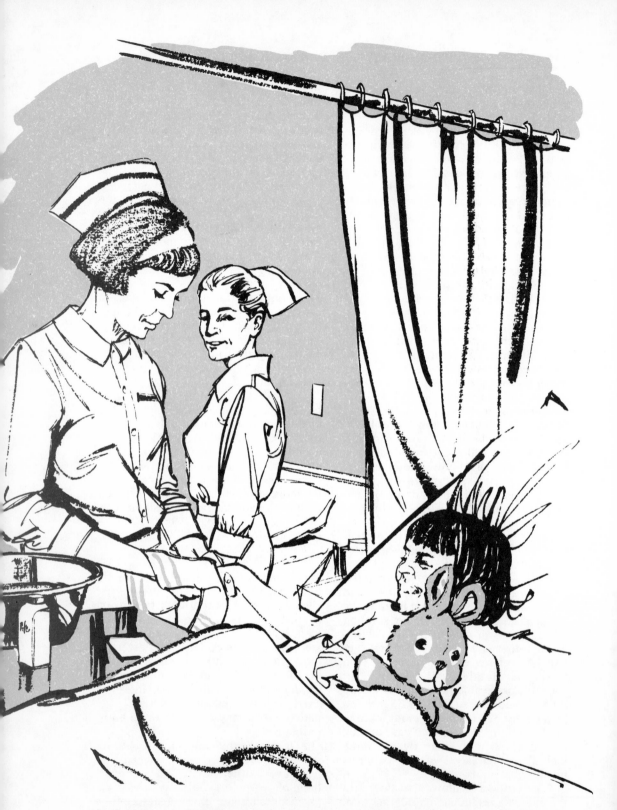

In bathing a bed patient the procedure begins with the face, neck, and `ears, and progresses to the arms and hands, each part being thoroughly dried in turn.

The bath is usually best given in the morning, about an hour after breakfast, just before the bed is remade. If possible, keep two single blankets as bath blankets. Loosen the bedding at the foot, and remove the spread and the blankets, spreading them over the backs of chairs to air. Place one bath blanket over the upper sheet, and, holding it at the top with one hand, draw the sheet out from below with the other. Arrange the other blanket under the patient by turning him first to one side and then to the other, the same as you would to place the lower sheet in bed making. This puts the patient between two bath blankets with little danger of chilling. When this method is not convenient, an old sheet or an extra bath towel may be used instead of the lower blanket to protect the bedding from dampness.

Have at the bedside a basin of water at about 100° F. (38° C.) a teakettle of hotter water, two washcloths, a face towel, one or two bath towels, soap, nail file, scissors, rubbing alcohol, talcum powder, and the patient's clean gown and bed linen. The room and the patient should both be warm before the bath is begun. If necessary, put a heating pad or hot water bottle at the patient's feet.

With the patient between the two bath blankets, as mentioned above, remove the pajamas or other sleeping attire. First bathe the face, the neck, and the ears, using care that the water does not drip; then dry thoroughly. Next, the arms, one at a time. With a bath towel spread underneath, bathe each arm with soapy water. Rinse with the second washcloth and then dry. Bathe the chest and the abdomen, then each thigh and leg. Placing a bath towel on the bed, set the washbowl with only a little water in it on the towel, and, flexing the knees, put the feet, one at a time, into the bowl and bathe them. Next, turning the patient on his side, bathe his back and hips with firm circular strokes, and dry.

Dry each part thoroughly before proceeding to the next. Use soap freely, but see that the skin is well rinsed. Empty and refill the basin frequently. The parts sometimes slighted in bathing are the armpits, the navel, the inner thighs, and between the toes. A bath is not complete unless the genitals and rectal area are thoroughly cleansed. If the patient is able, he should be provided with a washcloth and should bathe these areas himself.

The patient's back and hips should be rubbed with alcohol, especially all points of pressure. A light general rub with talcum powder after the alcohol rub adds to the patient's comfort.

When the bath is completed, the bed can be made before the patient is turned back so that one turn will suffice. One should not forget to keep the fingernails and toenails clean and trimmed.

To replace the pajama top or nightgown, gather it up in such a way that it forms a circle and place it on the chest, with the folds of the back just beneath the chin. After slipping on both sleeves, lift the patient's head and slip the garment over the head, drawing it down carefully over the shoulders and under the hips.

To replace the bottom portion of pajamas, have the patient lie on his back. Introduce his feet into the leg portions of the pajamas. Then, with the patient's knees bent, pull the garment over his knees and as far as possible on the thighs. Have the patient raise his hips while the body of the garment is slipped under his buttocks.

Administration of Medicine

All medicines must be given on the order of the patient's doctor and according to the directions on the labels of the containers. Follow all directions carefully, such as "Always give with milk" or "Do not take on an empty stomach," etc. Medicines in liquid form must be accurately measured. A medicine glass with a graduated scale, or a specially designed measuring spoon, are convenient. When measuring out medicine, have your mind on nothing else. First read the label, then

433

shake the bottle thoroughly to mix the contents, and read the label again. Remove the cap and pour the medicine into the medicine glass or measuring spoon. Hold the bottle with the label side up to prevent soiling the label while pouring. Replace the cap and read the label again before administering the medicine. Pills or capsules should be handed to the patient in a small dish or a teaspoon.

An unconscious patient should have liquid medicine dropped far back on his tongue to compel swallowing. But tablets, capsules, or powders should never be administered by mouth to someone who is unconscious, as they may cause choking or suffocation.

Acid medicines and those containing iron should be administered through a drinking tube to prevent injury to the teeth. In administering oils, such as castor oil, first rinse the glass in very cold water, leaving a little water in the bottom; then add the dose of oil and a little more water. The cold water prevents the oil from sticking to the teeth and tongue and enables the patient to take it in one swallow. Sucking a lemon or an orange immediately afterward takes away the taste of oil. Glasses, spoons, and tubes should always be well cleansed after use.

As grave results may follow mistakes in giving medicines, one cannot be too careful. Here are a few suggestions: (1) Never give medicine from an unlabeled box or bottle. (2) Never give medicine selected in the dark. (3) Never leave medicine within the reach of children or uncooperative patients. (4) Never leave disinfectants standing in glasses or near medicines. (5) If for any reason a dose of medicine has been omitted, do not increase the next dose.

Diet

The patient's physician should be consulted in regard to the patient's diet. If no dietary suggestions have been made, provide the most wholesome food in moderate amounts at regular mealtimes. In certain diseases special instructions must be heeded. The following principles and instructions are given as suggestions to supplement the physician's directions and may need to be modified accordingly:

In acute illnesses, beginning as they often do with headache, fever, nausea, vomiting, and perhaps a sore throat, it is best to withhold all food for the first twelve to twenty-four hours, or until a doctor is called. Give freely of water, either hot or cold as preferred by the patient. When the patient is nauseated, sipping water may prove helpful.

During illness, give only such nourishments as will not overtax the digestive system. Such foods should be chosen as are easy to take, to digest, and assimilate. A liquid diet is best adapted to fever conditions. Fruit juices, especially orange or grapefruit juice, make a cooling and refreshing beverage. In acute fevers of long duration, resulting in much wasting of tissues, liquids containing a higher percentage of food elements should be given. Milk, gruels, soups, broths, and malted milk give both nutrition and variety. Milk contains several food elements in a suitable combination, is easily digested, and agrees with most patients.

Liquid foods should be administered every four hours—about half a pint at each feeding. Water should be given freely between feedings. For a person who can take a soft diet, milk and cream toasts, soft-poached eggs, soft custards, well-cooked cereals, ice cream, and similar foods may be given. Consideration should be given to the patient's likes and dislikes—within reason, however. During convalescence, make additions to the diet gradually until a normal diet is reached. When the patient's appetite becomes good again, the danger of overfeeding should be recognized. Overweight should be avoided.

While a person is sick, usually an effort should be made to foster the appetite. Food should be served with regularity, as the desire for food may disappear with long waiting. The patient should not be kept waiting for breakfast until the family has been served and the morning duties done. A weak patient awakening very early in the morning will often go back to sleep after a hot drink. A glass of hot milk at night may induce sleep.

The manner in which food is served has much to do with its palatability. All dishes and linen must be clean. Have the patient eat at a table when possible. When fed in bed, the tray should not be overloaded, and the foods should be arranged for the patient's convenience in eating. It is better to serve a second course than to overload the tray. Aim to make the tray look attractive.

Cups and dishes should not be so full that the contents are likely to be spilled in handling. Hot foods should be served hot, and cold foods cold. The food should be of the best quality and properly seasoned. It should be tasted before being served so that any defects may be detected. (This should not be done in the presence of the patient or with the patient's spoon.) Hot liquids should be tested, but the helper should not blow on them to cool them.

Variety stimulates the appetite, but variety from meal to meal is more desirable than a great variety at one meal. Large servings of food do not tempt sick people. It is far better to serve a second helping of a pleasing dish than for the patient to be discouraged by an unduly large portion.

Before the tray is brought, the patient should be placed in a comfortable position, one in which he will not tire before the meal is ended. A helpless patient must be assisted in eating. Liquid foods may be served through a drinking tube. If giving a drink from a glass, raise the patient by slipping an arm beneath the pillow and lifting. This method is much better than lifting the head alone. When feeding a patient from a spoon, place a napkin under his chin and sit by the bedside. Allow plenty of time between mouthfuls. The patient should never feel hurried at his meals.

Home Care for Contagious Diseases

Infectious dieases that can be transmitted from person to person are called contagious or communicable diseases. The contagious diseases are often spoken of as "childhood diseases" because children are affected more frequently than adults.

As with many other diseases, contagious diseases are caused by the entry of germs and viruses into the body. These are easily carried by "droplet infection." They ride as passengers on tiny droplets of moisture expelled from a person's mouth during a sneeze or vigorous cough. A box of paper tissues should always be on hand. All persons are advised to cover the mouth and nose with a tissue or handkerchief at the time of sneezing or coughing. This precaution is doubly important for the patient with a contagious disease. The nurse or helper in attendance should instruct the patient to cover all sneezes and coughs; he should also try to remain out of the path of the current of air coming from the patient's nose and mouth. If the patient does not cooperate by covering his mouth and nose when sneezing, it may even be advisable for the helper to wear a surgical mask while caring for the patient.

Infectious agents may also be carried by the patient's sputum, by discharges from his nose and open wounds, and by the urine and feces. More will be said about these matters in the paragraph dealing with the disposal of wastes.

Hand Washing and Nail Care. In the routine care of a patient, it is the attendant's hands which become contaminated first. Without proper cleansing, the hands readily carry infectious agents from the patient to objects about the room and to other parts of the house. Anyone caring for a sick person should develop the firm habit of not touching his own face and hair.

Hands should be carefully washed after each contact with a person suffering from an infectious disease, preferably with warm running water and plenty of soap. Time should be taken to work the suds in between the fingers and high onto the wrist. Fingernails should be given careful attention by cleaning beneath them with an orange stick or other blunt instrument while

435

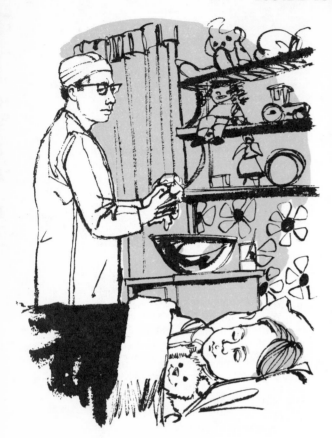

the hands are being washed. Paper towels are preferable for drying because they are disposable. When frequent washings irritate the skin of the hands, a mild hand lotion may be applied after each washing.

Wearing a Gown. It is easy for the helper's clothes to become contaminated while waiting on a patient. Without precaution, this may lead to the spread of the infection to other persons. The usual method of precaution is for the helper to wear a covering garment (gown) whenever he comes in contact with the patient or the patient's bedclothing. It is not necessary, of course, to put on a gown simply to hand the patient a book or a drink of water.

The gown need not be the same type as is worn in a hospital. It should have long sleeves, however, and should fully

cover the helper. A "model's coat" or full covering apron is quite suitable. It should be left hanging near the door in the patient's room when the helper leaves so as to be easily available when he returns. The helper should wash his hands, of course, each time after the gown is removed. In case only a short-sleeved gown is available, the hands and forearms, up to the elbows, need to be washed thoroughly.

Care of the Patient's Dishes. All food remaining on the patient's dishes should be discarded at once. If the discarded food is to be placed in the garbage can, it should be placed in a plastic sack which is then closed tightly before being tossed into the garbage can. This precaution prevents flies and other insects from making contact with the germs that the food fragments may carry.

Many people prefer to save time and effort by using disposable plastic or paper dishes as well as plastic spoons, forks, and knives. These can then be discarded after use. If the patient's dishes are to be washed, they should be washed separately either in an automatic dishwasher or by hand, with abundant soap and detergent. After the usual washing, they should be stacked in a position that permits them to drain and then rinsed with boiling water, following which they should merely drain dry rather than being dried by a dish towel. After they are dry, they may be safely returned to the dish cupboard along with other household dishes.

Disposal of Wastes. For discharges from the patient's nose, mouth, or infected wounds, the safest method of disposal is to collect them in paper tissue and to keep the accumulation in a tightly closed plastic sack to be taken out later and burned.

Urine and feces from the patient can be safely flushed down the toilet, provided the home has a properly functioning septic tank or is connected to a city sewer system in which the sewage is scientifically treated. Such material should never be discarded into a stream or a lake. Under other circumstances, the patient's urine and feces should be chemically treated with a disinfectant before being emptied. Disinfectants, as phenol or cresol, are available at the drugstore. The urine and feces should remain in contact with the disinfectant solution for an hour before being finally emptied. Care should be used to keep the bottle of disinfectant out of the reach of children, for it is poison.

The Patient's Laundry. The patient's laundry, including bedclothing, bed linen, and towels, should be washed as soon as possible after removal from the sick room. It should be washed separately from other laundry, but may be washed in the washing machine or by whatever other method is usual. The water used should be hot, and abundant soap or detergent should be used. Pieces of laundry heavily contaminated by the patient's discharges should be boiled for five minutes before being washed in the usual manner. If the household wash is sent to a commercial laundry, that from the patient's room should be packaged separately and this package plainly labeled to warn that it contains contaminated articles.

Returning the Sick Room to General Use. Even after a patient with a contagious disease has recovered, the organisms associated with his illness may linger in the sick room. Thus, certain precautions should be taken before the sick room is returned to general use. Woodwork, the bare portion of the floor, and furniture should be washed with soap and water and the room aired for several hours. A carpet cleaner, such as can be rented, can be used to clean thoroughly the carpet or rugs. Articles such as toys, hot water bottles, and heating-pad covers should be washed and placed in the sunshine to dry. Bedclothing, throw rugs, drapes, and other articles not easily washable should be aired in the sunlight for six hours or more. Utensils used in the sick room should be washed carefully with soap and water and, if they will not be damaged by the heat, placed in actively boiling water for at least five minutes. If a nondisposable thermometer has been used to take the patient's temperature, it should be washed with soap or detergent and cool water, soaked in alcohol (rubbing alcohol is suitable) for 30 minutes, rinsed, and dried.

Importance of Good Nursing

The healing processes of the body afflicted by disease or injury are greatly influenced by the patient's mental attitude. The patient's comfort and feeling of hopefulness depend largely on the helper's or nurse's diligent and intelligent care and cheerful manner. Many times this type of care is much more effective in promoting recovery than what the physician is able to do. Good nursing care should also be provided to the patient with a progressive disease expected to be fatal. One should remember that all will eventually die—it is only a matter of difference in time. Remember the golden rule: How would I wish to be treated in the same situation?

The successful helper will learn to anticipate the needs of the patient and to see little things to do for his comfort without being asked. He will not allow the patient to be wearied by visitors or annoyed by gossip. Frequent rubbing of the back, hips, and heels with alcohol, then dusting with talcum powder, will help to prevent bedsores. If the patient is feverish or restless in the afternoon, rubbing the back and legs or sponging with alcohol is soothing. Heavy covers may be responsible for much restlessness.

The evening must be free from excitement, and early preparations should be made for the night's rest. If the helper sleeps in the room, he should prepare his own bed and then make the following preparations for the patient: Wash the face and hands, cleanse the mouth, brush the hair, and change the gown if indicated. A hot footbath may quiet the patient. Having him go to the toilet or use the bedpan may induce

437

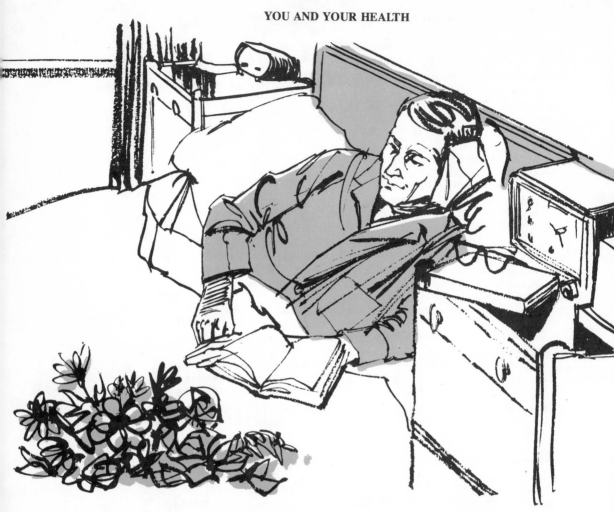

A cheerful atmosphere in the sickroom aids in recovery from disease.

sleep by relieving discomfort.

Turn the patient on his side, and brush the bed free from crumbs or any other small objects that may have been left in it. A small whisk broom is excellent for this purpose. Loosen the lower sheet, pull it smooth, and retuck it under the mattress; then do the same on the opposite side of the bed. Rub the back and hips, using firm circular strokes to the general area, and finish with long, soothing strokes down the spine. Remove the pillows, and shake and readjust them. Loosen the covers at the foot. Adjust the patient's sleeping attire; straighten the upper sheet and the blankets and tuck them in again, allowing plenty of freedom. Ask

the patient if there is anything more that he wants. Then, turning out or adjusting the light, say Good night and leave the room so that the patient may go to sleep. This prevents his lying awake expecting your return or thinking that something more is to be done.

When the patient does not change his position in bed because of weakness or the lack of feeling in the skin, then it is most important for the helper to move him frequently so as to prevent pressure sores. Pressure sores are preventable. The patient may be turned to either side, to a face-down position, or to intermediate positions. Any one position should be maintained no longer than two hours. Air pillows and sheepskin pads are very helpful.

The following counsel on care of patients in the home, published years ago, has an up-to-date ring and provides an excellent summary:

"Those who minister to the sick should understand the importance of careful attention to the laws of health. Nowhere is obedience to these laws more important than in the sickroom. Nowhere does so much depend upon faithfulness in little things on the part of the attendants. In cases of serious illness, a little neglect, a slight inattention to a patient's special needs or dangers, the manifestation of fear, excitement, or petulance, even a lack of sympathy, may turn the scale that is balancing life and death, and cause to go down to the grave a patient who otherwise might have recovered.

"The efficiency of the nurse depends, to a great degree, upon physical vigor. The better the health, the better will she be able to endure the strain of attendance upon the sick, and the more successfully can she perform her duties. Those who care for the sick should give special attention to diet, cleanliness, fresh air, and exercise. . . .

"Where the illness is serious, requiring the attendance of a nurse night and day, the work should be shared by at least two efficient nurses, so that each may have opportunity for rest and for exercise in the open air. . . .

"Nurses, and all who have to do with the sickroom, should be cheerful, calm, and self-possessed. All hurry, excitement, or confusion, should be avoided. Doors should be opened and shut with care, and the whole household be kept quiet. In cases of fever, special care is needed when the crisis comes and the fever is passing away. Then constant watching is often necessary. Igno-

rance, forgetfulness, and recklessness have caused the death of many who might have lived had they received proper care from judicious, thoughtful nurses."—E. G. White, *The Ministry of Healing,* pp. 219-222.

Anticipating the possible need of having to care for a sick relative in the home or even in preparation for a specific need, it is recommended that advantage be taken of courses offered in home nursing by the American Red Cross or other community or church agencies. Really almost every homemaker will become a home nurse sometime. In any specific problem, help is available from community agencies such as the Public Health Department, the Visiting Nurses' Association, or homecare facilities associated with medical centers.

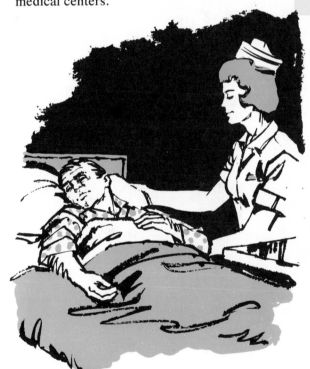

Simple Home Treatments

It is inconceivable that every slight ache or pain be reason for calling a doctor. Such a practice would result in an impossible situation. It is reasonable that people use domestic remedies for relief from obviously minor symptoms. Actually such a practice is encouraged by the medical profession. But medical help should certainly be sought when a symptom is severe, when it persists, when it returns frequently, or when any doubt arises as to its significance. Such symptoms should be considered as warning signals of an abnormality that needs professional attention.

The knowledge and practice of healthful living habits will do much in preventing disease conditions with their unpleasant symptoms. It is best to eat the apple a day that keeps the doctor away. One of the main objectives of these three volumes is to acquaint the reader with the principles of healthful living and thus to minimize the necessity of treatment of any kind. But illnesses and injuries do occur, and for minor ones every householder should be equipped to administer simple remedies.

Unfortunately, wall cabinets in many homes are stocked with medicines for headache, acid stomach, sleeplessness, et cetera; and members of the family tend to use these rather indiscriminately. Self-medication is encouraged by advertisements on television and radio, in the press, and in the drugstore. People are filling themselves with chemicals that actually cause damage to the body's tissues.

In contrast to medication by drugs, there are available to all, simple treatments which do not leave residuals in the body. These consist of the rational use of natural remedies such as water, light, controlled exercise, and rest. With these remedies, as with the use of drugs, self-treatment should be restricted to only minor symptoms which do not warrant calling for medical help, to temporary emergency situations when waiting for the doctor, or to treatment done under medical direction. The results of these treatments depend on the natural physiological response of the body to its surroundings and to its own activity. It should be understood that any major treatment suggested here should be carried out with the approval of the patient's physician.

Hydrotherapy

Among the simple drugless methods of treating disease or simple injuries, the use of heat and cold ranks high in importance. Heat or cold may be easily applied with the use of that most common substance, water, in one of its three states—liquid, vapor (steam), and solid (ice). The use of water in treatment is called "hydrotherapy." Only a few of the simplest treatments can be considered here. None of these require hospital equipment. While these simple treatments can be given in the home, careful observation of all details of instruction is necessary, for even these simple treatments wrongly applied may do harm. Usually, anything with potential for good may do harm when wrongly used.

Characteristic Effects of Heat and Cold. When one bathes his face with cold water or takes a quick dip or plunges into cold water, after the first shock there comes a delightful feeling of invigoration, with quickened circulation and soon a glow of warmth in the skin. A concomitant result is greater energy for either muscular or brain work, all normal body activities being stimulated. These changes that result from a brief application of cold water to the skin are spoken of as reaction.

People in vigorous health usually react well to cold water, especially after they have become accustomed to its use. The process of becoming accustomed to it may need to be quite gradual, but the health and vigor that result are well worth the time and effort necessary to acquire them, especially in the case of a weakly person.

In treating the sick by the use of hydrotherapy, securing a reaction is important, for upon this depends success in stimulating the activity of the organs not working normally. It may be difficult to secure a good reaction. The patient's circulation may be poor, or he may chill readily. The cold water may have to be applied to only one part of his body at a time, after a hot application has first warmed the skin or while hot applications are being administered to other parts of his body; and the cold application may have to be made with energetic rubbing. In case of chilliness, hot applications sufficient even to produce sweating must be used before a cold application so that the patient will react properly. This is most important and must not be forgotten, especially with such diseases as colds, influenza, and pneumonia.

Internal congestion may be relieved by hot applications over a fairly large skin area as the blood is drawn to the skin surface. This effect results from the attempt of the body to get rid of the heat thus applied. Cold application used for a comparatively long time on a relatively small area of skin will reduce swelling and congestion in the surface area and in the deep structures. The effect on the underlying organs is produced by the nerve connections between specific skin areas and specific organs.

Thus heat alone may be used in treating deep congestions or inflammations, such as lung congestion and pleurisy. The ice bag alone may be used, as with an acute, severely inflamed breast; or, better still, the ice bag may be applied directly over the inflamed part, and hot applications at a distance, as with acute appendicitis—the ice bag over the appendix and hot applications to the legs and feet. Of course, even if appendicitis is suspected the physician should be called. When the head is hot and throbbing, a hot footbath together with cold cloth to the head helps greatly. When the lungs are congested, a hot footbath and very hot fomentations over the congested part draw the blood to the surface and to the feet. An ice bag applied to the chest over the heart, in case of heart disease with a rapid pulse, slows the heartbeat and increases its force. Again, the physician should be called when heart disease is suspected.

Hot applications alternating with cold promptly increase the number of red and white blood cells in active circulation, and a series of such treatments, together with fresh air, sunshine, and nourishing food, are helpful in treating anemia and other diseases of the blood. Alternate hot and cold applications are often beneficial in treating local infection.

In giving treatments, seemingly small details are of great importance, and to disregard them may not only nullify the benefit to the patient but actually harm him. Be sure to follow directions carefully. Remember that chilling the patient may cause harm; but, on the other hand, the cold water must be used cold, or little good will be accomplished. Hot applications must be hot, not lukewarm; and mere complaint that they are hot is not sufficient reason for cooling them before they are applied. Burning can be prevented, as will be explained later.

When applying heat, great care must be exercised to avoid damage to a part with poor blood vessels—a point particularly true of the feet. Direct heat application to a part acutely inflamed and swollen should be avoided—direct cold may be much better. The effects of hot and cold water on the body can be clearly demonstrated, but the exact explanation of how these effects take place may not be fully understood. The important thing is that they do occur.

"Heat" and "cold" are comparative terms, and must be defined. This cannot be done with accuracy, since various people differ in their toleration to heat and cold. The temperature sensation produced by water varies according to the condition of the skin, its previous temperature, the vigor of blood circulation, and the season of the year. Testing the temperature of water to be used in hydrotherapy, therefore, should be done with a thermometer as well as with the hand.

Equipment Needed for Home Hydrotherapy. Only simple appliances are needed for giving water treatments in the home. Substitutes may be used in emergencies, but it is much better to provide the things listed below:

1. One set of six cloths, wool or half wool, each at least 30 x 36 inches (75 x 90 cm.) in size. An old part-woolen bed blanket cut in four pieces makes four good cloths. These when heated as described in the following procedures are called "fomentations."

2. Two rough friction mitts, without fingers, made from rough toweling or wash cloths.

3. Two hot-water bottles, rubber preferred.

4. One rubber ice bag.

5. One bath thermometer.

6. Two elliptical foot tubs about 16 inches (40 cm.) long and 10 inches (25 cm.) deep.

7. Pans, kettles, towels, sheets, and blankets such as are usually found in the home.

8. Two large, deep metal or plastic cans or buckets. These should be about 12 inches (30 cm.) in diameter and 16 inches (40 cm.) deep.

Fomentations

A fomentation is a local application of moist heat by means of cloths (largely wool) wrung from boiling water or heated in a steam chest.

Articles Needed. Provide a deep dishpan or a large kettle of water to be kept actively boiling, a cover to retain the heat, a set of six fomentation cloths, several Turkish towels, a hand towel, a sheet, a bowl of cold water or ice water, and a table.

The Patient and the Bed. See that all clothing is removed so that it doesn't become damp from perspiration. Cover the patient with a sheet plus other covering to keep him warm. See especially that the feet are warm and that they are kept so during the treating. A hot footbath should be given or hot-water bottles put to the feet, this beginning before the fomentations and continuing all the time that the fomentations are being applied.

Protect the bedding by a blanket or sheet folded lengthwise and placed under the patient. After applying the fomentation, cover it with a dry cloth or newspaper in order to protect the bedding above it.

Preparation of the Fomentation. If possible, the hot-water kettle and the table should be near the bed, and the preparation of the fomentation should be done quickly so that loss of heat before application will be minimal. Three cloths are necessary for each fomentation if they are to be very hot, one for the dry covering and two to be wrung from boiling water for the inside moist part. If less heat is required, one inside cloth may be sufficient. Two such sets of cloths are necessary so that one fomentation can be in preparation while the other is in use.

Spread out on the table the cloth for the dry covering. Then fold together in three thicknesses the cloth or cloths to be used inside, so as to make a long, narrow piece. Immerse this folded cloth, except the two ends which are held in the hands, in the boiling water. Leave until thoroughly soaked with boiling water, then wring quickly by firm twisting and pulling until water no longer drips from it. If held up by one end, the folded cloth will quickly untwist to its original one-third width. Place this across the middle of the dry fomentation cloth already spread out on the table. Fold the dry ends of the inside cloth over its damp center and then fold the dry outer cloth about the damp inner one. In the folding, the fomentation should be made the right size and shape to fit the part to be treated. It should be large enough to extend slightly beyond the boundaries of this area.

Procedure. The fomentation should lie in close contact with the skin and should be renewed in five minutes or less. If necessary, it may be laid over a dry Turkish towel to temper the heat. If unbearably hot, lift the fomentation slightly for a few seconds and rub with the hand the part under it, or remove the moisture on the patient's skin by firm rubbing once or twice with a dry towel wrapped about the hand. Always protect the area being treated from chilling by keeping it covered with a dry fomentation cloth or dry towel when the fomentation is not actually being applied.

To renew the fomentation, prepare another similar one and have it ready to apply immediately upon removing the previous one. At the time of exchange the skin should be dried quickly by using a towel, because moisture remaining on the skin makes it harder for the patient to endure the heat of the newly prepared fomentation.

Unless otherwise directed, three successive applications should be made, covering a period of from ten to fifteen minutes. After the last one is finished, the part should immediately be given a very brief rub with a cold, wet towel or with rubbing alcohol. Dry the skin thoroughly, but quickly, and cover the patient at once to avoid chilling.

Precautions. In cases of unconsciousness, paralyzed sensation, diabetes, dropsy, or poor blood vessels, especially in the feet, great care must be taken to avoid burning. The fomentation should be slightly raised at frequent intervals and the hand of the attendant thrust beneath it to test its heat in such cases. This heat testing should be done in as brief a period as possible, however, so as to avoid chilling.

In case of free perspiration, a general cold friction, a wet hand rub, a wet towel rub, or an alcohol rub should be given following the last of the three fomentations.

Apply cold compresses to the head throughout the time of applying fomentations to any other part of the body. In heart disease, usually in high fever, and with a rapid pulse from any cause, an ice bag should be placed over the heart.

In order to relieve pain, the fomentation must be very hot, as hot as can be borne, and should be renewed as soon as it ceases to feel hot. In cases of severe pain, the cold application at the close should be omitted, the treated part being dried and immediately covered with flannel or other dry covering. A test of the efficacy of fomentations is the redness of the skin after completion of the treatment.

If it is not certain that fomentations can be given without chilling the patient, do not give them at all. Moist

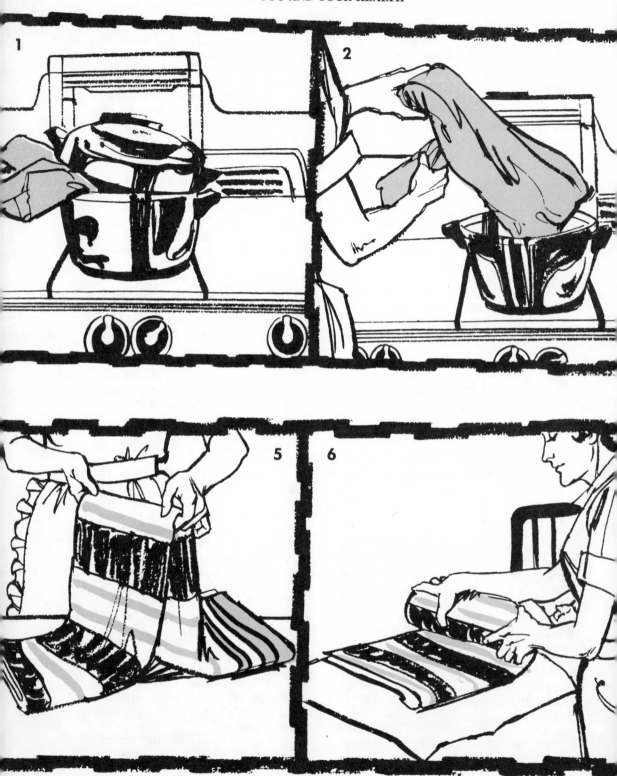

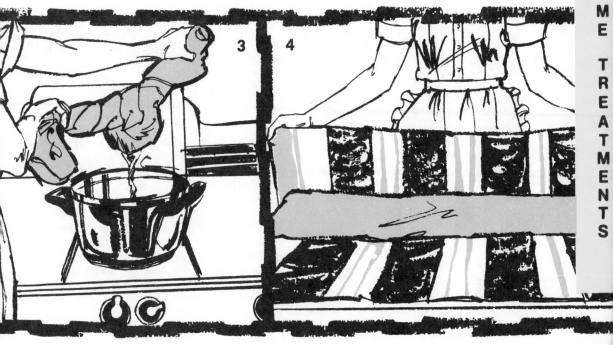

Local treatment by fomentation involves application of moist heat by means of cloths wrung from boiling water, procedure as follows, steps numbered to correspond with numbers on the drawings:

1. Immerse folded cloth to be used inside pack in a pan of boiling water, leaving ends hanging over the edge to be kept dry.

2. Leave until thoroughly soaked; then remove by grasping dry ends.

3. Twist and pull cloth to wring out as much of the water as possible.

4. Hold twisted cloth up by one end to allow it to untwist. Then place it across dry fomentation cloth spread out on the table.

5. Fold the dry outer cloth about the damp inner one to make the pack, which is now ready to be applied to patient.

6. Place fomentation pack in close contact with patient's skin, with a dry towel spread underneath if pack is unbearably hot, and leave it applied for about five minutes.

heat applied by means of a hot-water bottle laid over two thicknesses of moist Turkish toweling is a fair substitute.

Various Forms. Applied to the throat and upper chest, fomentations help in relieving sore throat, tonsillitis, cough, bronchitis, lung congestion, et cetera.

When applied to the throat only, the hot cloth should be folded so as to be about eight inches (20 cm.) wide. To protect the lower part of the face, a Turkish towel may be placed across the neck, under the fomentation. The heat pack should be tucked up close below the ears. For the chest only, the fomentation should be folded nearly square

445

and as large as possible. For pleurisy, it should be applied to the side of the chest under the arm, from breastbone to spine; for the kidneys and for lumbago, across the small of the back. For the spine, it should be long and narrow, about six inches (15 cm.) wide. Fomentations to the spine help to promote sleep, and for this purpose they should be only moderately hot. For the knee, the cloth may be folded as for the spine, and, being drawn under the joint, the two ends are wrapped about the front of it, one above the other. The use of two fomentations, one behind and one in front of the knee, at the same time, tucked in snugly to exclude air, may be fully as effective as the single fomentation wrapped around the joint and more comfortable.

Sometimes it is desirable to apply a fomentation to the eye or to some other small area. The full-sized fomentation cloth cannot be used in such cases. A thick pad composed of thirty to fifty layers of gauze, dipped in very hot water and squeezed almost dry, is a good substitute. Since such small fomentations lose heat rapidly, they should be changed every minute or two. Small fomentations are frequently called hot compresses.

Another form of fomentation has been called the revulsive compress, and is given with the following addition: A hand towel is wrung from cold water and spread over the skin surface immediately after the removal of each fomentation. It is pressed firmly against the skin, turned over, again pressed firmly over the skin, and removed. A smooth piece of ice may be rubbed over the skin after each fomentation instead of applying a cold compress. The skin must be quickly wiped dry before heat is again applied.

Alternate hot and cold to the spine, with fomentations as the source of heat, acts as a stimulant and tonic, being used in the case of colds, bronchitis, and similar ailments after the acute stage is past. To the abdomen, it is useful in stimulating the flow of digestive juices and the movements of the stom-ach and bowels. In treating the chest, the abdomen, the neck, or a joint, for the cold part of the treatment use a cloth wrung from cold water rather than a piece of ice.

There are two modifications of the fomentation available commercially. One is the Hydrocollator ®, which consists of material that holds water sewn into pads of convenient size. These pads are heated in a container of water operated electrically and controlled by a thermostat. When taken out of the water these pads will hold heat for a prolonged time; they do not drip water. They should be covered with toweling and applied to the part to be heated. These hot packs have certain advantages because of ease of preparation, but they also have disadvantages, such as not being easily molded to the part being treated, and being heavy.

Another modification of the fomentation available commercially is an electrically heated pad (Thermophore ®), so designed that moisture from the body accumulates during the application and thus simulates the condition of a cloth fomentation. Special precautions must be taken with its use. A special switch which must be actively pressed during the application is a safety feature.

Local Cold Applications

Cold Compress. This is a local application of cold by means of a cloth wrung from cold water. Hand towels or ordinary cotton cloths may be used. These should be folded to the desired size, and wrung from cold water, preferably ice water. The wringing should be barely sufficient to prevent dripping. As a continuous cold application, the compress must be changed frequently, always before it becomes warm to any great extent. The thicker the compress, the less frequently will it require changing. Cold compresses may be applied to the head, the neck, over the heart or the lungs, to the abdomen, the spine, or other parts. (See paragraph at the end of this subsection for conditions in which cold applications may be used.)

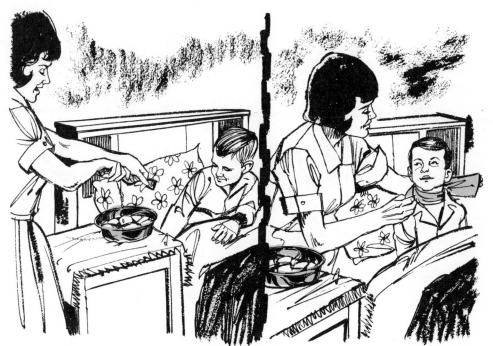

Cold compress: Cloth is wrung dry from ice water and applied firmly to part to be treated.

When applied to the head, they should be pressed down firmly on the surface, especially over the forehead and temples. The pillow should be protected by a rubber cloth, an oilcloth, a plastic sheet, or a towel. When compresses are applied to the abdomen, the bedding and the patient's garments should be protected by Turkish towels.

Ice Pack. For this, finely chipped ice is wrapped in water-repellent 100 percent wool flannel. The pack thus formed tends not to drip water and may be left in place for thirty minutes. It is usually best to cover the area to be treated with toweling. Care must be taken not to permit soaking next to the skin, since this may cause injury to the skin. The bedding should be protected with waterproof material. The ice pack may be renewed after a few minutes interval.

Ice Bag. The ice bag is a waterproof

bag usually made of flexible rubber, with a large screw cap for introducing finely chipped ice. When the bag is filled with ice, there should be just enough water in it to permit expelling all of the air before screwing the cap on tight. The bag should be so filled that it is quite flat and easily molded over the part to be treated. It must be covered with one or more layers of toweling.

Local cold applications may be used for cooling inflamed areas such as an acutely inflamed joint or a sprained ankle. They may be given for their reflex effect on deeper structures, such as over the heart in a rapid heartbeat associated with a high fever, to the forehead in the case of headache, or to the abdomen in acute appendicitis. Of course one should remember the potential dangers in these conditions if medical attention is not sought.

Alternate Hot and Cold Arm Bath

To give this treatment to an infected

447

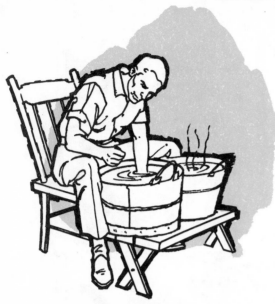

Alternate hot and cold baths aid in combating infection in arm or hand.

hand or arm, use two foot tubs, one with water as hot as can be borne (temperature to be gradually raised) and the other with ice water having pieces of ice in it. Immerse the hand and arm in the hot water for three to four minutes and then in the cold for thirty to sixty seconds. Continue these alternations for thirty to forty minutes, finishing with the cold. Hot water should be added to keep the temperature as hot as can be borne. The procedure should be repeated two to four times daily. Do not rub the part. Massage should be avoided in infections.

Alternate Hot and Cold Foot (Leg) Bath

Use two foot tubs of water deep enough to cover the ankles, one as hot as can be borne (temperature to be gradually raised) and the other as cold as possible with pieces of ice floating in it. Immerse the feet in the hot water for two minutes and then in the cold for fifteen to thirty seconds. Continue the alternation for fifteen to twenty minutes. Finish with the cold, and wipe the feet dry.

The alternate hot and cold footbath is

a powerful stimulant to the circulation in the feet. For this reason, the lessening of congestion in the upper part of the body secured by its use is decided and enduring. It is especially useful in congestive headache, in which case a cold compress should be applied to the head, or to the head and neck, at the same time. It is also useful in treating infections of the feet, in which case it should be given several times a day and continued for at least half an hour each time. In case of infection, do not rub the part. For leg bath, use deep wide buckets or deep metal cans.

Hot Footbath

The hot footbath is one of the most useful of all water treatments. Its chief use is as a preliminary or adjunct to some other treatment. It may be given with the patient lying down or sitting. A large pail may be used, but more convenient is a tub of elliptical shape, about sixteen inches long and ten inches deep.

If the footbath is given in bed, protect the bedding with a plastic sheet or newspapers. Cover the patient with a blanket or sheet, tucking the covering about his legs and the foot tub so as to prevent the circulation of air.

The water should rise above the ankles. The bath should begin at a temperature of about 104° F. (40° C.), and should be gradually increased by pouring in hot water as fast as can be borne, to a maximum of about 112° F. (44° C.), as the patient can bear it. Always take the feet out of the bath when adding hot water. The attendant's hands should always cradle the feet as they are again lowered into the water. Excess water has to be dipped out of the tub. The bath may be continued from ten minutes to half an hour. At the close the feet should receive a brief pour or dash of cold water and be thoroughly dried with brisk rubbing.

It is often necessary to use a cold compress to the head if the footbath is very hot, is continued for a long time, or is given with the patient sitting up, and in all cases where there is a ten-

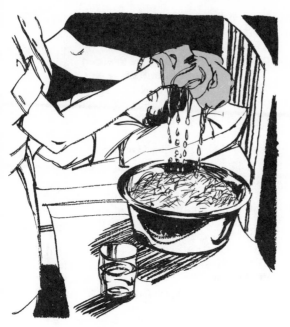

dency to faintness. This cold compress not only helps to prevent faintness, but it minimizes the likelihood of headache after the treatment.

Definite caution should be given against applying heat to the feet in the presence of poor blood vessels, as in thromboangiitis obliterans (Buerger's disease) and where there is acute swelling as in acute sprain and early acute arthritis.

The hot footbath draws blood from all other parts of the body, especially congested areas, by dilating the skin blood vessels of the feet and to a lesser extent those of the whole body. The cold pour given at the close helps to maintain the blood in the feet.

Cold Mitten Friction

Provide a bowl or pail of very cold water or ice water, a sheet, three Turkish towels, two friction mitts made of some coarse material such as Turkish toweling, and compresses for the head and neck. The mitts are preferably in the form of simple sacks, large enough to reach well above the wrist.

The patient should feel warm before this treatment. He should be warmly covered, with his feet warm. If they are cold, warm them and keep them so with a hot foot bath or hot-water bottles. The cold mitten friction may be a stimulating conclusion of a heating treatment.

Bare one part of the body at a time. Do not expose a part longer than necessary, dry quickly and thoroughly, and cover at once with warm, dry covering. Before beginning the regular part of the treatment, bathe the patient's face and neck with cold water, or apply cold compresses to the head and neck. This is especially important in treating patients with heart disease. In this condition, an ice bag should be placed over the heart before the treatment is begun.

Beginning with the right arm, place one towel under the arm and another around the shoulder to protect the bed and the patient. With the mitts on the hands, dip them into the cold water and shake or squeeze out the excess of

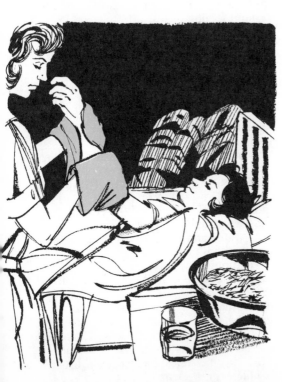

The cold mitten friction to the skin may provide a stimulating conclusion to a heat treatment.

449

water. While the patient holds the arm upward at an angle of about 45 degrees, rub the arm and hand with rapid to-and-fro movements till they are in a glow. Quickly remove the mitts, dropping them into the bowl, and cover the entire arm with one of the Turkish towels. Dry by friction outside the towel, and then rub with the towel until the arm is thoroughly dry and well reddened. Treat the left arm in the same manner.

Now, covering the rest of the body, bare the chest and abdomen. Tuck a Turkish towel snugly under each side along the trunk and over the arms. Rub the chest with a mitt dipped in cold water in a way similar to that in which the arms were rubbed. Then cover the entire chest with one of the Turkish towels and have the patient grasp the two upper corners of it as they lie near the shoulders. Rub briskly with downward strokes over the towel. Then, wrapping the towel neatly about your hand, again rub the entire surface, around the shoulders and down the sides, so as to dry thoroughly all parts that have been wet.

Cover the chest and expose the right leg and thigh. Bend the knee and place a Turkish towel under its whole length. Place another towel around the upper thigh at the groin. Begin the friction with the foot and leg. Dip the mitts again for the thigh. In like manner treat the left leg and thigh, after the right leg and thigh have been thoroughly dried.

Have the patient turn over and lie on a pillow placed under the chest. Treat the back in the same manner as the front of the trunk. To dry, cover the entire back with a Turkish towel, have the patient hold the upper corners of it in the same manner as for the chest, rub with downward strokes over the towel, and wrap the towel around your hand and rub the surface of the skin again until it is thoroughly dry and aglow.

The important factors in giving a successful cold mitten friction are: See that the friction is firm enough and brisk enough to make the skin glow; and be sure that the subsequent drying is done with speed and force enough to maintain this glow. To vary the severity and the tonic effects, the temperature of the water may be lowered, more may be left in the mitts, the mitts may be dipped more times in treating each part, or the friction may be given more vigorously.

The Heating Compress

A heating compress is a moderately moist but thin cold compress so covered that warming soon occurs. Its end results are an application of mild, moist heat to the body. It is most commonly applied to the throat or a joint. To apply a heating compress use several thicknesses of gauze or one or more thicknesses of linen or cotton cloth wrung firmly out of cold water, and so perfectly covered with dry flannel as to prevent the circulation of air around the moist area. This will cause an accumulation of body heat and a rather prompt feeling of warmth.

The patient must not be chilly but generally warm before applying the compress, since its effectiveness depends on a good warming reaction to the cold application. In case warming does not occur within one or two minutes, this effect should be hastened by applying some form of heat, as a hot footbath.

A heating compress is usually left in place for several hours, between other treatments, or overnight. If left on overnight, it will probably be dry by morning. On removal of the compress, the part should be rubbed briefly with cold water and dried by rubbing vigorously with a towel.

Heating compresses may be applied to the neck, the foot, the ankle, the knee, the hand, or the wrist. Rarely more than two thicknesses of gauze need be used. Cotton padding may be needed to help secure close application of the compress to the skin surface. This may be held in place by a broad bandage or a strip of cloth. In rheumatic fever, the joint may be rubbed with methyl salicylate before the heating compress is applied. This drug helps to relieve the pain; and because of its action as a counterirritant, the heating effect is increased.

In applying a heating compress to the throat, one should use four to six thicknesses of cheesecloth or two or three thicknesses of some other cotton cloth, about three inches wide and long enough to encircle the neck. Wet this and squeeze it dry enough to prevent dripping, then wrap it around the neck. Then wrap on two thicknesses of flannel wide enough to cover the neck from the chin to the shoulders and long enough to encircle the neck and lap over. The skin of the neck should be rubbed with cold water immediately after the removal of the compress in the morning and then thoroughly dried.

The heating throat compress is a useful treatment for acute pharyngitis, laryngitis, tonsillitis, or any other disease condition causing acute sore throat or hoarseness.

The heating compress can be applied in a similar manner to large surfaces of the body, as the chest and the abdomen. Since in this case a large surface of the body has to react to the cold application, one must be especially sure that the patient does not become chilled. It may be advisable to use some preheating procedure as a hot footbath or even a fomentation to the area being treated. Always the dry covering should extend two or more inches beyond the wet one. The edges of this covering must be pulled firmly so that air will not enter. One may use safety pins to help keep the edges snug.

In the case of the abdominal application, the inside moist layer consists of one thickness of linen or cotton cloth or four thicknesses of gauze, about eight inches wide and long enough to go about one and a half times around the body. The outer flannel covering should be about twelve inches wide and about the same length as the inner layer. In applying it, the dry flannel is placed across the bed, and the cloth or

gauze, wrung nearly dry from cold water, placed over its center lengthwise. The patient now lies back on the bandage so that the lower edge will be below the upper edge of the hipbones. Each end of the wet cloth or gauze is pulled tightly across the abdomen and tucked under the opposite side. Both ends of the dry flannel are then folded tightly over these and securely fastened with safety pins.

The moist abdominal heating compress has been found useful in indigestion, and in neurasthenia, insomnia, constipation, and other maladies. It is best worn at night.

The heating compress may be applied to the chest but especially in this case great care needs to be taken to avoid chilling by making sure that the body is warm before the application and that the edges of the dry cover are pulled close to the skin. The shape of the chest makes this more difficult.

The heating compress, when used for a patient under a physician's care, is to be given only with the physician's knowledge and consent.

Rubs and Sponges

Sponging consists of the application of a liquid by means of a sponge, a washcloth, or the bare hand, in which the chief effect is derived from the liquid itself, little friction being needed. When the bare hand is used, the treatment is often called a "rub," though little real rubbing is done.

In using cool or tepid water to reduce fever, a washcloth may be used. It is squeezed out enough to prevent dripping, and considerable time is spent on each part of the body, going back and forth over the part until it is perceptibly cooler. Each part is dried lightly, without rubbing. Hot sponging is used in fevers where there is chilliness, the same methods being followed as with cool or tepid sponging, except that less water is applied.

The alcohol rub or sponge is a popular means of finishing a sweating bath,

451

for quieting purposes at night, or for reducing fever. Wood alcohol should never be used. Rubbing alcohol, as sold in drugstores, will do.

Showers and Sprays

Showers and sprays consist of water, at various or varying temperatures, falling upon or dashed against the body. Understandably, they can be given only to ambulatory patients and where equipment is available to adjust temperature to the desired degree and keep it there, or to change it from hot to cold and back again within a few seconds' time. When there is a stall shower in the home, sprays can be given with significant effectiveness. An over-tub shower is usually not very satisfactory because of the cramped quarters and danger from falling. The thermostat for the water tank should be set quite high; this makes it possible to change hot shower temperature quickly to cold by turning the hot valve to "off," without greatly decreasing the force of the water. During the giving of shower treatment, no faucets in the rest of the house should be used lest such use might change the proportion of hot and cold water in the shower and thus modify the temperature of the water striking the patient's skin.

Alternate Hot and Cold Shower or Spray. Adjust the temperature of the water until it feels moderately warm. While standing in the shower, raise the temperature of the water fairly rapidly until it is as hot as can be borne. Stand under this hot shower about three minutes; then turn the hot water off and stand under the cold shower about half a minute. Again raise the temperature fairly rapidly until it is as hot as can be borne. The treatment should consist of three or four changes from hot to cold and back again, ending with the cold. Then dry by rubbing with a coarse Turkish towel. The alternate hot and cold shower is a strong stimulant to the circulation.

Cold Shower or Spray. Adjust the temperature of the water until it feels comfortably warm, stand under the shower for ten to twenty seconds, turn off the hot water while standing under the shower and let the cold water run for about one minute, then turn off the shower and dry the body by brisk rubbing with a coarse Turkish towel. The temperature of the air in the room should be about 75° F. (24° C.), and, if necessary, the feet should be warmed by means of a hot footbath before beginning the cold shower. The cold shower is a brisk tonic for those who can stand it without becoming chilled. The cold may be continued longer as one becomes accustomed to it. This or the cold tub bath is a good tonic measure for the normal person.

Hot Shower or Spray. Adjust the water temperature to a comfortable warmth. While standing under the shower, gradually raise the temperature until it is as hot as can be borne. Stand there from five to ten minutes. Then turn the hot water off and the cold water on full force for no more than ten seconds. Then dry the body. The hot shower is an effective skin cleanser, and will cause free perspiration unless it is comparatively brief. Avoid becoming chilled as long as any noticeable perspiring persists. Also be on guard against the possibility of lightheadedness or even fainting due to a drop in blood pressure. Because of this danger, an attendant should remain near during the treatment.

Tub Baths

It is desirable to have a tub five and a half or six feet long, so that the body can be completely immersed. It is especially important that the temperature of the water be tested with a bath thermometer. The tub in the ordinary home is shorter than the above-indicated length, but it can still be used with fair results. In such a case the patient has to bend his knees while lying down.

Cold Tub Bath. For a cold tub bath the temperature should range from 50°

to 70° F. (10 to 21° C.) and the time from a few seconds to several minutes, depending on the temperature and effect desired. It is necessary to employ brisk rubbing constantly or at brief intervals to prevent chilling if the bath lasts more than a few seconds. The patient's face should be bathed in cold water before he enters the bath. It is important to make sure that the skin is warm before the bath is given.

When a brief cold bath is given to a patient with a normal temperature, the effect is that of a tonic or stimulant. The temperature of the bath may be lowered on successive occasions and the length of the application increased as the patient's tolerance improves. Should he feel chilly after the treatment, it is because the water was so cold or the duration of the bath so long as to exceed his personal tolerance. The cold bath is a good health-promoting measure for the normal person. The cold rubbing bath, continued over a longer period of time, is an efficient method of reducing temperature, but it should be given under the direction of a physician.

Graduated Tub Bath. The graduated tub bath provides an effective means of lowering the body temperature of a patient with fever. It may be continued until the patient's temperature is lowered by as much as two or three degrees F. (one or two degrees C.), but not longer than a half hour. It should begin at about 97° F. (36° C.) or a little lower than the patient's mouth temperature. The skin must be warm at the beginning. Apply cold compresses to the head. Gradually reduce the temperature of the bath water to about 86° F. (36° C.). When it has been brought below 90° F. (32° C.), or if the patient feels chilly or shows gooseflesh, he should be rubbed constantly to keep the blood in the skin, and thus prevent or overcome chilling. The patient's pulse and mouth temperature should be closely watched during the bath, the temperature being checked every five minutes. On removal from the bath, im-

mediately wrap the patient in a sheet, drying him quickly. If after the bath there is gooseflesh or chilliness, rub the skin briskly with your hands until the blood returns.

Hot Tub Bath. For a hot tub bath, water temperature should range from 100° to 109° F. (38° to 42° C.) and the time from five to twenty minutes. Give cold water freely to drink. Keep the head cool with cold compresses. If necessary, apply an ice bag to the heart and one to the back of the neck. It is usually wise to begin the bath at about 98° F. (37° C.), gradually raising the temperature to the desired level by adding hot water and letting out water as necessary. Always use a bath thermometer and stir the water well as hot water is added. The treatment may be finished by cooling the bath, or by a cold pour or shower given briefly immediately after the patient rises from the bath, the patient's body being then dried with brisk rubbing.

The effect varies with the tempera-

The hot half bath may be used to treat certain pelvic complaints.

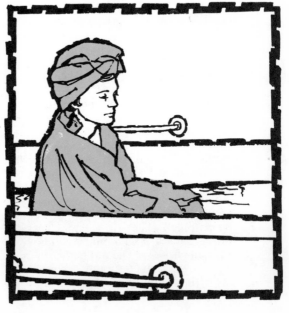

ture of the water and the duration of the bath. If it is much prolonged or if the temperature is very high, the body temperature is raised and profuse sweating is produced. Hot tub baths may be used as a preparation for cold treatment.

In giving the patient a bath hot enough and long enough to raise his body temperature perceptibly, the attendant should remain nearby because there is some danger that the patient might faint, especially when he stands up. Since most of the body is immersed in hot water, the body has little ability to protect itself from overheating. The attendant should take the patient's mouth temperature every five or ten minutes. The hot bath should be used only with the knowledge of the physician. It may be of value in such conditions as arthritis.

Hot Half Bath. The usual bathtub in the home is well suited for the hot half bath, since the patient sits up in the tub with only his legs and hips in the water. This bath provides a good method of applying the temperature effect of the water to the hip region for certain pelvic complaints. Fill the tub with enough water to reach nearly to the patient's waist. The temperature of the water should be about 101° F. (38° C.) at the beginning of the bath, and should be gradually raised over a period of about five minutes by drawing out some of the water and running in hot water until the temperature reaches toleration (not more than 112° F. [44° C.]). A bath thermometer must be used, and the water must be kept circulating by using the hand and thermometer as a paddle. Continue the bath for five to twenty minutes or more; it may be ended by dashing cold water over the patient's hips and drying quickly.

Throughout the time of the bath the patient's shoulders may be protected by a folded sheet or a large Turkish towel, and a cold compress may be kept on his head. The hot half bath may be used to produce a moderate artificial fever. It is safer to use for this purpose

than the hot tub bath since a large part of the body is out of the water. This permits the body to protect itself from overheating. Still care should be taken lest the patient faint, especially when he stands up. He should not be left alone.

Neutral Tub Bath. For a neutral tub bath, water temperature should range from 94° to 97° F. (34° to 36° C.), and the time from fifteen minutes to three or four hours, usually twenty to thirty minutes. Wet the forehead and the face with cool water. Cool the bath slightly at the close. Dry the patient with a sheet immediately after the bath. Avoid unnecessary rubbing, and do not excite the patient in any other way, as this destroys the quieting effect. The neutral bath is given for sedative purposes. In cooler weather it may be necessary to employ the upper limit of the stated temperature range. The air of the bathroom should be warm; and, if the bath is much prolonged, stretch a sheet over the tub. This bath may be a useful means of the treatment of nervous tension.

Dry Heat

Electric Heating Pad. The best pads are made with controls that permit three or more degrees of heat. For prolonged applications of unvarying dry heat, there is no better apparatus than such a pad. It should be applied over a dry cover or cloth. In chronic arthritis, it can give much relief; and it can be used in all other conditions for which dry heat is suitable. Applied over a wet compress (see **The Heating Compress** earlier in this chapter), it produces much the same effect as a protracted fomentation. The wet compress is composed of several thicknesses of gauze or a double thickness of cotton cloth, wrung out of tap water and placed in direct contact with the patient's skin. A sheet of rubber or some other waterproof material must be placed between the wet compress and the heating pad so as to prevent short-circuiting the wires in the pad by moisture. A special patented electric heating pad is the Thermophore ®, which is designed to retain body moisture and thus act more like a fomentation. Great caution must be taken to prevent skin burning, especially when there is poor circulation or poor skin sensation, or when the patient is not fully conscious or may fall asleep. The patient must be able to discontinue the heat application himself. The Thermophore ® is supplied with a switch which must be actively pressed for operation—as a safety feature.

Hot-Water Bottle. Most hot-water bottles are made of rubber. They should be partly filled with very hot water, never with boiling water, and wrapped in cloth, preferably flannel or a Turkish towel. When properly wrapped, hot-water bottles will hold a useful degree of heat for an hour or more. The safe heat for a hot-water bottle can be tested by holding it against the cheek. An ordinary rubber bottle has a capacity of about two quarts. When not in use, the bottle should be hung bottom up and with the stopper out. It should never be left doubled sharply on itself, as it is likely to crack at the fold.

Hot-water bottles, even as electric heating pads, can be dangerous if not used with proper caution. For this reason they are not used in many hospitals. The patient must be able to take the responsibility to control their use since they are usually left with the patient and not continually watched by the attendant as with most other heat applications.

Radiant Heat. In many cases, particularly with neuralgia, neuritis, arthritis, and sinusitis, radiant heat from some red-hot source is one of the most effective forms of dry heat.

Units to provide radiant heat can be obtained from hospital supply stores. A good simple source of such heat is an inexpensive electrical appliance such as a bathroom heater—the kind without a fan. Another good kind is an infrared

bulb, for sale in most department stores and drugstores. Such a bathroom heater can be set on a chair beside the bed and the distance from the part of the body to be treated adjusted so that the heat is nearly as great as the patient can bear.

Heat can be applied with such an apparatus for half an hour or longer at a time without injury, if properly watched. The treatment can safely be repeated several times a day. In treating a case of sinusitis, thick pads of wet gauze should be laid over the eyes to protect them from the heat while it is falling on the rest of the face and forehead.

Radiant heaters are easy to use and have the advantage of permitting observation of the part under treatment during the application. Precautions that have already been mentioned for other heat applications must be followed. Remember that the patient should not be left alone with the heater unless he can be fully relied upon to control the treatment. There must be good sensation and good circulation in the part of the body being treated. Caution, of course, must be taken to prevent accidental igniting of flammable material.

Light Treatments

Visible, infrared, and ultraviolet light; X rays, diathermy, and radio waves are all basically the same, the difference being their respective ranges of wavelength. But they differ greatly in their effects on the human body. Certain ultraviolet wavelengths are strong in producing a sunburn; others help prevent the disease called rickets. Infrared rays heat the skin, diathermy energy heats the deep body tissues, and even radio waves will heat the body if they are strong enough.

Ultraviolet radiation sources usually throw off comparatively few visible light rays and practically no heat rays at all. The invisible effects are not apparent to the patient at the time of the treatment, the reddening and tanning effect on the skin being considerably delayed. The "burn" that may follow such a treatment, like a sunburn, may be severe enough to be painful or even harmful before the patient realizes that anything is happening. Therefore quartz-light or any other ultraviolet-light treatments should be given only by experienced people. The eyes are especially susceptible to the "burn." They must always be covered during the exposure.

The effects of the various forms of radiation we have briefly presented leave the door open for pseudoscientists and quacks to spread inflated ideas about the value of radiation and for the manufacturers of various types of ultraviolet and colored lamps to make unwarranted claims for their products. Anybody considering the use of a lamp with the hope of obtaining radiation therapy other than that obtainable from radiant heat should consult his physician.

These warnings should not be construed as denying the value of ultraviolet rays. When these rays fall upon the bare skin, they lead to the formation of vitamin D in it, a vitamin essential to health and one which ordinary food may not supply in sufficient quantities. Sunlight, however, normally supplies the body's needs for vitamin D adequately, either by direct exposure of the skin or by irradiation of the food supply.

Ultraviolet rays also have a strong bactericidal effect. In other and not so well understood ways they promote general health and increase resistance to disease. Controlled sunbaths may be of great value to sick persons who are confined. If it is impossible or not feasible to obtain these desirable effects by means of sunbaths, then consideration may be given to some other reliable source of ultraviolet rays. The best results, however, can be obtained with safety only if a physician and a qualified physical therapist closely supervise the treatment.

Sunbaths

The sunbath has a definite place as a simple home treatment. There are cer-tain principles and precautions that should be followed, however. For these the reader is referred to the previous discussion on light treatments.

A sunbath is best taken in the morning when the air is clear and the heat not too great. In the summer it may be taken as early as seven o'clock. In cooler weather, it may be taken later in the forenoon. Care must be taken to prevent overheating or chilling.

In order to avoid sunburn, it is necessary to start with a short exposure and to increase the time gradually on following days. To secure the benefit of the ultraviolet rays of the sun, it is essential that the sunlight fall upon the naked skin with no glass or screen intervening. The head, however, should preferably not be exposed. The eyes should be protected by the use of glasses or covered with cloth. If desired, a cold compress may be applied to the forehead, but this is not often necessary. The sunbath can with benefit be followed by a cool shower, a cold mitten friction, or an alcohol rub.

Following a sunbath, there should be a feeling of well-being. Headache, fatigue, and nausea are symptoms of overexposure. They give warning that the duration of subsequent sunbaths should be reduced. Later they may be gradually increased again.

The first exposure to the sun may be three to five minutes on the front of the body and the same time on the back except the head. The time may be increased one to three minutes each day until the total time of a single treatment is from half an hour to an hour. The length of the sunbath may be increased still further upon a physician's advice. Sunbaths, however, must not be used in cases of pulmonary tuberculosis. Since there are other conditions and certain medicines which may sensitize the body to ultraviolet light, the patient's physician should be consulted.

Massage

Massage is a system of remedial or hygienic manipulations of the body tissues with the hand or some instrument.

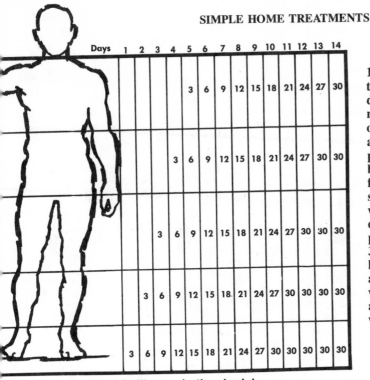

Days	1	2	3	4	5	6	7	8	9	10	11	12	13	14
				3	6	9	12	15	18	21	24	27	30	
			3	6	9	12	15	18	21	24	27	30	30	
		3	6	9	12	15	18	21	24	27	30	30	30	
	3	6	9	12	15	18.	21	24	27	30	30	30	30	
	3	6	9	12	15	18	21	24	27	30	30	30	30	30

Modified Rollier sunbath schedule

1. This sunbath begins at the feet, exposure the first day 3 minutes front and 3 minutes back. 2. The second day the legs from the ankles to the knees are exposed 3 minutes front and back, and the feet 6 minutes front and back. 3. The schedule is continued in this way until on the fourteenth day the whole body is exposed 30 minutes front and 30 minutes back, or one hour in all. From now on, any increase over an hour would be 3 minutes front and 3 minutes back, of the whole body each day.

It consists of rubbing, stroking, kneading, vibrating, or tapping. Although it is natural for a person to rub a part that may feel uncomfortable, the procedures of massage for the treatment of disease or injury are too complicated for a person to administer unless he has had proper training in an accredited institution. Massage by a well-trained therapist should be given only with the consent of the patient's doctor; even then it may have to be done with special precautions.

Exercise

Exercise is necessary for the maintenance of health. This fact becomes clearly evident when a healthy individual is made bedfast, let us say, by a fractured leg. He will lose strength and weight. Just as in health, so in disease, the need of exercise persists, and activity should be maintained as much as the disease condition will allow. In addition to fulfilling this need, exercise may also be used as treatment. Exercise benefits the body in several ways, the by-products adding up to effective therapy.

Exercise stimulates the circulation to the active part. Thus controlled exercise may be used to improve the flow of blood in a leg which may be suffering for want of blood, as in Buerger's disease.

The heart is also stimulated by general muscular activity. Under close medical supervision controlled exercise and, therefore, controlled heart activity is beneficial in the prevention and treatment of heart failure.

The return of blood from the extremities is furthered by the pumping action resulting from muscle contraction. For this reason when a person is confined to bed, it is desirable for him to move his legs occasionally—if this is permitted.

Because the body responds to the need of more oxygen for the muscles during muscular activity, more breathing is required. Exercise may be used as a means to accomplish deeper breathing.

457

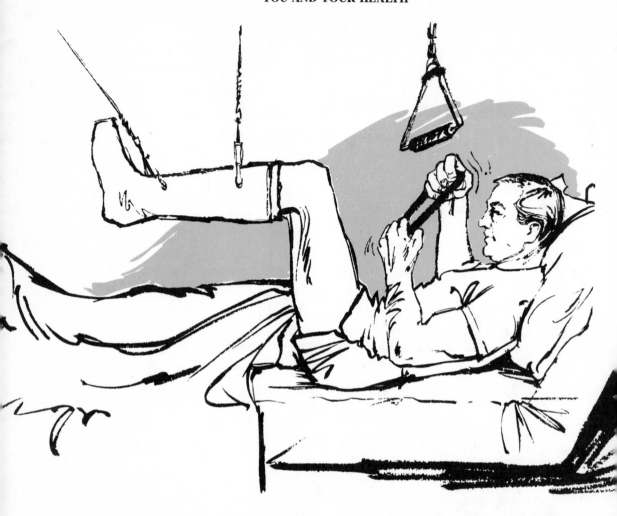

Active muscles require more food than muscles at rest. Thus exercise may be employed as a means of stimulating appetite. It also furthers elimination.

The proper amount of physical activity will encourage sleep. In many cases sleeplessness can be relieved by a good walk before bedtime.

The yawn and the stretch of the limbs observed in both animals and man are nature's automatic method to keep the muscles from tightening or stiffening up. In a number of diseases there is a special tendency for the muscles to tighten. These include arthritis, poliomyelitis, stroke, and injury to the spinal cord. Muscles that cannot be stretched out tend to become shortened, with a tendency toward deformities. When it is painful to move a part, or to stretch naturally, the part is likely to be held in the position least painful. This limiting of the movements of a part over a long period will result in muscle shortening and even in deformity. If in arthritis all joints are moved throughout their complete range only once a day, shortening deformities will not occur.

Contracting the muscles with force develops their strength. In order for this to be most effective, one needs to follow the principles of body building as done by athletes. That is, the movements must be done regularly and daily over a long period of time, also with gradual increase of force and duration. By this means muscle tissue, blood circulation, the heart, the organs of breathing, and the organs of digestion will be benefited.

Heavy resistive exercises, gradually increased to develop strength, have a special application in improving joint stability, as with a weak knee or ankle. Such exercises are also of value in treating paralyses of individual muscles by developing the strength of neighboring muscles which can assist in movement.

Habitually poor posture may result in muscle tightening and even in deformities, especially when there is also a tendency to arthritis. Use of exercises to strengthen certain muscles and to stretch others, plus a growing sense of what correct posture is, will help in improving and in maintaining good posture. Good posture helps to retain and improve general health.

Exercises of a specific nature may be prescribed by the physician. For the performance of these the guidance of a physical or occupational therapist may be needed. On the other hand, the need for exercise and the desired type of activity may be so obvious and simple that the patient needs no special guidance except his own judgment. In general, a program of exercise should be associated with a purpose or goal and, when finished, with a sense of accomplishment. It is better to link exercise with a hobby than simply to go through the movements. Such satisfying activities as gardening, building, exploring, and picture taking, when associated with proper activity and good posture, are better than simple weight lifting or throwing a ball.

The use of exercise as a treatment procedure has been only introduced here. Detailed material for a specific problem should be requested from the doctor in charge of the case. One should remember that with some disease conditions exercise should be done with caution and under the surveillance of the physician, especially in cases where heart disease is involved.

Rest and Relaxation

Rest alternating with activity, relaxation alternating with work, sleep alternating with wakefulness are cycles necessary for normal life and health. A correct relationship between the opposing states must be maintained. Obviously in conditions of injury or disease this relationship becomes more important than in health, assuming therapeutic importance.

When a part is injured, it will likely be held motionless, as when a broken arm is put in a cast. After the bone is sufficiently healed, the limb is taken out of the cast for regulated exercises. Exercise of the muscles, such as by tensing one against the other, is usually desirable even while the part is in the cast.

It may be said that a patient suffers from overwork, though usually this is not a correct statement. More likely he needs a review of his daily program so that wasted movements can be saved, thus permitting time for rest periods and for adequate hours of sleep.

The "overworked" patient may not realize that most of his muscles are kept in a constant state of tension. By learning how to relax unnecessary muscle tension, he may accomplish even more than before but with less fatigue. Relaxation of muscle tension may stop such complaints as headache, nervousness, acid stomach, palpitation, and fatigue, which often result from psychological stress.

What some may consider to be rest may actually include a large component of psychic strain or emotional tension. After a hard day's work one may choose to look for several hours at television shows. Although a pleasing diversion, such activity may not be conducive to muscular relaxation or to restful sleep during the remaining hours of the night.

The periods of rest may be many, but short, and still be restful. The extreme illustration of this is the heart muscle. Although it necessarily works sixty minutes out of each hour and twenty-four hours a day, it may actually rest longer than the body as a whole, for it rests between heartbeats for a longer time than it works while beating. One should look for opportunity for rest periods during the day even though they might be short.

For the person who is "overworked," arranging to get away and loaf for several days may not be the best answer. The needed "rest" may be provided best by devoting a day to swimming or mountain climbing.

"Rest" has its hazards. Some of these were pointed out in the paragraphs on exercise. Another important hazard is psychological. The idea of the need for rest may become so dominant in the mind of a patient that without any real physical abnormality he who was originally normal may now become an invalid.

In Conclusion

In this chapter we have briefly described various simple treatments that can be given in the home with simple equipment and with untrained help and even by the patient himself. Many times the reader will appreciate that the careful application of common sense is all that is really required in the administration of these treatments. On the other hand, common sense may clearly indicate that help by professionally trained people, such as physical and occupational therapists, is needed. One of the most important things to learn is when one should call the physician.

Notes

Notes

Notes

Notes

HUMAN ANATOMY

FULL-COLOR PLATES WITH FOUR IN TRANSPARENT

"TRANS-VISION"® SHOWING STRUCTURES OF THE HUMAN TORSO

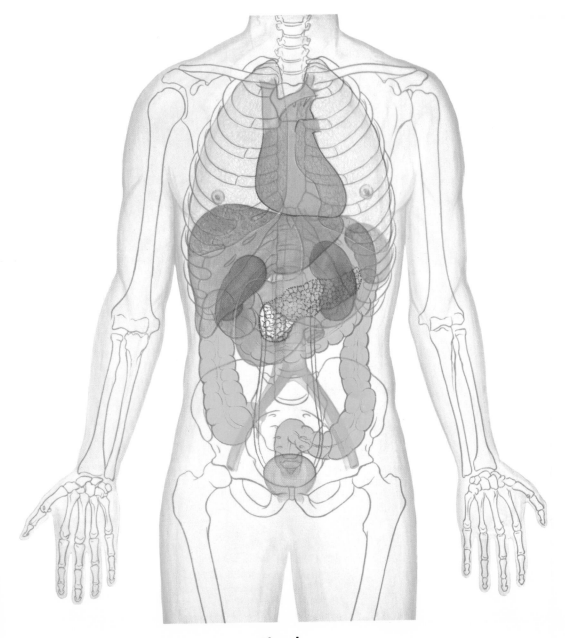

Plate I

ERNEST W. BECK, medical illustrator

in collaboration with

HARRY MONSEN , Ph.D.

Professor of Anatomy, College of Medicine, University of Illinois

Plate II

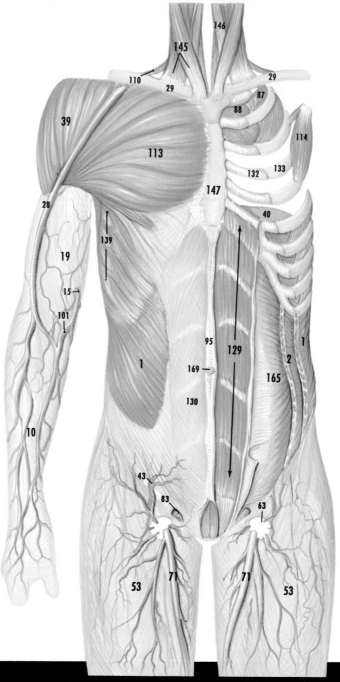

Plate III

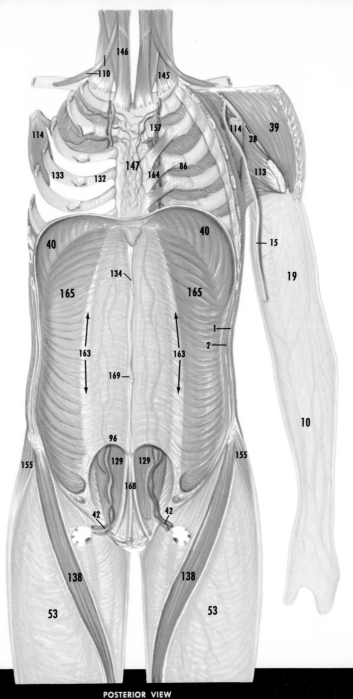

POSTERIOR VIEW

1. Abdominal oblique muscle, external
2. Abdominal oblique muscle, internal
10. Antebrachial fascia
15. Basilic vein
19. Brachial fascia
28. Cephalic vein
39. Deltoid muscle
40. Diaphragm
42. Epigastric artery and vein, deep inferior
53. Fascia of the thigh

86. Intercostal artery and vein
96. Linea semicircularis
110. Omohyoid muscle
113. Pectoralis major muscle
114. Pectoralis minor muscle
129. Rectus abdominis muscle
132. Rib (costal) cartilage
133. Rib
134. Round ligament of the liver
138. Sartorius muscle
145. Sternocleidomastoid muscle

146. Sternohyoid muscle
147. Sternum
155. Tensor fascia lata muscle
157. Thoracic artery and vein, internal
163. Transversalis fascia
164. Transverse thoracic muscle
165. Transversus abdominis muscle
168. Umbilical ligaments
169. Umbilicus

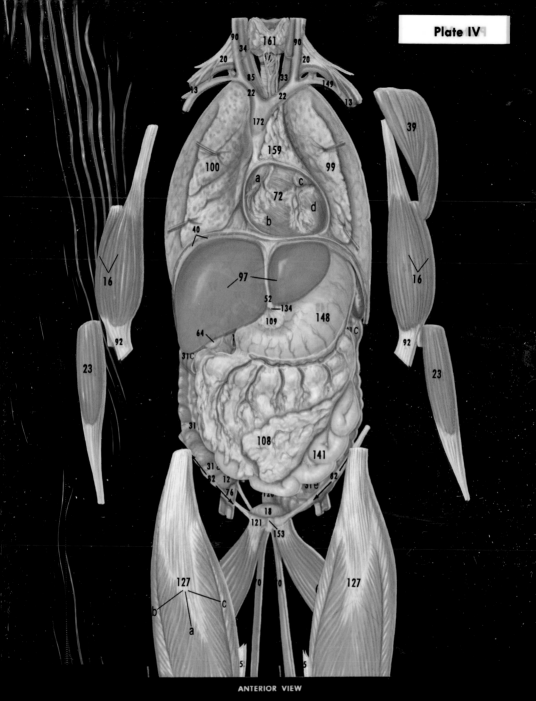

Plate IV

ANTERIOR VIEW

5. Adductor canal
13. Axillary artery and vein
16. Biceps brachii muscle
20. Brachial nerve plexus
22. Brachiocephalic vein
23. Brachioradialis muscle
33. Common carotid artery, left
34. Common carotid artery, right
39. Deltoid muscle

40. Diaphragm
52. Falciform ligament
64. Gallbladder
72. Heart:
   a. Right auricle
   b. Right ventricle
   c. Left auricle
   d. Left ventricle
85. Innominate (brachiocephalic) artery
90. Jugular vein, internal
92. Lacertus fibrosus

97. Liver
99. Lung, left
100. Lung, right
108. Omentum, greater
109. Omentum, lesser
127. Quadriceps femoris muscle:
   a. Rectus femoris
   b. Vastus lateralis
   c. Vastus medialis
134. Round ligament
141. Small intestine

148. Stomach
149. Subclavian artery and vein
159. Thymus gland
161. Thyroid gland
172. Vena cava, superior

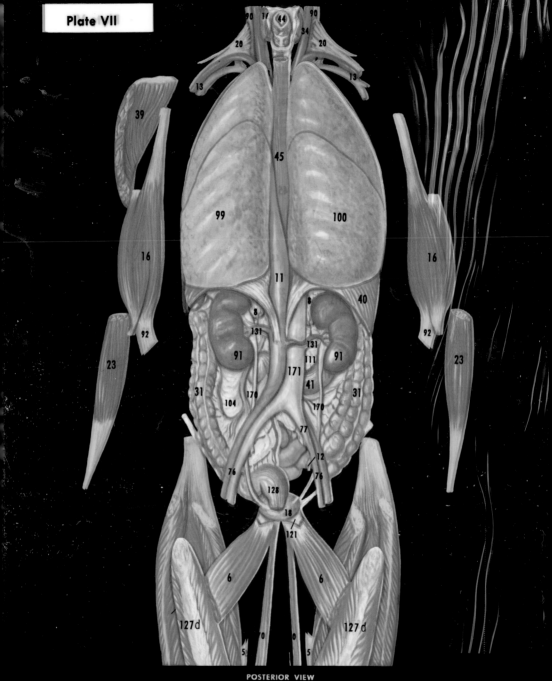

Plate VII

POSTERIOR VIEW

6. Adductor longus muscle
8. Adrenal (suprarenal) gland
11. Aorta
12. Appendix, vermiform
18. Bladder, urinary
31. Colon (large intestine)
40. Diaphragm
41. Duodenum
44. Epiglottis

45. Esophagus
70. Gracilis muscle
76. Iliac artery and vein, external
77. Iliac artery and vein, right common
91. Kidney
99. Lung, left
100. Lung, right

104. Mesentery
111. Pancreas
121. Pubic bone
127. Quadriceps femoris muscle: d. Vastus intermedius
128. Rectum
131. Renal artery and vein
170. Ureter
171. Vena cava, inferior

Plate VIII

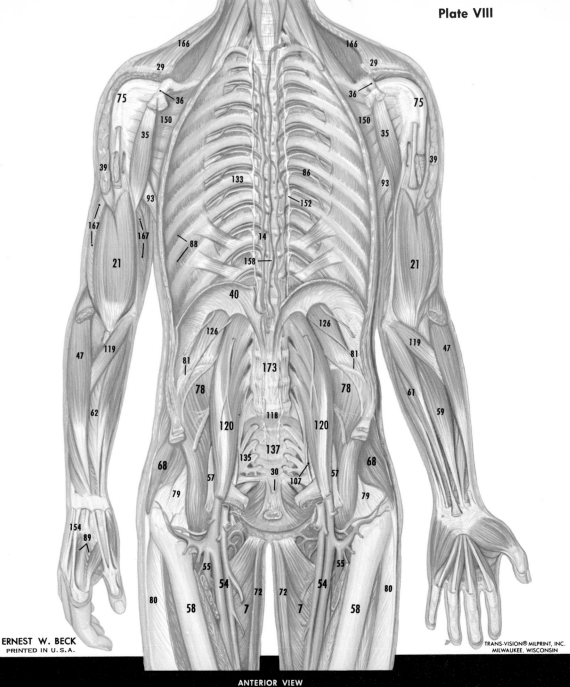

ANTERIOR VIEW

7. Adductor magnus muscle
14. Azygos veins
21. Brachialis muscle
29. Clavicle
30. Coccyx
35. Coracobrachialis muscle
36. Coracoid process of the scapula
39. Deltoid muscle
40. Diaphragm
47. Extensor carpi radialis longus muscle
54. Femoral artery and vein

55. Femoral artery, deep
57. Femoral nerve
58. Femur
59. Flexor carpi radialis muscle
61. Flexor digitorum profundus muscle
62. Flexor digitorum superficialis muscle
68. Gluteus medius muscle
75. Humerus
78. Iliacus muscle
79. Iliofemoral ligament
80. Iliotibial tract
81. Ilium

86. Intercostal artery, vein and nerve
88. Intercostal muscle, internal
89. Interosseous muscles, dorsal
93. Latissimus dorsi muscle
107. Obturator nerve
118. Promontory
119. Pronator teres muscle
120. Psoas muscles (major and minor)
126. Quadratus lumborum muscle

133. Rib
135. Sacral nerves
137. Sacrum
150. Subscapularis muscle
152. Sympathetic (autonomic) nerve chain
154. Tendons of extensor muscles of hand
158. Thoracic duct
166. Trapezius muscle
167. Triceps brachii muscle
173. Vertebral column

ERNEST W. BECK
PRINTED IN U.S.A.

TRANS-VISION® MILPRINT, INC.
MILWAUKEE, WISCONSIN

Plate IX

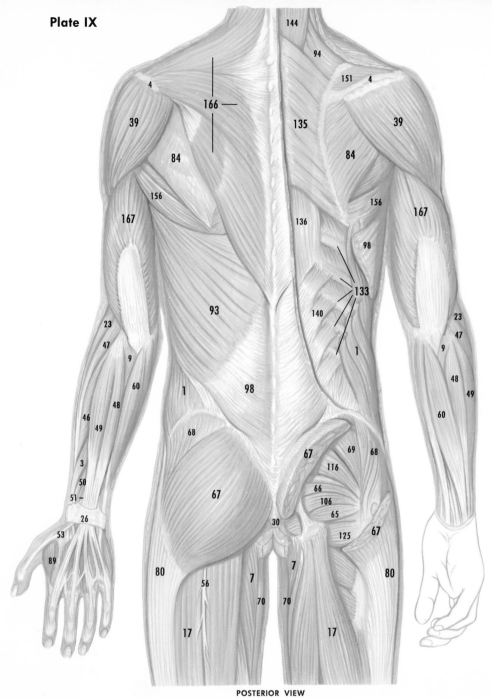

POSTERIOR VIEW

1. Abdominal oblique muscle, external
3. Abductor pollicis longus muscle
4. Acromion process of the scapula
7. Adductor magnus muscle
9. Anconeus muscle
17. Biceps femoris muscle
23. Brachioradialis muscle
26. Carpal ligament, dorsal
30. Coccyx
39. Deltoid muscle
46. Extensor carpi radialis brevis muscle

47. Extensor carpi radialis longus muscle
48. Extensor carpi ulnaris muscle
49. Extensor digitorum communis muscle
50. Extensor pollicis brevis muscle
51. Extensor pollicis longus muscle
56. Femoral cutaneous nerve, posterior
60. Flexor carpi ulnaris muscle
65. Gemellus inferior muscle

66. Gemellus superior muscle
67. Gluteus maximus muscle
68. Gluteus medius muscle
69. Gluteus minimus muscle
70. Gracilis muscle
80. Iliotibial tract
84. Infraspinatus muscle
89. Interosseous muscle, dorsal
93. Latissimus dorsi muscle
94. Levator scapulae muscle
98. Lumbodorsal fascia

106. Obturator internus muscle
116. Piriformis muscle
125. Quadratus femoris muscle
133. Ribs (VII-XII)
135. Rhomboideus muscle
136. Erector spinae muscle
140. Serratus posterior inferior muscle
144. Splenius capitis muscle
151. Supraspinatus muscle
156. Teres major muscle
166. Trapezius muscle
167. Triceps brachii muscle

Plate X

BONES AND SINUSES OF THE SKULL

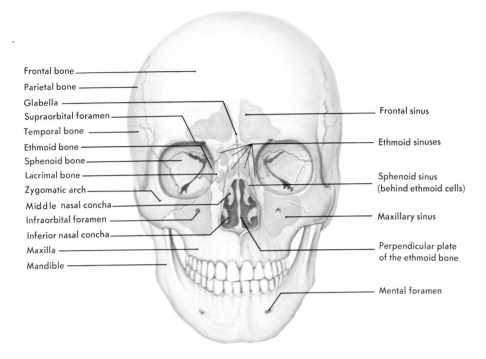

Frontal bone
Parietal bone
Glabella
Supraorbital foramen
Temporal bone
Ethmoid bone
Sphenoid bone
Lacrimal bone
Zygomatic arch
Middle nasal concha
Infraorbital foramen
Inferior nasal concha
Maxilla
Mandible

Frontal sinus
Ethmoid sinuses
Sphenoid sinus
(behind ethmoid cells)
Maxillary sinus
Perpendicular plate
of the ethmoid bone
Mental foramen

HEMISECTION OF THE HEAD AND NECK

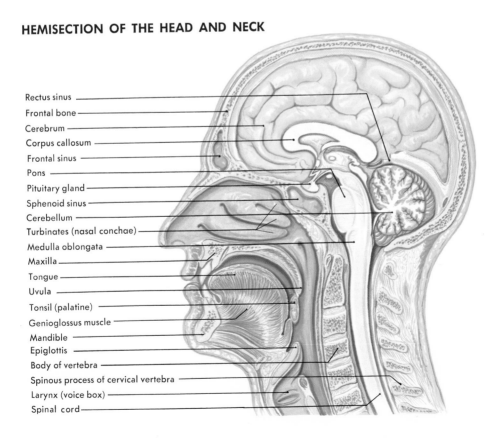

Rectus sinus
Frontal bone
Cerebrum
Corpus callosum
Frontal sinus
Pons
Pituitary gland
Sphenoid sinus
Cerebellum
Turbinates (nasal conchae)
Medulla oblongata
Maxilla
Tongue
Uvula
Tonsil (palatine)
Genioglossus muscle
Mandible
Epiglottis
Body of vertebra
Spinous process of cervical vertebra
Larynx (voice box)
Spinal cord

Plate XI

ANATOMY OF THE EAR

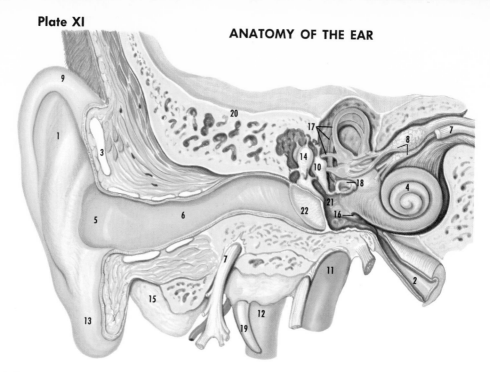

1. Anthelix
2. Auditory tube
3. Cartilage
4. Cochlea
5. Concha
6. External acoustic meatus
7. Facial nerve
8. Ganglia of the vestibular nerve
9. Helix
10. Incus (anvil)
11. Internal carotid artery
12. Internal jugular vein
13. Lobe
14. Malleus (hammer)
15. Mastoid process
16. Round window
17. Semicircular canals
18. Stapes (stirrup)
19. Styloid process
20. Temporal bone
21. Tympanic cavity
22. Tympanic membrane (eardrum)

ANATOMY OF THE EYE

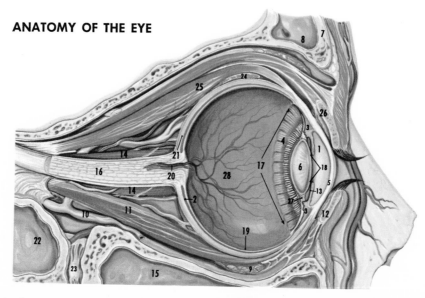

1. Aqueous chamber
2. Choroid
3. Ciliary muscle
4. Ciliary processes
5. Cornea
6. Crystalline lens
7. Frontal bone
8. Frontal sinus
9. Inferior oblique muscle
10. Inferior ophthalmic vein
11. Inferior rectus muscle
12. Inferior tarsus
13. Iris
14. Lateral rectus muscle
15. Maxillary sinus
16. Optic nerve
17. Ora serrata
18. Pupil of the iris
19. Retina
20. Retinal artery and vein
21. Sclera
22. Sphenoid sinus
23. Pterygopalatine ganglion
24. Superior oblique muscle
25. Superior rectus muscle
26. Superior tarsus
27. Suspensory ligament
28. Vitreous chamber

Plate XII

SCHEMATIC BODY CELL

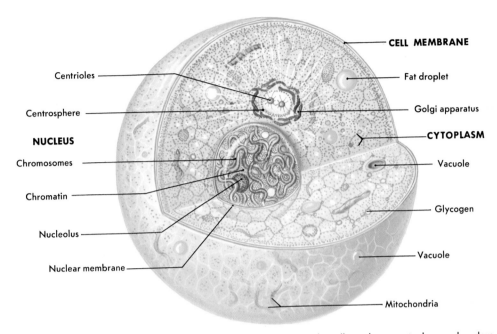

CELL MEMBRANE

Centrioles

Centrosphere

Fat droplet

Golgi apparatus

NUCLEUS

CYTOPLASM

Chromosomes

Vacuole

Chromatin

Glycogen

Nucleolus

Nuclear membrane

Vacuole

Mitochondria

Every living cell, regardless of its shape or size, has three main parts: the cell membrane, cytoplasm, and nucleus. Together they constitute protoplasm. Billions of such cells as shown above make up the tissues of our bodies.

TYPES OF CELLS

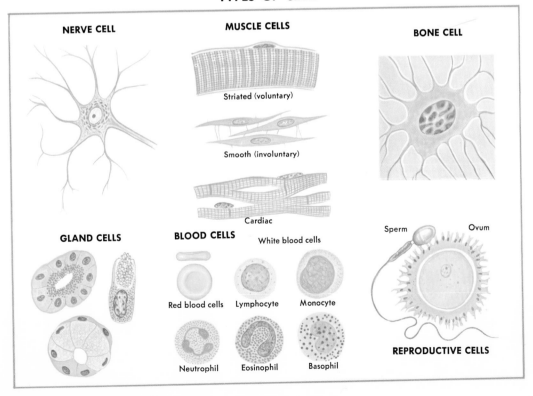

NERVE CELL

MUSCLE CELLS

BONE CELL

Striated (voluntary)

Smooth (involuntary)

Cardiac

GLAND CELLS

BLOOD CELLS

White blood cells

Sperm   Ovum

Red blood cells   Lymphocyte   Monocyte

Neutrophil   Eosinophil   Basophil

REPRODUCTIVE CELLS

Plate XIII

SKELETON

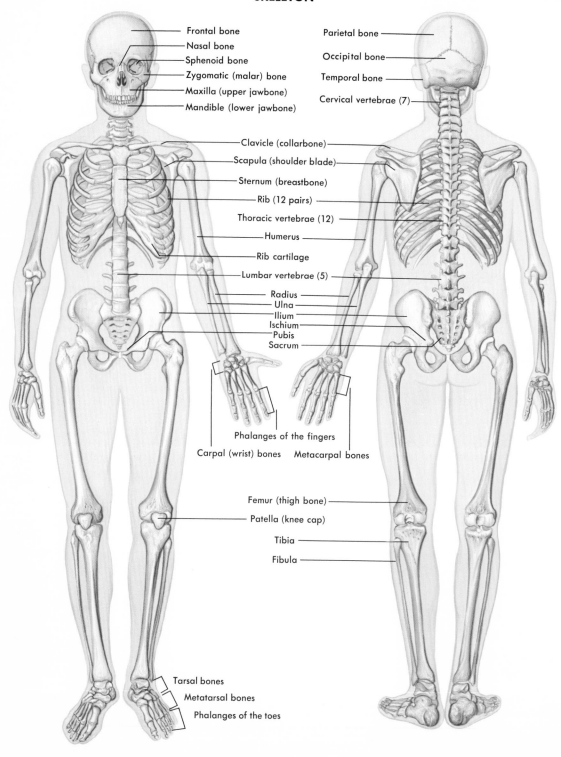

Frontal bone
Nasal bone
Sphenoid bone
Zygomatic (malar) bone
Maxilla (upper jawbone)
Mandible (lower jawbone)

Parietal bone
Occipital bone
Temporal bone
Cervical vertebrae (7)

Clavicle (collarbone)
Scapula (shoulder blade)
Sternum (breastbone)
Rib (12 pairs)
Thoracic vertebrae (12)
Humerus
Rib cartilage
Lumbar vertebrae (5)
Radius
Ulna
Ilium
Ischium
Pubis
Sacrum

Phalanges of the fingers
Carpal (wrist) bones   Metacarpal bones

Femur (thigh bone)
Patella (knee cap)
Tibia
Fibula

Tarsal bones
Metatarsal bones
Phalanges of the toes

Plate XIV

FEMALE PELVIC ORGANS

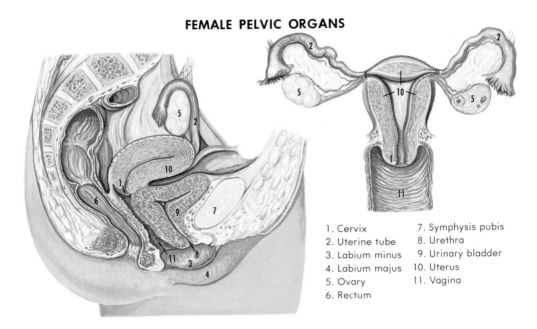

1. Cervix
2. Uterine tube
3. Labium minus
4. Labium majus
5. Ovary
6. Rectum
7. Symphysis pubis
8. Urethra
9. Urinary bladder
10. Uterus
11. Vagina

MALE PELVIC ORGANS

SECTION THROUGH PENIS

SCHEME OF DUCT ARRANGEMENT IN THE TESTIS AND EPIDIDYMIS

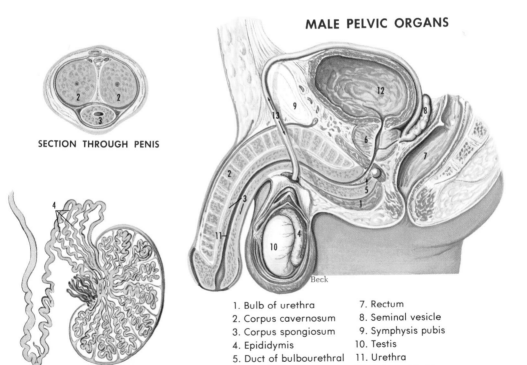

Beck

1. Bulb of urethra
2. Corpus cavernosum
3. Corpus spongiosum
4. Epididymis
5. Duct of bulbourethral gland
6. Prostate gland
7. Rectum
8. Seminal vesicle
9. Symphysis pubis
10. Testis
11. Urethra
12. Urinary bladder
13. Ductus deferens

Plate XV

LYMPHATIC ORGANS

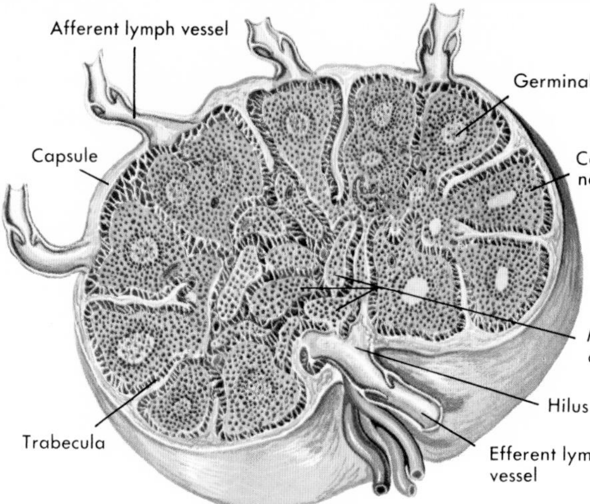

Afferent lymph vessel

Germinal center

Capsule

Cortical nodules

Medullary cords

Hilus

Trabecula

Efferent lymph vessel

LYMPH NODE

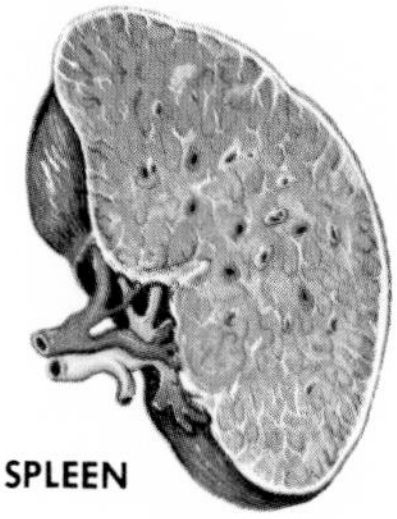

SPLEEN

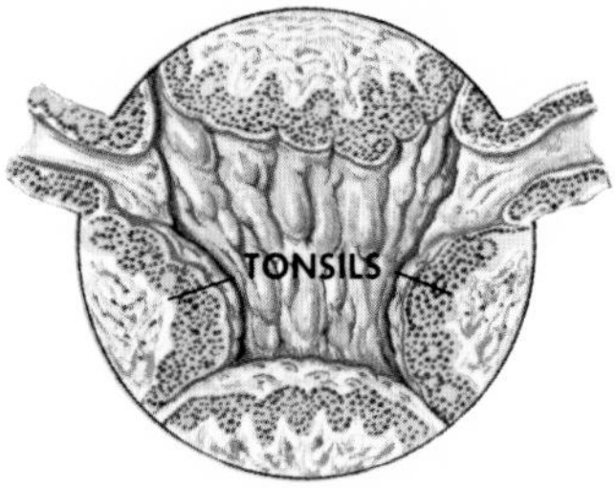

TONSILS

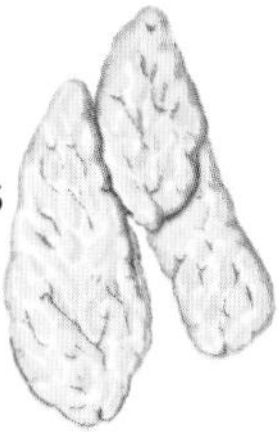

THYMUS

LYMPHATIC VESSELS

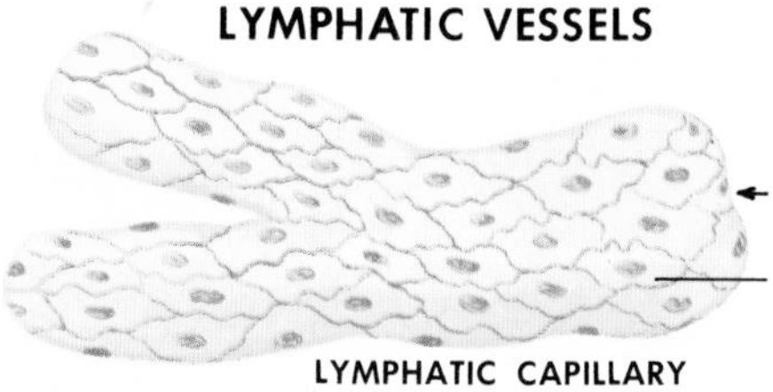

← Closed end

Single layer of endothelial cells

LYMPHATIC CAPILLARY

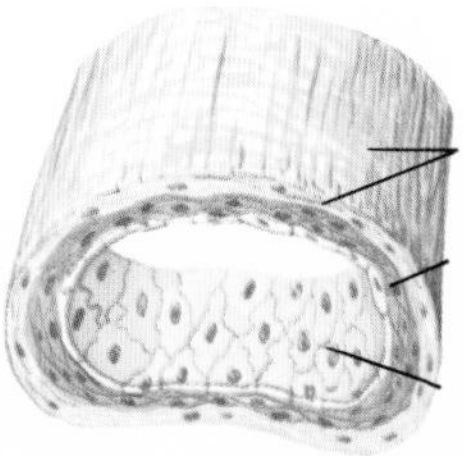

Outer coat (fibrous tissue)

Middle coat (muscle layer)

Inner coat (endothelial cells)

LARGE LYMPHATIC VESSEL

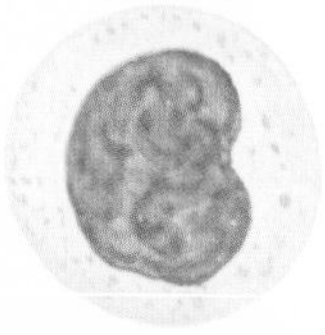

Monocyte

Lymphocyte

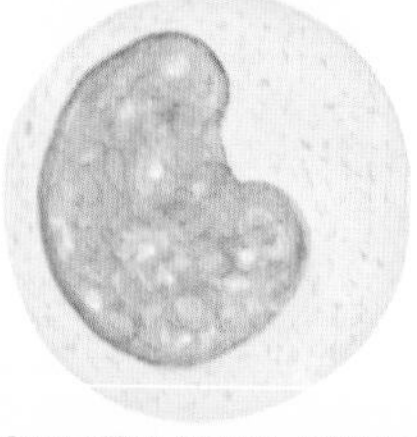

FREE CELLS OF THE LYMPHATIC SYSTEM

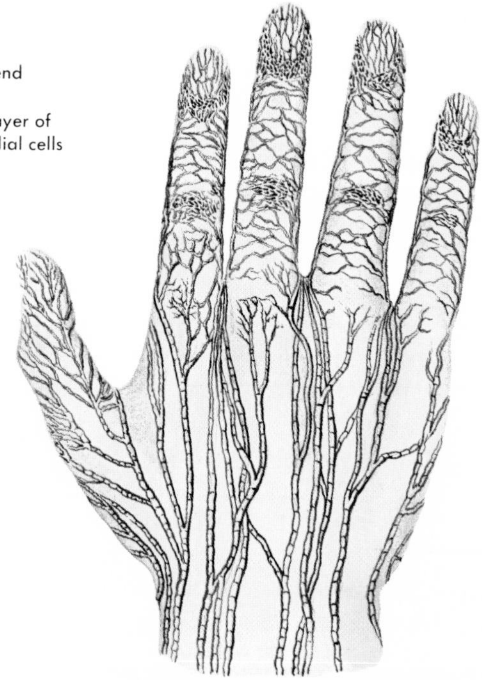

LYMPHATICS OF THE HAND

Illustrated Study
of Cells

In diagnosing an illness the doctor frequently calls for laboratory tests, which could include microscopic examination of blood cells or of tissue samples obtained from organs suspected of being diseased. Because many systemic diseases produce unique effects on the blood and on the tissues, such tests give clues to possible infection or to incipient stages of abnormalities such as cancer or degenerative diseases.

Normal cells and abnormal cells often look so near alike that it takes a trained eye to detect malformation or disease. A physician skilled in recognizing specific changes produced by disease is called a pathologist, and the method of removing a small portion of tissue for special study, a biopsy examination.

The following magnifications show what a doctor sees when he looks through a microscope at normal and abnormal cells and tissues. They are not medical drawings but illustrations showing actual tissue mounted on glass slides by a special technique known as microtomy.

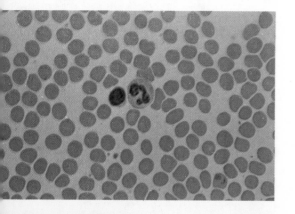

A microscopic view of a normal blood preparation in which occasional white blood cells are seen among numerous red blood cells. Seen here, a lymphocyte (dark cell) and a neutrophilic granulocyte.

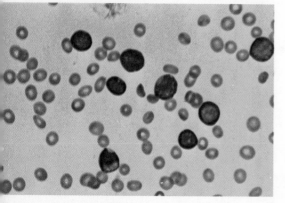

A microscopic view of a blood preparation in a case of lymphocytic leukemia. In this disease lymphocytes increase tremendously.

A microscopic view showing gland tissue of the normal breast during pregnancy.

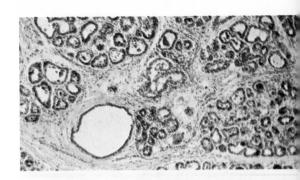

A microscopic view of a small area of breast tissue showing clusters of cells of a malignant tumor (carcinoma).

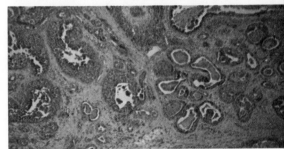

A microscopic view of a small portion of a carcinoma of the breast (a malignant tumor). The tumor cells manifest a tendency to invade the adjacent tissue.

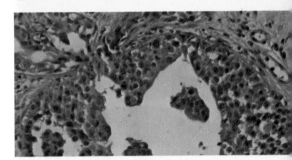

A microscopic view of a normal small artery showing its scalloped lining and the surrounding narrow layer of smooth muscle. During life, the pressure of blood within the artery smooths out the scallops of the lining. The pointer indicates the layer of smooth muscle that forms most of the artery's wall.

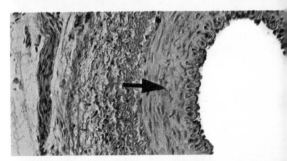

A microscopic view of a coronary artery in which the passageway for blood has been almost occluded by arteriosclerosis.

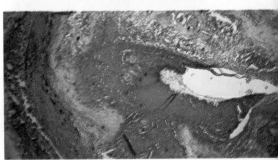

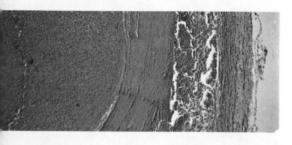

A microscopic view of a section of the wall of a vein which contains a thrombus—material consisting mostly of clotted blood.

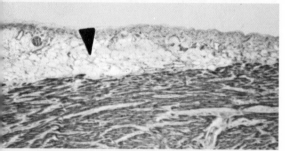

A microscopic view of a portion of the wall of a normal heart showing its external surface. The arrow indicates a delicate layer of fat just beneath the heart's outer wall.

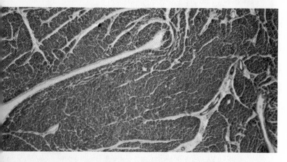

A microscopic view of a small portion of the wall of the normal heart showing its lining membrane as it extends between two folds of muscle tissue.

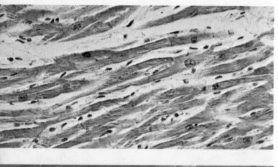

A microscopic view of the muscle contained in the wall of a normal heart.

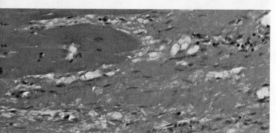

A microscopic view of a portion of the heart wall in which healing has occurred following a typical "heart attack" caused by the occlusion of a branch of a coronary artery. The lighter areas consist of scar tissue; the darker structures are remaining heart muscle fibers.

A microscopic view of normal lung tissue. The arrow points to a bronchiole, which represents the final branching of the system of tubes which bring air into the lung.

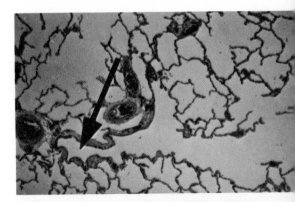

A microscopic view of a small area of lung tissue indicating how carbon which is inhaled remains in the lung tissue. Inasmuch as carbon is insoluble and inert, these deposits remain for the duration of life.

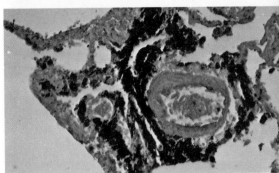

A high-power microscopic view of an area of lung which has been invaded by a bronchiogenic carcinoma—the highly malignant tumor which is so commonly caused by the use of cigarettes.

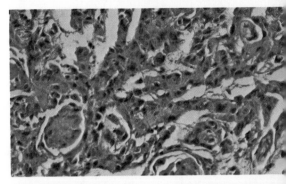

Microscopic view of an area of lung which has become involved in bronchopneumonia. Notice that the air sacs have become filled with defense cells and tissue debris.

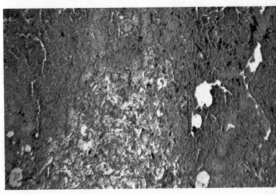

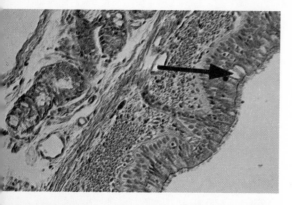

A microscopic view of a portion of the wall of the normal trachea. The epithelium lining the trachea is equipped with tiny villi—fingerlike structures which, by their waving action, sweep out foreign material which has been carried in by the inhaled air. The arrow indicates two goblet cells which produce mucus. In the deeper areas are glands which also produce mucus.

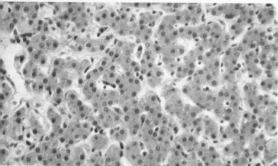

A microscopic view of normal liver tissue. During life the cords of liver cells are bathed by the blood which routinely passes through the liver.

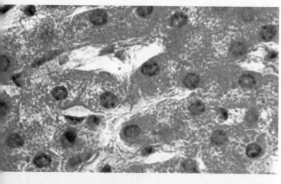

A high-power microscopic view of normal liver tissue showing the individual cells.

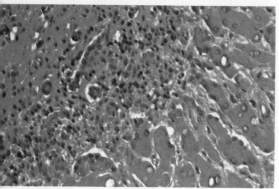

A microscopic view of liver tissue in cirrhosis. In this disease, large areas of normal tissue are replaced by dense scarlike tissue.

A microscopic view of normal skin from the palm of the hand. The two heavy bands at the left constitute the epidermis, the intermediate zone of tissue arranged as a "feltwork" is the dermis, and the looser tissue at the right is the subcutaneous area. The arrow indicates the duct of a sweat gland spiraling to the surface.

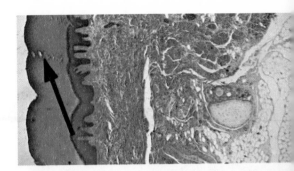

A microscopic view of normal thin skin such as occurs on the arm. The arrow points to the duct of a sweat gland. To the extreme right is the root of a hair. Left of the hair root and continuing to the free surface is a portion of a hair follicle with its associated sebaceous gland.

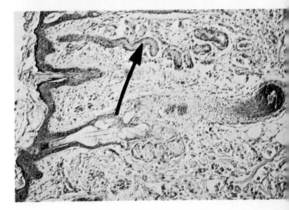

A microscopic view of thin skin in which there is a beginning basal cell carcinoma (skin cancer) at the left.

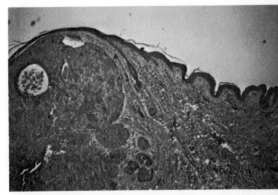

A microscopic view of a portion of a basal cell carcinoma of the skin showing how the cell groups of this tumor tend to invade the deeper dermal tissues.

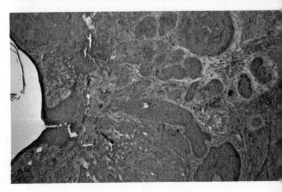

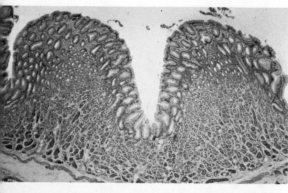

A low-power microscopic view of the normal glandular membrane of the stomach.

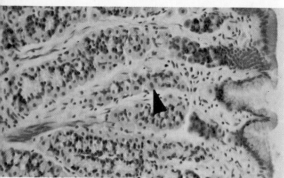

A microscopic view of the glandular membrane which lines the stomach and produces gastric juice. Arrow points to a "parietal cell" which produces hydrochloric acid.

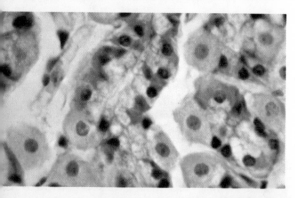

A high magnification of some of the gland cells in the lining of the stomach. The large, conspicuous cells are the "parietal cells" which produce hydrochloric acid.

A low-power microscopic view of the lining membrane of the stomach showing an area in which an ulcer has developed.

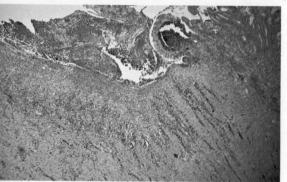

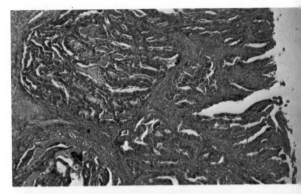

A microscopic view of a portion of the glandular lining of the stomach which has become involved by a malignant tumor.

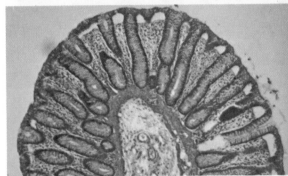

A low-power microscopic view of a fold of the mucosa lining the normal large intestine. Many tube-shaped glands are present.

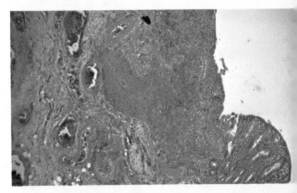

A low-power microscopic view of the large intestine in a case of ulcerative colitis. Notice that a portion of the glandular lining has been destroyed.

A microscopic view of a beginning carcinoma in the large intestine. As yet the malignant tumor has not invaded the adjacent deeper tissues and is therefore called a "carcinoma in situ."

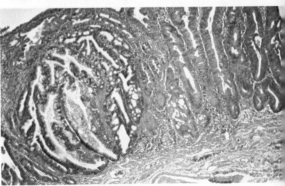

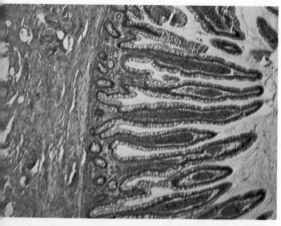

A microscopic view of the elaborate membrane lining the normal small intestine. The fingerlike extensions are called villi.

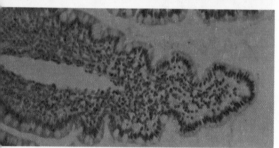

A high magnification of the villi which occur in the lining of the small intestine. Many of the cells covering a villus secrete mucus. At the center of each villus is a lacteal vessel which carries away the fatty component of the food as it is absorbed.

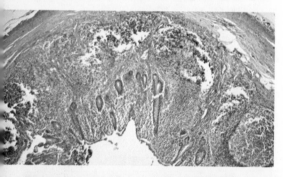

A low-power microscopic view of a sector of the wall of a normal appendix.

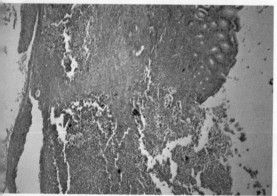

A microscopic view of a portion of the wall of the appendix in a case of acute appendicitis. The tissue is inflamed and fragile.

A low-power microscopic view of the cortical region of a normal kidney showing both glomeruli and tubules.

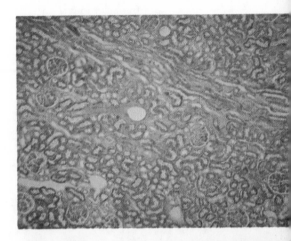

A high magnification of the cortical region of normal kidney tissue. The arrow points to that part of a glomerulus at which the tiny blood vessels enter and leave.

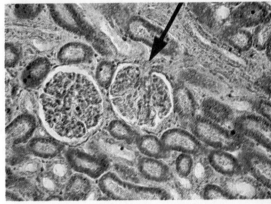

A microscopic view of the medullary region of a normal kidney showing the minute parallel tubules.

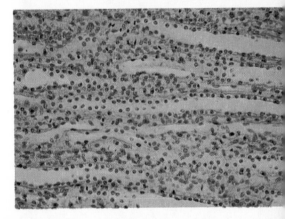

A microscopic view of the medullary region of a normal kidney showing the minute parallel tubules.

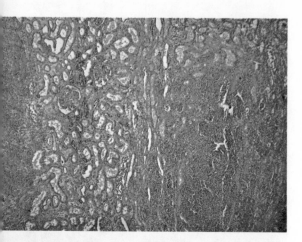

A microscopic view of kidney tissue in active pyelonephritis.

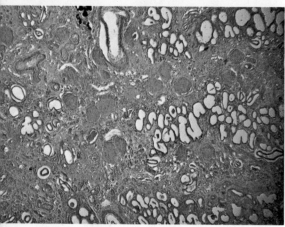

A microscopic view of kidney tissue in chronic glomerulonephritis.

Photo and Illustrations

Credits for photos and illustrations used in Volume 3 of *You and Your Health:*

Sandoz Pharmaceuticals, pages 12, 80; Lederle Laboratories, pages 14, 46, 92, 104; Lucille Innes, pages 15, 18, 20, 21, 39, 90, 99 (lower), 100, 106, 107, 130, 240, 370; James Converse, pages 16, 83, 99 (upper), 118, 152, 157, 192, 194, 216, 224, 322, 349, 352, 356, 357, 358 (lower), 359, 360, 361, 365, 374, 376, 377, 378, 379, 383, 384, 388, 389, 391, 392, 394, 395, 408, 411, 416, 424, 425, 428 (lower), 429, 432, 436, 438, 439, 444, 445, 447, 448, 449, 453, 457, 458; Robert Eldridge, pages 24 (upper), 48, 114, 351, 358 (upper), 428 (upper); Kelly Solis-Novarro, pages 24 (lower), 26, 57, 117, 154, 160 (top), 231 (lower); United Press International, pages 25, 215, 295; Public Health Service Audiovisual Facility, pages 28, 29, 55, 59, 190, 191, 198 (lower), 207, 231 (upper), 247, 249, 251, 253, 254, 256, 259, 260, 261, 262, 265, 266, 271, 273, 275, 277, 279, 281, 283, 289, 291, 302, 304, 306, 314, 317, 323; Chas. Pfizer & Co., Inc., pages 34, 160, 306, 308, 309, 310, 311, 312; Margery Gardephe, pages 36, 37, 41, 94, 95, 103, 135, 147; F. Netter, M.D., © Ciba, pages 69, 197, 300, 321; D. Tank, pages 85, 123, 135, 142, 204, 234, 326, 332 (upper), 337, 343, 422; Joan Walter, page 86; The Upjohn Company, pages 97, 159, 165, 169, 217; Ichiro Nakashima, pages 112, 121, 125, 139, 241, 243, 245, 375, 400, 404, 427; Howard Larkin, pages 146, 148, 234; Doho Chemical Company, page 161; Review & Herald Publishing Association, page 164; Elias A. Papazian, page 172; Three Lions, Inc., pages 172 (inset), 367 (insets); American Cancer Society, page 176; Gene Ahrens, page 198 (upper); Lester Quade, pages 226, 237; Eric Kreye, pages 234, 268; A. Devaney, Inc., page 242; Loma Linda School of Medicine, pages 247, 250; Joe Maniscalco, pages 257, 363, 413; Black Star, page 282; Clay Adams, pages 284, 285; Paul R. Nelson, Samuel Myslis, Robert H. Wright, page 296; Ron Polacsek, page 332 (lower).

General Index

(All numbers along with entries refer to pages in one of the three volumes. All cross references refer to other entries in this index)